AMERICAN ACADEMY
OF OPHTHALMOLOGY®
Protecting Sight. Empowering Lives.

2 | Fundamentals and Principles of Ophthalmology

Last major revision 2019–2020

2022–2023
BCSC
Basic and Clinical Science Course™

EB
Published after collaborative review with the European Board of Ophthalmology subcommittee

The American Academy of Ophthalmology is accredited by the Accreditation Council for Continuing Medical Education (ACCME) to provide continuing medical education for physicians.

The American Academy of Ophthalmology designates this enduring material for a maximum of 15 *AMA PRA Category 1 Credits*™. Physicians should claim only the credit commensurate with the extent of their participation in the activity.

Originally released June 2019; reviewed for currency August 2021; CME expiration date: June 1, 2023. *AMA PRA Category 1 Credits*™ may be claimed only once between June 1, 2019, and the expiration date.

BCSC® volumes are designed to increase the physician's ophthalmic knowledge through study and review. Users of this activity are encouraged to read the text and then answer the study questions provided at the back of the book.

To claim *AMA PRA Category 1 Credits*™ upon completion of this activity, learners must demonstrate appropriate knowledge and participation in the activity by taking the posttest for Section 2 and achieving a score of 80% or higher. For further details, please see the instructions for requesting CME credit at the back of the book.

The Academy provides this material for educational purposes only. It is not intended to represent the only or best method or procedure in every case, nor to replace a physician's own judgment or give specific advice for case management. Including all indications, contraindications, side effects, and alternative agents for each drug or treatment is beyond the scope of this material. All information and recommendations should be verified, prior to use, with current information included in the manufacturers' package inserts or other independent sources, and considered in light of the patient's condition and history. Reference to certain drugs, instruments, and other products in this course is made for illustrative purposes only and is not intended to constitute an endorsement of such. Some material may include information on applications that are not considered community standard, that reflect indications not included in approved FDA labeling, or that are approved for use only in restricted research settings. **The FDA has stated that it is the responsibility of the physician to determine the FDA status of each drug or device he or she wishes to use, and to use them with appropriate, informed patient consent in compliance with applicable law.** The Academy specifically disclaims any and all liability for injury or other damages of any kind, from negligence or otherwise, for any and all claims that may arise from the use of any recommendations or other information contained herein.

Cover image: From BCSC Section 12, *Retina and Vitreous.* Confocal scanning laser ophthalmoscopy multicolor fundus image (30° field of view) of a healthy eye. *(Courtesy of Lucia Sobrin, MD.)*

FSC
www.fsc.org
MIX
Paper from responsible sources
FSC® C001701

Printed in China.

Basic and Clinical Science Course

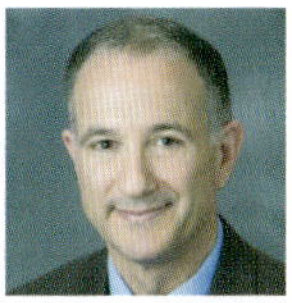

Christopher J. Rapuano, MD, Philadelphia, Pennsylvania
Senior Secretary for Clinical Education

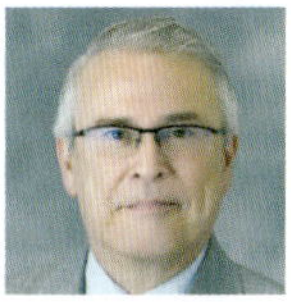

J. Timothy Stout, MD, PhD, MBA, Houston, Texas
Secretary for Lifelong Learning and Assessment

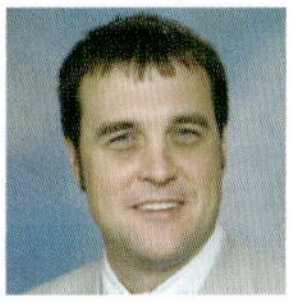

Colin A. McCannel, MD, Los Angeles, California
BCSC Course Chair

Section 2

Faculty for the Major Revision

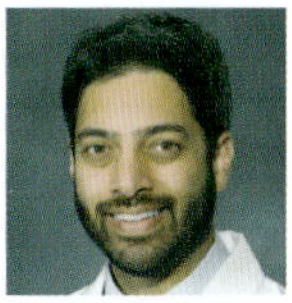

Vikram S. Brar, MD
Chair
Richmond, Virginia

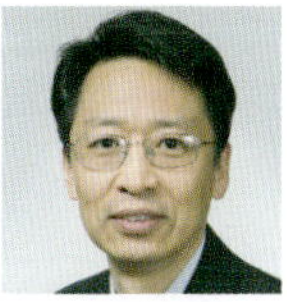

Simon K. Law, MD
Los Angeles, California

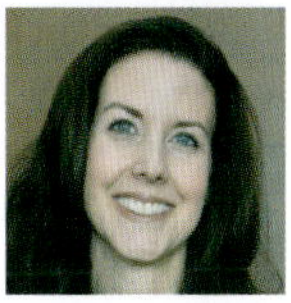

Jennifer L. Lindsey, MD
Nashville, Tennessee

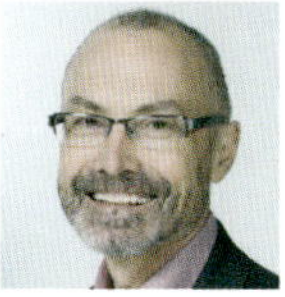

David A. Mackey, MD
Perth, Western Australia

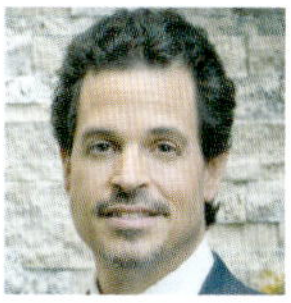

Robert L. Schultze, MD
Slingerlands, New York

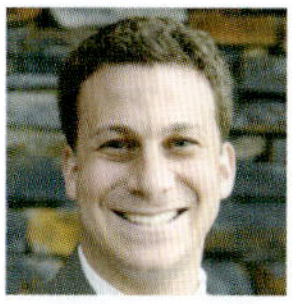

Evan Silverstein, MD
Richmond, Virginia

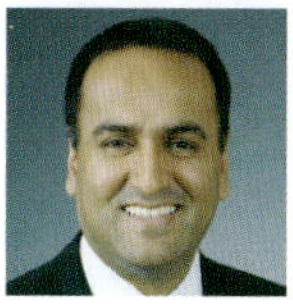

Ravi S. J. Singh, MD
Shawnee Mission, Kansas

The Academy wishes to acknowledge the following consultant for his work on Chapter 18: Michael D. Abràmoff, MD, PhD, Iowa City, Iowa

The Academy wishes to acknowledge the following committees for review of this edition:

Committee on Aging: Elliot H. Sohn, MD, Iowa City, Iowa

Vision Rehabilitation Committee: Mona A. Kaleem, MD, Ellicott City, Maryland

Practicing Ophthalmologists Advisory Committee for Education: Bradley D. Fouraker, MD, *Primary Reviewer* and *Chair,* Tampa, Florida; Alice Bashinsky, MD, Asheville, North Carolina; David J. Browning, MD, PhD, Charlotte, North Carolina; Cynthia S. Chiu, MD, Oakland, California; Steven J. Grosser, MD, Golden Valley, Minnesota; Stephen R. Klapper, MD, Carmel, Indiana; Troy M. Tanji, MD, Waipahu, Hawaii; Michelle S. Ying, MD, MSPH, Ladson, South Carolina

The Academy also wishes to acknowledge the following committee for assistance in developing Study Questions and Answers for this BCSC Section:

Self-Assessment Committee: Deepa Abraham, MD, Seattle, Washington; William R. Barlow, MD, Salt Lake City, Utah; William L. Becker, MD, St Louis, Missouri; Michele M. Bloomer, MD, San Francisco, California; John J. Chen, MD, PhD, Rochester, Minnesota; Zelia M. Correa, MD, Baltimore, Maryland; Deborah M. Costakos, MD, Milwaukee, Wisconsin; Theodore Curtis, MD, Mount Kisco, New York; Laura C. Fine, MD, Boston, Massachusetts; Robert E. Fintelmann, MD, Phoenix, Arizona; Jeffrey M. Goshe, MD, Cleveland, Ohio; Mark Greiner, MD, Iowa City, Iowa; Paul B. Griggs, MD, Seattle, Washington; David R. Hardten, MD, Minnetonka, Minnesota; Rachel M. Huckfeldt, MD, Boston, Massachusetts; Sarah S. Khodadadeh, MD, Vero Beach, Florida; Douglas R. Lazzaro, MD, Brooklyn, New York; Amanda C. Maltry, MD, Minneapolis, Minnesota; Brian Privett, MD, Cedar Rapids, Iowa; Sunita Radhakrishnan, MD, San Mateo, California; Jordan J. Rixen, MD, Lincoln, Nebraska; Mark I. Salevitz, MD, Scottsdale, Arizona; Ravi S. J. Singh, MD, Shawnee Mission, Kansas; Mitchell B. Strominger, MD, Reno, Nevada; Janet Y. Tsui, MD, Santa Clara, California; Ari L. Weitzner, MD, New York, New York; Zoë R. Williams, MD, Rochester, New York; Kimberly M. Winges, MD, Portland, Oregon

EB

European Board of Ophthalmology: Peter J. Ringens, MD, PhD, *EBO Chair for BCSC Section 2* and *EBO-BCSC Program Liaison,* Maastricht, Netherlands

Financial Disclosures

Academy staff members who contributed to the development of this product state that within the 24 months prior to their contributions to this CME activity and for the duration of development, they have had no financial interest in or other relationship with any entity that produces, markets, resells, or distributes health care goods or services consumed by or used in patients, or with any competing commercial product or service.

The authors and reviewers state that within the 24 months prior to their contributions to this CME activity and for the duration of development, they have had the following financial relationships:*

Dr Browning: Aerpio Therapeutics (S), Alcon Laboratories (S), Alimera Sciences (C), Emmes (S), Genentech (S), Novartis Pharmaceuticals (S), Ohr Pharmaceuticals (S), Pfizer (S), Regeneron Pharmaceuticals (S), Springer (P), Zeiss (O)

Dr Correa: Castle Biosciences (C)

Dr Fintelmann: Alphaeon (O), Strathspey Crown (O)

Dr Fouraker: Addition Technology (C, L), Alcon Laboratories (C, L), OASIS Medical (C, L)

Dr Goshe: Carl Zeiss Meditec (L)

Dr Grosser: InjectSense (O), Ivantis (O)

Dr Hardten: Allergan (C, L, S), Avedro (C), Eye Surgical Instruments (C, O), Johnson & Johnson (C), Oculus (L), Optical Systems Design (C, O), TLC Vision (C)

Dr Huckfeldt: AGTC (S), MeiraGTx (S), Spark Therapeutics (S)

Dr Klapper: AdOM Advanced Optical Technologies (O)

Dr Privett: Omeros (O)

Dr Radhakrishnan: Netra Systems (C, O)

Dr Schultze: Alcon Laboratories (L), Bausch + Lomb Surgical (L), Novartis Alcon Pharmaceuticals (L), Sun Pharmaceuticals (L)

Dr Silverstein: I-See Vision Technology (O); Welch Allyn (C)

Dr Sohn: GlaxoSmithKline (S), Oxford Biomedical (S), Regeneron (S), Sanofi Fovea (S)

The other authors and reviewers state that within the 24 months prior to their contributions to this CME activity and for the duration of development, they have had no financial interest in or other relationship with any entity that produces, markets, resells, or distributes health care goods or services consumed by or used in patients, or with any competing commercial product or service.

* C = consultant fee, paid advisory boards, or fees for attending a meeting; E = employed by or received a W2 from a commercial company; L = lecture fees or honoraria, travel fees or reimbursements when speaking at the invitation of a commercial company; O = equity ownership/stock options in publicly or privately traded firms, excluding mutual funds; P = patents and/or royalties for intellectual property; S = grant support or other financial support to the investigator from all sources, including research support from government agencies, foundations, device manufacturers, and/or pharmaceutical companies

Recent Past Faculty

Michael H. Goldstein, MD
Alon Kahana, MD, PhD
William R. Katowitz, MD
Lawrence M. Levine, MD

In addition, the Academy gratefully acknowledges the contributions of numerous past faculty and advisory committee members who have played an important role in the development of previous editions of the Basic and Clinical Science Course.

American Academy of Ophthalmology Staff

Dale E. Fajardo, EdD, MBA, *Vice President, Education*
Beth Wilson, *Director, Continuing Professional Development*
Denise Evenson, *Director, Brand & Creative*
Ann McGuire, *Acquisitions and Development Manager*
Stephanie Tanaka, *Publications Manager*
Susan Malloy, *Acquisitions Editor and Program Manager*
Jasmine Chen, *Manager of E-Learning*
Lana Ip, *Senior Designer*
Beth Collins, *Medical Editor*
Eric Gerdes, *Interactive Designer*
Lynda Hanwella, *Publications Specialist*
Debra Marchi, *Permissions Assistant*

American Academy of Ophthalmology
655 Beach Street
Box 7424
San Francisco, CA 94120-7424

Contents

Introduction to the BCSC

The Basic and Clinical Science Course (BCSC) is designed to meet the needs of residents and practitioners for a comprehensive yet concise curriculum of the field of ophthalmology. The BCSC has developed from its original brief outline format, which relied heavily on outside readings, to a more convenient and educationally useful self-contained text. The Academy updates and revises the course annually, with the goals of integrating the basic science and clinical practice of ophthalmology and of keeping ophthalmologists current with new developments in the various subspecialties. To address an important and timely issue, Chapter 18, Digital Ophthalmology, has been added to Section 2. This is a preview of the chapter on this topic that will appear in the 2023–2024 major revision.

The BCSC incorporates the effort and expertise of more than 100 ophthalmologists, organized into 13 Section faculties, working with Academy editorial staff. In addition, the course continues to benefit from many lasting contributions made by the faculties of previous editions. Members of the Academy Practicing Ophthalmologists Advisory Committee for Education, Committee on Aging, and Vision Rehabilitation Committee review every volume before major revisions. Members of the European Board of Ophthalmology, organized into Section faculties, also review each volume before major revisions, focusing primarily on differences between American and European ophthalmology practice.

Organization of the Course

The Basic and Clinical Science Course comprises 13 volumes, incorporating fundamental ophthalmic knowledge, subspecialty areas, and special topics:

1 Update on General Medicine
2 Fundamentals and Principles of Ophthalmology
3 Clinical Optics and Vision Rehabilitation
4 Ophthalmic Pathology and Intraocular Tumors
5 Neuro-Ophthalmology
6 Pediatric Ophthalmology and Strabismus
7 Oculofacial Plastic and Orbital Surgery
8 External Disease and Cornea
9 Uveitis and Ocular Inflammation
10 Glaucoma
11 Lens and Cataract
12 Retina and Vitreous
13 Refractive Surgery

References

Readers who wish to explore specific topics in greater detail may consult the references cited within each chapter and listed in the Basic Texts section at the back of the book.

These references are intended to be selective rather than exhaustive, chosen by the BCSC faculty as being important, current, and readily available to residents and practitioners.

Multimedia

This edition of Section 2, *Fundamentals and Principles of Ophthalmology,* includes videos related to topics covered in the book and interactive content, or "activities," developed by members of the BCSC faculty. The videos and activities are available to readers of the print and electronic versions of Section 2 (www.aao.org/bcscvideo_section02) and (www.aao.org/bcscactivity_section02). Mobile device users can scan the QR codes below (a QR-code reader may need to be installed on the device) to access the videos and activities.

Videos

Activities

Self-Assessment and CME Credit

Each volume of the BCSC is designed as an independent study activity for ophthalmology residents and practitioners. The learning objectives for this volume are given on pages 1 and 2. The text, illustrations, and references provide the information necessary to achieve the objectives; the study questions allow readers to test their understanding of the material and their mastery of the objectives. Physicians who wish to claim CME credit for this educational activity may do so online by following the instructions at the end of the book.*

Conclusion

The Basic and Clinical Science Course has expanded greatly over the years, with the addition of much new text, numerous illustrations, and video content. Recent editions have sought to place greater emphasis on clinical applicability while maintaining a solid foundation in basic science. As with any educational program, it reflects the experience of its authors. As its faculties change and medicine progresses, new viewpoints emerge on controversial subjects and techniques. Not all alternate approaches can be included in this series; as with any educational endeavor, the learner should seek additional sources, including Academy Preferred Practice Pattern Guidelines.

The BCSC faculty and staff continually strive to improve the educational usefulness of the course; you, the reader, can contribute to this ongoing process. If you have any suggestions or questions about the series, please do not hesitate to contact the faculty or the editors. The authors, editors, and reviewers hope that your study of the BCSC will be of lasting value and that each Section will serve as a practical resource for quality patient care.

*This activity meets the Self-Assessment CME requirements defined by the American Board of Ophthalmology (ABO). Please be advised that the ABO is not an accrediting body for purposes of any CME program. ABO does not sponsor this or any outside activity, and ABO does not endorse any particular CME activity. Complete information regarding the ABO Self-Assessment CME Maintenance of Certification requirements is available at https://abop.org/maintain-certification/cme-self-assessment/.

Objectives

Upon completion of BCSC Section 2, *Fundamentals and Principles of Ophthalmology,* the reader should be able to

- identify the bones making up the orbital walls and the orbital foramina
- identify the origin and pathways of cranial nerves I–VII
- identify the origins and insertions of the extraocular muscles
- describe the distribution of the arterial and venous circulations of the orbit and optic nerve
- describe the anastomoses in the orbit between the external and internal carotid arteries
- describe the venous drainage of the eyelids and orbit, as well as the cavernous sinus
- describe the structural–functional relationships of the outflow pathways for aqueous humor of the eye
- identify various ocular tissues and describe their function and ultrastructural details
- describe the elements of the visual cycle and phototransduction cascade and their relation to vision and inherited retinal diseases
- state the events of embryogenesis that are important for the subsequent development of the eye and orbit
- identify the roles of growth factors, homeobox genes, and neural crest cells in the genesis of the eye
- describe the sequence of events in the differentiation of the ocular tissues during embryonic and fetal development of the eye
- draw a pedigree and identify the main patterns of inheritance
- describe the organization of the human genome and the role of genetic mutations in health and disease

- explain how appropriate diagnosis and management of genetic diseases can lead to better patient care
- describe the role of the ophthalmologist in the provision of genetic counseling as well as the indications for ordering genetic testing and referring patients for gene therapy
- discuss the biochemical composition of the various parts of the eye and the eye's secretions
- list the various functions of the retinal pigment epithelium, such as phagocytosis, vitamin A metabolism, and maintenance of retinal adhesion
- describe the role of free radicals and antioxidants in the eye
- describe the phases of clinical trials in relation to drug approval by the US Food and Drug Administration
- describe the features of the eye that facilitate or impede drug delivery
- describe the basic principles of ocular pharmacokinetics, pharmacodynamics, and pharmacogenetics
- describe the basic principles underlying the use of autonomic therapeutic agents in a variety of ocular conditions
- list the indications, contraindications, mechanisms of action, and adverse effects of various drugs used in the management of glaucoma
- describe the mechanisms of action of antibiotic, antiviral, and antifungal medications
- describe the mechanisms of action, delivery, and side effects of drugs used in corticosteroid and immunomodulatory therapy
- describe available anti–vascular endothelial growth factor agents
- describe the anesthetic agents used in ophthalmology and methods of their delivery
- describe the basic principles of and indications for neuroimaging and ophthalmic ultrasonography as they relate to common ophthalmic and neuro-ophthalmic conditions

PART I

Anatomy

CHAPTER 1

Orbit and Ocular Adnexa

This chapter includes a related activity, which can be accessed by scanning the QR code provided in the text or going to www.aao.org/bcscactivity_section02.

Highlights

- The shortest, most direct path to the optic nerve is along the medial wall.
- Emissary channels in the medial wall of the orbit can facilitate the spread of infection from the ethmoid sinus into the orbit.
- The lesser wing of the sphenoid bone houses the optic canal.
- Fractures of the orbital floor can involve the infraorbital groove, which contains the infraorbital nerve, and should be suspected in cases of orbital trauma associated with infraorbital hypoesthesia.
- An imaginary line drawn externally between the extraocular muscle insertions approximates the ora serrata internally.
- At the annulus of Zinn, the medial and superior rectus muscles are adjacent to the optic nerve sheath. Because of this anatomical relationship, patients with retrobulbar optic neuritis experience pain with eye movement.
- The eyelid vasculature includes multiple sites of anastomoses between the external and internal carotid arteries.

Orbital Anatomy

Orbital anatomy, pathology, and changes associated with aging are discussed in detail in BCSC Section 7, *Oculofacial Plastic and Orbital Surgery.*

Dimensions of the Adult Orbit

Each eye lies within a bony orbit, the volume of which is slightly less than 30 mL. Each orbit is pear shaped; the optic nerve represents the stem. The orbital entrance averages approximately 35 mm in height and 45 mm in width and is widest approximately 1 cm behind the anterior orbital margin. The depth of the orbit, measured from the orbital entrance to the orbital apex, varies from 40 to 45 mm, depending on whether the measurement is made along the lateral wall or the medial wall. Race and sex affect each of these measurements.

Bony Orbit

The bony orbit surrounds the globe and helps protect it from blunt injury. Seven bones make up the bony orbit (Fig 1-1; also see Chapter 1 in BCSC Section 7, *Oculofacial Plastic and Orbital Surgery*):

- frontal bone
- zygomatic bone
- maxillary bone
- ethmoid bone

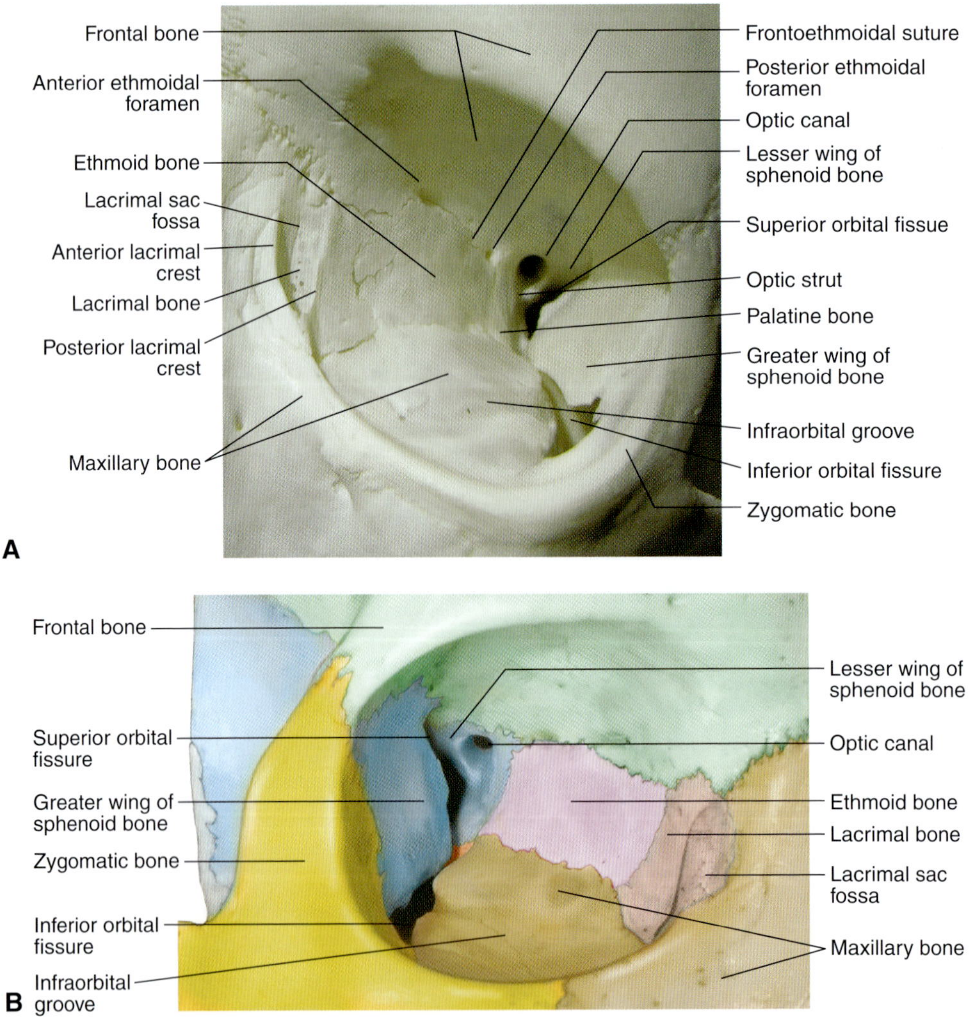

Figure 1-1 **A,** Anatomy of the left orbit in a human skull. **B,** Color diagram of bones of the right orbit. The infraorbital groove leads to the anterior infraorbital canal and houses the infraorbital nerve. *(Part A courtesy of Alon Kahana, MD, PhD; part B illustration by Dave Peace.)*

- sphenoid bone (greater and lesser wings)
- lacrimal bone
- palatine bone

Orbital Margin

The orbital margin, or rim, forms a quadrilateral spiral whose superior margin is formed by the frontal bone, which is interrupted medially by the supraorbital notch (Fig 1-2). The medial margin is formed above by the frontal bone and below by the posterior lacrimal crest of the lacrimal bone and the anterior lacrimal crest of the maxillary bone. The inferior margin derives from the maxillary and zygomatic bones. Laterally, the zygomatic and frontal bones complete the rim.

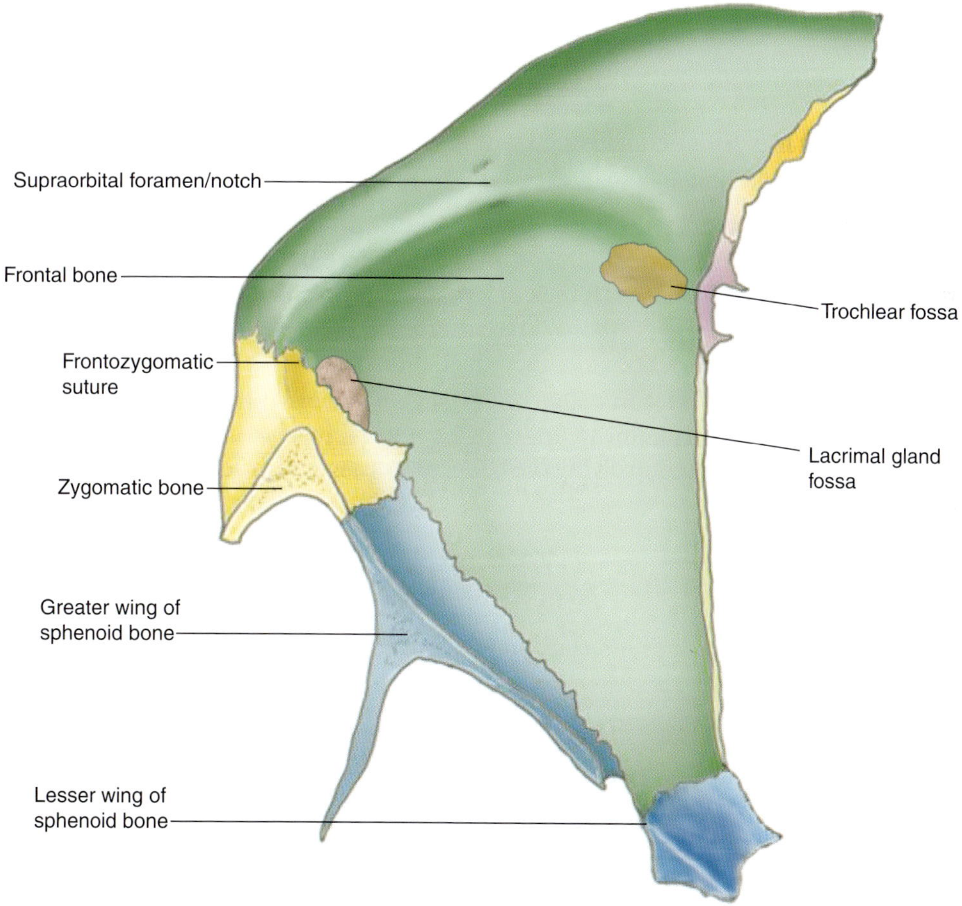

Figure 1-2 Right orbital roof. The orbital roof is composed of 2 bones: (1) the orbital plate of the frontal bone; and (2) the lesser wing of the sphenoid bone. The frontal sinus lies within the anterior orbital roof. The supraorbital foramen/notch, located within the medial one-third of the superior orbital rim, transmits the supraorbital nerve, a terminal branch of the frontal nerve of the ophthalmic division of cranial nerve V (CN V_1). Medially, the frontal bone forms the roof of the ethmoid sinus and extends to the cribriform plate. *(Illustration by Dave Peace.)*

Orbital Roof

The orbital roof is formed from 2 bones (see Fig 1-2):

- orbital plate of the frontal bone
- lesser wing of the sphenoid bone

The fossa for the lacrimal gland, lying anterolaterally behind the zygomatic process of the frontal bone, resides within the orbital roof. Medially, the trochlear fossa is located on the frontal bone approximately 4–5 mm from the orbital margin and is the site of the pulley of the superior oblique muscle, where the trochlea, a curved plate of hyaline cartilage, is attached.

Medial Orbital Wall

The medial wall of the orbit is formed from 4 bones (Fig 1-3):

- frontal process of the maxillary bone
- lacrimal bone
- orbital plate of the ethmoid bone
- lesser wing of the sphenoid bone

The ethmoid bone makes up the largest portion of the medial wall. The fossa for the lacrimal sac is formed by the frontal process of the maxillary bone and the lacrimal bone. Below, the fossa is continuous with the bony nasolacrimal canal, which extends into the inferior meatus (the space beneath the inferior turbinate) of the nose.

The orbital plate of the ethmoid bone, which forms part of the medial orbital wall, is a paper-thin structure—hence its name, *lamina papyracea*—and is the most common site of fracture following blunt trauma to the orbit. The medial wall has 2 foramina, which can act as conduits for processes involving the ethmoid sinus to enter the orbit.

> **CLINICAL PEARL**
>
> The most direct path to the optic nerve is along the medial wall: this is relevant for surgical procedures such as enucleation or optic nerve sheath decompression.

Orbital Floor

The floor of the orbit, which is the roof of the maxillary antrum (or sinus), is composed of 3 bones (Fig 1-4):

- orbital plate of the maxillary bone
- palatine bone
- orbital plate of the zygomatic bone

The infraorbital groove traverses the floor and descends anteriorly into the infraorbital canal. Both the groove and the canal house the infraorbital nerve (maxillary division of the trigeminal nerve, V_2), which emerges at the infraorbital foramen, below the orbital

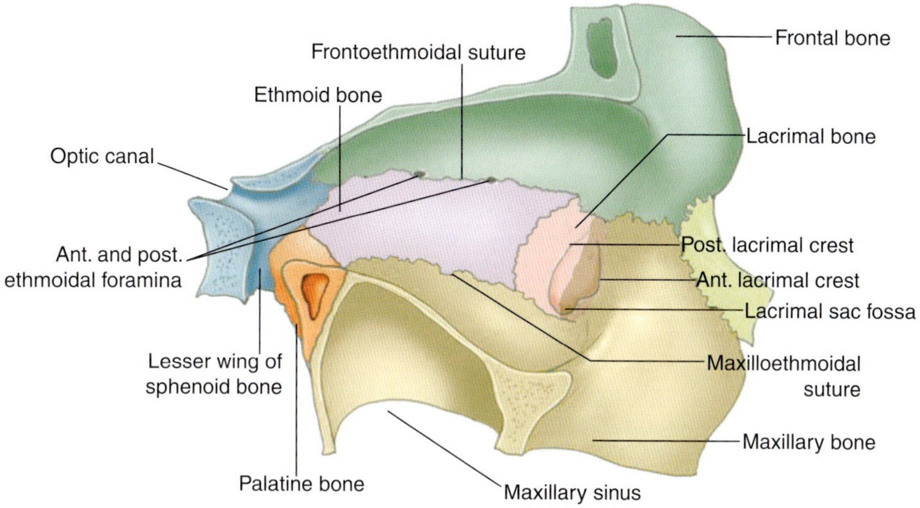

Figure 1-3 Right medial orbital wall. The medial orbital wall is formed by 4 bones: (1) maxillary (frontal process); (2) lacrimal; (3) lesser wing of the sphenoid bone; and (4) orbital plate of the ethmoid. The largest component of the medial wall is the lamina papyracea of the ethmoid bone. Superiorly, the anterior and posterior foramina at the level of the frontoethmoidal suture transmit the anterior and posterior ethmoidal arteries, respectively. The anterior medial orbital wall includes the fossa for the lacrimal sac, which is formed by both the maxillary and lacrimal bones. The lacrimal bone is divided by the posterior lacrimal crest. The anterior part of the lacrimal sac fossa is formed by the anterior lacrimal crest of the maxillary bone. *(Illustration by Dave Peace.)*

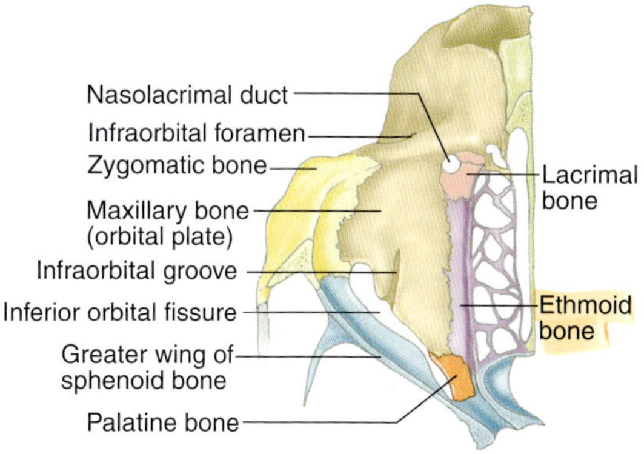

Figure 1-4 Left orbital floor. The orbital floor is composed of 3 bones: (1) maxillary bone; (2) orbital plate of zygomatic bone; and (3) palatine bone. The nasolacrimal duct sits in the anterior middle area of the orbital floor, medial to the origin of the inferior oblique muscle. *(Illustration by Dave Peace.)*

margin of the maxillary bone. For this reason, patients evaluated for orbital floor fractures should also be assessed for infraorbital hypoesthesia.

Arising from the floor of the orbit just lateral to the opening of the nasolacrimal canal is the inferior oblique muscle, the only extraocular muscle that does not originate from the orbital apex. The floor of the orbit slopes downward approximately 20° from posterior to anterior. Before puberty, the orbital floor bones are immature and more prone to "trapdoor"-type fractures and secondary muscle entrapment.

Wei LA, Durairaj VD. Pediatric orbital floor fractures. *J AAPOS.* 2011;15(2):173–180.

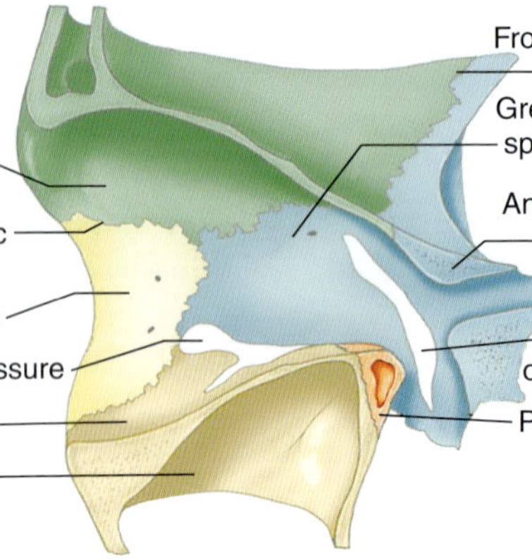

Figure 1-5 Right lateral orbital wall. The lateral orbital wall is formed by the zygomatic bone and the greater wing of the sphenoid bone. The junction between the lateral orbital wall and the roof is represented by the frontosphenoid suture. Posteriorly, the wall is bordered by the inferior and superior orbital fissures. The sphenoid wing makes up the posterior portion of the lateral wall and separates the orbit from the middle cranial fossa. Medially, the lateral orbital wall ends at the inferior and superior orbital fissures. *(Illustration by Dave Peace.)*

Lateral Orbital Wall

The thickest and strongest of the orbital walls, the lateral wall is formed from 2 bones (Fig 1-5):

- zygomatic bone
- greater wing of the sphenoid bone

The lateral orbital tubercle *(Whitnall tubercle),* a small elevation of the orbital margin of the zygomatic bone, lies approximately 11 mm below the frontozygomatic suture. This important landmark is the site of attachment for the following structures:

- check ligament of the lateral rectus muscle
- suspensory ligament of the eyeball (Lockwood suspensory ligament)
- lateral canthal tendon
- lateral horn of the levator aponeurosis

Orbital Foramina, Ducts, Canals, and Fissures

Foramina

The *optic foramen* is the entry point to the optic canal, which leads from the middle cranial fossa to the apex of the orbit (see Fig 1-1). The optic canal is directed forward, laterally, and somewhat downward and conducts the optic nerve, the ophthalmic artery, and sympathetic fibers from the carotid plexus. The optic canal passes through the lesser wing of the sphenoid bone.

The *supraorbital foramen* (which, in some individuals, is a notch instead of a foramen) is located at the medial third of the superior margin of the orbit. It transmits blood vessels and the supraorbital nerve, which is an extension of the frontal nerve, a branch of the ophthalmic division (V_1) of cranial nerve V (CN V, the trigeminal nerve). The *anterior ethmoidal foramen* is located at the frontoethmoidal suture and transmits the anterior ethmoidal vessels and nerve. The *posterior ethmoidal foramen* lies at the junction of the roof and the medial wall of the orbit and transmits the posterior ethmoidal vessels and nerve through the frontal bone (see Fig 1-3). The *zygomaticotemporal and zygomaticofacial foramina* lie in the portion of the lateral orbital wall formed by the zygomatic bone and transmit vessels and branches of the zygomatic nerve (see Fig 1-5).

Nasolacrimal duct

The nasolacrimal duct travels inferiorly from the lacrimal sac fossa into the inferior meatus of the nose (see Figs 1-4, 1-40).

Infraorbital canal

The infraorbital canal continues anteriorly from the infraorbital groove and exits 4 mm below the inferior orbital margin. From there it transmits the infraorbital nerve, a branch of V_2 (the maxillary division of CN V) (see Fig 1-1).

Fissures

The *superior orbital fissure* (Fig 1-6; see also Fig 1-1) is located between the greater and lesser wings of the sphenoid bone and lies lateral to and partly above and below the optic foramen. It is approximately 22 mm long and is spanned by the tendinous ring formed by the common origin of the rectus muscles *(annulus of Zinn)*. Above the ring, the superior orbital fissure transmits the following structures (Fig 1-7):

- lacrimal nerve of CN V_1
- frontal nerve of CN V_1
- CN IV (trochlear nerve)
- superior ophthalmic vein

Within the ring or between the heads of the rectus muscle are the following (see Fig 1-7):

- superior and inferior divisions of CN III (the oculomotor nerve)
- nasociliary branch of CN V_1, which also carries the postganglionic sympathetic fibers en route to the ciliary ganglion
- CN VI (the abducens nerve)

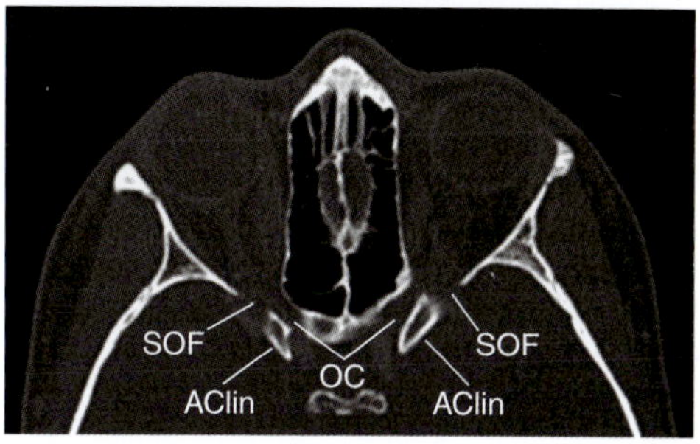

Figure 1-6 Axial computed tomography scan of the orbits. The superior orbital fissure (SOF) passes above and below the plane of the optic canal (OC) and is commonly mistaken for the OC. The OC lies in the same plane as the anterior clinoid processes (AClin) and may be cut obliquely in scans so that the entire canal length does not always appear. *(Courtesy of William R. Katowitz, MD.)*

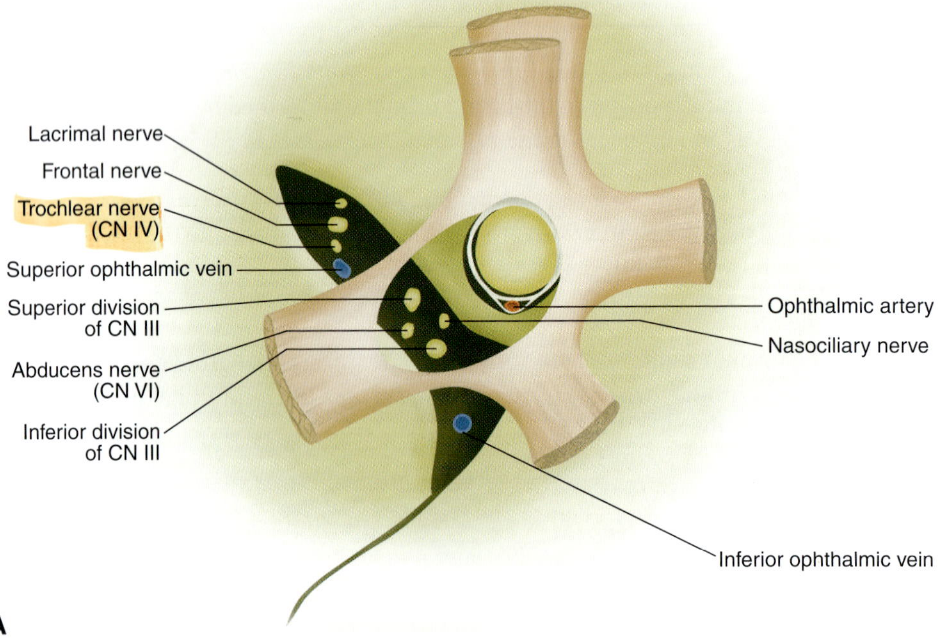

Figure 1-7 **A,** Anterior view of the right orbital apex showing the distribution of the nerves as they enter through the superior orbital fissure and optic canal. This view also shows the annulus of Zinn, the fibrous ring formed by the origin of the 4 rectus muscles.

(Continued)

The course of the inferior ophthalmic vein is variable, and it can travel within or below the ring as it exits the orbit.

The *inferior orbital fissure* lies just below the superior fissure, between the lateral wall and the floor of the orbit, providing access to the pterygopalatine and inferotemporal fossae (see Fig 1-1). Therefore, it is close to the foramen rotundum and the pterygoid canal. The inferior orbital fissure transmits the infraorbital and zygomatic branches of CN V_2, an orbital nerve from the pterygopalatine ganglion, and the inferior ophthalmic vein. The inferior ophthalmic vein connects with the pterygoid plexus before draining into the cavernous sinus.

Periorbital Sinuses

The periorbital sinuses have a close anatomical relationship with the orbits (Fig 1-8). The medial walls of the orbits, which border the nasal cavity anteriorly and the ethmoid sinus and sphenoid sinus posteriorly, are almost parallel. In adults, the lateral wall of each orbit forms an angle of approximately 45° with the medial plane. The lateral walls border the middle cranial, temporal, and pterygopalatine fossae. Superior to the orbit are the anterior cranial fossa and the frontal sinus. The maxillary sinus and the palatine air cells are located inferiorly.

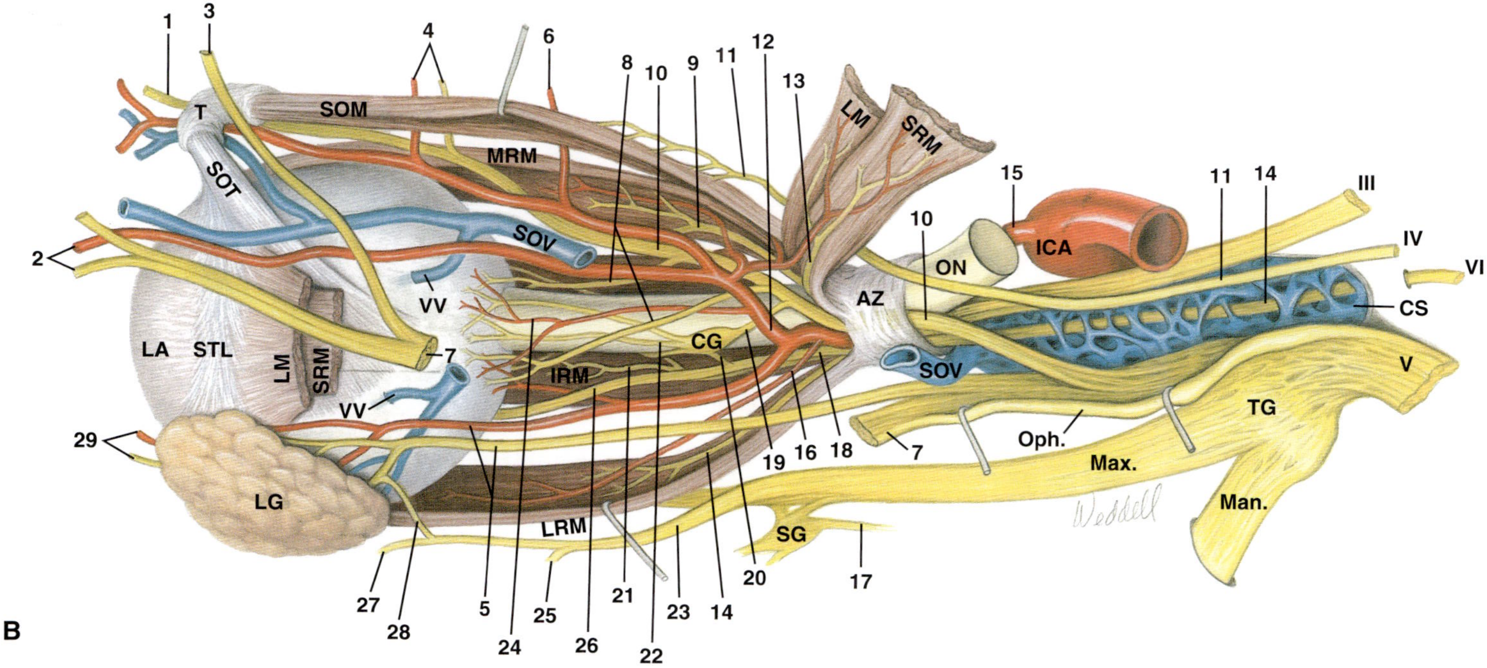

Figure 1-7 *(continued)* **B,** Top view of the left orbit. AZ, annulus of Zinn; CG, ciliary ganglion; CS, cavernous sinus; ICA, internal carotid artery; IRM, inferior rectus muscle; LA, levator aponeurosis; LG, lacrimal gland; LM, levator muscle; LRM, lateral rectus muscle; Man., mandibular nerve; Max., maxillary nerve; MRM, medial rectus muscle; ON, optic nerve; Oph., ophthalmic nerve; SG, sphenopalatine ganglion; SOM, superior oblique muscle; SOT, superior oblique tendon; SOV, superior ophthalmic vein; SRM, superior rectus muscle; STL, superior transverse ligament; T, trochlea; TG, trigeminal (gasserian) ganglion; VV, vortex veins; 1, infratrochlear nerve; 2, supraorbital nerve and artery; 3, supratrochlear nerve; 4, anterior ethmoid nerve and artery; 5, lacrimal nerve and artery; 6, posterior ethmoid artery; 7, frontal nerve; 8, long ciliary nerves; 9, branch of CN III to medial rectus muscle; 10, nasociliary nerve; 11, CN IV; 12, ophthalmic (orbital) artery; 13, superior ramus of CN III; 14, CN VI; 15, ophthalmic artery, origin; 16, anterior ciliary artery; 17, vidian nerve; 18, inferior ramus of CN III; 19, sensory branches from ciliary ganglion to nasociliary nerve; 20, motor (parasympathetic) nerve to ciliary ganglion from nerve to inferior oblique muscle; 21, branch of CN III to inferior rectus muscle; 22, short ciliary nerves; 23, zygomatic nerve; 24, posterior ciliary arteries; 25, zygomaticofacial nerve; 26, nerve to inferior oblique muscle; 27, zygomaticotemporal nerve; 28, lacrimal secretory nerve; 29, lacrimal artery and nerve terminal branches. *(Part A illustration by Cyndie C.H. Wooley. Part B reproduced from Stewart WB, ed.* Ophthalmic Plastic and Reconstructive Surgery. *4th ed. San Francisco: American Academy of Ophthalmology Manuals Program; 1984.)*

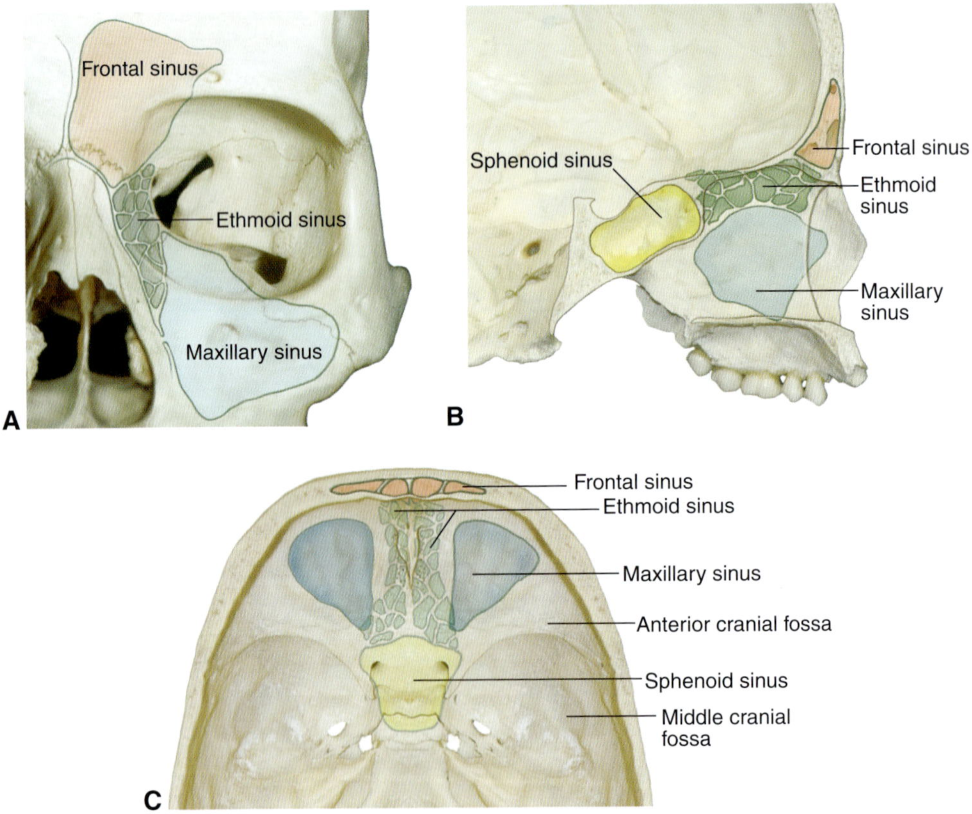

Figure 1-8 Coronal **(A)**, sagittal **(B)**, and axial **(C)** views of the anatomical relationship of the 4 periorbital sinuses. *(Illustrations by Dave Peace.)*

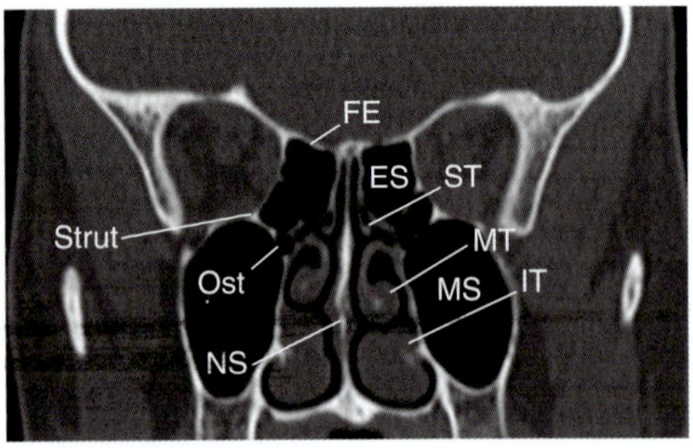

Figure 1-9 Coronal computed tomography scan of the orbits and sinuses showing the maxillary and ethmoid sinuses. ES = ethmoid sinus; FE = fovea ethmoidalis; IT = inferior turbinate; MS = maxillary sinus; MT = middle turbinate; NS = nasal septum; Ost = ostium of the maxillary sinus; ST = superior turbinate; Strut = inferomedial orbital strut. *(Courtesy of William R. Katowitz, MD.)*

The inferomedial orbital strut is located along the inferonasal orbit, where the orbital bones slope from the floor to the medial wall. This region is significant because of its proximity to the ostium of the maxillary sinus (Fig 1-9). In addition, the *fovea ethmoidalis,* which forms the roof of the ethmoid sinuses, is a lateral extension of the cribriform plate. The locations of the periorbital sinuses and their relation to anatomical features of the skull are indicated in Figure 1-8 and discussed further in BCSC Section 7, *Oculofacial Plastic and Orbital Surgery.*

CLINICAL PEARL

When lacrimal surgery is planned, it is important to identify the fovea ethmoidalis to prevent inadvertent cerebral spinal fluid leakage as well as intracranial injury.

Gospe SM 3rd, Bhatti MT. Orbital anatomy. *Int Ophthalmol Clin.* 2018;58(2):5–23.
Zide BM, Jelks GW. *Surgical Anatomy Around the Orbit: The System of Zones.* Philadelphia: Lippincott Williams & Wilkins; 2015.

Cranial Nerves

Six of the 12 cranial nerves (CN II–VII) directly innervate the eye and periocular tissues. Because certain tumors affecting CN I (the olfactory nerve) can give rise to important ophthalmic signs and symptoms, it is imperative that ophthalmologists be familiar with the anatomy of this nerve. Chapter 3 discusses CN I–VII in greater depth; also see BCSC Section 7, *Oculofacial Plastic and Orbital Surgery,* and Section 5, *Neuro-Ophthalmology.*

Ciliary Ganglion

The ciliary ganglion is located approximately 1 cm in front of the annulus of Zinn, on the lateral side of the ophthalmic artery, between the optic nerve and the lateral rectus muscle (Fig 1-10). It receives 3 roots:

- A long (10–12-mm) *sensory root* arises from the nasociliary branch of CN V_1 and contains sensory fibers from the cornea, the iris, and the ciliary body.
- A short *motor root* arises from the inferior division of CN III. It carries preganglionic parasympathetic fibers from the Edinger-Westphal nucleus. The fibers of the motor root synapse in the ganglion, and the postganglionic fibers carry parasympathetic axons to supply the iris sphincter.
- A *sympathetic root* carries postganglionic fibers originating from the superior cervical ganglion, from which they course superiorly with the internal carotid artery. In the cavernous sinus, the sympathetic fibers leave the carotid artery to temporarily join the abducens nerve before entering the orbit either with the nasociliary branch of CN V_1 or as an individual root. The sympathetic root enters the orbit through the superior orbital fissure within the tendinous ring, passes through the ciliary ganglion without synapse, and innervates blood vessels of the eye, as well as the dilator muscle of the pupil. Fibers destined for the Müller muscle travel along the frontal and lacrimal branches of CN V_1.

Branches of the Ciliary Ganglion

Only the parasympathetic fibers synapse in the ciliary ganglion. The sympathetic fibers are postganglionic from the superior cervical ganglion and pass through it without

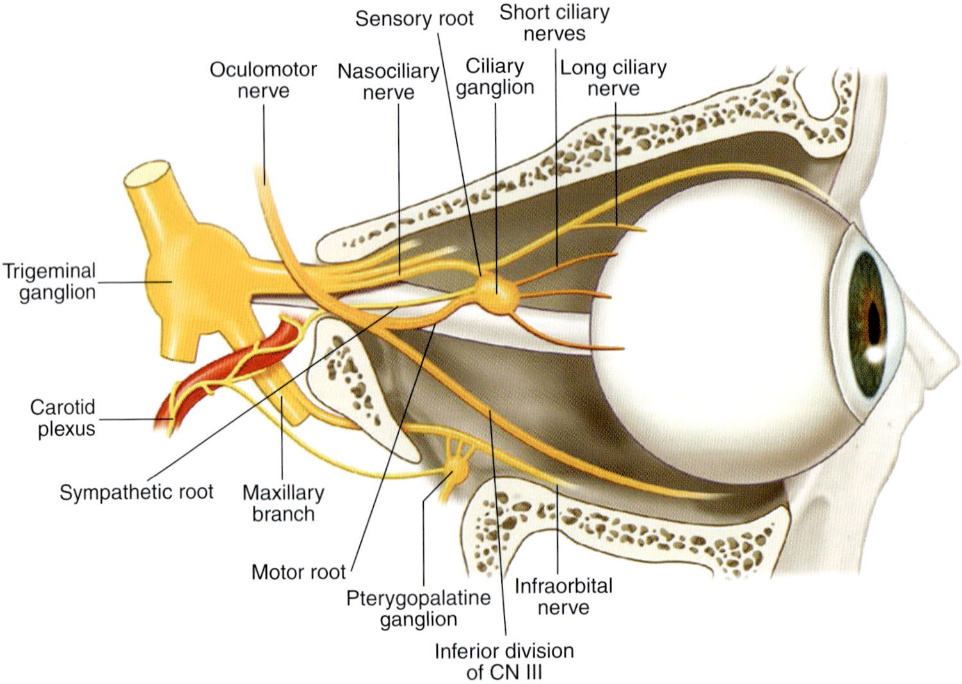

Figure 1-10 Ciliary ganglion. Schematic of the lateral orbit with ciliary ganglion. Note the 3 roots: (1) sensory root, which carries sensation from the globe to the trigeminal ganglion via the nasociliary nerve; (2) sympathetic root carrying postganglionic sympathetic fibers from the superior cervical ganglion and carotid plexus; (3) motor root carrying preganglionic parasympathetic fibers from the inferior division of the oculomotor nerve. *(Modified with permission from Levin LA, Nilsson SFE, Ver Hoeve J, Wu SM.* Adler's Physiology of the Eye. *11th ed. Philadelphia: Elsevier/Saunders; 2011:364.)*

synapsing. Sensory fibers from cell bodies in the trigeminal ganglion carry sensation from the eye, orbit, and face. Together, the nonsynapsing sympathetic fibers; the sensory fibers; and the myelinated, fast-conducting postganglionic parasympathetic fibers form the short ciliary nerves (see also Chapter 3, Fig 3-18).

Short Ciliary Nerves

There are 2 groups of short ciliary nerves, totaling 6–10, which arise from the ciliary ganglion (see Fig 1-10). They travel on both sides of the optic nerve and, together with the long ciliary nerves, pierce the sclera around the optic nerve (see Fig 1-19). Both long and short ciliary nerves pass anteriorly between the choroid and the sclera to the ciliary muscle, where they form a plexus that supplies the cornea, the ciliary body, and the iris. The long ciliary nerves, which arise directly from the nasociliary branch of CN V_1 (ophthalmic division of the trigeminal neve), are sensory nerves. The short ciliary nerves are both sensory and motor nerves, carrying autonomic fibers to the pupil and ciliary muscles (see Chapter 3).

Extraocular Muscles

There are 7 extraocular muscles (Figs 1-11 through 1-14, Table 1-1, Activity 1-1):

- medial rectus
- lateral rectus
- superior rectus
- inferior rectus
- superior oblique
- inferior oblique
- levator palpebrae superioris

ACTIVITY 1-1 Interactive model of the extraocular muscles.
Activity developed by Mary A. O'Hara, MD.
Access all Section 2 activities at www.aao.org/bcscactivity_section02.

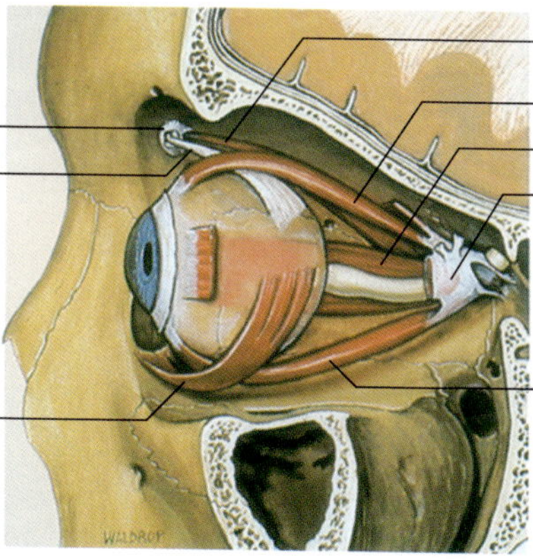

Figure 1-11 Extraocular muscles, lateral composite (sagittal) view of the left eye. *(Reproduced with permission from Dutton JJ.* Atlas of Clinical and Surgical Orbital Anatomy. *Philadelphia: Saunders; 1994.)*

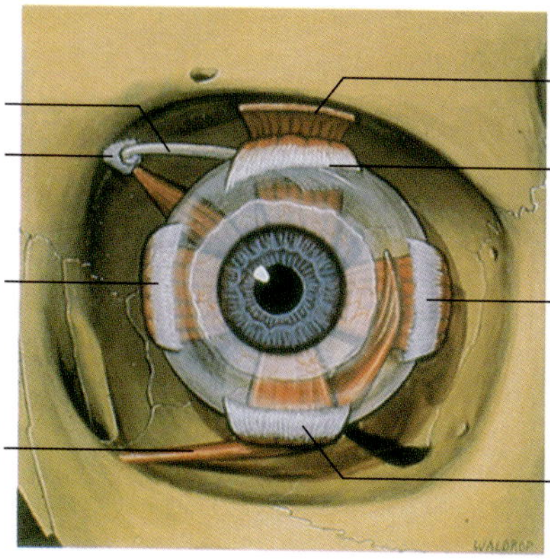

Figure 1-12 Extraocular muscles, frontal view of the left eye, coronal plane. *(Reproduced with permission from Dutton JJ.* Atlas of Clinical and Surgical Orbital Anatomy. *Philadelphia: Saunders; 1994.)*

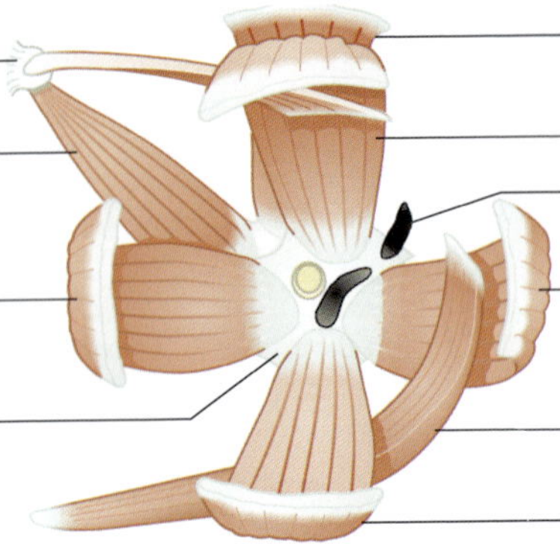

Figure 1-13 Extraocular muscles, frontal view, left eye, with globe removed. *(Reproduced with permission from Dutton JJ.* Atlas of Clinical and Surgical Orbital Anatomy. *Philadelphia: Saunders; 1994.)*

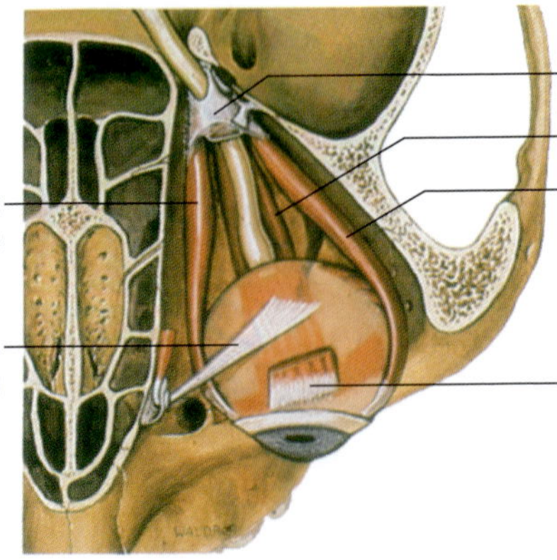

Figure 1-14 Extraocular muscles, superior composite (axial) view. *(Reproduced with permission from Dutton JJ.* Atlas of Clinical and Surgical Orbital Anatomy. *Philadelphia: Saunders; 1994.)*

Extraocular Muscle Origins

The annulus of Zinn consists of superior and inferior orbital tendons and is the origin of the 4 rectus muscles (Fig 1-15). The upper tendon gives rise to the entire superior rectus muscle, as well as portions of the lateral and medial rectus muscles. The inferior tendon gives rise to the entire inferior rectus muscle and portions of the medial and lateral rectus muscles. The levator palpebrae superioris muscle arises from the lesser wing of the sphenoid bone, at the apex of the orbit, just superior to the annulus of Zinn (see the section "Levator palpebrae superioris muscle" later in the chapter).

The superior oblique muscle originates from the periosteum of the body of the sphenoid bone, above and medial to the optic foramen. The inferior oblique muscle originates anteriorly, from a shallow depression in the orbital plate of the maxillary bone, at the anteromedial corner of the orbital floor, near the fossa for the lacrimal sac. From its origin, the inferior oblique muscle then extends posteriorly, laterally, and superiorly to insert into the globe (see Table 1-1).

Table 1-1 Comparison of the Extraocular Muscles

Muscle	Origin	Insertion	Size	Blood Supply	Nerve Supply
Medial rectus	Annulus of Zinn	Medially, in horizontal meridian 5.5 mm from limbus	40.8 mm long; tendon: 3.7 mm long, 10.3 mm wide	Medial (inferior) muscular branch of ophthalmic artery	Inferior division of CN III (oculomotor)
Inferior rectus	Annulus of Zinn at orbital apex	Inferiorly, in vertical meridian 6.5 mm from limbus	40 mm long; tendon: 5.5 mm long, 9.8 mm wide	Medial (inferior) muscular branch of ophthalmic artery and infraorbital artery	Inferior division of CN III (oculomotor)
Lateral rectus	Annulus of Zinn spanning the superior orbital fissure	Laterally, in horizontal meridian 6.9 mm from limbus	40.6 mm long; tendon: 8 mm long, 9.2 mm wide	Lateral (superior) muscular branch of ophthalmic artery and lacrimal artery	CN VI (abducens)
Superior rectus	Annulus of Zinn at orbital apex	Superiorly, in vertical meridian 7.7 mm from limbus	41.8 mm long; tendon: 5.8 mm long, 10.6 mm wide	Lateral (superior) muscular branch of ophthalmic artery	Superior division of CN III (oculomotor)
Superior oblique	Medial to optic foramen, between annulus of Zinn and periorbita	To trochlea, through pulley, just behind orbital rim, then hooking back under superior rectus, inserting posterior to center of rotation	40 mm long; tendon: 20 mm long, 10.8 mm wide	Lateral (superior) muscular branch of ophthalmic artery	CN IV (trochlear)
Inferior oblique	From a depression on orbital floor near orbital rim (maxilla)	Posterior inferotemporal quadrant at level of macula; posterior to center of rotation	37 mm long; tendon: 1 mm long, 9.6 mm wide at insertion	Medial (inferior) muscular branch of ophthalmic artery and infraorbital artery	Inferior division of CN III (oculomotor)
Levator palpebrae superioris	Lesser wing of sphenoid bone	Trochlea, supraorbital notch, superior tarsus, lateral orbital tubercle, posterior lacrimal crest	60 mm long; muscle: 40 mm, tendon: 14–20 mm	Branches of the ophthalmic artery	Superior division of CN III (oculomotor)

CN = cranial nerve.

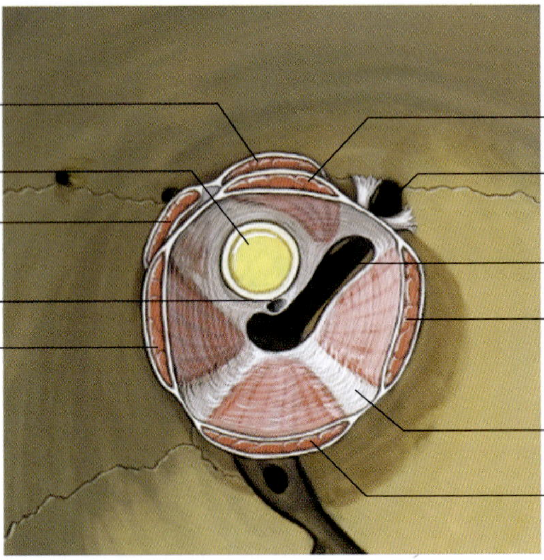

Figure 1-15 Origin of the extraocular muscles. All extraocular muscles, except the inferior oblique, originate in the orbital apex. The 4 rectus muscles share a common fibrotendinous ring known as the *annulus of Zinn*. Note that the superior rectus and medial rectus are juxtaposed to the optic nerve sheath; this is the reason that patients with retrobulbar optic neuritis experience pain with movement of the eye. *(Reproduced with permission from Dutton JJ.* Atlas of Clinical and Surgical Orbital Anatomy. *2nd ed. Philadelphia: Elsevier/Saunders; 2011, Fig 3-8.)*

Extraocular Muscle Insertions

The 4 rectus muscles insert anteriorly on the globe. Starting at the medial rectus muscle and proceeding to the inferior rectus, lateral rectus, and superior rectus muscles, the muscle insertions lie progressively farther from the limbus. An imaginary curve drawn through these insertions creates a spiral, called the *spiral of Tillaux* (Fig 1-16). The relationship between the muscle insertions and the location of the ora serrata is clinically important. A misdirected suture passed through the insertion of any extraocular muscle could perforate the retina.

The superior oblique muscle, after passing through the trochlea in the superomedial orbital rim, inserts onto the sclera superiorly, under the insertion of the superior rectus. The inferior oblique muscle inserts onto the sclera in the posterior inferotemporal quadrant.

Extraocular Muscle Distribution in the Orbit

See Figures 1-12 through 1-14 for the arrangement of the extraocular muscles within the orbit. Note the relationship between the oblique extraocular muscles and the superior, medial, and inferior rectus muscles. See Chapter 17 for additional figures depicting the location of the extraocular muscles within the orbit and their relationship to surrounding structures, along with corresponding computed tomography and magnetic resonance imaging scans.

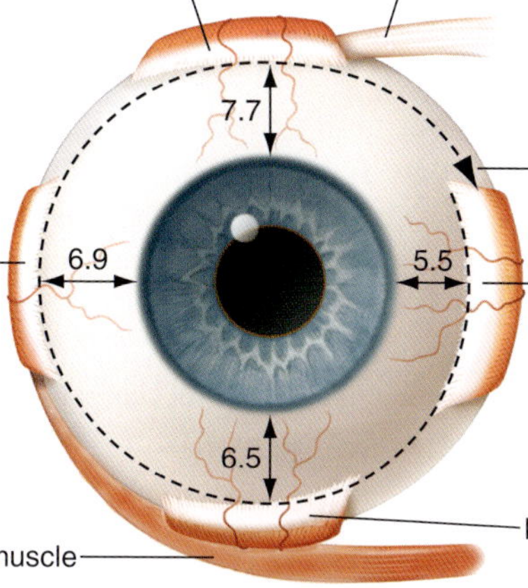

Figure 1-16 The medial rectus tendon is closest to the limbus, and the superior rectus tendon is farthest from it. By connecting the insertions of the tendons beginning with the medial rectus, then the inferior rectus, then the lateral rectus, and finally the superior rectus, a spiral (known as the *spiral of Tillaux*) is obtained. Measurements are in millimeters. The anterior ciliary arteries are also shown. *(Illustration by Christine Gralapp.)*

Blood Supply to the Extraocular Muscles

The extraocular muscles are supplied by the following (see Table 1-1):

- muscular branches of the ophthalmic artery
- infraorbital artery
- lacrimal artery

The muscular branches of the ophthalmic artery give rise to the anterior ciliary arteries and can be divided into lateral (superior) and medial (inferior) branches. Each rectus muscle has 1–4 anterior ciliary arteries, which eventually pass through the muscle belly; penetrate the sclera, anastomosing with the major arterial circle; and contribute to the blood supply of the anterior segment (see Fig 1-22). The lateral rectus muscle receives part of its blood supply from the lacrimal artery; the inferior oblique and inferior rectus muscles receive part of their blood supply from the infraorbital artery (see Figs 1-17, 1-21).

Innervation of the Extraocular Muscles

The lateral rectus muscle is innervated by CN VI (the abducens nerve). The superior oblique muscle is innervated by CN IV (the trochlear nerve). CN III (the oculomotor nerve) has superior and inferior divisions: the upper division innervates the levator palpebrae superioris and superior rectus muscles, and the lower division innervates the medial rectus, inferior rectus, and inferior oblique muscles (see Table 1-1).

Fine Structure of the Extraocular Muscles

In the extraocular muscles, the ratio of nerve fibers to muscle fibers is very high (1:3–1:5) compared with the ratio of nerve axons to muscle fibers in skeletal muscle (1:50–1:125). This high ratio enables precise control of ocular movements. The fibers of the extraocular muscles are a mixture of (1) slow, tonic-type fibers, which are innervated by multiple grapelike nerve endings *(en grappe)* and are useful for smooth-pursuit movements; and (2) fast, twitch-type fibers, which have platelike nerve endings *(en plaque)* and aid in rapid saccadic movements of the eye.

Porter JD, Baker RS, Ragusa RJ, Brueckner JK. Extraocular muscles: basic and clinical aspects of structure and function. *Surv Ophthalmol.* 1995;39(6):451–484.

Vascular Supply and Drainage of the Orbit

Posterior and Anterior Ciliary Arteries

Approximately 16–20 short posterior ciliary arteries and 6–10 short ciliary nerves enter the globe in a ring around the optic nerve (Figs 1-17, 1-18, 1-19). Usually, 2 long posterior ciliary arteries and 2 long ciliary nerves enter the sclera on either side of the optic nerve, close to the horizontal meridian. They course anteriorly in the suprachoroidal space, terminating at the major arterial circle of the iris.

The posterior ciliary vessels originate from the ophthalmic artery and supply the entire uvea, the cilioretinal arteries, the sclera, the margin of the cornea, and the adjacent conjunctiva. Occlusion of the posterior ciliary vessels (as in giant cell arteritis) may have profound consequences for the eye, such as anterior ischemic optic neuropathy.

The anterior ciliary arteries also arise from the ophthalmic artery and usually supply (in pairs) the superior, medial, and inferior rectus muscles (Figs 1-20, 1-21). After emerging from the surface of the rectus muscles, the anterior ciliary vessels perforate the sclera anterior to the rectus muscle insertions, where they anastomose with the long posterior ciliary arteries at the major arterial circle of the iris.

Within the eye, the posterior ciliary vessel forms the intramuscular circle of the iris, branches of which supply the major arterial circle (which is usually discontinuous). This circle lies within the apex of the ciliary muscle, which it supplies together with the iris (Fig 1-22). The iris vessels have a radial arrangement that, in lightly pigmented blue irises, is visible upon slit-lamp examination. This radial arrangement can be distinguished from the irregular new iris vessels formed in rubeosis iridis.

Vortex Veins

The vortex veins drain the venous system of the choroid, ciliary body, and iris (see Fig 1-19). Each eye contains 4–7 (or more) veins. One or more veins are usually located in each quadrant and exit 14–25 mm from the limbus, between the rectus muscles. The ampullae of the vortex veins are 8–9 mm from the ora serrata and are visible by indirect ophthalmoscopy. A circle connecting these ampullae corresponds roughly to the equator and

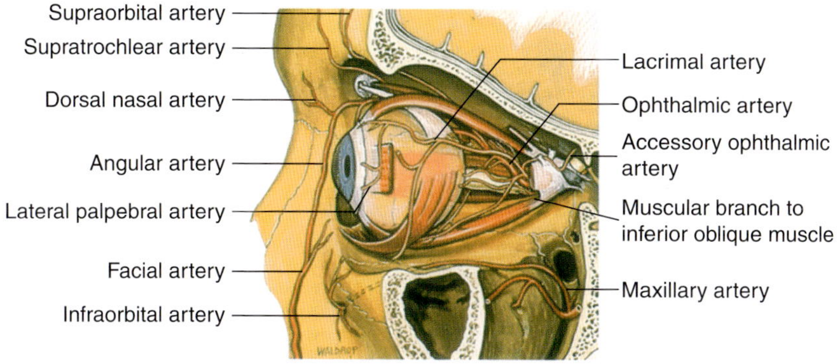

A

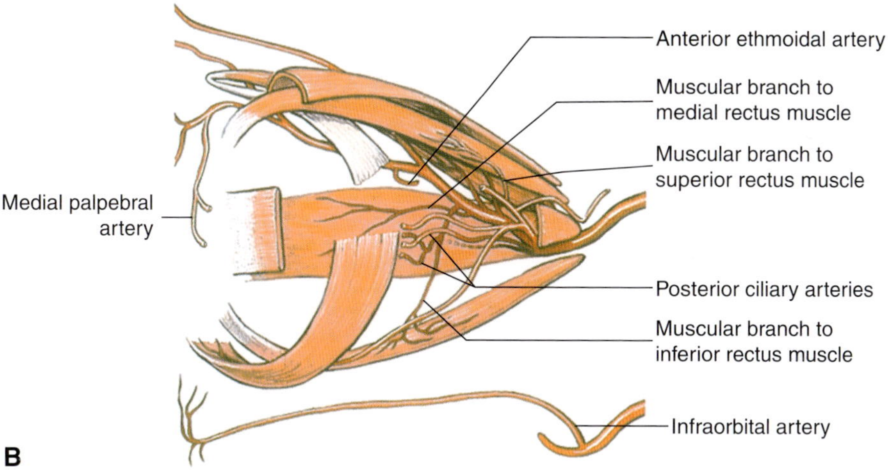

B

Figure 1-17 Orbital arteries. **A,** Lateral (sagittal) view with extraocular muscles, composite view. **B,** Central dissection. *(Reproduced with permission from Dutton JJ.* Atlas of Clinical and Surgical Orbital Anatomy. *Philadelphia: Saunders; 1994.)*

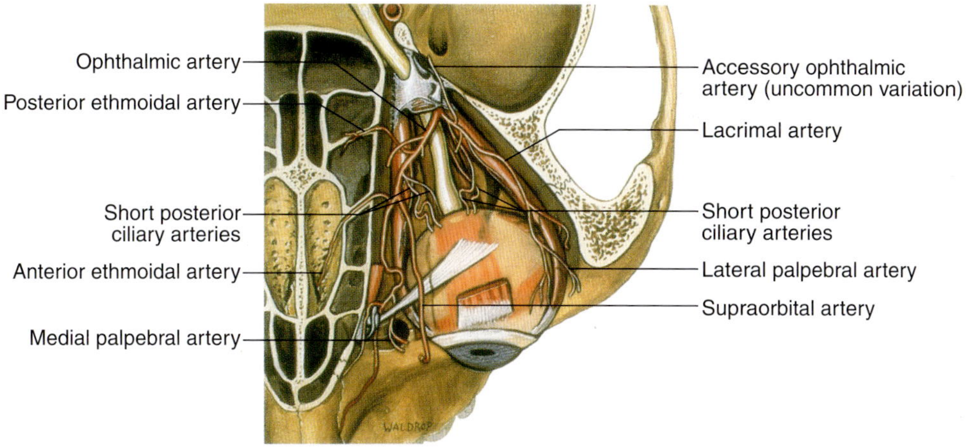

Figure 1-18 Orbital arteries, superior composite (axial) view. *(Modified with permission from Dutton JJ.* Atlas of Clinical and Surgical Orbital Anatomy. *Philadelphia: Saunders; 1994.)*

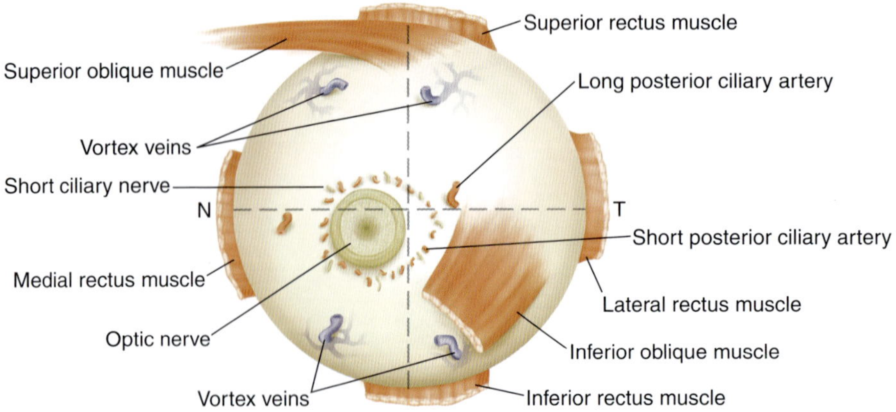

Figure 1-19 Posterior view of the right globe. There are 2 long posterior ciliary arteries and 16–20 short posterior ciliary arteries. N = nasal; T = temporal. *(Modified by Cyndie C.H. Wooley from an illustration by Thomas A. Weingeist, PhD, MD.)*

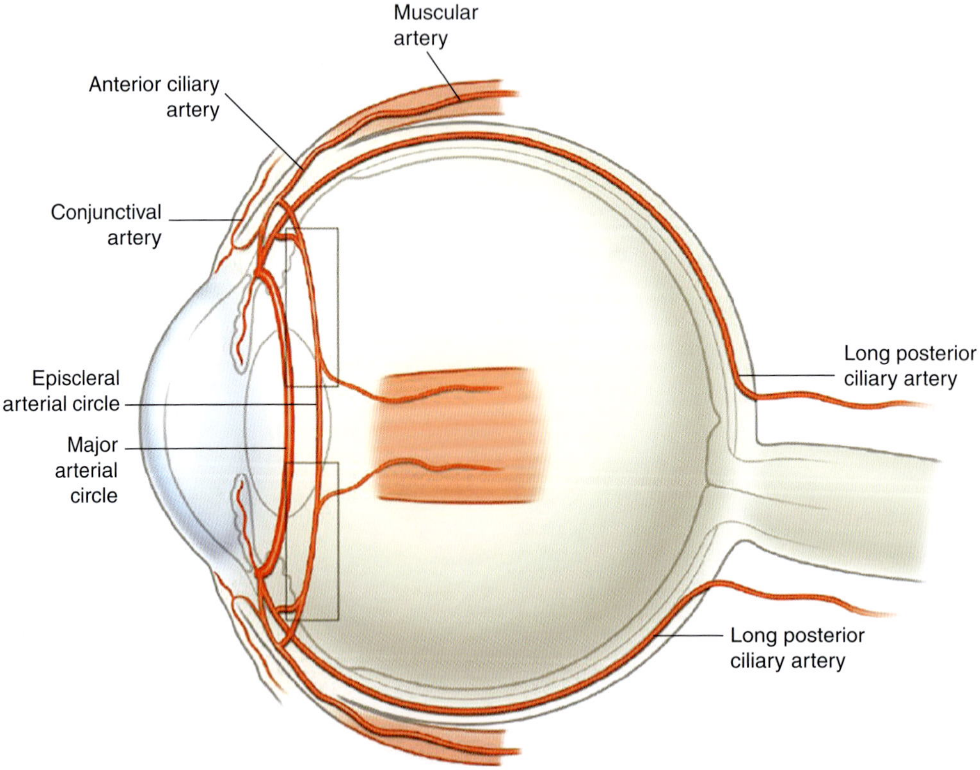

Figure 1-20 Schematic of the anastomoses between the anterior and posterior ciliary circulation. The long posterior ciliary arteries travel in the suprachoroidal space, where they terminate at the major arterial circle of the iris. The anterior ciliary arteries emerge from the surface of the rectus muscles to penetrate the sclera and join the posterior ciliary arteries at the major arterial circle of the iris. The episcleral arterial circle runs on the surface of the sclera, connecting the anterior ciliary arteries. *(Modified with permission from Levin LA, Nilsson SFE, Ver Hoeve J, Wu SM.* Adler's Physiology of the Eye. *11th ed. Philadelphia: Elsevier/Saunders; 2011, Fig 4.35.)*

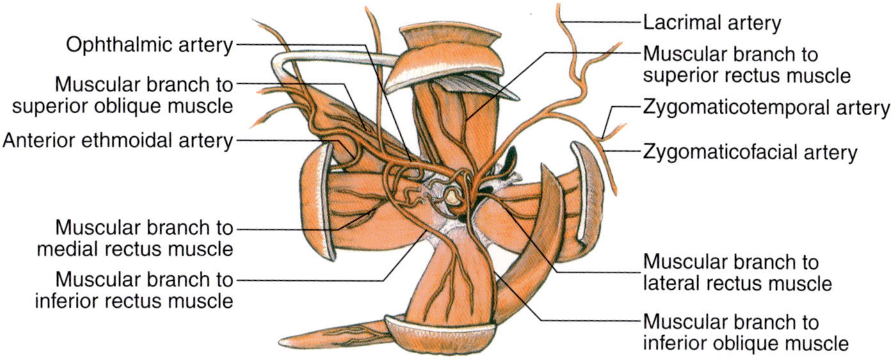

Figure 1-21 Orbital arteries, frontal view with extraocular muscles. *(Reproduced with permission from Dutton JJ.* Atlas of Clinical and Surgical Orbital Anatomy. *Philadelphia: Saunders; 1994.)*

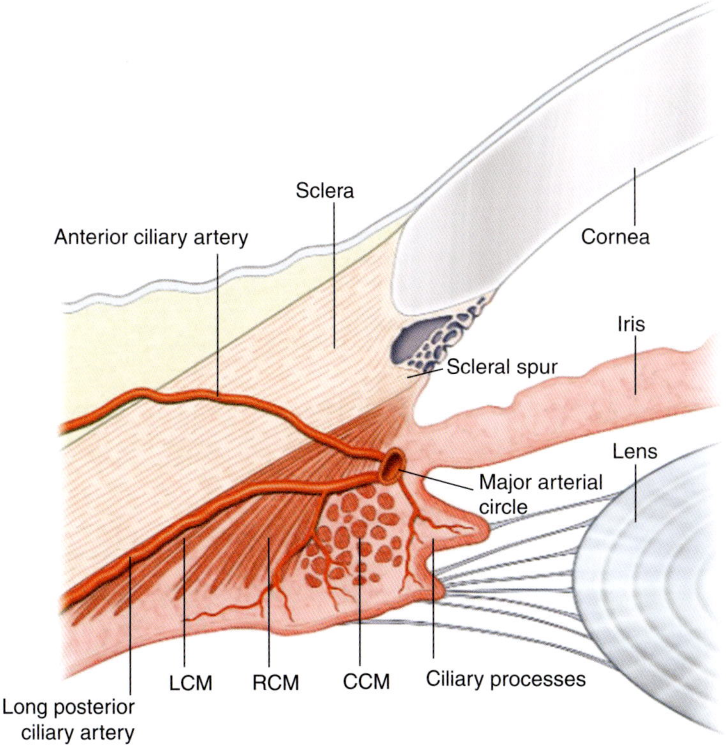

Figure 1-22 Anastomosis of the anterior and posterior ciliary circulation. CCM = circular ciliary muscle; LCM = longitudinal ciliary muscle; RCM = radial ciliary muscle. *(Reproduced with permission from Levin LA, Nilsson SFE, Ver Hoeve J, Wu SM.* Adler's Physiology of the Eye. *11th ed. Philadelphia: Elsevier/Saunders; 2011:276.)*

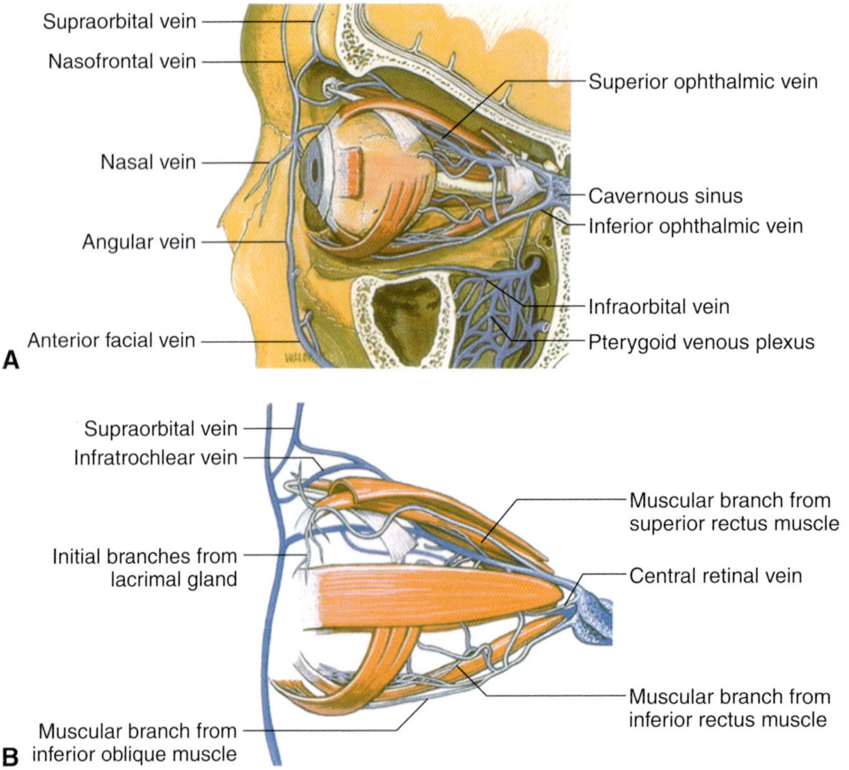

Figure 1-23 Orbital veins, lateral (sagittal) view. **A,** Composite view. Note the eventual connection of the facial venous system with the cavernous sinus. **B,** Central dissection. *(Reproduced with permission from Dutton JJ.* Atlas of Clinical and Surgical Orbital Anatomy. *Philadelphia: Saunders; 1994.)*

divides the central or posterior fundus from the peripheral or anterior portion. The vortex veins join the orbital venous system after leaving the eye (Fig 1-23).

Eyelids

The *palpebral fissure* is the exposed ocular surface between the upper and lower eyelids (Fig 1-24). Normally, the adult fissure is 27–30 mm long and 8–11 mm wide. The upper eyelid, which is more mobile than the lower, can be raised 15 mm by the action of the levator palpebrae superioris muscle alone and can be raised another 1–2 mm by the action of the Müller muscle. If the frontalis muscle of the brow is used, the palpebral fissure can be widened an additional 2 mm. See also BCSC Section 7, *Oculofacial Plastic and Orbital Surgery.*

Anatomy

Though small in surface area, the eyelid is complex in its structure and function. When the anatomy of the upper eyelid is described, it is helpful to divide it into distinct segments

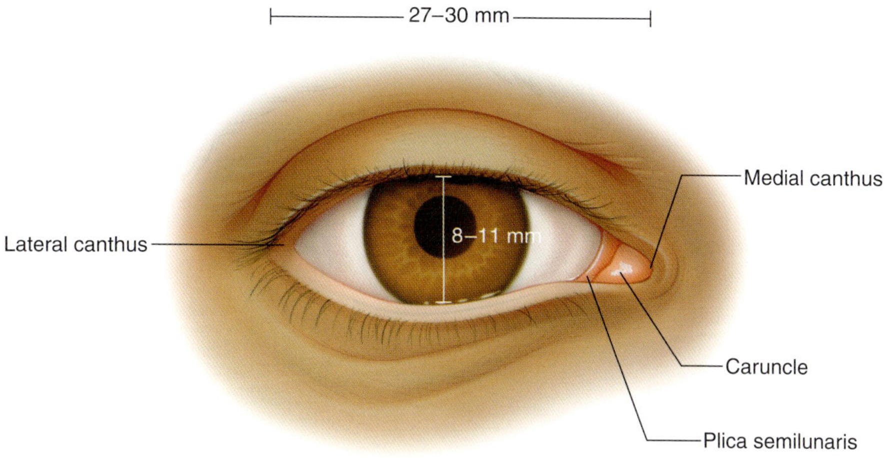

Figure 1-24 Landmarks of the external eye. *(Illustration by Christine Gralapp.)*

from the dermal surface inward. These segments include the following structures (Fig 1-25; see also Figs 1-26 through 1-34):

- skin and subcutaneous connective tissue
- muscles of protraction (orbicularis oculi muscle, the main protractor)
- orbital septum
- orbital fat
- muscles of retraction (levator palpebrae superioris, Müller muscle, capsulopalpebral fascia, inferior tarsal muscle)
- tarsus
- conjunctiva

Eyelid skin and subcutaneous connective tissue

The eyelid skin, the thinnest in the body, contains fine hairs, sebaceous glands, and sweat glands. A superior eyelid crease is present near the upper border of the tarsus, where the levator aponeurosis establishes its first insertional attachments. In many individuals of Asian descent, there are few attachments of the levator aponeurosis to the skin near the upper tarsal border, and the superior eyelid crease is minimal or absent. Figure 1-26 depicts the 2 major racial variations in eyelid anatomy.

The loose connective tissue of the eyelid contains no fat. Blood or other fluids can accumulate beneath the skin and cause rapid and dramatic swelling of the eyelids.

The eyelid margin contains several important landmarks (Fig 1-27). A small opening, the *punctum* of the canaliculus, presents medially at the summit of each lacrimal papilla. The superior punctum, normally hidden by slight internal rotation, is located more medially than the inferior punctum, which is usually apposed to the globe and is not normally visible without eversion.

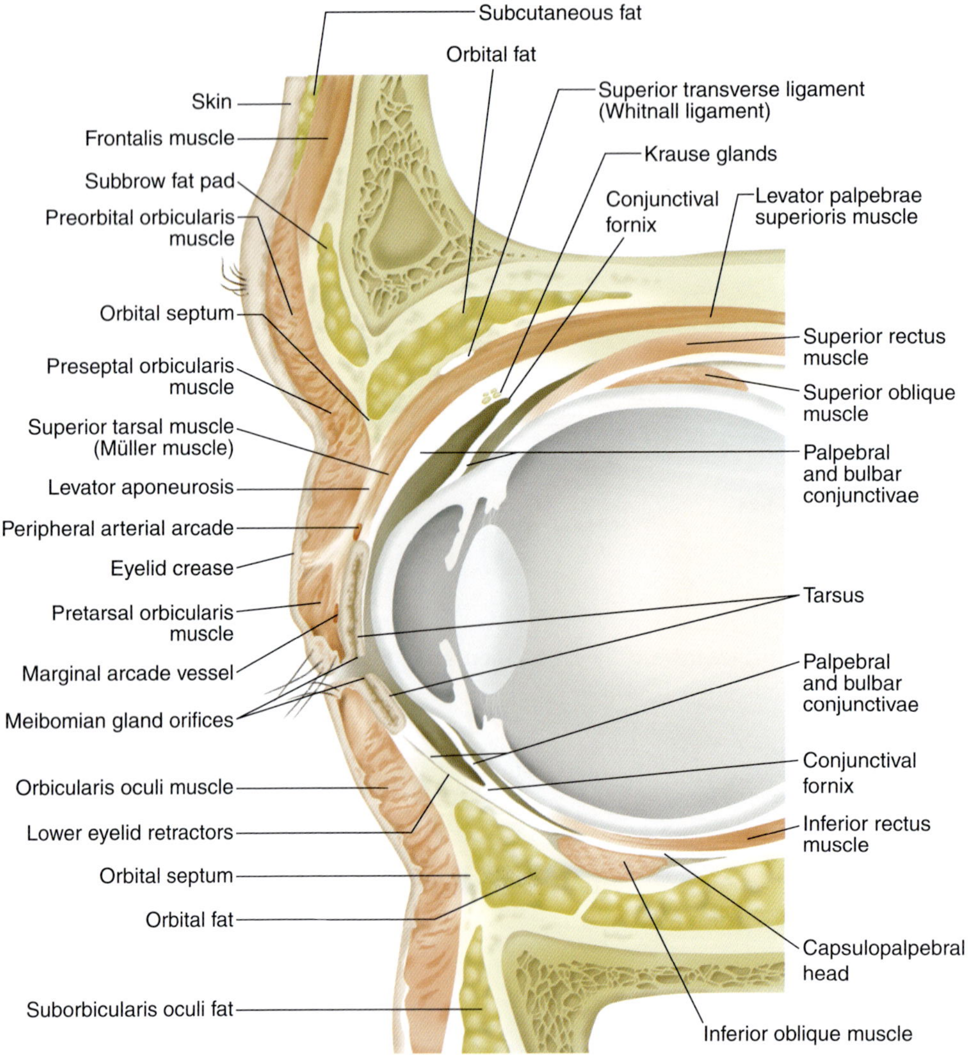

Figure 1-25 Eyelid anatomy: schematic cross section of the upper and lower eyelid area. *(Modified from Stewart WB.* Surgery of the Eyelid, Orbit, and Lacrimal System. *Ophthalmology Monograph 8, vol 2. San Francisco: American Academy of Ophthalmology; 1994:23, 85. Illustration by Cyndie C.H. Wooley.)*

Along the entire length of the free margin of the eyelid is the delicate *gray line* (or *intermarginal sulcus*), which corresponds histologically to the most superficial portion of the orbicularis oculi muscle, the muscle of Riolan, and to the avascular plane of the eyelid. Anterior to this line, the eyelashes (or cilia) arise, and behind this line are the openings of the meibomian (or tarsal) glands just anterior to the mucocutaneous junction.

The eyelashes are arranged in 2 or 3 irregular rows along the anterior dermal edge of the eyelid margin. They are usually longer and more numerous on the upper eyelid than on the lower one. The margins contain the *glands of Zeis,* which are modified sebaceous

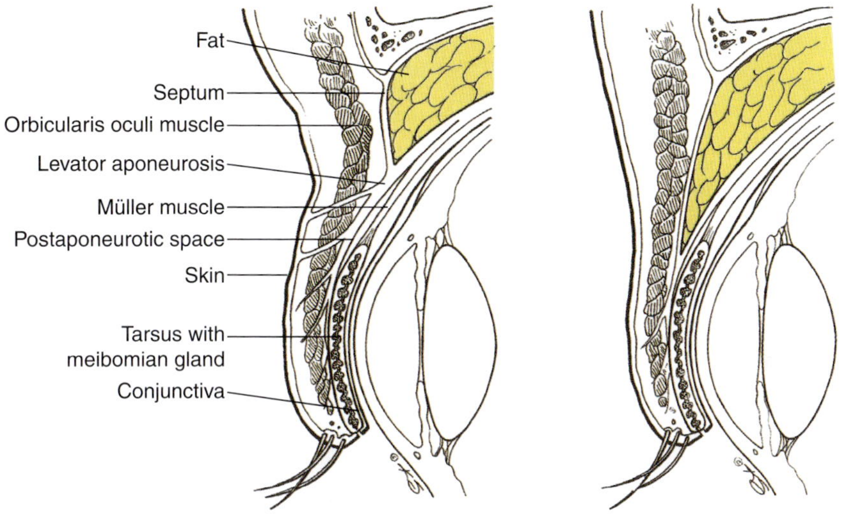

Figure 1-26 Racial variations in eyelid anatomy. Variant I *(left):* the orbital septum inserts onto the levator aponeurosis above the tarsus. Variant II (Asian, *right*): the orbital septum inserts onto the levator aponeurosis between the eyelid margin and the superior border of the tarsus, and there are fewer aponeurotic attachments to the skin. *(Modified with permission from Katowitz JA, ed.* Pediatric Oculoplastic Surgery. *Philadelphia: Springer-Verlag; 2002.)*

glands associated with the cilia, and the *glands of Moll,* which are apocrine sweat glands in the skin (see Fig 1-27; Table 1-2).

Muscle of protraction: orbicularis oculi muscle

The *orbicularis oculi muscle,* the main protractor of the eyelid, is arranged in several concentric bands around the palpebral fissure and can be divided into orbital and palpebral (preseptal and pretarsal) parts (Fig 1-28). Innervation occurs by CN VII (the facial nerve). The orbital part inserts in a complex way into the medial canthal tendon and into other portions of the orbital margin and the corrugator supercilii muscle. The orbital part acts as a sphincter and functions solely during voluntary closure of the eye.

The palpebral orbicularis oculi muscle functions both voluntarily and involuntarily in spontaneous and reflex blinking. The preseptal and pretarsal portions unite along the superior palpebral furrow. The pretarsal orbicularis muscle adheres firmly to the tarsus; a portion of it attaches to the anterior lacrimal crest and the posterior lacrimal crest (sometimes called the *Horner muscle*) and plays a role in tear drainage. Orbicularis fibers extend to the eyelid margin, where there is the small bundle of striated muscle fibers called the *muscle of Riolan* (Fig 1-29; see also Fig 1-27B).

Orbital septum

The *orbital septum* is a thin sheet of connective tissue that encircles the orbit as an extension of the periosteum of the roof and the floor of the orbit (Fig 1-30). Superiorly, the septum is attached firmly to the periosteum of the superior half of the orbital margin, at the arcus marginalis. It passes medially in front of the trochlea and continues along

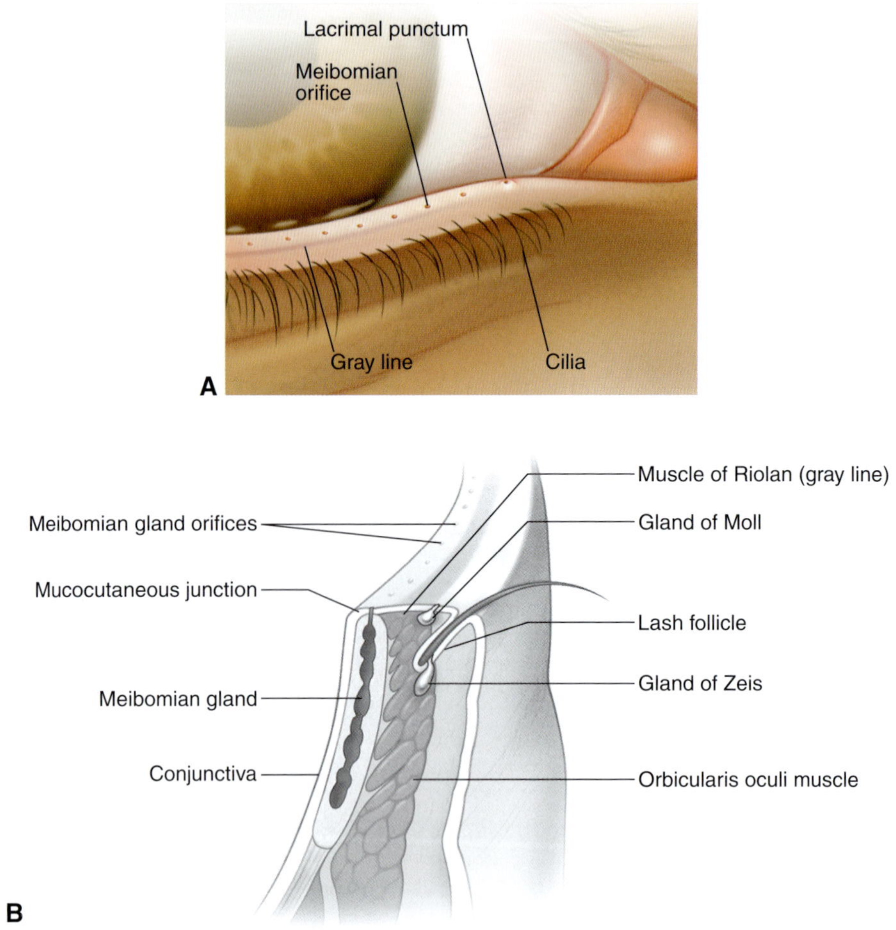

Figure 1-27 Anatomical landmarks of the lower eyelid margin. **A,** The gray line, or intermarginal sulcus, is visible between the bases of the cilia and the orifices of the meibomian glands. The lower eyelid has been slightly everted to clearly expose the inferior lacrimal punctum. **B,** Cross section of the lower eyelid margin. *(Illustrations by Christine Gralapp.)*

Table 1-2 Glands of the Eye and Adnexa

Glands	Location	Secretion	Content
Lacrimal	Orbital gland	Exocrine	Aqueous
	Palpebral gland	Exocrine	Aqueous
Accessory lacrimal	Plica, caruncle	Exocrine	Aqueous
Krause	Eyelid	Exocrine	Aqueous
Wolfring	Eyelid	Exocrine	Aqueous
Meibomian	Tarsus	Holocrine	Oil
Zeis	Follicles of cilia	Holocrine	Oil
	Eyelid, caruncle	Holocrine	Oil
Moll	Eyelid	Apocrine	Sweat
Goblet cell	Conjunctiva	Holocrine	Mucus
	Plica, caruncle	Holocrine	Mucus

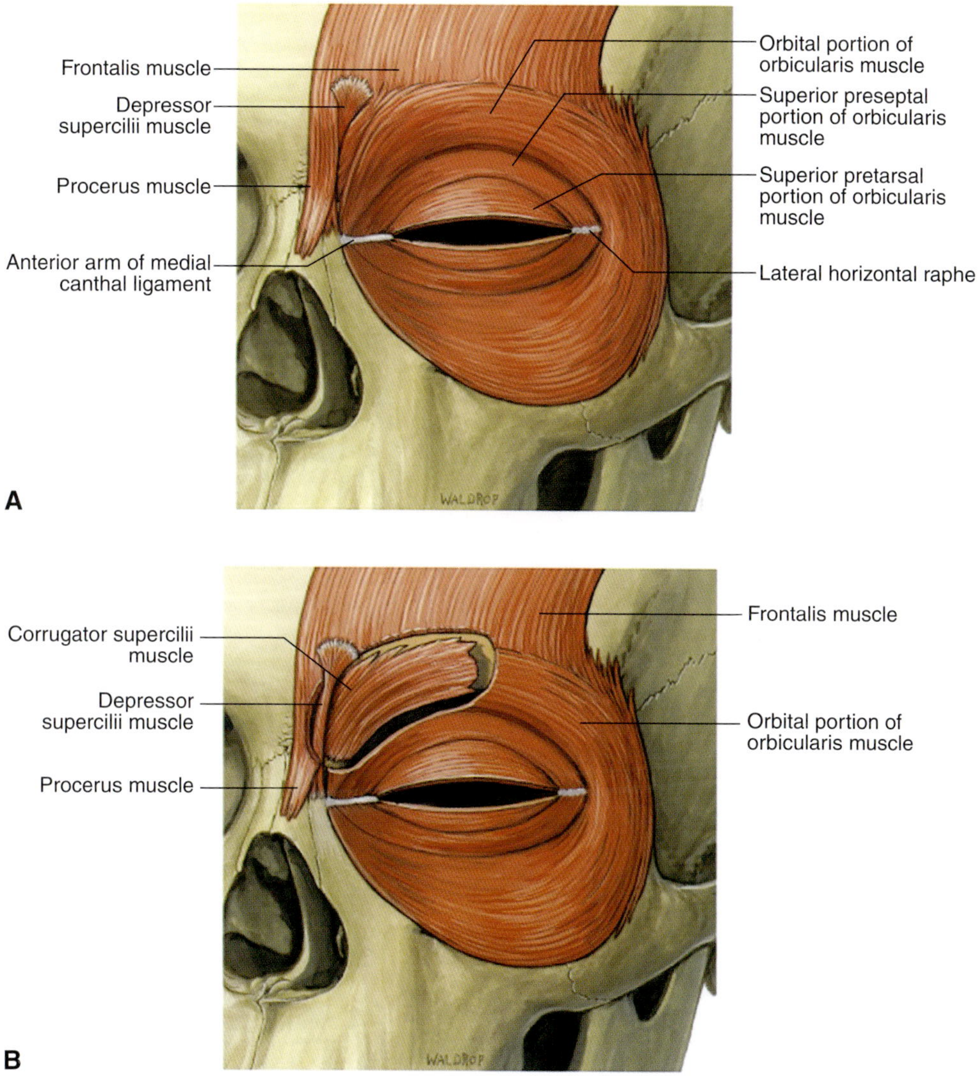

Figure 1-28 The 3 parts of the orbicularis oculi muscle. **A,** Orbital, preseptal, and pretarsal. Note the relationship of the orbicularis oculi with the frontalis, depressor supercilii, and procerus muscles. **B,** The corrugator supercilii muscle with a segment of the orbital portion of the orbicularis oculi muscle removed. *(Modified with permission from Dutton JJ.* Atlas of Clinical and Surgical Orbital Anatomy. *2nd ed. Philadelphia: Elsevier/Saunders; 2011, Figs 8-12, 8-13.)*

the medial margin of the orbit, along the margin of the frontal process of the maxillary bone, and onto the inferior margin of the orbit. Centrally, the orbital septum attaches to the aponeurosis of both the upper and lower eyelids. The septum delimits the anterior or posterior spread of edema, inflammation, or blood. Clinical examples include preseptal cellulitis, orbital cellulitis, and retrobulbar hemorrhage.

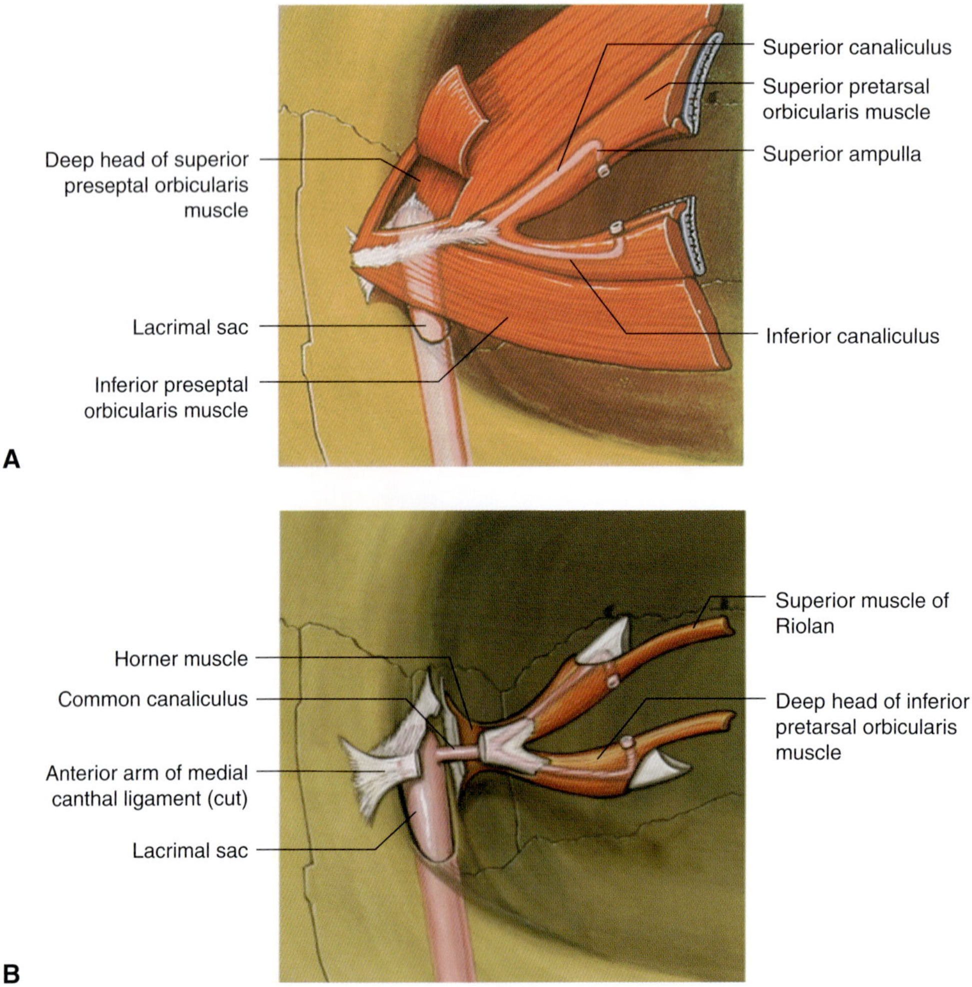

Figure 1-29 Lacrimal drainage system. **A,** Superficial extensions of the orbicularis oculi muscle. **B,** Deep head of the orbicularis oculi muscle; superficial components are reflected. *(Part A reproduced with permission from Dutton JJ.* Atlas of Clinical and Surgical Orbital Anatomy. *Philadelphia: Saunders; 1994. Part B reproduced with permission from Dutton JJ.* Atlas of Clinical and Surgical Orbital Anatomy. *2nd ed. Philadelphia: Elsevier/Saunders; 2011, Fig 9-3.)*

Orbital fat

Posterior to the septum lie the orbital (preaponeurotic) fat pads, 2 behind the superior septum and 3 behind the inferior septum (see Fig 1-30).

CLINICAL PEARL

In patients with periorbital lacerations, the presence of orbital fat indicates violation of the orbital septum.

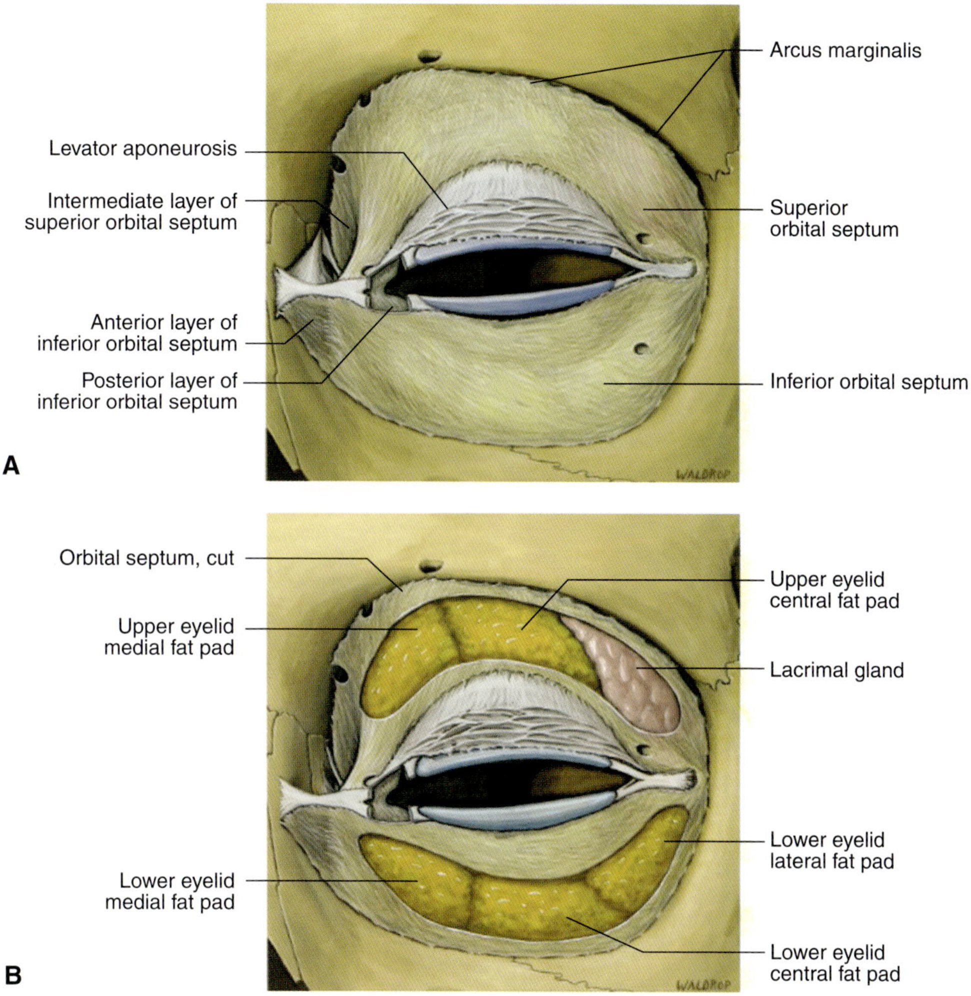

Figure 1-30 Orbital septum. **A,** The orbital septum arises from the periosteum of the bones of the orbital margin and inserts on the aponeurosis of the upper and lower eyelids. **B,** Preaponeurotic fat pads. *(Modified with permission from Dutton JJ.* Atlas of Clinical and Surgical Orbital Anatomy. *2nd ed. Philadelphia: Elsevier/Saunders; 2011, Figs 8-8, 8-9.)*

Muscles of retraction: upper eyelid

In the upper eyelid, the retractors are the *levator palpebrae superioris muscle* with its aponeurosis and the *Müller muscle (superior tarsal muscle).*

Levator palpebrae superioris muscle The levator palpebrae superioris muscle originates from the lesser wing of the sphenoid bone (see Fig 1-25). The body of the levator muscle overlies the superior rectus as it travels anteriorly toward the eyelid (Fig 1-31). The muscle itself, which is 40 mm long, is innervated by the superior division of CN III, and its action can lift the upper eyelid 15 mm.

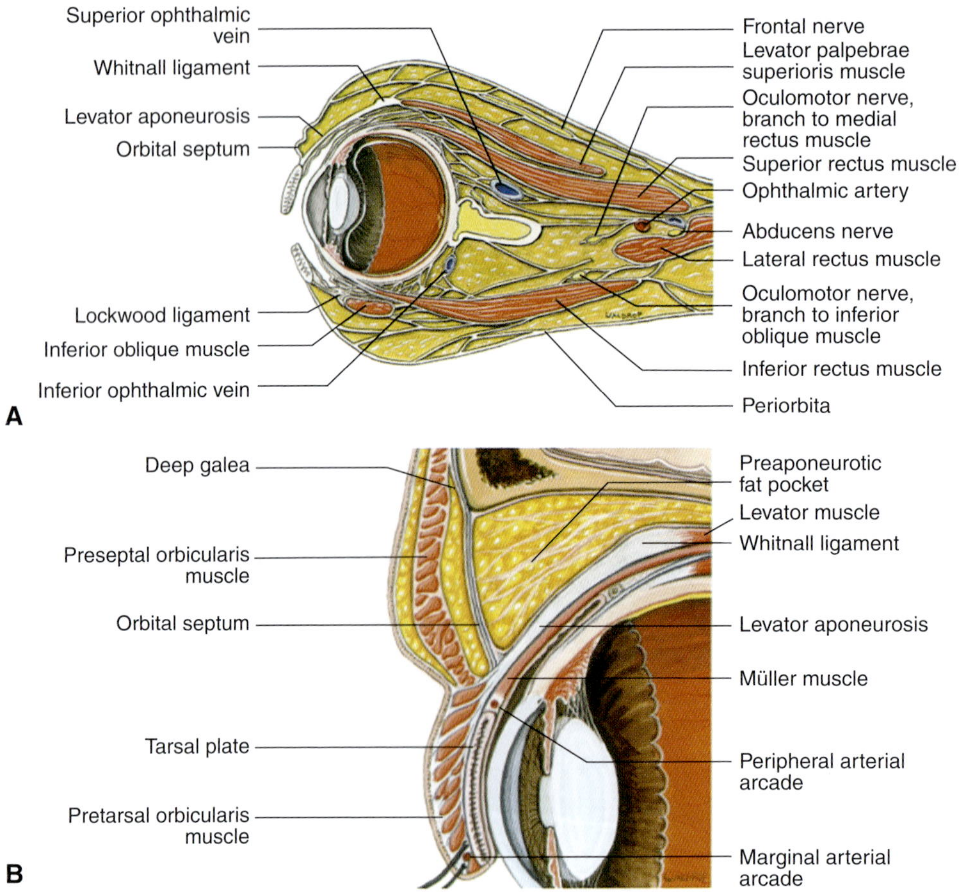

Figure 1-31 Levator palpebrae superioris muscle. Note the levator muscle's transition into the aponeurosis at the Whitnall ligament **(A)** and the aponeurosis passing through the pretarsal orbicularis muscle to the eyelid skin **(B).** *(Modified with permission from Dutton JJ.* Atlas of Clinical and Surgical Orbital Anatomy. *2nd ed. Philadelphia: Elsevier/Saunders; 2011, Figs 7-11, 8-15.)*

The *Whitnall (superior transverse) ligament* is formed by a condensation of tissue surrounding the levator muscle (Fig 1-32; see also Fig 1-31). It provides support for the upper eyelid and surrounding tissues. At the Whitnall ligament, the levator muscle transitions into the aponeurosis anteriorly and the Müller (superior tarsal) muscle posteriorly. The Whitnall ligament is also where the levator muscle's anterior–posterior vector changes to superior–inferior, toward the aponeurosis.

The *levator aponeurosis,* the tendon of the levator muscle, is 14–20 mm in length and has many attachments to the eyelid and surrounding orbit (see Figs 1-31, 1-32). Anteriorly, it passes through the orbicularis oculi muscle and inserts subcutaneously to produce the superior eyelid crease (see Fig 1-26). Posteriorly, the levator aponeurosis inserts into the surface of the tarsus. The aponeurosis forms its firmest attachments on the anterior aspect of the tarsus, approximately 3 mm superior to the eyelid margin. The aponeurosis

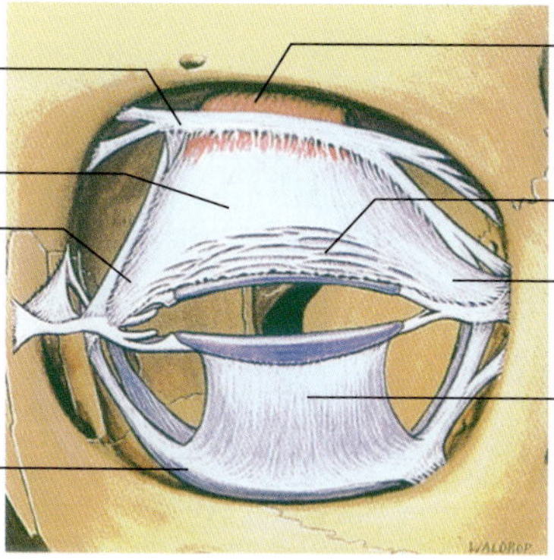

Figure 1-32 Levator aponeurosis and the Whitnall ligament. Note the medial and lateral horns of the aponeurosis and the suspensory ligament of Lockwood. *(Modified with permission from Dutton JJ.* Atlas of Clinical and Surgical Orbital Anatomy. *Philadelphia: Saunders; 1994.)*

also inserts into the trochlea of the superior oblique muscle and into the fibrous tissue bridging the supraorbital foramen/notch. The lateral horn of the aponeurosis divides the lacrimal gland into orbital and palpebral lobes and inserts at the lateral orbital tubercle. The medial horn inserts at the posterior lacrimal crest. Aponeurotic attachments also exist with the conjunctiva of the upper fornix and the orbital septum.

Müller muscle The Müller (superior tarsal) muscle originates from the undersurface of the levator palpebrae superioris muscle in the upper eyelid. This smooth muscle is innervated by the sympathetic nervous system, and its action is responsible for 1–2 mm of upper eyelid lift. The Müller muscle attaches to the upper border of the upper tarsus and to the conjunctiva of the upper fornix (see Fig 1-31B).

Muscles of retraction: lower eyelid

In the lower eyelid, the retractors are the *capsulopalpebral fascia,* which is analogous to the levator aponeurosis in the upper eyelid, and the *inferior tarsal muscle.* The inferior tarsal muscle arises from the capsulopalpebral head of the inferior rectus muscle in the lower eyelid. Like the Müller muscle, the inferior tarsal muscle is smooth muscle, but it is much weaker. It attaches to the lower border of the lower tarsus.

The inferior equivalent to the Whitnall ligament is the suspensory *ligament of Lockwood,* a fusion of the sheath of the inferior rectus muscle, the inferior tarsal muscle, and the check ligaments of the medial and lateral rectus muscles (see Fig 1-32). This ligament provides support for the globe and the anteroinferior orbit.

CLINICAL PEARL

The fusion of the sheath of the inferior rectus muscle, the Lockwood ligament, and the inferior tarsal muscle is an important consideration in surgery, because an operation on the inferior rectus muscle may be associated with palpebral fissure changes.

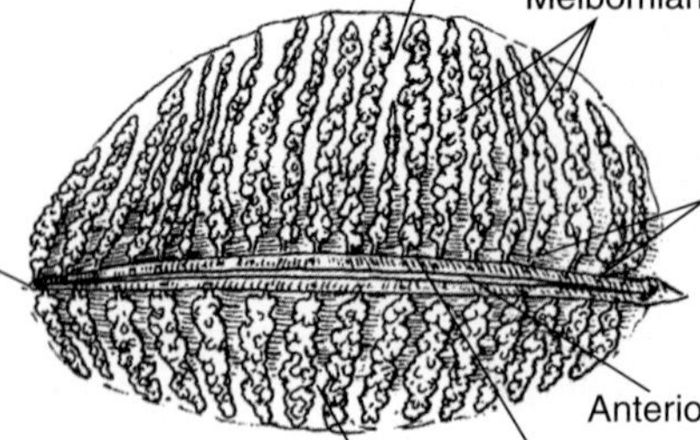

Figure 1-33 Posterior view of the eyelids with the palpebral fissure nearly closed. Note the meibomian (tarsal) glands with their short ducts and orifices. The palpebral conjunctiva has been removed to show these glands in situ. *(Modified with permission from Snell RS, Lemp MA.* Clinical Anatomy of the Eye. *Boston: Blackwell; 1989.)*

Tarsus

The *tarsal plates* consist of dense connective tissue, not cartilage. They are attached to the orbital margin by the medial and lateral canthal tendons (see Figs 1-25, 1-31B). Although the upper and lower tarsal plates are similar in width (29 mm) and thickness (1 mm), the height of the upper tarsus (11 mm) is almost 3 times greater than that of the lower tarsus (4 mm).

The *meibomian glands* (also called *tarsal glands*) are modified holocrine sebaceous glands that are oriented vertically in parallel rows through the tarsus (Fig 1-33; see also Figs 1-26, 1-27). Their distribution and number within the eyelid can be observed by infrared imaging of the eyelid (Fig 1-34). A single row of 30–40 meibomian orifices is present in the upper eyelid, but there are only 20–30 orifices in the lower eyelid. Oil (meibum) from meibomian orifices forms a reservoir on the skin of the eyelid margin and is spread onto the tear film with each blink. Alterations in meibomian gland lipid composition and secretion play a role in dry eye. Aging is associated with an alteration in the lipid profile of meibum and with meibomian gland loss.

Arita R, Itoh K, Inoue K, Amano S. Noncontact infrared meibography to document age-related changes of the meibomian glands in a normal population. *Ophthalmology.* 2008;115(5):911–915.

Sullivan BD, Evans JE, Dana MR, Sullivan DA. Influence of aging on the polar and neutral lipid profiles in human meibomian gland secretions. *Arch Ophthalmol.* 2006;124(9):1286–1292.

Conjunctiva

The palpebral (tarsal) conjunctiva is a transparent vascularized membrane consisting of nonkeratinized stratified squamous epithelium that lines the inner surface of the eyelids. Continuous with the conjunctival fornices (cul-de-sacs), it merges with the bulbar conjunctiva (covering the anterior portion of the sclera) before terminating at the limbus (Fig 1-35). The conjunctiva is discussed further later in the chapter.

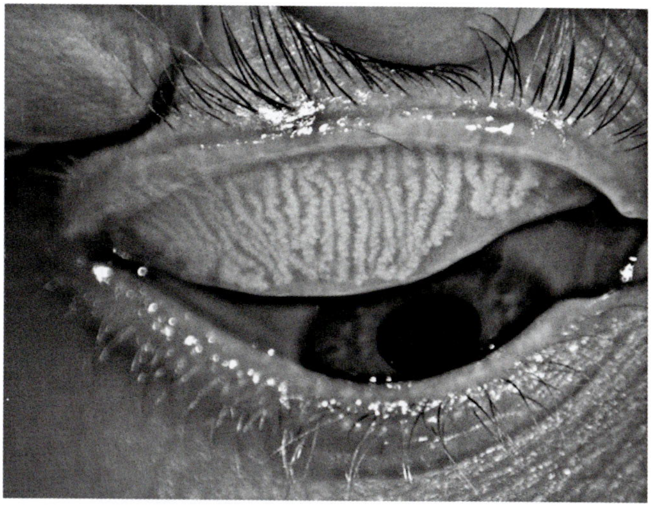

Figure 1-34 Infrared meibography image of the upper eyelid demonstrates normal meibomian gland architecture. *(Courtesy of Mina Massaro-Giordano, MD.)*

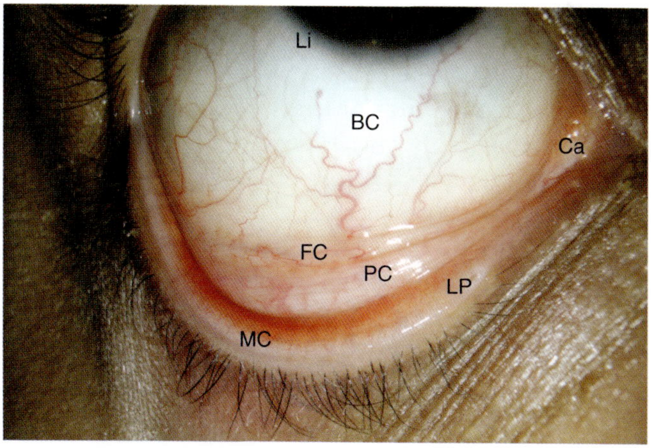

Figure 1-35 The different parts of the conjunctiva are depicted in this photograph: limbus (Li), bulbar conjunctiva (BC), forniceal conjunctiva (FC), palpebral conjunctiva (PC), and marginal conjunctiva (MC). Additional structures shown are the caruncle (Ca) and the lacrimal punctum (LP). *(Courtesy of Vikram S. Brar, MD.)*

Vascular Supply of the Eyelids

The blood supply of the eyelids is derived from the facial system, which arises from the external carotid artery, and the orbital system, which originates from the internal carotid artery along branches of the ophthalmic artery. Thus, the eyelid vasculature represents an anastomosis of the external and internal carotid arteries (Fig 1-36).

The *marginal arterial arcade* is located 3 mm from the free border of the eyelid, just above the ciliary follicles. It is either between the tarsal plate and the orbicularis oculi

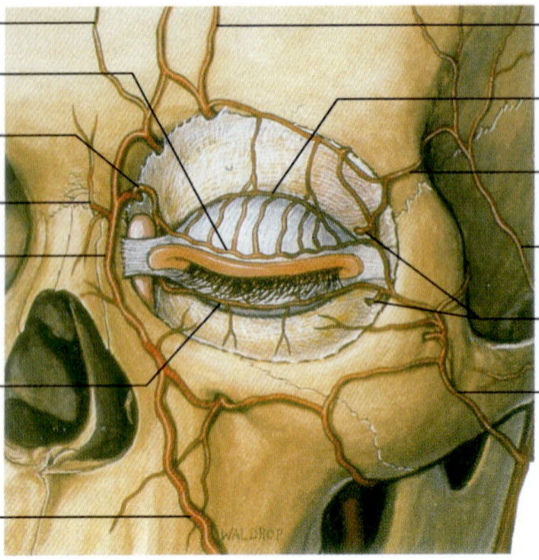

Figure 1-36 Arterial supply of the eyelids. Note the numerous locations where arteries emerging from the orbit anastomose with branches of the facial artery. The facial artery gives rise to the angular artery as it travels superiorly, lateral to the nose. The angular artery serves as an important landmark in dacryocystorhinostomy. *(Reproduced with permission from Dutton JJ.* Atlas of Clinical and Surgical Orbital Anatomy. *Philadelphia: Saunders; 1994.)*

muscle or within the tarsus. A smaller *peripheral arterial arcade* runs along the upper margin of the tarsal plate anterior to the Müller muscle. The superficial temporal artery is a terminal branch of the external carotid artery; BCSC Section 5, *Neuro-Ophthalmology,* discusses the anterior circulation in greater detail. The venous drainage system of the eyelids can be divided into 2 components: a superficial (or pretarsal) system, which drains into the internal and external jugular veins, and a deep (or posttarsal) system, which flows into the cavernous sinus. Thus, the venous circulation of the eyelid connects the face with the cavernous sinus, providing a route for the spread of infection.

Lymphatics of the Eyelids

Lymphatic vessels are present in the eyelids, the conjunctiva, and the orbit. Lymphatic drainage from the eyelids parallels the course of the veins (Fig 1-37).

There are 2 groups of lymphatics:

- a medial group that drains into the submandibular lymph nodes
- a lateral group that drains into the superficial preauricular lymph nodes

CLINICAL PEARL

Clinically, swelling of the lymph nodes is a diagnostic sign of several external eye infections, including adenoviral conjunctivitis and Parinaud oculoglandular syndrome.

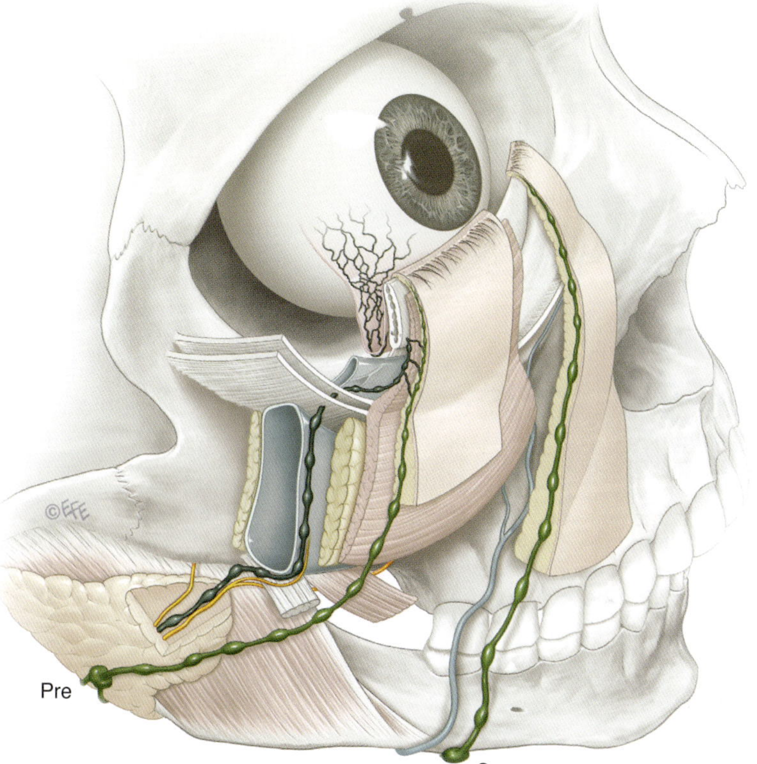

Figure 1-37 Lymphatic drainage *(green)* of the eyelid and conjunctiva. The medial drainage is received by the submandibular lymph node (Sm); the lateral drainage, by the preauricular lymph node (Pre). *(Illustration by Levent Efe Medical Illustration Studios.)*

Lacrimal Glands and Excretory System

Lacrimal Gland

The main lacrimal gland is located in a shallow depression within the orbital part of the frontal bone. The gland is separated from the orbit by fibroadipose tissue and is divided into 2 parts, orbital and palpebral lobes, by the lateral horn of the levator aponeurosis (Fig 1-38). When the upper eyelid is everted, the smaller palpebral lobe can be seen in the superolateral conjunctival fornix. An isthmus of glandular tissue may exist between the palpebral lobe and the larger orbital lobe.

A variable number of thin-walled excretory ducts, blood vessels, lymphatics, and nerves pass from the orbital lobe into the palpebral lacrimal gland. The ducts continue downward, and about 12 of them empty into the conjunctival fornix approximately 5 mm above the superior margin of the upper tarsus.

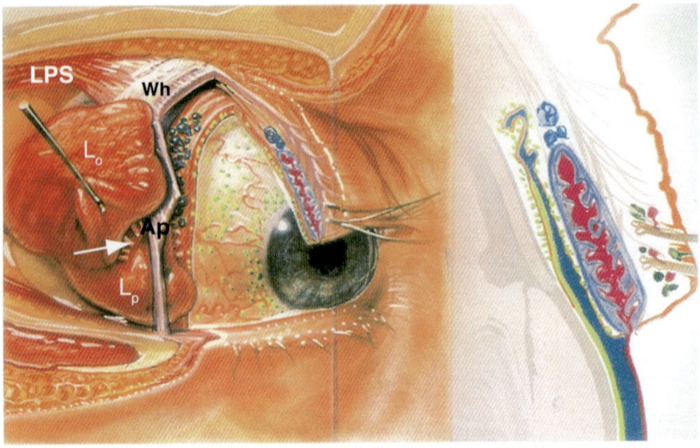

Figure 1-38 The lacrimal secretory system. The conjunctival and tarsal mucin-secreting goblet cells *(green)* contribute to the mucoaqueous and glycocalyx components of the tear film. The accessory lacrimal exocrine glands of Krause and Wolfring are present in the subconjunctival tissues *(blue)* and contribute to the aqueous component of the tear film. Oil-producing meibomian glands and palpebral glands of Zeis and Moll are shown in pink. The orbital lobe of the lacrimal gland (L_o) and the palpebral lobe of the lacrimal gland (L_p) are separated by the lateral horn of the levator aponeurosis (Ap). The tear ducts *(arrow)* from the orbital portion traverse the palpebral portion. The levator palpebrae superioris (LPS) muscle and the Whitnall ligament (Wh) are also shown. *(Modified with permission from Zide BM, Jelks GW.* Surgical Anatomy of the Orbit. *New York: Raven; 1985.)*

CLINICAL PEARL

Because the lacrimal excretory ducts of the orbital and palpebral lobes pass through the palpebral portion of the gland, biopsy of the lacrimal gland is usually performed on the orbital portion to avoid sacrificing the ducts.

The lacrimal glands are exocrine glands that produce a serous secretion. The body of each gland contains 2 cell types (Fig 1-39):

- glandular epithelial cells, which line the lumen of the gland
- myoepithelial cells, which surround the parenchyma and are covered by a basement membrane

Lacrimal secretions comprise the aqueous component of the tear film and include lysozymes, lactoferrin, and immunoglobulin A. The lacrimal gland undergoes structural and functional alterations with age, which may play a role in acquired dry eye.

The lacrimal artery, a branch of the ophthalmic artery, supplies the gland with blood. The lacrimal gland receives secretomotor cholinergic, vasoactive intestinal polypeptide (VIP)-ergic, and sympathetic nerve fibers in addition to sensory innervation via the lacrimal nerve (from CN V_1). The gland's extremely complex neuroanatomy governs both reflex and psychogenic stimulation (see BCSC Section 5, *Neuro-Ophthalmology*).

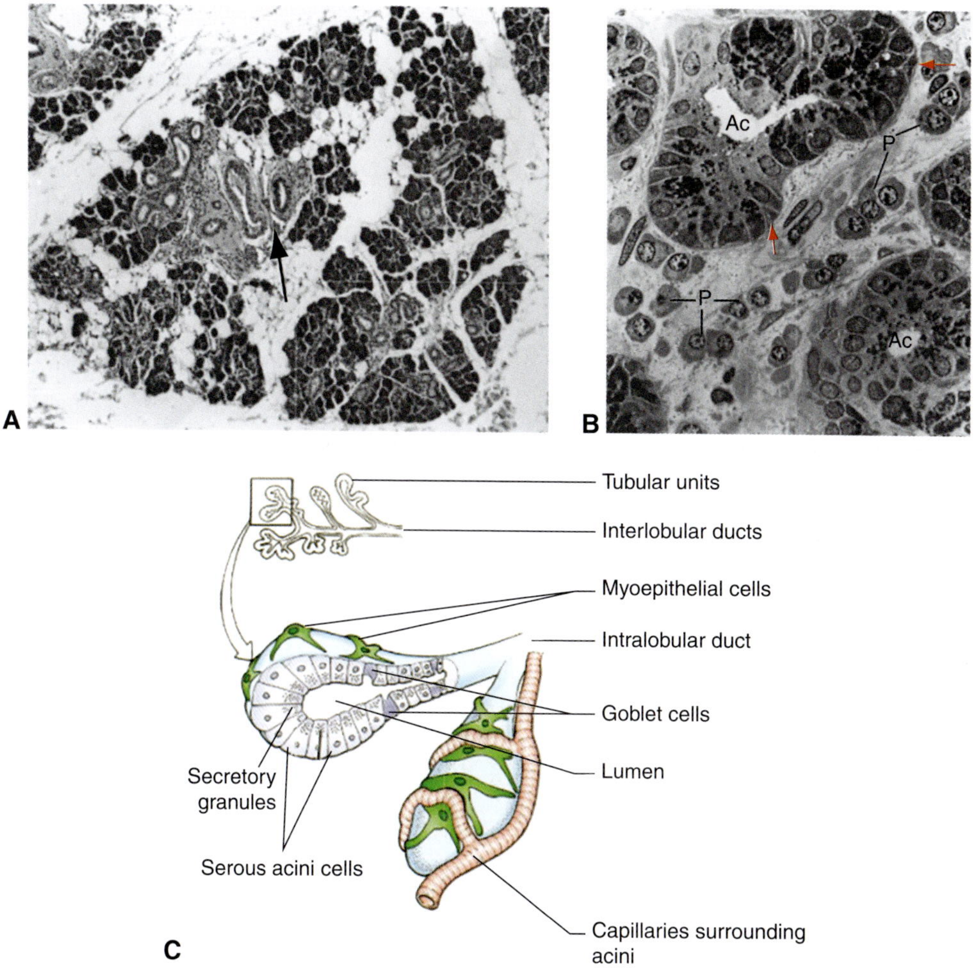

Figure 1-39 Lacrimal gland lobule. **A,** Low magnification of lacrimal gland lobule demonstrating its central duct *(arrow)*. **B,** Histologic section of the lacrimal gland demonstrating acinar units (Ac) made up of a central lumen surrounded by glandular epithelial cells with secretory granules. *Arrows* indicate surrounding myoepithelial cells. The stroma contains blood vessels and numerous plasma (P) cells that produce immunoglobulin A. **C,** Schematic of the lacrimal lobule. *(Modified with permission from Forrester JV, Dick AD, McMenamin PG, Roberts F, Pearlman E.* The Eye: Basic Sciences in Practice. *4th ed. Edinburgh: Elsevier; 2016:90.)*

Rocha EM, Alves M, Rios JD, Dartt DA. The aging lacrimal gland: changes in structure and function. *Ocul Surf.* 2008;6(4):162–174.

Accessory Glands

The accessory lacrimal *glands of Krause* and *Wolfring* are located at the proximal margin of the tarsus or in the fornices. They are cytologically identical to the main lacrimal gland and receive similar innervation (see Figs 1-25, 1-38). These glands account for approximately 10% of the total lacrimal secretory mass.

Lacrimal Excretory System

The lacrimal drainage system includes the upper and lower puncta, the lacrimal canaliculi, the lacrimal sac, and the nasolacrimal duct (Fig 1-40). The *lacrimal puncta* are small (roughly 0.3 mm in diameter) openings on the eyelid margin, located at the extreme nasal border of the eyelids at their junction with the inner canthus (see Fig 1-27A). The inferior punctum is approximately 6.5 mm from the medial canthus; the superior punctum is 6.0 mm from it. The lower eyelid punctum sits closer to the corneal limbus because of the growth of the maxillary sinus, which draws the lower eyelid punctum laterally. The puncta are directed posteriorly into the tear lake at the inner canthus. The ampulla is a slight dilation at the angle of the canaliculus, just beyond the punctum.

These openings lead to the *lacrimal canaliculi,* the *lacrimal sac,* and finally the *nasolacrimal duct,* which, in turn, leads to the nose. In 90% of people, the canaliculi join to form a common canaliculus prior to entering the lacrimal sac. Fibers of the tarsal orbicularis oculi muscles surround the canalicular system and lacrimal sac, driving the tears into

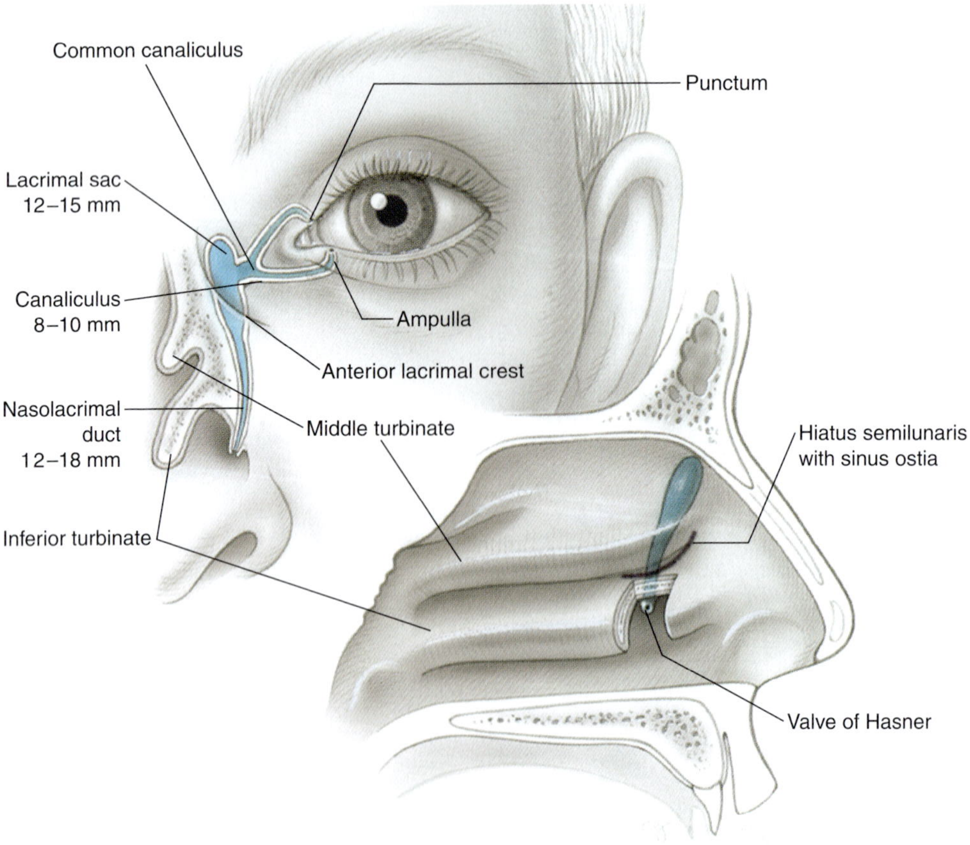

Figure 1-40 Lacrimal excretory system. The measurements given are for adults. *(Illustration by Christine Gralapp.)*

the system and down the duct with blinking (see Fig 1-29). A persistent membrane over the valve of Hasner is often associated with tearing and discharge in infants with nasolacrimal duct obstruction.

The lacrimal puncta and the canaliculi are lined with nonkeratinized stratified squamous epithelium that merges with the epithelium of the eyelid margins. Near the lacrimal sac, the epithelium differentiates into 2 layers:

- a superficial columnar layer
- a deep, flattened cell layer

Goblet cells and occasionally cilia are present. In the canaliculi, the substantia propria consists of collagenous connective tissue and elastic fibers. The wall of the lacrimal sac resembles adenoid tissue and has a rich venous plexus and many elastic fibers.

For further discussion, see BCSC Section 7, *Oculofacial Plastic and Orbital Surgery.*

Conjunctiva

The conjunctiva can be divided into 3 geographic zones: palpebral (tarsal), forniceal, and bulbar (see Fig 1-35). The *palpebral conjunctiva* begins at the mucocutaneous junction of the eyelid and covers the lid's inner surface. This part adheres firmly to the tarsus. The tissue becomes redundant and freely movable in the fornices *(forniceal conjunctiva),* where it becomes enmeshed with fibrous elements of the levator aponeurosis and the Müller muscle in the upper eyelid. In the lower eyelid, fibrous expansions of the inferior rectus muscle sheath fuse with the inferior tarsal muscle, the equivalent of the Müller muscle. The conjunctiva is reflected at the cul-de-sac and attaches to the globe. The delicate *bulbar conjunctiva* is freely movable but fuses with the Tenon capsule as it inserts into the limbus.

Anterior ciliary arteries supply blood to the bulbar conjunctiva. The palpebral conjunctiva is supplied by branches of the marginal arcades of the eyelids. The superior peripheral arcade, running along the upper border of the eyelid, sends branches proximally to supply the forniceal conjunctiva and then the bulbar conjunctiva, as do the posterior conjunctival arteries. The limbal blood supply derives from the ciliary arteries through the anterior conjunctival arteries. The vascular watershed between the anterior and posterior territories lies approximately 3–4 mm from the limbus.

The innervation of the conjunctiva is derived from the ophthalmic division of CN V.

The conjunctiva is a mucous membrane consisting of nonkeratinized stratified squamous epithelium with numerous goblet cells and a thin, richly vascularized substantia propria containing lymphatic vessels, plasma cells, macrophages, and mast cells. A lymphoid layer extends from the bulbar conjunctiva to the subtarsal folds of the eyelids. In places, specialized aggregations of *conjunctiva-associated lymphoid tissue (CALT)* correspond to *mucosa-associated lymphoid tissue (MALT)* elsewhere and comprise collections of T and B lymphocytes underlying a modified epithelium. These regions are concerned with antigen processing.

The thickness of the conjunctival epithelium varies from 2 to 5 cells. The basal cells are cuboidal and evolve into flattened polyhedral cells as they reach the surface. The goblet cells (unicellular mucous glands) are concentrated in the inferior and medial portions of the conjunctiva, especially in the region of the caruncle and plica semilunaris. They are sparsely distributed throughout the remainder of the conjunctiva and are absent in the limbal region. For further discussion of the limbus, see Chapter 8.

Caruncle

The caruncle is a small, fleshy, ovoid structure attached to the inferomedial side of the plica semilunaris (see Figs 1-24, 1-35). As a piece of modified skin, it contains sebaceous glands and fine, colorless hairs. The surface is covered by nonkeratinized stratified squamous epithelium.

Plica Semilunaris

The plica semilunaris is a narrow, highly vascular, crescent-shaped fold of the conjunctiva located lateral to and partly under the caruncle (see Fig 1-24). Its lateral border is free and separated from the bulbar conjunctiva, which it resembles histologically. The epithelium of the plica is rich in goblet cells. The plica's stroma contains fat and some nonstriated muscle. The plica is a vestigial structure analogous to the nictitating membrane, or third eyelid, of dogs and other animals.

Tenon Capsule

The Tenon capsule *(fascia bulbi)* is an envelope of elastic connective tissue that fuses posteriorly with the optic nerve sheath and anteriorly with a thin layer of tissue, the *intermuscular septum,* located 3 mm posterior to the limbus. The Tenon capsule is the cavity within which the globe moves. It is composed of compactly arranged collagen fibers and a few fibroblasts.

The Tenon capsule is thickest in the area of the equator of the globe. Connections between the Tenon capsule and the periorbital tissues help suspend the globe in the orbit. The extraocular muscles penetrate this connective tissue approximately 10 mm posterior to their insertions. The connective tissues form sleeves around the penetrating extraocular muscles, creating pulleys suspended from the periorbita. These pulleys stabilize the position of the muscles relative to the orbit during eye movements. The pulleys are connected to one another and to the Tenon fascia by connective tissue bands (Fig 1-41). Age-related connective tissue degeneration can lead to acquired strabismus. Loss of Tenon capsule with age can also lead to conjunctivochalasis (redundant folds of conjunctiva between the globe and the eyelid margin).

Demer JL. Mechanics of the orbita. *Dev Ophthalmol.* 2007;40:132–157.

Rutar T, Demer JL. "Heavy eye" syndrome in the absence of high myopia: a connective tissue degeneration in elderly strabismic patients. *J AAPOS.* 2009;13(1):36–44.

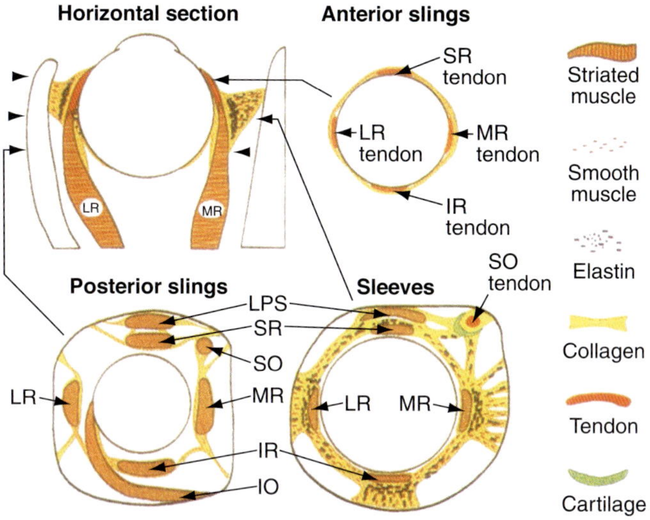

Figure 1-41 Schematic representation of the orbital connective tissues. IR = inferior rectus; LPS = levator palpebrae superioris; LR = lateral rectus; MR = medial rectus; SO = superior oblique; SR = superior rectus. *(Reproduced with permission from Demer JL, Miller JM, Pouken V, Vinters HV, Glasgow BJ. Evidence for fibromuscular pulleys of the recti extraocular muscles.* Invest Ophthalmol Vis Sci. *1995;36(6):1125. © Association for Research in Vision and Ophthalmology.)*

CHAPTER 2

The Eye

This chapter includes related videos, which can be accessed by scanning the QR codes provided in the text or going to www.aao.org/bcscvideo_section02.

Highlights

- Hemidesmosomes anchor the basal corneal epithelial cells to the Bowman layer. Disruption at this level can lead to scarring and recurrent erosion syndrome.
- In addition to housing corneal stem cells, the limbus is the site of passage of the collector channels that link the Schlemm canal to aqueous veins.
- The sclera is an avascular tissue with 2 overlying vascular layers (deep and superficial) in the episclera. Clinically, *episcleritis* refers to inflammation in the superficial layer, and scleritis involves the deep layer.
- The classification of uveitis, established by the 2005 SUN (Standardization of Uveitis Nomenclature) Working Group, is based on the primary site of inflammation within the zones of the uvea: anterior, intermediate, posterior, and all zones (panuveitis).
- The blood–ocular barrier prevents extravasation of intravascular contents into the eye. It consists of intercellular junctions of adjacent cells at various locations in the eye: the blood–aqueous barrier and the blood–retina barrier (inner and outer).
- Optical coherence tomography (OCT) has greatly enhanced visualization, as well as our understanding, of ophthalmic structures in the anterior and posterior segments. In addition, OCT angiography provides details of the microvasculature of the retina not previously seen on fluorescein angiography.
- The retina has a dual circulation, with the inner retina perfused by the retinal vessels seen on routine examination of the fundus and the outer retina perfused by the choroid.

Introduction

The eye is a fascinating and complex organ, an anatomical window into the nervous and vascular systems that can reveal systemic disease. More than 80% of our sensory input comes through sight. This chapter discusses the anatomy of the major parts of the human eye. The reader is encouraged to consult other volumes in the BCSC series for further discussion of many of the topics presented in this chapter.

Topographic Features of the Globe

The eyeball, or globe, is not a true sphere. The radius of curvature of the prolate (polar radius greater than equatorial radius, or "pointy") cornea is 8 mm, smaller than that of the sclera, which is 12 mm. This makes the globe an oblate "squashed" spheroid (equatorial radius greater than polar radius). The anteroposterior diameter of the adult eye is approximately 23–25 mm. The average transverse diameter of the adult eye is 24 mm (Fig 2-1).

The eye contains 3 compartments: the anterior chamber, the posterior chamber, and the vitreous cavity. The anterior chamber, the space between the iris and the cornea, is filled with aqueous fluid. Anterior chamber depth varies among individuals and in regional populations; the average depth is 3.11 mm. The average volume of the anterior chamber is 220 μL. The posterior chamber is the anatomical portion of the eye posterior to the iris and anterior to the lens and vitreous face. It is also filled with aqueous fluid and has an average volume of 60 μL. The largest compartment is the vitreous cavity, which makes up more than two-thirds of the volume of the eye (5–6 mL) and contains the vitreous gel (also called *vitreous, vitreous body,* or *vitreous humor*). The total volume of the average adult eye is approximately 6.5–7.0 mL (Table 2-1).

The eyeball is composed of 3 concentric layers: an outer protective layer, a middle vascular layer, and an inner neural layer. The outermost layer consists of the clear *cornea* anteriorly and the opaque white *sclera* posteriorly. This corneoscleral layer is composed of collagen and protects the internal ocular tissues.

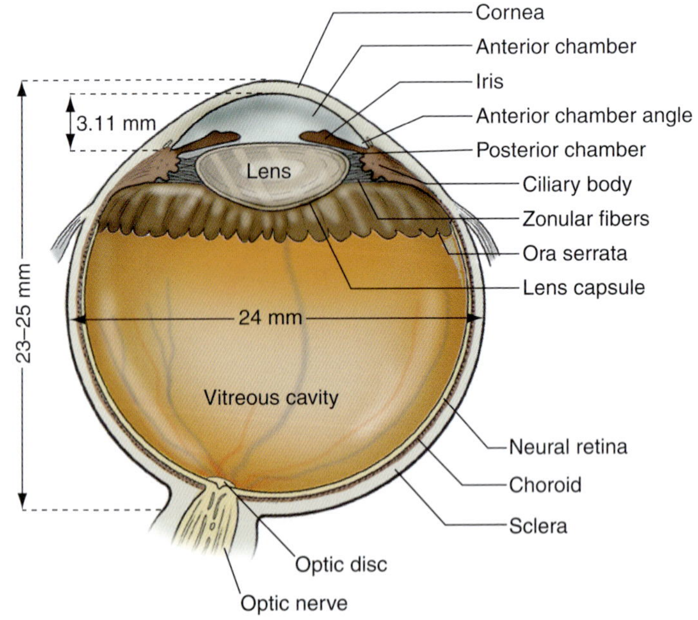

Figure 2-1 Sagittal section of the eye with absent vitreous and major structures identified. Dimensions are approximate and are average for the normal adult eye. *(Illustration by Christine Gralapp.)*

Table 2-1 Dimensions and Contents of the Adult Eye

	Anterior Chamber	Posterior Chamber	Vitreous Cavity	Eye as a Whole
Average depth (emmetropic eye)	3.11 mm (ranges from 1.5[a] to 4 mm)	0.52 mm	16.5 mm	23.5 mm (ranges from 19.5 to 26.5 mm)
Volume	220 µL	60 µL	5 to 6 mL	6.5 to 7 mL
Contents	Aqueous	Aqueous	Vitreous	

[a] Below 2.5 mm the risk of angle closure increases.

The cornea occupies the center of the anterior pole of the globe. Because the sclera and conjunctiva overlap the cornea anteriorly, slightly more above and below than medially and laterally, the cornea appears elliptical when viewed from the front. The *limbus,* which borders the cornea and the sclera, is blue-gray and translucent.

The middle layer of the globe, the *uvea,* consists of the choroid, ciliary body, and iris. Highly vascular, it serves nutritive and supportive functions, supplying oxygen to the outer retina and producing aqueous humor.

The innermost layer is the *retina.* This photosensitive layer contains the photoreceptors and neural elements that initiate the processing of visual information.

Other important surface features of the globe, such as the vortex veins, the posterior ciliary artery and nerves, and extraocular muscle insertions are discussed in Chapter 1; the optic nerve and its surrounding meningeal sheaths are discussed in Chapter 3.

Precorneal Tear Film

The exposed surfaces of the cornea and bulbar conjunctiva are covered by the *precorneal tear film,* which was formerly described as having 3 layers: lipid (from meibomian glands), aqueous (from the lacrimal gland), and mucin (primarily from goblet cells). It is now thought of as a lipid layer with underlying uniform gel consisting of soluble mucus (secreted by conjunctival goblet cells), mixed with fluids and proteins (secreted by the lacrimal glands). A glycocalyx mediates the interaction of the mucoaqueous layer with surface epithelial cells of the cornea.

Maintenance of the precorneal tear film is vital for normal corneal function. The tear film does the following:

- provides lubrication for the cornea and conjunctiva
- facilitates the exchange of solutes, including oxygen
- contributes to the antimicrobial defense of the ocular surface
- serves as a medium to remove debris

Further, the air–tear film interface at the surface of the cornea constitutes a major refractive element of the eye, because of the difference in the refractive index of air and that of the tear film. Aberrations in the tear film result from a variety of diseases (eg, dry eye, blepharitis) that can profoundly affect the integrity of the ocular surface and consequently the patient's vision. See Chapter 7 for in-depth discussion of the tear film.

Cornea

The cornea is a clear avascular tissue consisting of 5 layers (Fig 2-2):

- epithelium
- Bowman layer
- stroma
- Descemet membrane
- endothelium

The cornea covers one-sixth of the surface of the globe. It has a refractive index of 1.376 and an average radius of curvature of 7.8 mm. With a power of 43.25 diopters (D), the cornea produces most of the eye's refractive power of 58.60 D. Oxygen from the air and

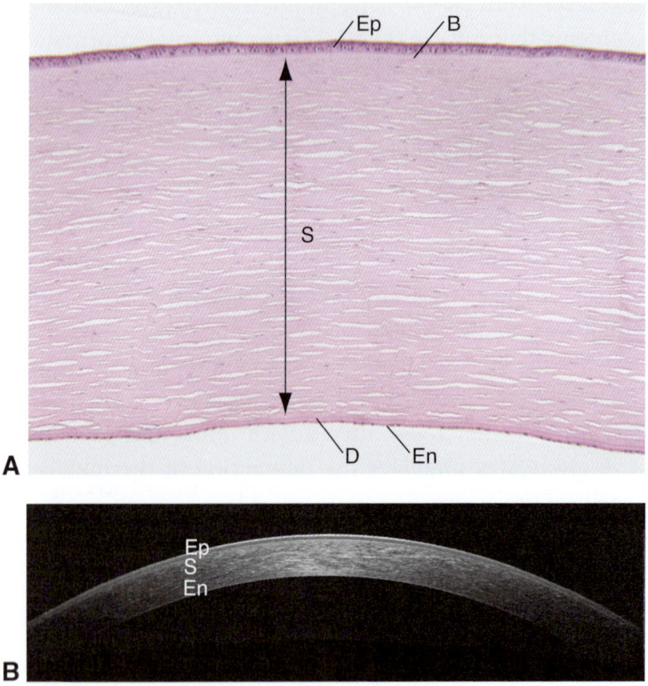

Figure 2-2 **A,** Histologic section showing the 5 layers of the cornea (thickness given within parentheses): epithelium (40–50 µm), Bowman layer (8–15 µm), stroma (470–500 µm), Descemet membrane (10–12 µm), and endothelium (4–6 µm). **B,** Anterior segment optical coherence tomography (AS-OCT) of the cornea. B = Bowman layer; D = Descemet membrane; En = endothelium; Ep = epithelium; S = stroma. *(Part A courtesy of George J. Harocopos, MD; part B courtesy of Vikram S. Brar, MD.)*

from the eyelid vasculature dissolves in tears and is transmitted to the cornea via the tear film. The cornea derives its macromolecules and nutrients from the aqueous humor.

Characteristics of the Central and Peripheral Cornea

In adults, the cornea measures about 12 mm in the horizontal meridian and about 11 mm in the vertical meridian. The central third of the cornea is nearly spherical and measures approximately 4 mm in diameter. Because the posterior surface of the cornea is more curved than the anterior surface, the central cornea is thinner (0.5 mm) than the peripheral cornea (1.0 mm). The cornea flattens in the periphery, with more extensive flattening nasally and superiorly than temporally and inferiorly. This topography is important in contact lens fitting. For additional discussion, see Chapter 2 in BCSC Section 8, *External Disease and Cornea,* and Chapter 6 in Section 3, *Clinical Optics and Vision Rehabilitation.*

Epithelium and Basal Lamina

The anterior surface of the cornea is covered by a lipophilic, nonkeratinized, stratified squamous epithelium that is composed of 4–6 cell layers and is typically 40–50 μm thick (Fig 2-3). The basal cells have a width of 12 μm and a density of approximately 6000 cells/mm^2. They are attached to the underlying basal lamina by hemidesmosomes. Trauma to the epithelium disrupting this layer can lead to recurrent corneal erosion due to improper re-formation of these hemidesmosomes.

Overlying the basal cell layer are 2 or 3 layers of polygonal "wing" cells. Superficial to these layers are 1–2 layers of corneal epithelial "surface" cells that are extremely thin (30 μm) and are attached to one another by tight junctions. The tight junctions allow the surface epithelial cells to act as a barrier to diffusion. Microvilli make the apical membranes of the surface cells highly irregular; however, the precorneal tear film renders the surfaces optically smooth.

Although the deeper epithelial cells are firmly attached to one another by desmosomes, they migrate continuously from the basal region toward the tear film, into which they are shed. They also migrate centripetally from their stem cell source at the limbus. Division of the slow-cycling stem cells gives rise to a progeny of daughter cells (transient amplifying cells), whose division serves to maintain the corneal epithelium (see also Chapter 8). Diffuse damage to the limbal stem cells (eg, by chemical burns or trachoma) leads to chronic epithelial surface defects.

Del Monte DW, Kim T. Anatomy and physiology of the cornea. *J Cataract Refract Surg.* 2011;37(3):588–598.

Bowman Layer

Beneath the basal lamina of the epithelium is the *Bowman layer,* or *Bowman membrane,* a tough layer consisting of randomly dispersed collagen fibrils. It is a modified region of the anterior stroma that is 8–15 μm thick (see Fig 2-2). Unlike the Descemet membrane, it is not restored after injury but is replaced by scar tissue.

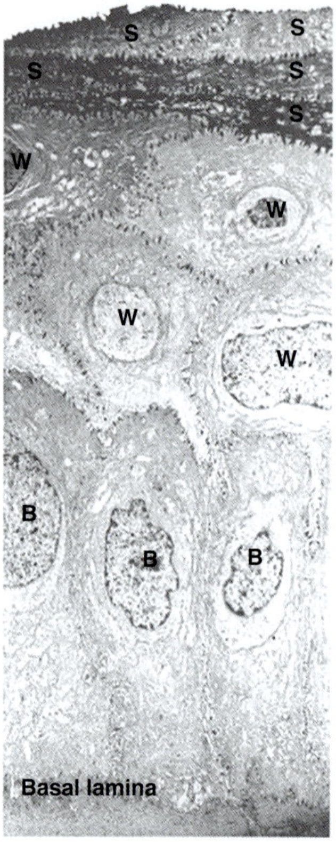

A

Figure 2-3 **A,** The corneal epithelium is composed of 4–6 cell layers that make up a stratified squamous epithelium, which is derived from the surface ectoderm. **B,** Schematic of the corneal epithelium demonstrating adhesion between cells and to the underlying basal lamina *(purple)* and Bowman layer via hemidesmosomes. B = basal cells; S = surface cells; W = wing cells. *(Reproduced with permission from Levin LA, Nilsson SFE, Ver Hoeve J, Wu SM.* Adler's Physiology of the Eye. *11th ed. Philadelphia: Elsevier/Saunders; 2011:94.)*

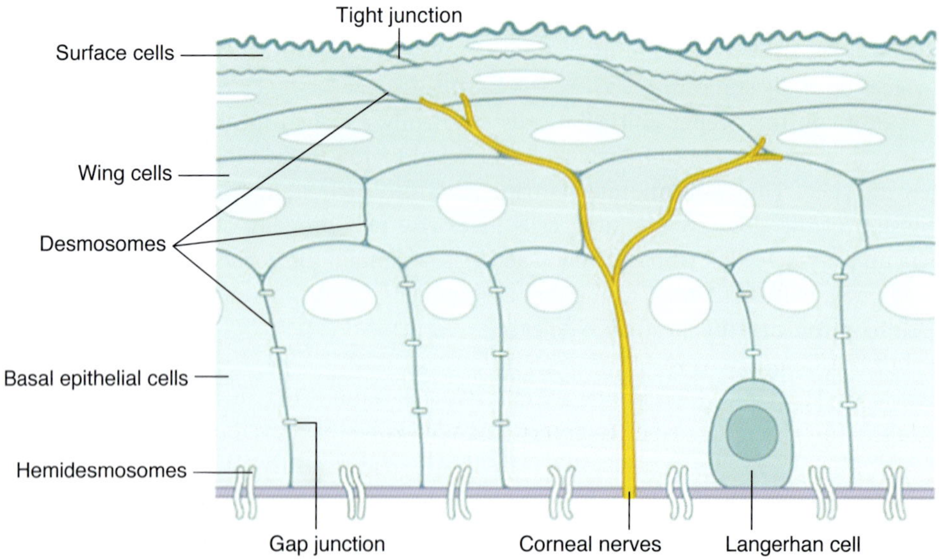

B

Stroma

The stroma constitutes approximately 90% of the total corneal thickness in humans (see Fig 2-2). It is composed of collagen-producing keratocytes, ground substance, and collagen lamellae. The collagen fibrils form obliquely oriented lamellae in the anterior third of the stroma (with some interlacing) and perpendicular lamellae in the less compact posterior two-thirds (see Chapter 8, Fig 8-3).

The corneal collagen fibrils extend across the entire diameter of the cornea, finally winding circumferentially around the limbus. The fibrils are remarkably uniform in size and separation, and this regularity helps determine the transparency of the cornea (see also Chapter 8). Separation of the collagen fibrils by edema leads to stromal clouding. The stroma's collagen types are I (predominant), III, IV, V, VI, XII, and XIV. Type VII forms the anchoring fibril of the epithelium. Natural crosslinking occurs with aging.

The ground substance of the cornea consists of proteoglycans that run along and between the collagen fibrils. Their glycosaminoglycan components (eg, keratan sulfate) are negatively charged and tend to repel each other—as well as draw in sodium and, secondarily, water—producing the swelling pressure of the stroma. The keratocytes lie between the corneal lamellae and synthesize both collagen and proteoglycans. Ultrastructurally, they resemble fibrocytes.

The cornea has approximately 2.4 million keratocytes, which occupy about 5% of the stromal volume; the density is higher anteriorly (1058 cells/mm^2) than posteriorly (771 cells/mm^2). Keratocytes are highly active cells rich in mitochondria, rough endoplasmic reticula, and Golgi apparatus. They have attachment structures, communicate through gap junctions, and have unusual fenestrations in their plasma membranes. Their flat profile and even distribution in the coronal plane ensure a minimum disturbance of light transmission.

Müller LJ, Pels L, Vrensen GF. Novel aspects of the ultrastructural organization of human corneal keratocytes. *Invest Ophthalmol Vis Sci.* 1995;36(13):2557–2567.

Mustonen RK, McDonald MB, Srivannaboon S, Tan AL, Doubrava MW, Kim CK. Normal human corneal cell populations evaluated by in vivo scanning slit confocal microscopy. *Cornea.* 1998;17(5):485–492.

Descemet Membrane

The basal lamina of the corneal endothelium, the *Descemet membrane,* is periodic acid–Schiff (PAS) positive (Fig 2-4). It is a true basement membrane, and its thickness increases with age. At birth, the Descemet membrane is 3–4 µm thick, increasing to 10–12 µm at adulthood. It is composed of an anterior banded zone that develops in utero (4.6 ± 0.4 µm thick) and a posterior nonbanded zone that is laid down by the corneal endothelium throughout life (average in adults is 11.8 ± 0.4 µm, increasing about 0.1 µm/year) (Fig 2-5). These zones provide a historical record of the synthetic function of the endothelium. Like other basal laminae, the Descemet membrane is rich in type IV collagen.

Peripheral excrescences of the Descemet membrane, known as *Hassall-Henle warts,* are common, especially among elderly people. Central excrescences (corneal guttae) also appear with increasing age.

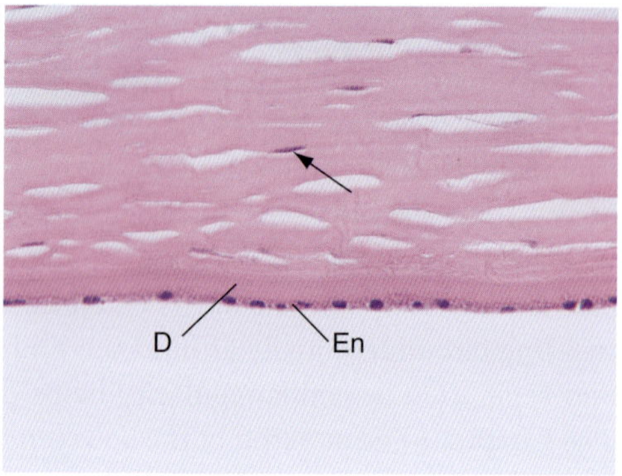

Figure 2-4 Histologic section of the posterior cornea. Higher magnification depicts the Descemet membrane (D) and endothelium (En). A keratocyte nucleus *(arrow)* is visible in the posterior stroma. *(Courtesy of George J. Harocopos, MD.)*

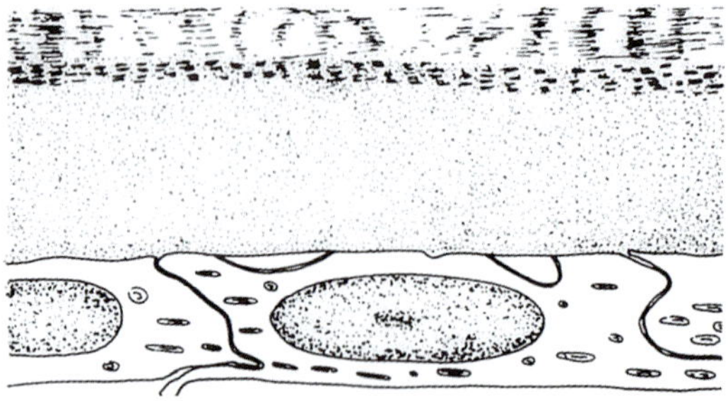

Figure 2-5 Corneal endothelium and the Descemet membrane. *(Illustration by Thomas A. Weingeist, PhD, MD.)*

Endothelium

The corneal endothelium is composed of a single layer of hexagonal cells derived from the neural crest (Fig 2-6). Therefore, the corneal endothelium is of neuroectodermal origin. In young adult eyes, approximately 500,000 cells are present, at a density of about 3000/mm^2 centrally and up to 8000/mm^2 peripherally. Mitosis of the endothelium is limited in humans, and the overall number of endothelial cells decreases with age.

The size, shape, and distribution of the endothelial cells can be observed by specular microscopy at the slit lamp. The apical surfaces of these cells face the anterior chamber; their basal surfaces secrete the Descemet membrane. Typically, young endothelial cells have large nuclei and abundant mitochondria. The active transport of ions by these cells leads to the transfer of water from the corneal stroma and the maintenance of stromal deturgescence and transparency.

Endothelial cell dysfunction and loss—through surgical injury, inflammation, or disease (eg, Fuchs endothelial corneal dystrophy)—may cause endothelial decompensation, stromal edema, and vision loss. Because endothelial mitosis is limited in humans, destruction of cells causes cell density to decrease and residual cells to spread and enlarge.

Zheng T, Le Q, Hong J, Xu J. Comparison of human corneal cell density by age and corneal location: an in vivo confocal microscopy study. *BMC Ophthalmol.* 2016;16:109.

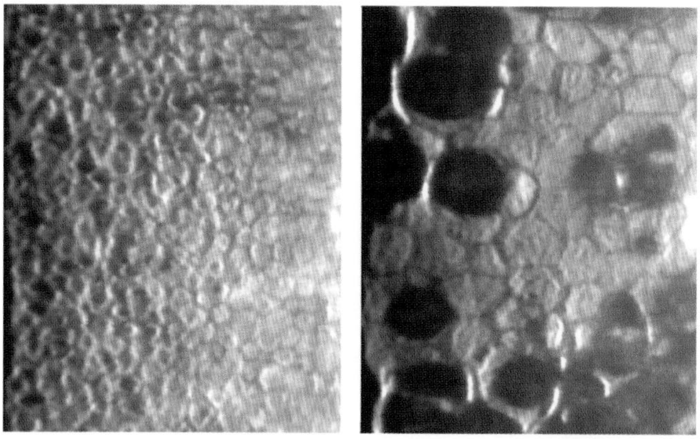

Figure 2-6 Specular microscopy of living corneal endothelium. Normal endothelium is shown on the left. Note the hexagonal shape of the endothelial cells. The corneal endothelium of a patient with Fuchs endothelial corneal dystrophy is shown on the right. Demonstrated are polymegathism (larger cells), pleomorphism (variability in size and shape of cells), and dark areas of endothelial cell loss (guttae). *(Courtesy of Preston H. Blomquist, MD.)*

Limbus

The transition zone between the peripheral cornea and the anterior sclera, known as the *limbus* (also called *corneoscleral junction* or *corneal limbus*), is defined differently by anatomists, pathologists, and clinicians. Though not a distinct anatomical structure, the limbus is important for 3 reasons: its relationship to the anterior chamber angle, its use as a surgical landmark, and its supply of corneal stem cells. The limbus is also the site of passage of the collector channel that links the Schlemm canal to aqueous veins.

The following structures are found at the limbus:

- conjunctiva and limbal palisades of Vogt, which house the corneal stem cells
- episclera (discussed later, under Sclera)
- junction of corneoscleral stroma
- aqueous outflow apparatus (collector channel)

The corneoscleral junction begins centrally in a plane connecting the end of the Bowman layer and the Schwalbe line, which is the termination of the Descemet membrane. Internally, its posterior limit is the anterior tip of the scleral spur (Fig 2-7). Pathologists consider the posterior limit of the limbus to be formed by another plane perpendicular to the surface of the eye, approximately 1.5 mm posterior to the termination of the Bowman layer in the horizontal meridian and 2.0 mm posterior in the vertical meridian, where there is greater scleral overlap (Fig 2-8).

The surgical limbus, an external landmark for incisions in cataract and glaucoma surgery, is sometimes referred to as the *gray* or *blue zone*. Its blue-gray appearance is due to the scattering of light through the oblique interface between cornea and sclera, which

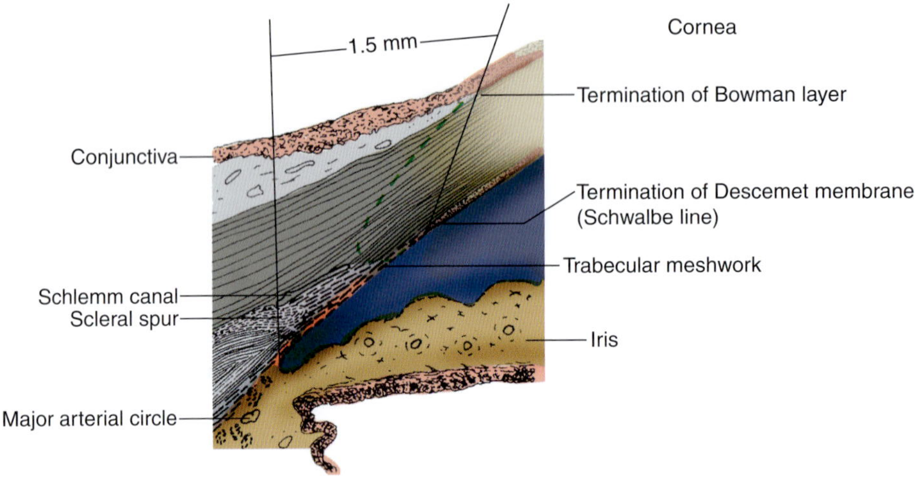

Figure 2-7 Anterior chamber angle and limbus, depicting the concept of the limbus. *Solid lines* represent the limbus as viewed by pathologists; the *green dotted line* represents the limbus as viewed by anatomists. *(Illustration by Thomas A. Weingeist, PhD, MD.)*

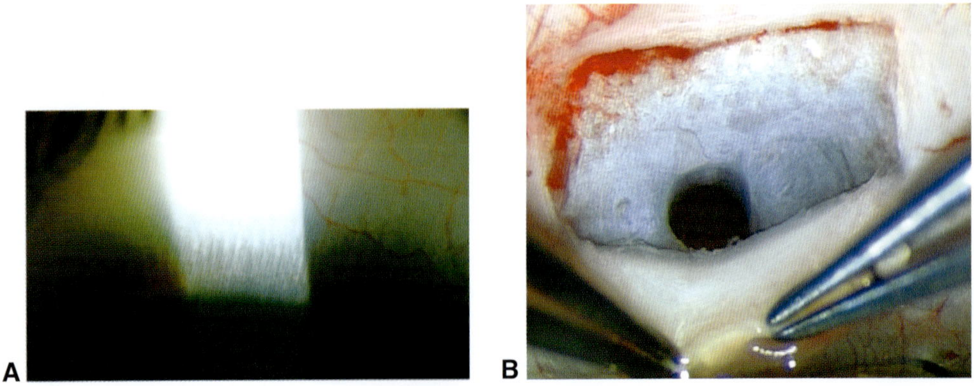

Figure 2-8 Limbus. **A,** Slit-lamp photograph showing the blue-gray corneoscleral limbus. The striations orthogonal to the cornea are the limbal palisades of Vogt, where the corneal stem cells reside. **B,** Photograph of limbus-based trabeculectomy. Note the blue-gray surgical limbus with corresponding sclerostomy. *(Part A courtesy of Cornea Service, Paulista School of Medicine, Federal University of São Paulo; part B courtesy of Keith Barton, MD, and reproduced with permission from Moorfields Eye Hospital.)*

occurs gradually over 1–2 mm (see Fig 2-8B). The posterior border of the blue-gray zone is a consistent external landmark that corresponds to the internal junction of cornea and sclera overlying the trabecular meshwork in all meridians.

Sclera

The sclera covers the posterior five-sixths of the surface of the globe, with an anterior opening for the cornea and a posterior opening for the optic nerve. The tendons of the rectus muscles insert into the superficial scleral collagen. The Tenon capsule covers the sclera and rectus muscles anteriorly, and both are overlain by the bulbar conjunctiva. The capsule and conjunctiva fuse near the limbus.

The sclera is thinnest (0.3 mm) just behind the insertions of the rectus muscles and thickest (1.0 mm) at the posterior pole around the optic nerve head. It is 0.4–0.5 mm thick at the equator and 0.6 mm thick anterior to the muscle insertions. Because of the thinness of the sclera, strabismus and retinal detachment surgery require careful placement of sutures.

CLINICAL PEARL

The most common sites of scleral rupture following blunt trauma are

- in the superonasal quadrant, near the limbus
- in a circumferential arc parallel to the corneal limbus opposite the site of impact
- behind the insertion of the rectus muscles

The sclera, like the cornea, is essentially avascular except for the vessels of the intrascleral vascular plexus, located just posterior to the limbus, and the episcleral vessels. The episcleral vessels have superficial and deep plexuses (Fig 2-9). The superficial plexus runs

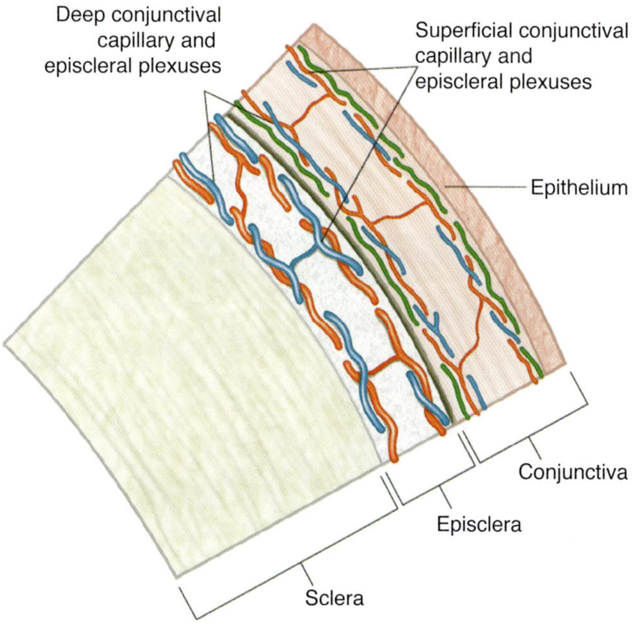

Figure 2-9 Episcleral vessels. The sclera is avascular but has overlying episcleral vessels, which are divided into superficial and deep plexuses. The organization of the conjunctival vasculature, which is also depicted, is similar to that of the episcleral vessels, with the addition of lymphatics, shown in green. *(Modified with permission from Levin LA, Nilsson SFE, Ver Hoeve J, Wu SM.* Adler's Physiology of the Eye. *11th ed. Philadelphia: Elsevier/Saunders; 2011:118–119.)*

beneath the Tenon capsule in a radial pattern; in episcleritis, it is this vascular plexus that is involved. The deep episcleral plexus rests on the surface of the sclera and is the layer involved in scleritis.

Numerous channels, or *emissaria,* penetrate the sclera (see Chapter 1, Figs 1-19, 1-20), allowing the passage of arteries, veins, and nerves:

- anterior emissaria: penetration of the anterior ciliary arteries anterior to the rectus muscle insertions
- middle emissaria: exit of vortex veins
- posterior emissaria: lamina cribrosa, penetration of the short and long posterior ciliary vessels and ciliary nerves

Extraocular extension of malignant melanoma of the choroid occurs by way of the middle emissaria.

Branches of the ciliary nerves that supply the cornea sometimes leave the sclera to form loops posterior to the nasal and temporal limbus. These nerve loops, called *Axenfeld loops,* are sometimes pigmented and, consequently, have been mistaken for uveal tissue or malignant melanoma (Fig 2-10).

Anterior to the rectus muscle insertions, the episclera consists of a dense vascular connective tissue that merges deeply with the superficial sclera and superficially with the Tenon capsule and the conjunctiva. The scleral stroma is composed of bundles of collagen, fibroblasts, and a moderate amount of ground substance.

Collagen fibers of the sclera vary in size and shape and taper at their ends, indicating that they are not continuous fibers as in the cornea. The inner layer of the sclera *(lamina fusca)* blends imperceptibly with the suprachoroidal and supraciliary lamellae of the uvea. The collagen fibers in this portion of the sclera branch and intermingle with the outer ciliary body and choroid. The opaque, porcelain-white appearance of the sclera contrasts markedly with the transparency of the cornea and is primarily due to 2 factors: the greater

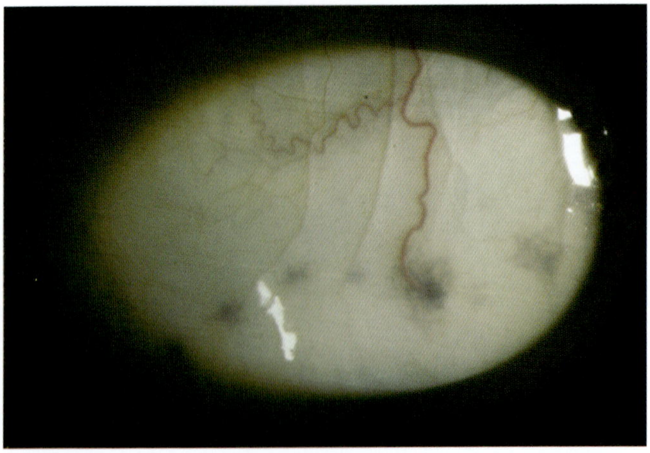

Figure 2-10 External photograph of Axenfeld nerve loops in an arc pattern roughly equidistant from the limbus. *(Reproduced with permission from Jesse Vislisel, MD; EyeRounds.org, University of Iowa. Photograph by Cindy Montague, CRA.)*

variation in collagen fibril separation and diameter, and the greater degree of fibril interweaving in the sclera (see also Chapter 8). In addition, the lack of vascular elements contributes to corneal clarity.

Anterior Chamber

The anterior chamber is bordered anteriorly by the cornea and posteriorly by the iris diaphragm and the pupil. The *anterior chamber angle,* which lies at the junction of the cornea and the iris, includes the following 5 structures (Figs 2-11 through 2-14):

- Schwalbe line
- Schlemm canal and trabecular meshwork (also see the section Trabecular Meshwork)
- scleral spur
- anterior border of the ciliary body (where its longitudinal fibers insert into the scleral spur)
- peripheral iris

The depth of the anterior chamber averages 3.0 mm but is deeper in aphakia, pseudophakia, and myopia and shallower in hyperopia. In the normal adult eye, the anterior chamber is deepest centrally and reaches its narrowest point slightly central to the angle recess.

The anterior chamber is filled with *aqueous humor,* which is produced by the ciliary epithelium in the posterior chamber. The fluid passes through the pupil aperture and drains by the trabecular pathway (ie, through the trabecular meshwork into the Schlemm canal) and the uveoscleral pathway (ie, the root of the iris and the ciliary body face, into

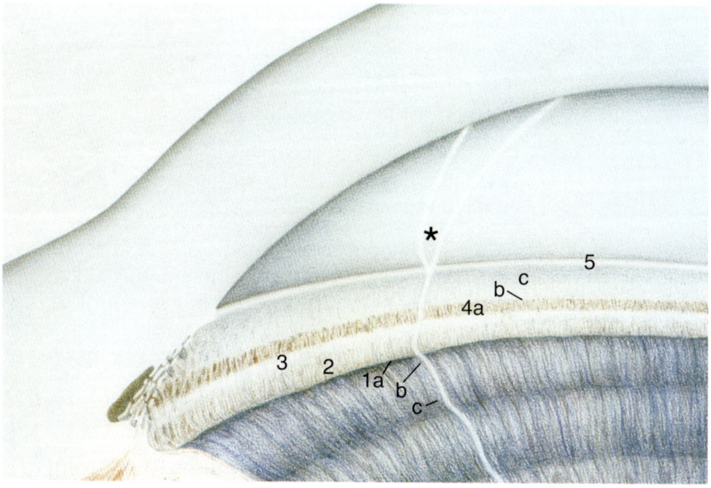

Figure 2-11 Structures of the anterior chamber angle. 1, Peripheral iris: a, insertion; b, curvature; c, angular approach. 2, Ciliary body band. 3, Scleral spur. 4, Trabecular meshwork: a, posterior; b, mid; c, anterior. 5, Schwalbe line. *(*),* Corneal optical wedge.

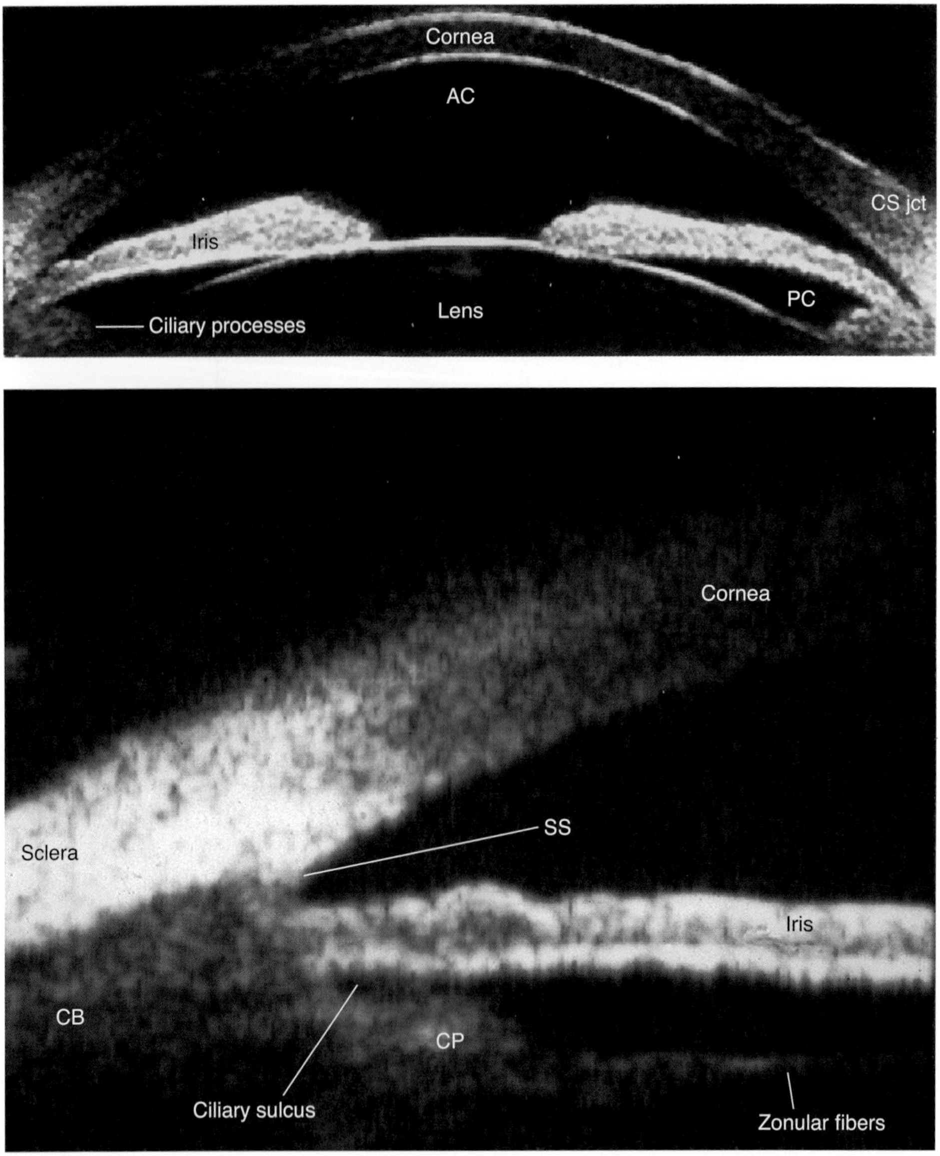

Figure 2-12 **A,** Ultrasound biomicroscopy composite image of the anterior segment, including the anterior chamber (AC). The iris is slightly convex, indicating mild pupillary block. The corneoscleral junction (CS jct), ciliary processes, and posterior chamber (PC) region are clearly imaged. The angle is narrow but open. Iris–lens contact is small. **B,** Ultrasound biomicroscopy image showing normal angle structures. CB = ciliary body; CP = ciliary processes; SS = scleral spur. *(Part A courtesy of Charles Pavlin, MD; part B courtesy of Ken K. Nischal, MD.)*

the suprachoroidal space). The uveoscleral pathway, thought to be influenced by age, accounts for up to 50% of aqueous outflow in young people. BCSC Section 10, *Glaucoma,* discusses the anterior chamber and aqueous humor in detail. High-resolution ultrasound biomicroscopy provides detailed 2-dimensional views of the anterior segment of the eye

A
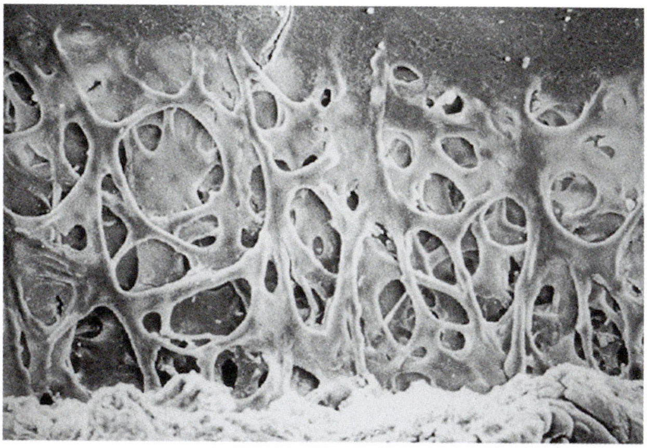

B
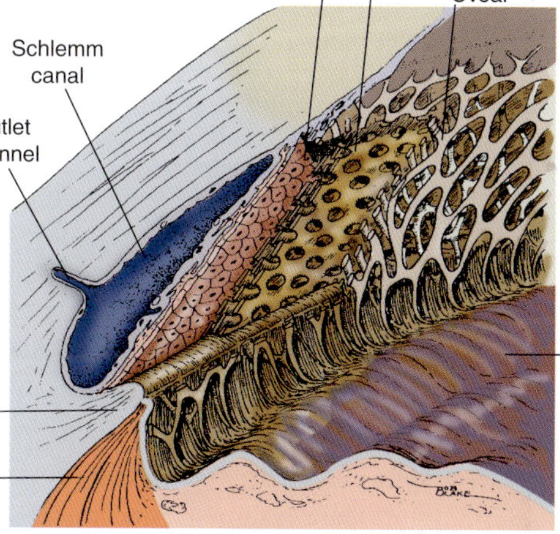

Figure 2-13 Trabecular meshwork. **A,** Electron micrograph with en face view of the trabecular meshwork from the anterior chamber. Note the decreasing space between trabecular beams in the deeper tissue planes. **B,** Layers of the trabecular meshwork: uveal, corneoscleral, and juxtacanalicular. The point of highest resistance to outflow is at the juxtacanalicular layer. The outlet channel traverses the limbus and drains into an aqueous vein. *(Part A reproduced with permission from Bowling B.* Kanski's Clinical Ophthalmology: A Systematic Approach. *8th ed. Oxford: Elsevier Limited; 2016:306. Part B modified with permission from Shields MB.* Textbook of Glaucoma. *3rd ed. Baltimore: Williams & Wilkins; 1992.)*

and is performed in vivo (see Fig 2-12), allowing the clinician to view the relationship of the structures in the anterior segment under different pathologic conditions (Video 2-1).

VIDEO 2-1 Imaging the anterior chamber angle.
Courtesy of Hiroshi Ishikawa, MD.
Access all Section 2 videos at www.aao.org/bcscvideo_section02.

The internal scleral sulcus accommodates the Schlemm canal externally and the trabecular meshwork internally. The Schwalbe line, the peripheral limit of the Descemet

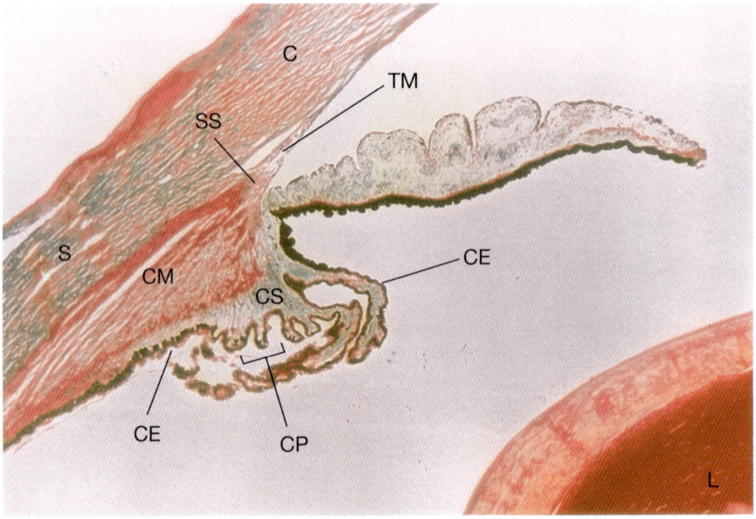

Figure 2-14 Anterior chamber angle, ciliary body, and peripheral lens. Note the triangular shape of the ciliary body. The ciliary muscle fibers (CM) appear red in contrast to the connective tissue. Note the longitudinal fibers inserting into the scleral spur (SS), which is clearly delineated from the ciliary muscle in the region of the trabecular meshwork (TM). The ciliary processes (CP) and ciliary stroma (CS) are lined by the double-layered ciliary epithelium (CE). The lens (L) is artifactually displaced posteriorly. (Masson trichrome stain ×8.) C = cornea; I = iris; S = sclera. *(Courtesy of Thomas A. Weingeist, PhD, MD.)*

membrane, forms the anterior margin of the sulcus; the scleral spur is its posterior landmark. The scleral spur receives the insertion of the longitudinal ciliary muscle, contraction of which opens up the trabecular spaces.

Myofibroblast-like scleral spur cells with contractile properties are disposed circumferentially within the scleral spur. They resemble mechanoreceptors, receive sensory innervation, and are connected by elastic tissue to the trabecular meshwork. In experiments, stimulation with vasoactive intestinal polypeptide (VIP) or calcitonin gene–related peptide (CGRP) causes an increase in outflow facility. Individual scleral spur cells are innervated by unmyelinated axons, the terminals of which contact the cell membranes of the spur cells without an intervening basal lamina. The nerve fibers in this region are immunoreactive for neuropeptide Y, substance P, CGRP, VIP, and nitrous oxide; therefore, they are mediated by sympathetic, sensory, and pterygopalatine nerve pathways. There are no cholinergic fibers in this region.

Myelinated nerve fibers extending forward from the ciliary region to the inner aspect of the scleral spur yield branches to the meshwork and to club-shaped endings in the scleral spur. These endings have the morphologic features of mechanoreceptors found elsewhere in the body, such as in the carotid artery. The endings are incompletely covered by a Schwann cell sheath and make contact with extracellular matrix materials such as elastin. Various functions have been proposed for these endings, including proprioception to the ciliary muscle, which inserts into the scleral spur; signaling contraction of the scleral spur cells; and baroreception in response to changes in intraocular pressure.

Tamm ER, Braunger BM, Fuchshofer R. Intraocular pressure and the mechanisms involved in resistance of the aqueous humor flow in the trabecular meshwork outflow pathways. *Prog Mol Biol Transl Sci.* 2015;134:301–314.

Trabecular Meshwork

The relationship of the trabecular meshwork and the Schlemm canal to other structures is complex because the outflow apparatus is composed of tissue derived from the cornea, sclera, iris, and ciliary body (see Figs 2-11, 2-13). The trabecular meshwork is a circular spongework of connective tissue lined by trabeculocytes. These cells have contractile properties, which may influence outflow resistance. They also have phagocytic properties. The meshwork is roughly triangular in cross section; the apex is at the Schwalbe line, and the base is formed by the scleral spur and the ciliary body.

The trabecular meshwork can be divided into 3 layers (see Fig 2-13):

- uveal trabecular meshwork
- corneoscleral meshwork
- juxtacanalicular meshwork, which is directly adjacent to the Schlemm canal

The uveal portion and the corneoscleral meshwork can be divided by an imaginary line drawn from the Schwalbe line to the scleral spur. The uveal meshwork lies internal and the corneoscleral meshwork external to this line.

Aging changes to the trabecular meshwork include increased pigmentation, decreased number of trabecular cells, and thickening of the basement membrane beneath the trabecular cells. Trabecular sheets thicken two- to threefold. Endothelial cellularity is lost, connective tissue increases, debris accumulates in the meshwork, and glycosaminoglycans accumulate in the extracellular space. These changes can increase resistance to aqueous outflow. Such changes are exaggerated in chronic open-angle glaucoma. This subject is covered in greater depth in BCSC Section 10, *Glaucoma.*

Uveal Trabecular Meshwork

The uveal meshwork faces the anterior chamber. It is composed of cordlike trabeculae and has fewer elastic fibers than does the corneoscleral meshwork. The trabeculocytes usually contain pigment granules. The trabecular apertures are less circular and larger than those of the corneoscleral meshwork.

Corneoscleral Meshwork

The corneoscleral meshwork consists of a series of thin, flat, perforated connective tissue sheets arranged in a laminar pattern. Each trabecular beam is covered by a monolayer of thin trabecular cells exhibiting multiple pinocytotic vesicles. The basal lamina of these cells forms the outer cortex of the trabecular beam; the inner core is composed of collagen and elastic fibers.

Juxtacanalicular Meshwork

The juxtacanalicular meshwork invests the entire extent of the Schlemm canal and forms its inner wall. On its trabecular aspect, between the outermost layers of the corneoscleral meshwork and the endothelial lining of the Schlemm canal, lies the *endothelial meshwork,* a multilayered collection of cells forming a loose network. Between these cells are spaces up to 10 µm wide through which aqueous humor can percolate to reach the endothelial lining of the Schlemm canal (Fig 2-15). This region of the drainage system contributes the most to outflow resistance, partly because the pathway is narrow and tortuous and partly because of the resistance offered by extracellular proteoglycans and glycoproteins.

Schlemm Canal

The Schlemm canal is a circular tube that closely resembles a lymphatic vessel. It is formed by a continuous monolayer of nonfenestrated endothelium and a thin connective tissue wall. The basement membrane of the endothelium is poorly defined. The lateral walls of the endothelial cells are joined by tight junctions. Micropinocytotic vesicles are present at the apical and basal surfaces of the cells. Larger vesicles (so-called giant vacuoles) have been observed along the internal canal wall (Fig 2-16). These vacuoles are lined by a single membrane, and their size and number are increased by a rise in intraocular pressure. They are thought to contribute to the pressure-dependent outflow of the aqueous humor. In one form of microinvasive glaucoma surgery (MIGS), a microstent is implanted in the Schlemm canal to bypass the trabecular meshwork, the point of greatest outflow resistance, thereby increasing aqueous outflow.

Collector Channels

Approximately 25–30 collector channels arise from the Schlemm canal (Fig 2-17) and drain into the deep and midscleral venous plexuses. Up to 8 of these channels drain directly into the episcleral venous plexus as aqueous veins (Fig 2-18), which are visible in the conjunctiva by biomicroscopy.

Uvea

The uvea (also called *uveal tract*) is the main vascular layer of the eye. It consists of 3 parts (Fig 2-19):

- iris
- ciliary body (located in the anterior uvea)
- choroid (located in the posterior uvea)

These structures are discussed separately in the next 3 sections.

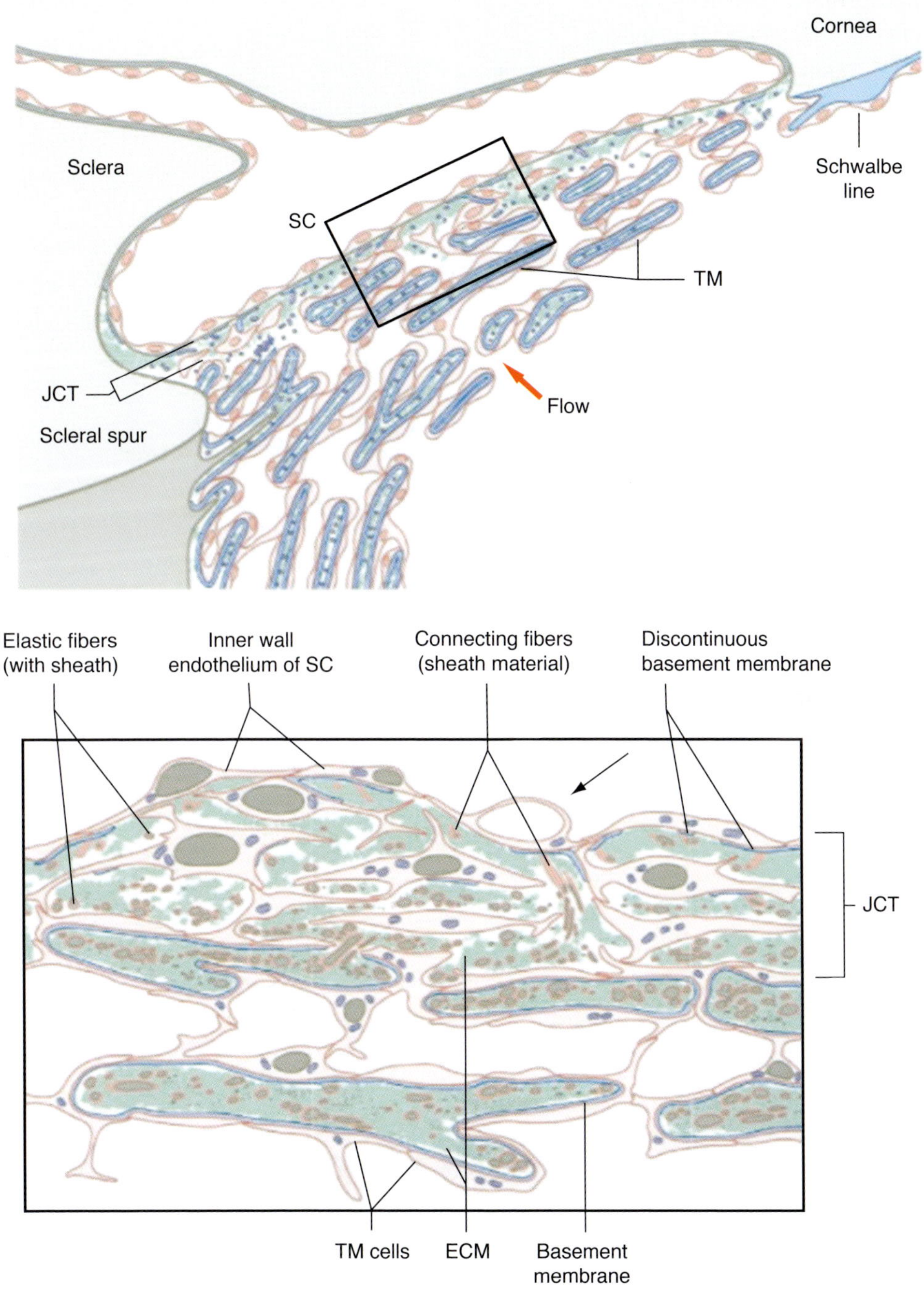

Figure 2-15 Relationship between the juxtacanalicular (JCT) meshwork and the Schlemm canal (SC). *Inset:* The endothelial meshwork (ECM) within the juxtacanalicular meshwork. Note the vacuole along the inner wall of the Schlemm canal *(black arrow).* TM = trabecular meshwork. *(Modified with permission from Levin LA, Nilsson SFE, Ver Hoeve J, Wu SM.* Adler's Physiology of the Eye. *11th ed. Philadelphia: Elsevier/Saunders; 2011:285.)*

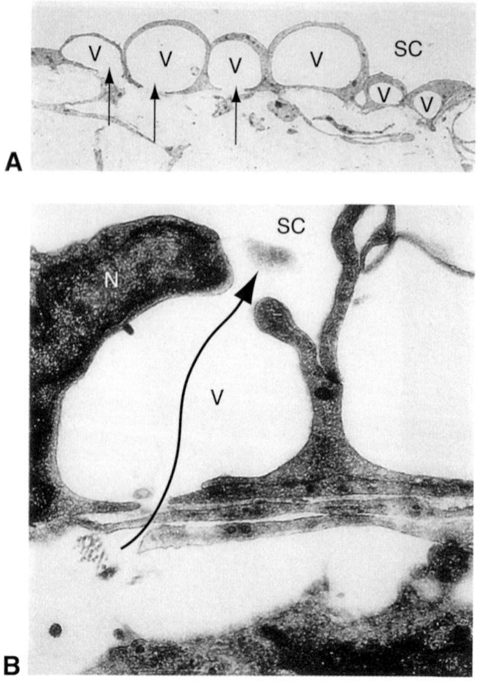

Figure 2-16 **A,** Low-magnification electron micrograph of the endothelial lining of Schlemm canal (SC), showing that most of the vacuolar configurations (V) at this level have direct communication *(arrows)* with the subendothelial extracellular spaces, which contain aqueous humor (×3970). **B,** Electron micrograph of a vacuolar structure that shows both basal and apical openings, thus constituting a vacuolar transcellular channel *(arrow).* Through this channel, the fluid-containing extracellular space on the basal aspect of the cell is temporarily connected with the lumen of the Schlemm canal, allowing bulk outflow of aqueous humor. N = indented nucleus of the cell (×23,825). *(Reproduced with permission from Tripathi RC. The functional morphology of the outflow systems of ocular and cerebospinal fluids.* Exp Eye Res. *1977;25(Suppl):65–116.)*

The uvea is firmly attached to the sclera at only 3 sites:

- scleral spur
- exit points of the vortex veins
- optic nerve

These attachments account for the characteristic anterior dome-shaped choroidal detachment.

The classification of uveitis, established by the 2005 SUN (Standardization of Uveitis Nomenclature) Working Group anatomical classification system, is based on the primary site of inflammation within the zones of the uvea:

- anterior: anterior chamber
- intermediate: vitreous
- posterior: choroid (primary or secondary from the retina)
- panuveitis: anterior chamber, vitreous, and retina or choroid

Uveitis is discussed extensively in BCSC Section 9, *Uveitis and Ocular Inflammation.*

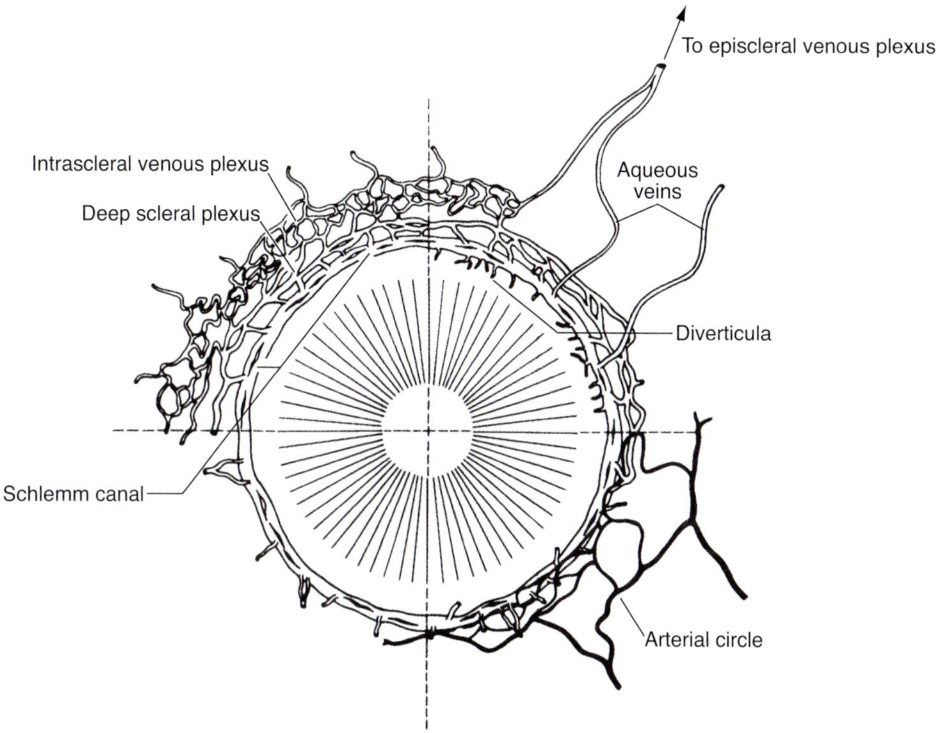

Figure 2-17 Schematic representation of the Schlemm canal and relationships of the arteriolar and venous vascular supply. For clarity, the various systems have been limited to only parts of the circumference of the canal. Small, tortuous, blind diverticula (so-called Sondermann channels) extend from the canal into the trabecular meshwork. Externally, the collector channels arising from the Schlemm canal anastomose to form the intrascleral and deep scleral venous plexuses. At irregular intervals around the circumference, aqueous veins arise from the intrascleral plexus and connect directly to the episcleral veins. The arteriolar supply closely approximates the canal, but no direct communication occurs between the two. *(Reproduced with permission from Tripathi RC, Tripathi BJ. Functional anatomy of the anterior chamber angle. In: Jakobiec FA, ed.* Ocular Anatomy, Embryology, and Teratology. *Philadelphia: Harper & Row; 1982:236.)*

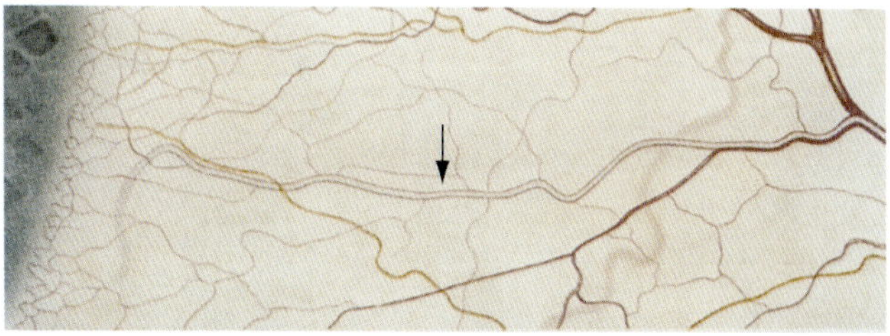

Figure 2-18 Aqueous vein *(arrow)*. Collector channels from the Schlemm canal drain into the episcleral venous plexus. With high magnification of the slit-lamp biomicroscope, they are visible near the limbus. Laminar flow and the mixing of aqueous and blood are visible. *(Reproduced with permission from Thiel R.* Atlas of Diseases of the Eye. *Amsterdam: Elsevier; 1963.)*

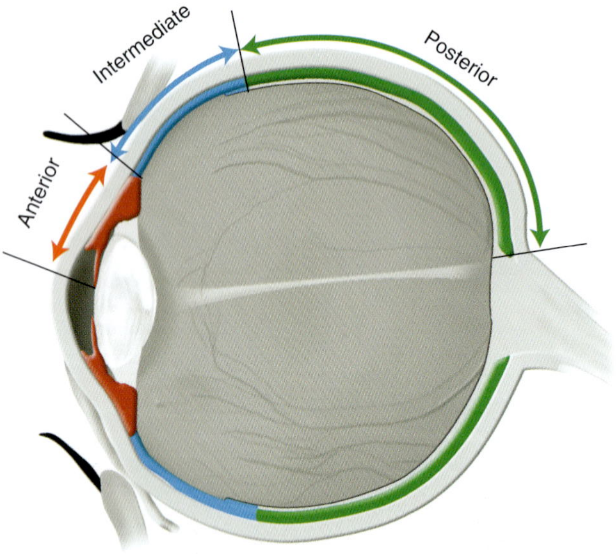

Figure 2-19 The uvea consists of the iris, ciliary body, and choroid. The classification of uveitis, established by the SUN (Standardization of Uveitis Nomenclature) Working Group, is based on the primary site of inflammation. Anterior uveitis *(red)* involves the iris and anterior ciliary body; intermediate uveitis *(blue)* involves the posterior ciliary body and the pars plana and/or the peripheral retina; posterior uveitis *(green)* involves the choroid, either primarily or secondarily from the retina. *(Illustration by Paul Schiffmacher.)*

Iris

The iris is the most anterior extension of the uvea (Figs 2-20, 2-21). It is made up of blood vessels and connective tissue, in addition to the melanocytes and pigment cells responsible for its distinctive color. The mobility of the iris allows the pupil to change size. During mydriasis, the iris is pulled into numerous ridges and folds; during miosis, its anterior surface is smoother.

The major structures of the iris are as follows:

- stroma
- vessels and nerves
- dilator muscle and anterior pigmented epithelium
- sphincter muscle
- posterior pigmented epithelium

Stroma

The iris stroma is composed of pigmented cells (melanocytes), nonpigmented cells, collagen fibers, and a matrix containing hyaluronic acid. The aqueous humor flows freely within the loose stroma along the anterior border of the iris, which contains multiple

A

B

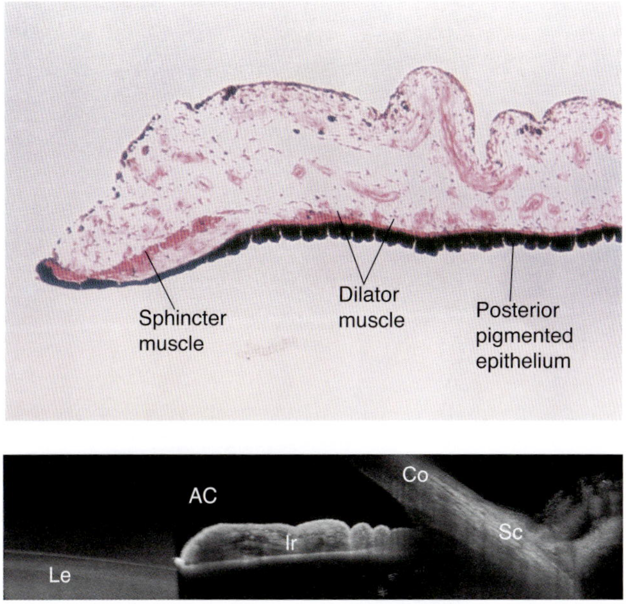

Figure 2-20 Iris. **A,** Histologic section of the iris showing the sphincter muscle, typically found within 1 mm of the pupil border. The dilator muscle, derived from the anterior pigmented layer of the iris epithelium, is found in the mid iris. **B,** AS-OCT scan of the iris. AC = anterior chamber; Co = cornea; Ir = iris; Le = lens; Sc = sclera. *(Part A courtesy of Thomas A. Weingeist, PhD, MD; part B courtesy of Vikram S. Brar, MD.)*

crypts and crevices that vary in size, shape, and depth. This surface is covered by an interrupted layer of connective tissue cells that merges with the ciliary body.

The overall structure of the iris stroma is similar in irides of all colors. Differences in color are related to the amount of pigmentation in the anterior border layer and the deep stroma. The stroma of blue irides is lightly pigmented, and brown irides have a densely pigmented stroma.

Vessels and Nerves

Blood vessels form the bulk of the iris stroma. Most follow a radial course, arising from the major arterial circle and passing to the center of the pupil. In the region of the *collarette* (the thickest portion of the iris), anastomoses occur between the arterial and venous arcades to form the minor vascular circle of the iris, which is often incomplete. The major arterial circle is located at the apex of the ciliary body, not the iris (see Chapter 1, Fig 1-20).

The diameter of the capillaries is relatively large. Their endothelium is nonfenestrated and is surrounded by a basement membrane, associated pericytes, and a zone of collagenous filaments. The intima has no internal elastic lamina. Myelinated and unmyelinated nerve fibers serve sensory, vasomotor, and muscular functions throughout the stroma.

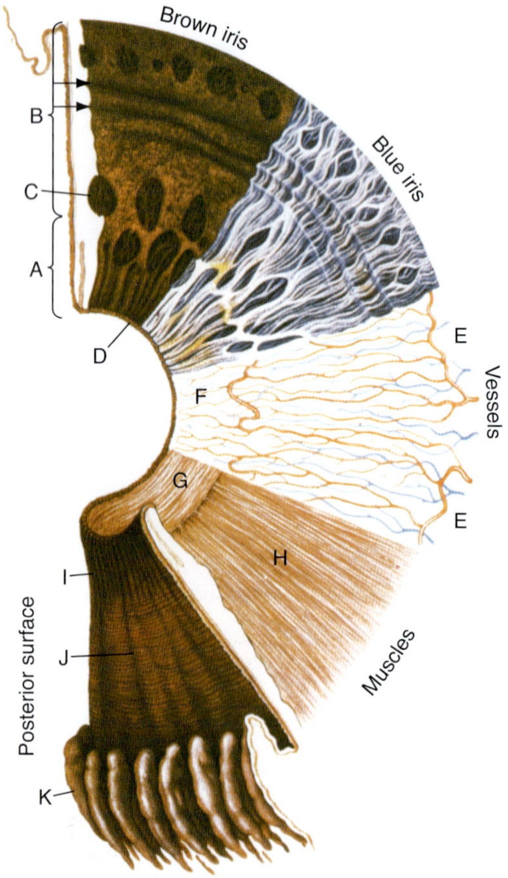

Figure 2-21 Composite drawing of the surfaces and layers of the iris, beginning at the upper left and proceeding clockwise. The iris cross section shows the pupillary (A) and ciliary (B) portions; the surface view shows a brown iris with its dense, matted anterior border layer. Circular contraction furrows are shown *(arrows)* in the ciliary portion of the iris. Fuchs crypts (C) are seen at either side of the collarette in the pupillary and ciliary portions and peripherally near the iris root. The pigment ruff is seen at the pupillary edge (D). The blue iris surface shows a less dense anterior border layer and more prominent trabeculae. The iris vessels are shown beginning at the major arterial circle in the ciliary body (E). Radial branches of the arteries and veins extend toward the pupillary region. The arteries form the incomplete minor arterial circle (F), from which branches extend toward the pupil, creating capillary arcades. The sector below demonstrates the circular arrangement of the sphincter muscle (G) and the radial processes of the dilator muscle (H). The posterior surface of the iris shows the radial contraction furrows (I) and the structural folds (J) of Schwalbe. Circular contraction folds are also present in the ciliary portion. The pars plicata of the ciliary body is shown at bottom (K). *(Reproduced with permission from Hogan MJ, Alvarado JA, and Weddell JE.* Histology of the Human Eye. *Philadelphia: WB Saunders; 1971.)*

Dilator Muscle and Anterior Pigmented Epithelium

The dilator muscle develops from the anterior pigmented epithelium and is derived from the neuroectoderm. It lies parallel and anterior to the posterior pigmented epithelium (Fig 2-22; see Fig 2-20). The smooth muscle cells contain fine myofilaments and melanosomes. The myofibrils are confined mainly to the basal portion of the cells and extend anteriorly into the

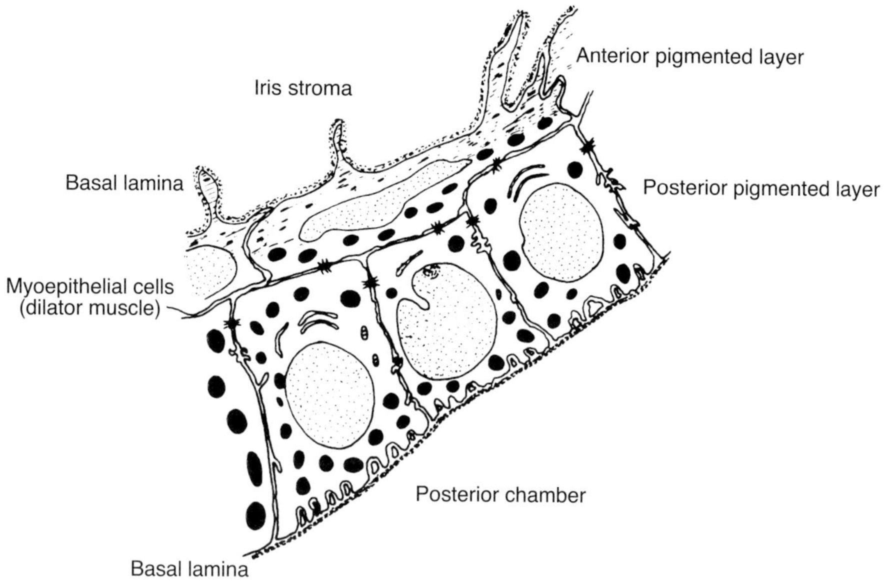

Figure 2-22 Anterior and posterior pigmented epithelia of the iris. The posterior pigmented epithelium is larger than the anterior epithelium and contains more pigment granules than does the latter. *(Illustration by Thomas A. Weingeist, PhD, MD.)*

iris stroma. The melanosomes and the nucleus are found in the apical region of each myoepithelial cell. The remaining anterior pigmented epithelium is smaller and less pigmented than its posterior counterpart, making it difficult to visualize even on histologic sections.

There is dual sympathetic and parasympathetic innervation. The dilator muscle contracts in response to sympathetic α_1-adrenergic stimulation; cholinergic parasympathetic stimulation may have an inhibitory role. See BCSC Section 5, *Neuro-Ophthalmology,* for additional discussion of physiology and pathology of the dilator muscle.

Sphincter Muscle

Like the dilator muscle, the sphincter muscle is derived from neuroectoderm. It is composed of a circular band of smooth muscle fibers and is located near the pupillary margin in the deep stroma, anterior to the posterior pigmented epithelium of the iris (see Fig 2-20). The sphincter muscle receives its primary innervation from parasympathetic nerve fibers that originate in the Edinger-Westphal nucleus and travel with the oculomotor nerve, and it responds pharmacologically to muscarinic stimulation. The reciprocal sympathetic innervation to the sphincter appears to serve an inhibitory role, helping relax the sphincter in darkness. See BCSC Section 5, *Neuro-Ophthalmology,* for additional discussion of physiology and pathology of the sphincter muscle.

Posterior Pigmented Epithelium

The posterior pigmented epithelium of the iris, also called *iris pigment epithelium (IPE),* is densely pigmented and appears velvety smooth and uniform. It is continuous with the nonpigmented epithelium of the ciliary body and thence with the neurosensory portion of the retina. The polarity of its cells is maintained from embryogenesis. The basal surface of the pigmented layer borders the posterior chamber. The apical surface faces the stroma and adheres to the anterior iris epithelium (see Fig 2-22).

The posterior pigmented epithelium of the iris curves around the pupillary margin and extends for a short distance onto the anterior border layer of the iris stroma as the pigment ruff. In rubeosis iridis, the pigmented epithelium extends farther onto the anterior surface of the iris, a condition called *ectropion.* The term *ectropion uveae,* which refers to an outfolding over the pupil of the IPE, is a misnomer because the IPE is derived from neuroectoderm (not neural crest) and therefore is not considered part of the uvea.

Wright KW, Strube YNJ, eds. *Pediatric Ophthalmology and Strabismus.* 3rd ed. Oxford: Oxford University Press; 2012.

Ciliary Body

The ciliary body, which is triangular in cross section, bridges the anterior and posterior segments of the eye (see Fig 2-14). The apex of the ciliary body is directed posteriorly toward the ora serrata. The base of the ciliary body gives rise to the iris. The only attachment of the ciliary body to the sclera is at its base, via its longitudinal muscle fibers, where they insert into the scleral spur.

The ciliary body has 2 principal functions: aqueous humor formation and lens accommodation. It also plays a role in the trabecular and uveoscleral outflow of aqueous humor.

Ciliary Epithelium and Stroma

The ciliary body is 6–7 mm wide and consists of 2 parts: the pars plana and the pars plicata. The *pars plana* is a relatively avascular, smooth, pigmented zone that is 4 mm wide and extends from the ora serrata to the ciliary processes. The safest posterior surgical approach to the vitreous cavity is through the pars plana, located 3–4 mm from the corneal limbus.

The *pars plicata* is richly vascularized and consists of approximately 70 radial folds, or *ciliary processes.* The zonular fibers of the lens attach primarily in the valleys of the ciliary processes but also along the pars plana (see Figs 2-21, 2-47).

The capillary plexus of each ciliary process is supplied by arterioles as they pass anteriorly and posteriorly from the major arterial circle; each plexus is drained by 1 or 2 large venules at the crest of each process. Sphincter tone within the arteriolar smooth muscle affects the capillary hydrostatic pressure gradient. In addition, sphincter tone influences whether blood flows into the capillary plexus or directly to the draining choroidal vein, bypassing the plexus completely. Neuronal innervation of the vascular smooth muscle and humoral vasoactive substances may be important in determining regional blood flow, capillary surface area available for exchange of fluid, and hydrostatic capillary pressure. All of these factors affect the rate of aqueous humor formation.

The ciliary body is lined by a double layer of epithelial cells: the inner, nonpigmented ciliary epithelium and the outer, pigmented ciliary epithelium (Fig 2-23). The basal lamina of the nonpigmented epithelium faces the posterior chamber, and the basal lamina of the outer pigmented epithelium is attached to the ciliary stroma and blood vessels. The nonpigmented and pigmented cell layers are oriented apex to apex and are fused by a complex system of junctions and cellular interdigitations. Along the lateral intercellular spaces, near the apical border of the nonpigmented epithelium, are tight junctions (zonulae occludentes) that maintain the blood–aqueous barrier. The basal lamina of the pigmented epithelium is thick and more homogeneous than that of the nonpigmented epithelium.

The pigmented epithelium is relatively uniform throughout the ciliary body. Each of its cuboidal cells has multiple basal infoldings, a large nucleus, mitochondria, an extensive endoplasmic reticulum, and many melanosomes. The nonpigmented epithelium tends to be cuboidal in the pars plana but columnar in the pars plicata. It also has multiple basal infoldings, abundant mitochondria, and large nuclei. The endoplasmic reticulum and Golgi complexes in these cells are important for aqueous humor formation.

The uveal portion of the ciliary body, the stroma, consists of comparatively large fenestrated capillaries, collagen fibers, and fibroblasts.

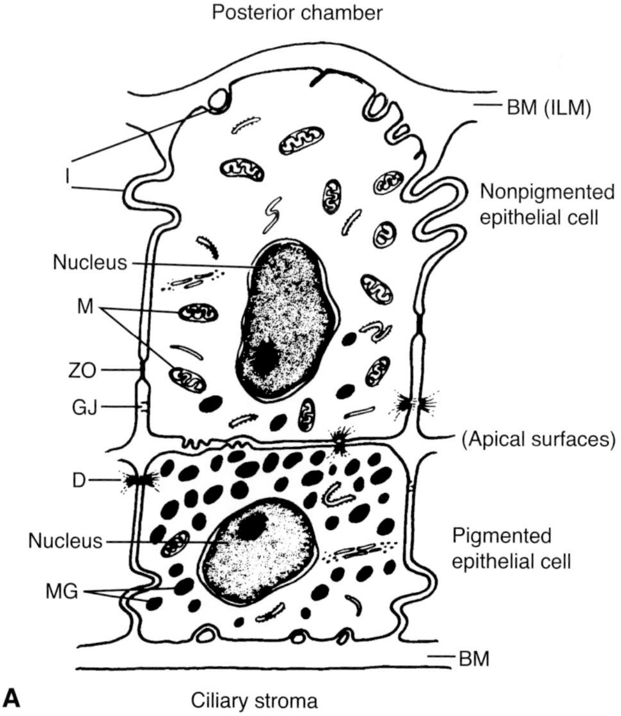

Figure 2-23 **A,** The 2 layers of the ciliary epithelium, showing apical surfaces in apposition to each other. Basement membrane (BM) lines the double layer and constitutes the internal limiting membane (ILM) on the inner surface. The nonpigmented epithelium is characterized by large numbers of mitochondria (M), zonula occludens (ZO), and lateral and surface interdigitations (I). The blood–aqueous barrier is established by the intercellular ZOs. The pigmented epithelium contains numerous melanin granules (MG). Additional intercellular junctions include desmosomes (D) and gap junctions (GJ).

(Continued)

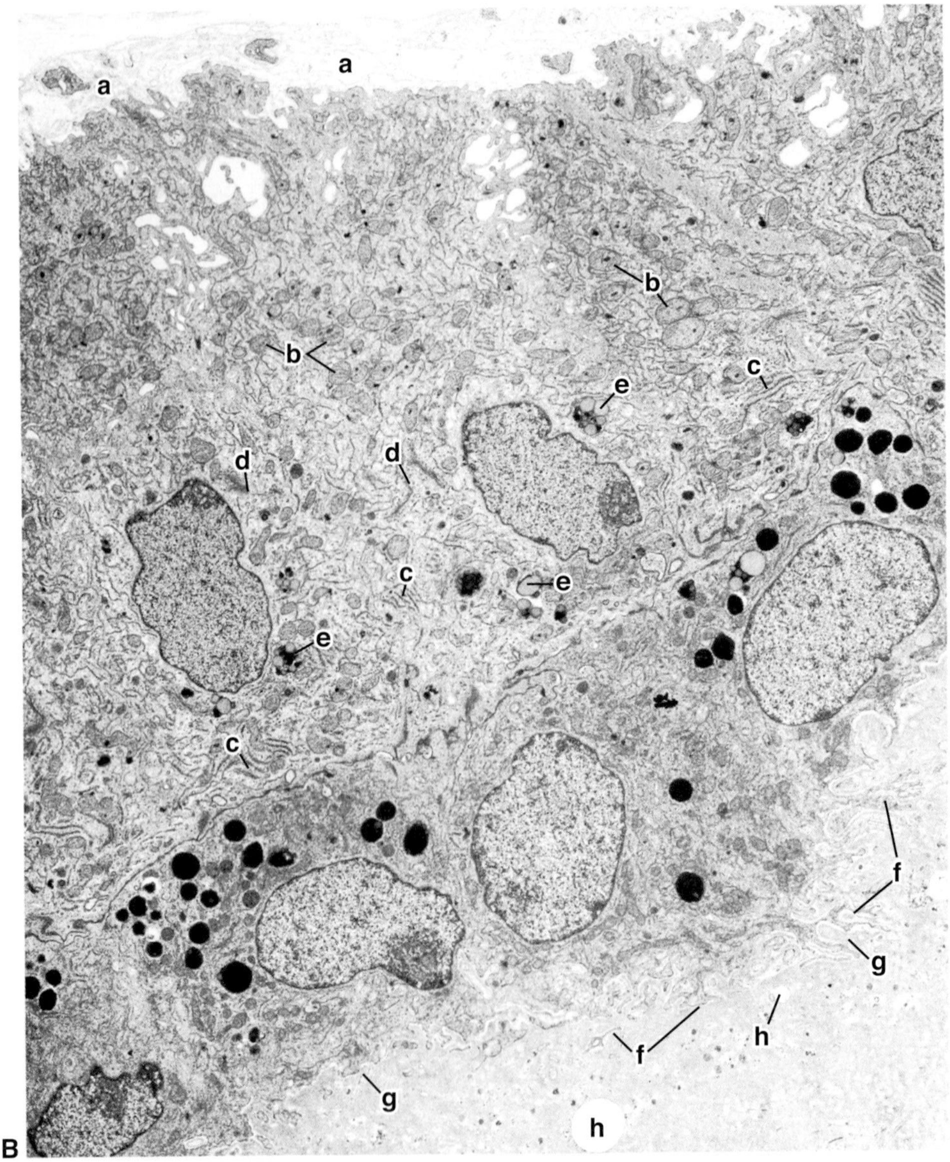

Figure 2-23 *(continued)* **B,** Pars plicata of the ciliary body showing the 2 epithelial layers in the eye of an older person. The nonpigmented epithelial cells measure approximately 20 µm high by 12 µm wide. The cuboidal pigmented epithelial cells are approximately 10 µm high. The thickened ILM (a) is laminated and vesicular; such thickened membranes are a characteristic of older eyes. The cytoplasm of the nonpigmented epithelium is characterized by its numerous mitochondria (b) and the cisternae of the rough-surfaced endoplasmic reticulum (c). A poorly developed Golgi apparatus (d) and several lysosomes and residual bodies (e) are shown. The pigmented epithelium contains many melanin granules, measuring about 1 µm in diameter and located mainly in the apical portion. The basal surface is rather irregular, having many fingerlike processes (f). The basement membrane of the pigmented epithelium (g) and a smooth granular material containing vesicles (h) and coarse granular particles are seen at the bottom of the figure. The appearance of the basement membrane is typical of older eyes and can be discerned with a light microscope (×5700). *(Part A reproduced with permission from Shields MB.* Textbook of Glaucoma. *3rd ed. Baltimore: Williams & Wilkins; 1992. Part B modified with permission from Hogan MJ, Alvarado JA, Weddell JE.* Histology of the Human Eye. *Philadelphia: Saunders; 1971:283.)*

The main arterial supply to the ciliary body comes from the anterior and long posterior ciliary arteries, which join to form a multilayered arterial plexus consisting of a superficial episcleral plexus; a deeper intramuscular plexus; and an incomplete major arterial circle often mistakenly attributed to the iris but actually located posterior to the anterior chamber angle recess, in the ciliary body (see Chapter 1, Figs 1-19, 1-20, 1-22). The major veins drain posteriorly through the vortex system, although some drainage also occurs through the intrascleral venous plexus and the episcleral veins into the limbal region.

Ciliary Muscle

The 3 layers of fibers in the ciliary muscle (Fig 2-24) are

- longitudinal
- radial
- circular

Most of the ciliary muscle is made up of the outer layer of longitudinal fibers that attach to the scleral spur. The radial muscle fibers arise in the midportion of the ciliary body, and the circular fibers are located in the innermost portion. Clinically, the 3 groups of muscle fibers function as a unit. Presbyopia is associated with age-related changes in the lens (discussed in the section Lens, later in this chapter) rather than in the ciliary muscle. Even

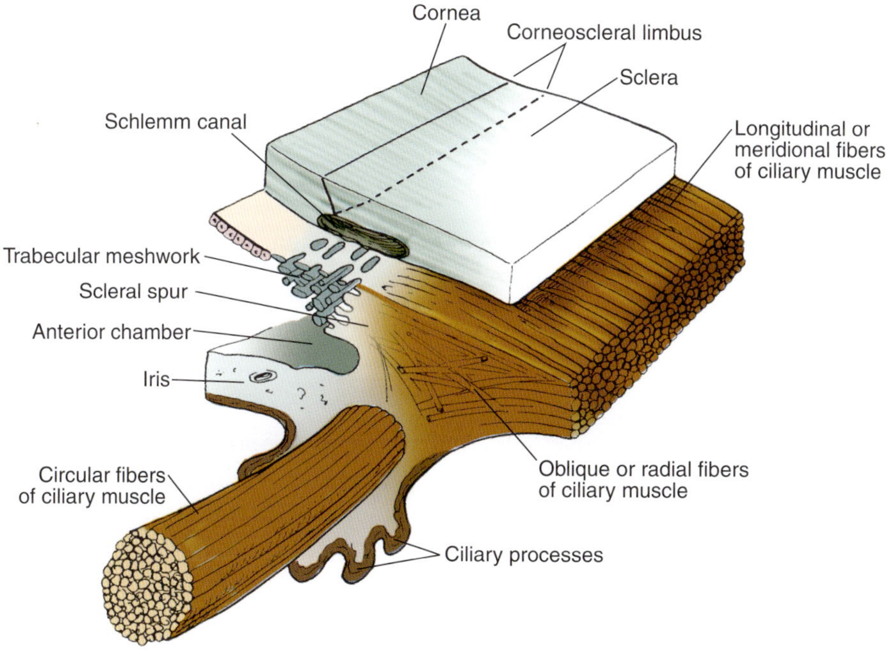

Figure 2-24 Schematic representation of the arrangement of the smooth muscle fibers in the ciliary body. Note the relationship of the ciliary body to the iris, the anterior chamber, the Schlemm canal, and the corneoscleral limbus. *(Modified with permission from Snell RS, Lemp MA.* Clinical Anatomy of the Eye. *Cambridge, MA: Blackwell Scientific Publications; 1989.)*

so, the muscle does change with age: the amount of connective tissue between the muscle bundles increases, and there is a loss of elastic recoil after contraction.

The ciliary muscle fibers behave like other smooth, nonstriated muscle fibers. Ultrastructural studies reveal that they contain multiple myofibrils with characteristic electron-dense attachment bodies, mitochondria, glycogen particles, and a prominent nucleus. The anterior elastic tendons insert into the scleral spur and around the tips of the oblique and circular muscle fibers as they insert into the trabecular meshwork. Both myelinated and unmyelinated nerve fibers are observed throughout the ciliary muscle.

Innervation is derived mainly from parasympathetic fibers of the third cranial nerve via the short ciliary nerves. Approximately 97% of these ciliary fibers are directed to the ciliary muscle, for accommodation, and about 3% are directed to the iris sphincter. Sympathetic fibers have also been observed and may play a role in relaxing the muscle. Cholinergic drugs contract the ciliary muscle. Because some of the muscle fibers form tendinous attachments to the scleral spur, their contraction increases aqueous flow by opening up the spaces of the trabecular meshwork.

Streeten BW. The ciliary body. In: Duane TD, Jaeger EA, eds. *Biomedical Foundations of Ophthalmology.* Philadelphia: Lippincott; 1995.

Supraciliary Space

The supraciliary space is a potential space located below the sclera and above the choroid and ciliary body. This space can expand to accommodate fluid (as for the delivery of drugs) or microstents (as in minimally invasive glaucoma surgery [MIGS]).

Brandão LM, Grieshaber MC. Update on minimally invasive glaucoma surgery (MIGS) and new implants. *J Ophthalmol.* 2013;2013:705915.

Choroid

The choroid, the posterior portion of the uvea, nourishes the outer portion of the retina (Fig 2-25). It averages 0.25 mm in thickness and consists of 3 layers of vessels:

- the choriocapillaris, the innermost layer
- a middle layer of small vessels (Sattler layer)
- an outer layer of large vessels (Haller layer)

Perfusion of the choroid comes both from the long and short posterior ciliary arteries and from the perforating anterior ciliary arteries. Venous blood drains through the vortex system. Blood flow through the choroid is high compared with that through other tissues. As a result, the oxygen content of choroidal venous blood is only 2%–3% lower than that of arterial blood.

Choriocapillaris and Choroidal Vessels

The choriocapillaris is a continuous layer of large capillaries (40–60 μm in diameter) lying in a single plane beneath the RPE (Fig 2-26). The vessel walls are extremely thin and

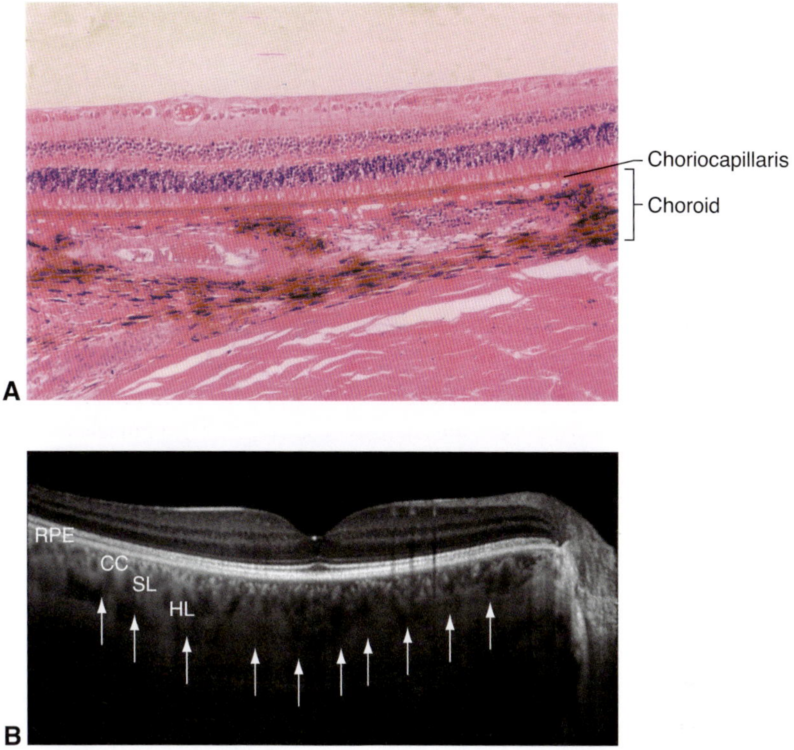

Figure 2-25 Choroid. **A,** Histologic section of the choroid; the choriocapillaris is just below the retinal pigment epithelium (RPE). Beneath the capillaries of the choriocapillaris are the larger middle (Sattler) and outer (Haller) vascular layers. There are scattered melanocytes within the choroid. **B,** OCT image of the choroid (bounded by the RPE and the choroid–sclera junction *[arrows]*) depicts the choriocapillaris (CC), Sattler layer (SL), and Haller layer (HL). *(Part A courtesy of Thomas A. Weingeist, PhD, MD; part B courtesy of Vikram S. Brar, MD.)*

contain multiple fenestrations, especially on the surface facing the retina (Fig 2-27). Pericytes are located along the outer wall.

The middle and outer layers of choroidal vessels are not fenestrated. The large vessels, typical of small arteries elsewhere, possess an internal elastic lamina and smooth muscle cells in the media. As a result, small molecules such as fluorescein, which diffuse across the endothelium of the choriocapillaris, do not leak through medium and large choroidal vessels.

Choroidal Stroma

Abundant melanocytes, as well as occasional macrophages, lymphocytes, mast cells, and plasma cells, appear throughout the choroidal stroma. The intercellular space contains collagen fibers and nerve fibers. In lightly pigmented eyes, pigmentation in the choroid is sparse compared with that of darkly pigmented eyes.

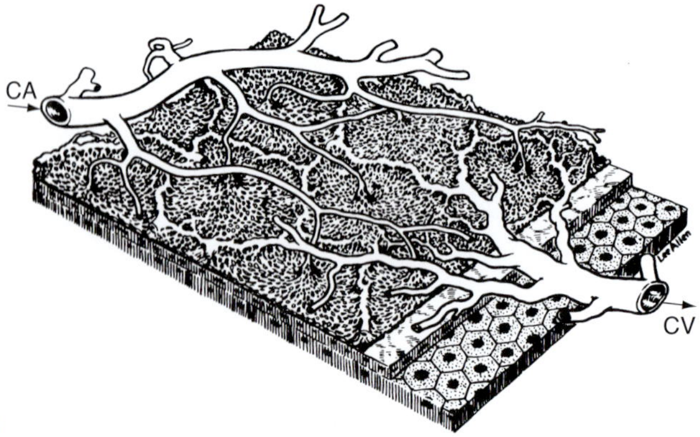

A

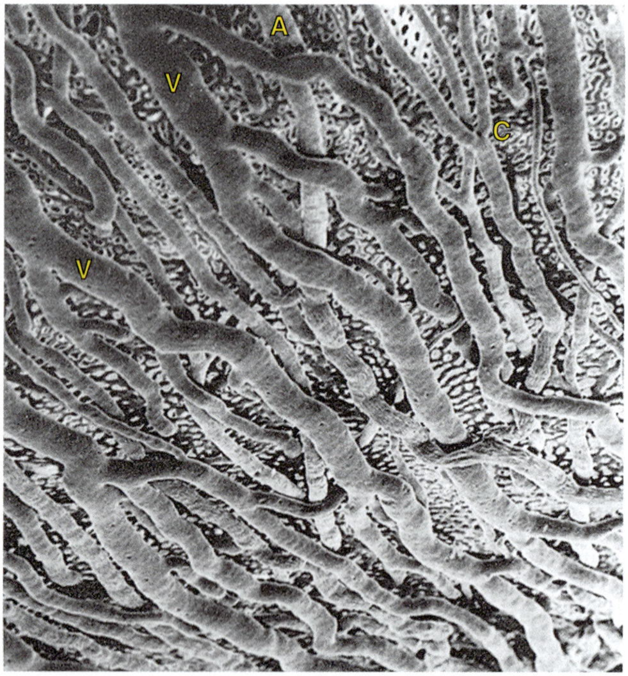

B

Figure 2-26 Lobular pattern of the choriocapillaris. **A,** Note that the RPE is internal to the choriocapillaris. **B,** Electron micrograph of the choriocapillaris and larger choroidal vessels. A = arteries; C = choriocapillaris; CA = choroidal arteriole; CV = choroidal venule; V = veins. *(Part A reproduced with permission from Hayreh SS. The choriocapillaris.* Albrecht Von Graefes Arch Klin Exp Ophthalmol. *1974;192(3):165–179. Part B courtesy of A. Fryczkowski, MD.)*

CLINICAL PEARL

Loss of melanin production within the RPE and melanocytes within the choroid and iris occurs in patients with ocular and oculocutaneous albinism. Lack of pigmentation within the posterior segment can impair uptake during laser photocoagulation.

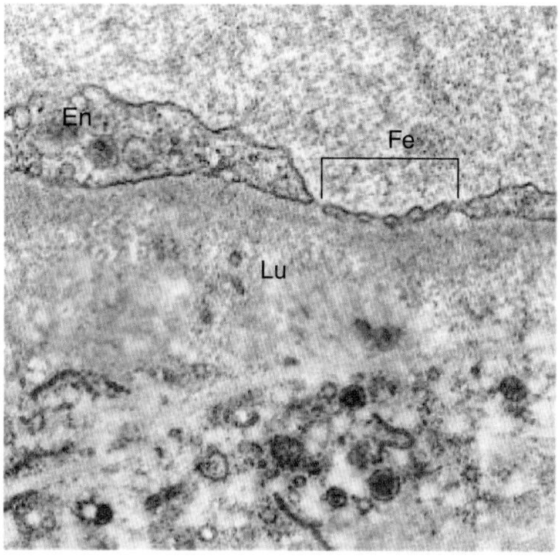

Figure 2-27 Electron micrograph of the choriocapillaris. Fenestrations of the vessel walls are depicted. En = endothelial cell; Fe = fenestrations; Lu = lumen. *(Adapted with permission from Spalton D, Hitchings R, Hunter P.* Atlas of Clinical Ophthalmology. *3rd ed. Oxford: Elsevier/Mosby; 2005:261.)*

Lens

The crystalline lens is a biconvex structure located directly behind the posterior chamber and pupil (Fig 2-28). The lens contributes 20.00 D of the 60.00 D of focusing power of the average adult eye. The equatorial diameter is 6.5 mm at birth; it increases in the first 2–3 decades of life and remains approximately 9–10 mm in diameter in adults. The anteroposterior width of the lens is approximately 3 mm at birth and increases after the second decade of life to approximately 6 mm by age 80 years. This growth is accompanied by a shortening of the anterior radius of curvature of the lens, which would increase its optical power if not for a compensatory change in the refractive gradient across the lens substance.

In youth, accommodation for near vision is achieved by ciliary muscle contraction, which moves the ciliary muscle mass forward and inward. This contraction relaxes zonular tension and allows the lens to assume a globular shape, causing its anterior radius of curvature to shorten (Fig 2-29). With age, accommodative power is steadily lost. At age 8 years, the power is 14.00 D. By age 28 years, the accommodative power decreases to approximately 9.00 D, and it decreases further to 1.00 D by age 64 years. Causes of this power loss include the increased size of the lens, altered mechanical relationships, and the increased stiffness of the lens nucleus secondary to changes in the crystalline proteins of the fiber cytoplasm. Other factors, such as alterations in the geometry of zonular attachments with age and changes in lens capsule elasticity, may also play a role.

The lens lacks innervation and is avascular. After regression of the hyaloid vasculature during embryogenesis, the lens depends solely on the aqueous and vitreous for its nourishment. From embryonic life on, it is entirely enclosed by a basal lamina, the lens capsule. See also BCSC Section 11, *Lens and Cataract.*

Capsule

The lens capsule is a product of the lens epithelium (see Fig 2-28). It is rich in type IV collagen and other matrix proteins. Synthesis of the anterior lens capsule (which overlies

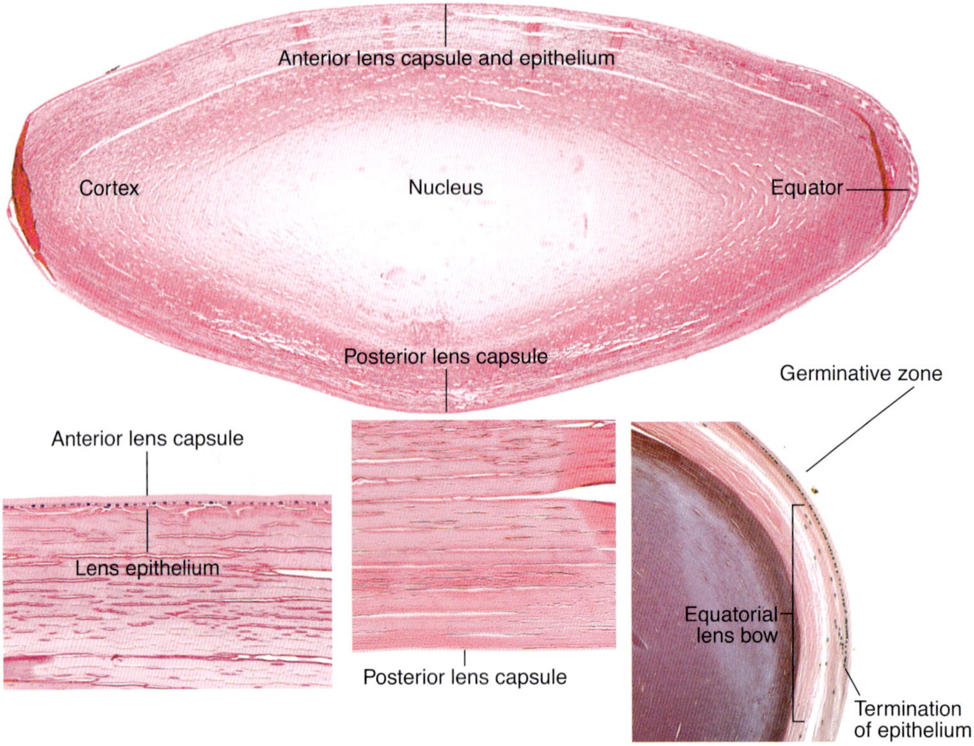

Figure 2-28 Microscopic appearance of the adult lens. *(Courtesy of Tatyana Milman, MD, except for lower right image, which is courtesy of Nasreen A. Syed, MD.)*

the epithelium) continues throughout life so that its thickness increases. Because there are no lens epithelial cells posteriorly, the thickness of the posterior capsule remains constant. Values of 15.5 μm for the thickness of the anterior capsule and 2.8 μm for the posterior capsule have been cited for the adult lens, although these values may vary among individuals and based on the location within the capsule.

Morphologically, the lens capsule consists of fine filaments arranged in lamellae, parallel to the surface (see Fig 2-29). The anterior lens capsule contains a fibrogranular material, identified as laminin, which is absent from the posterior capsule at the ultrastructural level. The thinness of the posterior capsule creates a potential for rupture during cataract surgery.

Epithelium

The lens epithelium lies beneath the anterior and equatorial capsule but is absent under the posterior capsule (see Fig 2-28). The basal aspects of the cells abut the lens capsule without specialized attachment sites. The apices of the cells face the interior of the lens, and the lateral borders interdigitate, with practically no intercellular space. Each cell contains a prominent nucleus but relatively few cytoplasmic organelles.

Regional differences in the lens epithelium are important. The central zone represents a stable population of cells whose numbers slowly decline with age. An intermediate

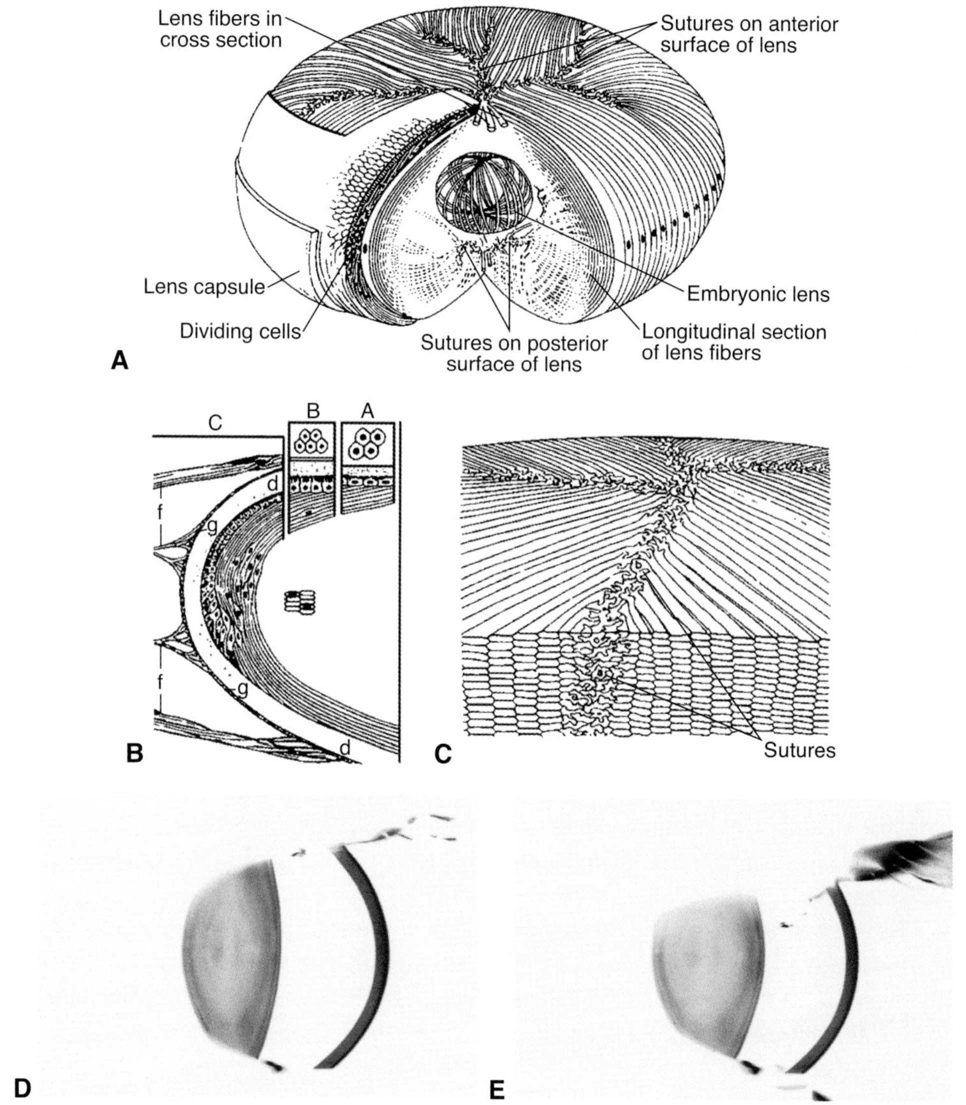

Figure 2-29 Organization of the lens. At areas where lens cells converge and meet, sutures are formed. **A,** Cutaway view of the adult lens showing an embryonic lens inside. The embryonal nucleus has a Y-shaped suture at both the anterior and posterior poles; in the adult lens cortex, the organization of the sutures is more complex. At the equator, the lens epithelium can divide, and the cells become highly elongated and ribbonlike, sending processes anteriorly and posteriorly. As new lens cells are formed, older cells come to lie in the deeper parts of the cortex. **B,** Cross section and corresponding surface view showing the difference in lens fibers at the anterior (A), intermediate (B), and equatorial (C) zones. The lens capsule, or basement membrane of the lens epithelium (d), is shown in relation to the zonular fibers (f) and their attachment to the lens (g). **C,** The diagram shows a closer view of lens sutures. **D** and **E,** Optical sections of the lens of a young adult human (25-year-old woman) demonstrated by Scheimpflug photography. The cornea is to the right. The lens is in the nonaccommodative state in part **D.** The lens is shown during accommodation in part **E.** Note that the anterior radius of curvature is shortened in the latter case. *(Parts A–C reproduced with permission from Kessel RG, Kardon RH.* Tissues and Organs: A Text-Atlas of Scanning Electron Microscopy. *San Francisco: WH Freeman; 1979. Parts D and E courtesy of Jane Koretz.)*

zone of smaller cells shows occasional mitoses. Peripherally in the equatorial lens bow area, there are meridional rows of cuboidal preequatorial cells that form the *germinative zone* of the lens (see Figs 2-28, 2-29). Here, cells undergo mitotic division, elongate anteriorly and posteriorly, and form the differentiated fiber cells of the lens. In the human lens, cell division continues throughout life and is responsible for the continued growth of the lens.

> **CLINICAL PEARL**
>
> Following phacoemulsification, residual germinative cells can cause posterior capsule opacification as a result of aberrant proliferation and cell migration.

Fibers

As new lens fibers form, they compact previously formed fibers, with the older layers toward the center, surrounding the central embryonic and fetal nuclei formed during embryonic development (see Fig 2-29). There is no definite morphologic distinction, but rather a gradual transition between the nucleus and cortex of the lens. The terms *endonucleus, nucleus, epinucleus,* and *cortex* refer to potential differences in appearance and behavior of the layers during surgical procedures.

In optical section with the slit lamp, lamellar zones of discontinuity are visible in the cortex. The fiber cells are hexagonal in cross section; have a spindle shape; and possess numerous interlocking, fingerlike projections. Apart from the most superficial cortical fibers, the cytoplasm is homogeneous and contains few organelles. The high refractive index of the lens results from the high concentration of lens crystallins (α, β, and γ) in the fiber cytoplasm.

Lens sutures are formed by the interdigitation of the anterior and posterior tips of the spindle-shaped fibers. In the fetal lens, this interdigitation forms the anterior Y-shaped suture and the posterior inverted Y–shaped suture. As the lens ages, further branches are added to the sutures; each new set of branch points corresponds to the appearance of a fresh optical zone of discontinuity.

Zonular Fibers

The lens is held in place by the system of zonular fibers *(zonule, suspensory ligament)* that originate from the basal laminae of the nonpigmented epithelium of the pars plana and pars plicata of the ciliary body. These fibers attach chiefly to the lens capsule anterior and posterior to the equator (Fig 2-30). Each zonular fiber is made up of multiple filaments of fibrillin that merge with the equatorial lens capsule. In Marfan syndrome, mutations in the fibrillin gene lead to weakening of the zonular fibers and subluxation of the lens.

When the eye is focused for distance, the zonule is under tension and the lens form is relatively flattened. During accommodation, contraction of the ciliary muscle moves the

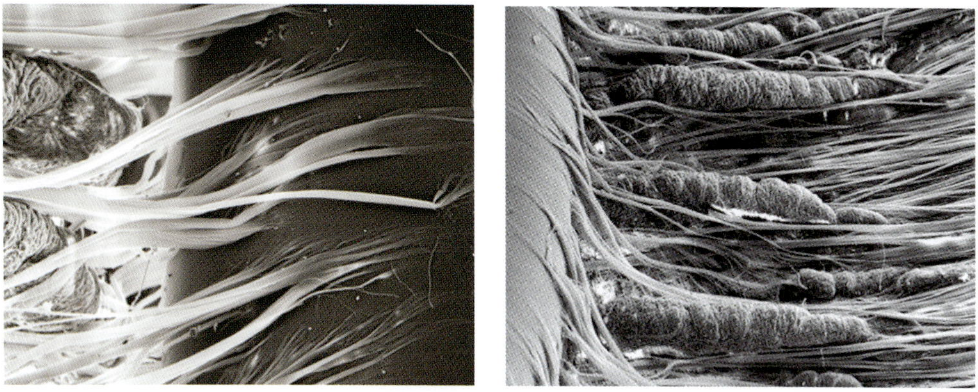

Figure 2-30 Zonular fibers. The zonular fibers insert into the lens capsule anterior and posterior to the equator. Note the ciliary processes between the zonular fibers. *(Courtesy of John Marshall.)*

proximal attachment of the zonule forward and inward, so the lens becomes more globular and the eye adjusts for near vision (Video 2-2).

VIDEO 2-2 Computer model of accommodation.
Courtesy of Daniel B. Goldberg, MD.

Bourge JL, Robert AM, Robert L, Renard G. Zonular fibers, multimolecular composition as related to function (elasticity) and pathology. *Pathol Biol* (Paris). 2007;55(7):347–359.

Goldberg DB. Computer-animated model of accommodation and presbyopia. *J Cataract Refract Surg.* 2015;41(2):437–445.

Streeten BW. Anatomy of the zonular apparatus. In: Duane TD, Jaeger EA, eds. *Biomedical Foundations of Ophthalmology.* Philadelphia: Harper & Row; 1992.

Retina

The *fundus oculi* is the part of the eye that is visible with ophthalmoscopy; it includes the retina, its vessels, and the optic nerve (the anterior surface of which is visible ophthalmoscopically as the *optic disc*). The reddish color of the fundus is due to the transmission of light reflected from the posterior sclera through the capillary bed of the choroid. The *macula* lies between the temporal vascular arcades. At the macula's center lies the *fovea* (Fig 2-31), which contains a specialized region in its center known as the *foveola*. The macula and fovea are discussed in greater detail later in the chapter. In the far periphery, the *ora serrata,* the junction between the retina and the pars plana, can be observed with gonioscopy or indirect ophthalmoscopy.

Embryologically, the retina and its underlying epithelial layer have a common origin, the optic vesicle (see Chapter 4). Thus, the retina can be described as having 2 parts: (1) the neurosensory retina, containing the photoreceptors, neurons, and other elements; and (2) the retinal pigment epithelium (RPE).

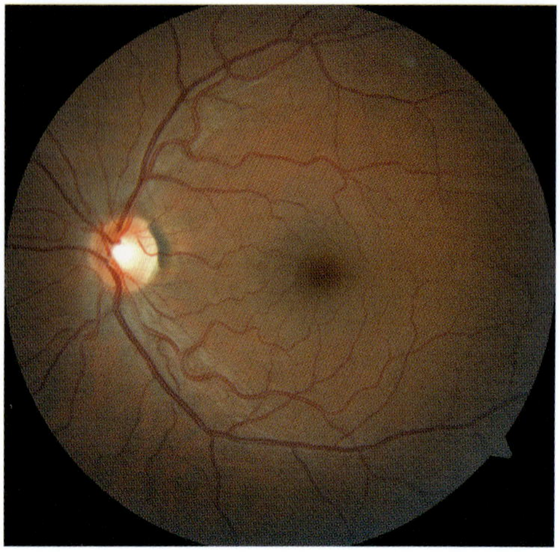

Figure 2-31 Retina. Fundus photograph of the posterior pole. The anatomical macula is bounded by the superior and inferior temporal vascular arcades. The central dark area comprises the fovea. *(Courtesy of Vikram S. Brar, MD.)*

Neurosensory Retina

The *neurosensory retina* is a thin, transparent structure that develops from the inner layer of the optic cup. The neurosensory retina is composed of neuronal, glial, and vascular elements (see Figs 2-33, 2-34).

In cross section, from inner to outer retina, the layers of the neurosensory retina are as follows (Fig 2-32):

- internal limiting membrane
- nerve fiber layer
- ganglion cell layer
- inner plexiform layer
- inner nuclear layer
- middle limiting membrane (see also Fig 1-4 in BCSC Section 12, *Retina and Vitreous*)
- outer plexiform layer (referred to as *Henle fiber layer* in the foveal region)
- outer nuclear layer
- external limiting membrane
- rod and cone inner segments
- rod and cone outer segments

These layers are discussed later in the chapter, in the section "Stratification of the neurosensory retina." The retina is discussed in depth in BCSC Section 12, *Retina and Vitreous.*

Neuronal elements

The photoreceptor layer of the neurosensory retina consists of highly specialized neuroepithelial cells called *rods* and *cones.* There are approximately 100–125 million rods and 6–7 million cones in the human retina, an approximate ratio of 20:1. Each photoreceptor cell consists of an outer segment and an inner segment. The outer segments,

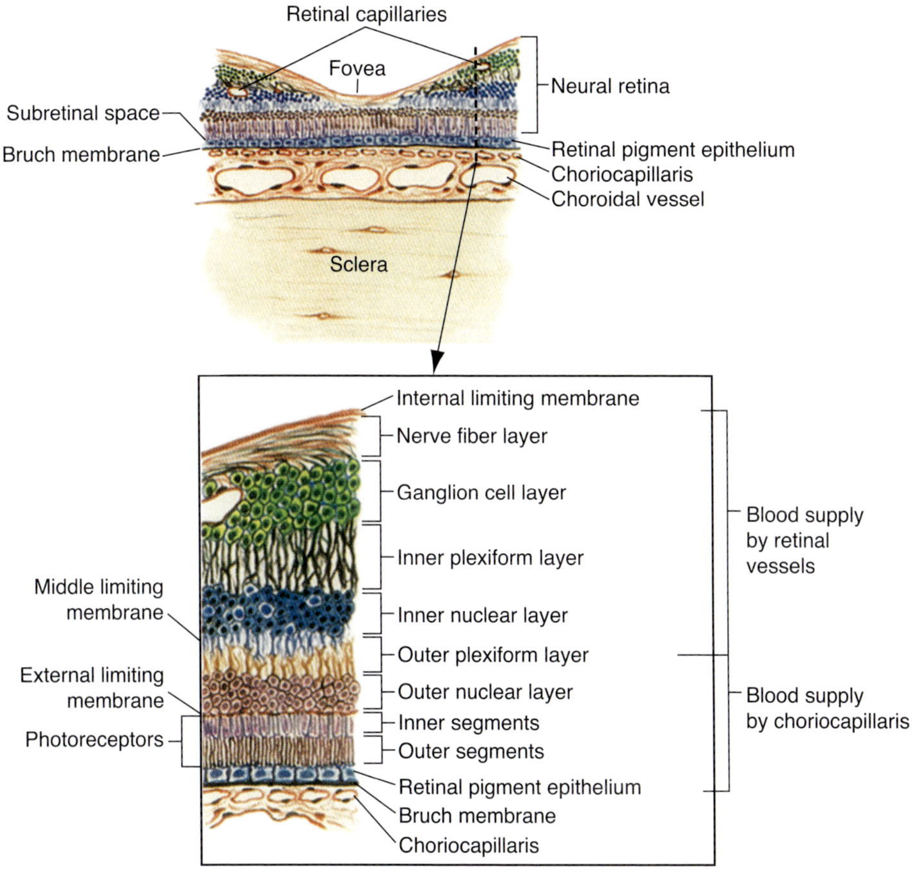

Figure 2-32 Cross section of the retina illustrating its layers and the approximate location of the blood supply to these layers. *(Modified with permission from D'Amico DJ. Diseases of the retina.* N Engl J Med. *1994;331:95–106.)*

surrounded by a mucopolysaccharide matrix, make contact with the apical processes of the RPE. Tight junctions or other intercellular connections do not exist between the photoreceptor cell outer segments and the RPE. The factors responsible for keeping these layers in apposition are poorly understood but probably involve active transport and other mechanisms, including van der Waals forces, oncotic pressure, and electrostatic forces.

The rod photoreceptor consists of an outer segment that contains multiple laminated discs resembling a stack of coins and a central connecting cilium (Fig 2-33). The microtubules of the cilium have a 9-plus-0 cross-sectional configuration rather than the 9-plus-2 configuration found in motile cilia. The rod inner segment is subdivided into 2 additional elements: an outer ellipsoid containing numerous mitochondria, and an inner myoid containing a large amount of glycogen; the myoid is continuous with the main cell body, where the nucleus is located. The inner portion of the cell contains the *synaptic body,* or *spherule,*

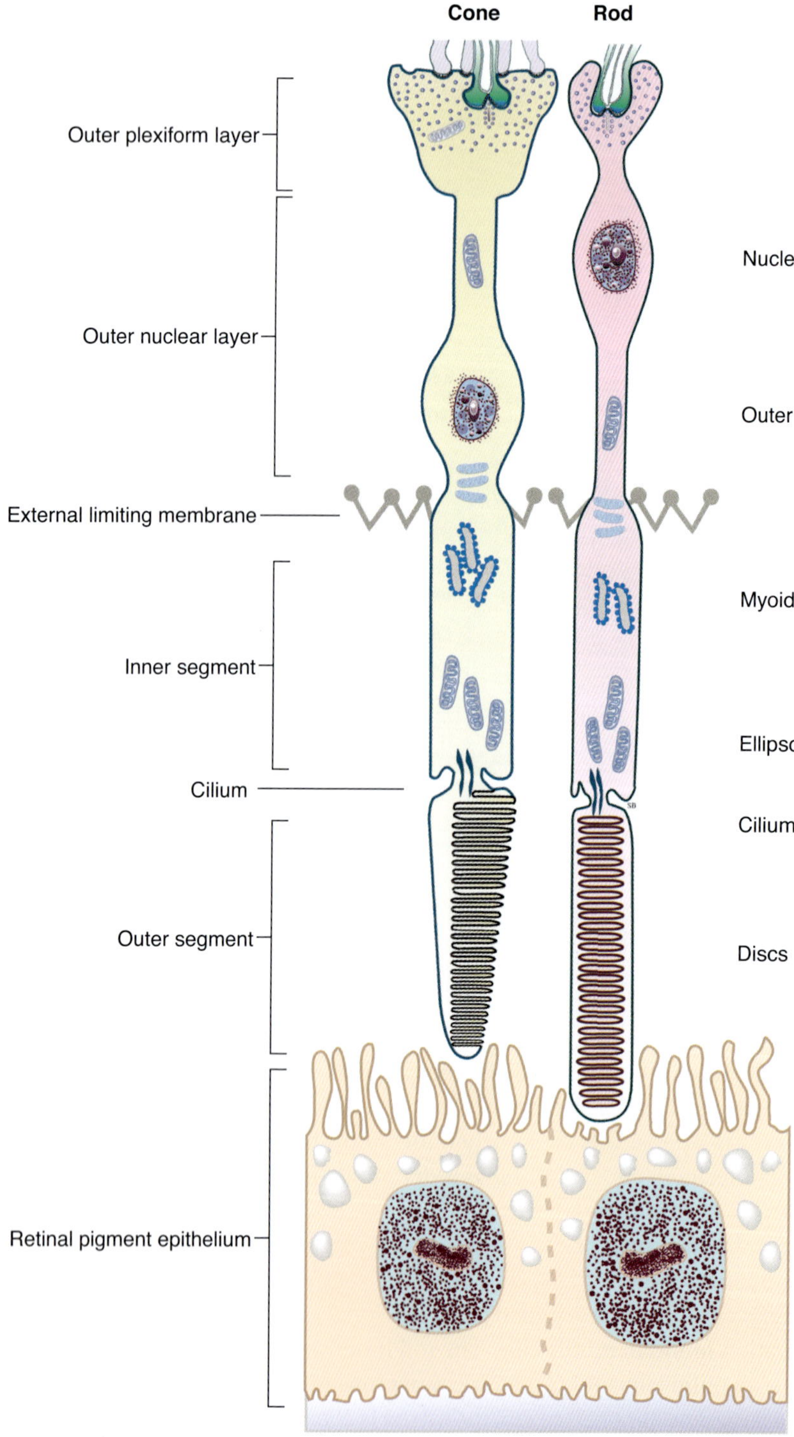

Figure 2-33 Rod and cone photoreceptor cells. *(Illustration by Sylvia Barker.)*

of the rod, which is formed by a single invagination that accommodates 2 horizontal-cell processes and 1 or more central bipolar dendrites (Fig 2-34). The outer segments of the cones have a different morphology depending on their location in the retina.

The extrafoveal cone photoreceptors of the retina have conical ellipsoids and myoids, and their nuclei tend to be closer to the external limiting membrane than are the nuclei of the rods. Although the structure of the outer segments of the rods and cones is similar, at least 1 important difference exists. Rod discs are not attached to the cell membrane; they are discrete structures. Cone discs are attached to the cell membrane and are thought to be renewed by membranous replacement (see Fig 2-33).

The cone *synaptic body,* or *pedicle,* is more complex than the rod spherule. Cone pedicles synapse with other rods and cones as well as with horizontal and bipolar cell processes (see Fig 2-34). Foveal cones have cylindrical inner segments similar to rods but otherwise are cytologically identical to extrafoveal cones.

Horizontal cells make synaptic connections with many rod spherules and cone pedicles; they also extend cell processes horizontally throughout the outer plexiform layer. *Bipolar cells* are oriented vertically. Their dendrites synapse with rod or cone synaptic bodies, and their axons make synaptic contact with ganglion cells and amacrine cells in the inner plexiform layer.

The axons of the ganglion cells bend to become parallel to the inner surface of the retina, where they form the nerve fiber layer and later the axons of the optic nerve. Each optic nerve has more than 1 million nerve fibers. The nerve fibers from the temporal retina follow an arcuate course around the macula to enter the superior and inferior poles of the optic nerve head. The papillomacular fibers travel straight to the optic nerve

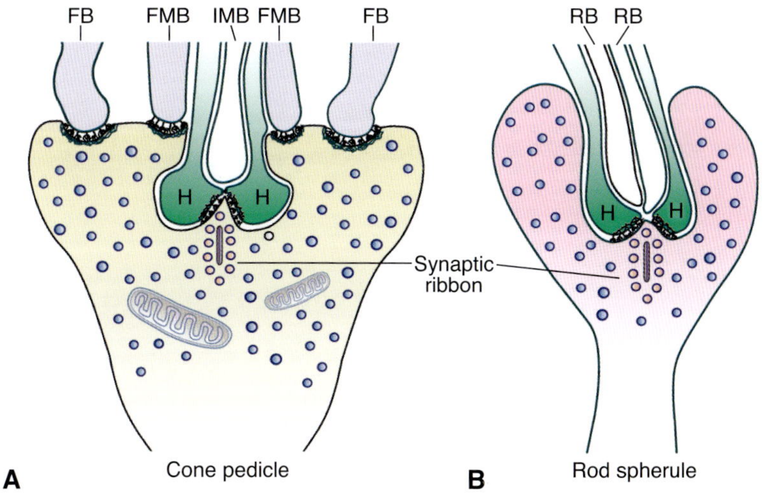

Figure 2-34 Synaptic bodies of photoreceptors. **A,** Cone pedicle with synapses to several types of bipolar cells. **B,** Rod spherule with synapses to bipolar cells. FB = flat bipolar; FMB = flat midget bipolar; H = horizontal cell processes; IMB = invaginating midget bipolar; RB = rod bipolar. *(Illustration by Sylvia Barker.)*

from the fovea. The nasal axons also pursue a radial course. The visibility of the nerve fibers is enhanced when they are viewed ophthalmoscopically using green (red-free) illumination.

The neuronal elements and their connections in the retina are highly complex (Fig 2-35). Many types of bipolar, amacrine, and ganglion cells exist. The neuronal elements of 100–125 million rods and 6–7 million cones are interconnected, and signal processing within the neurosensory retina is significant.

Glial elements

Müller cells are glial cells that extend vertically from the external limiting membrane inward to the internal limiting membrane (see Fig 2-35). Their nuclei are located in the inner nuclear layer. Müller cells, along with the other glial elements (the fibrous and protoplasmic astrocytes and microglia), provide structural support and nutrition to the retina and are crucial to normal physiology. In addition, they contribute to the inner blood–retina barrier.

Vascular elements

The retina is a highly metabolic structure, with the highest rate of oxygen consumption per unit weight in the body. The retinal blood vessels are analogous to the cerebral blood vessels and maintain the inner blood–retina barrier. This physiologic barrier is due to the single layer of nonfenestrated endothelial cells, whose intercellular junctions, under physiologic conditions, are impervious to tracer substances such as fluorescein

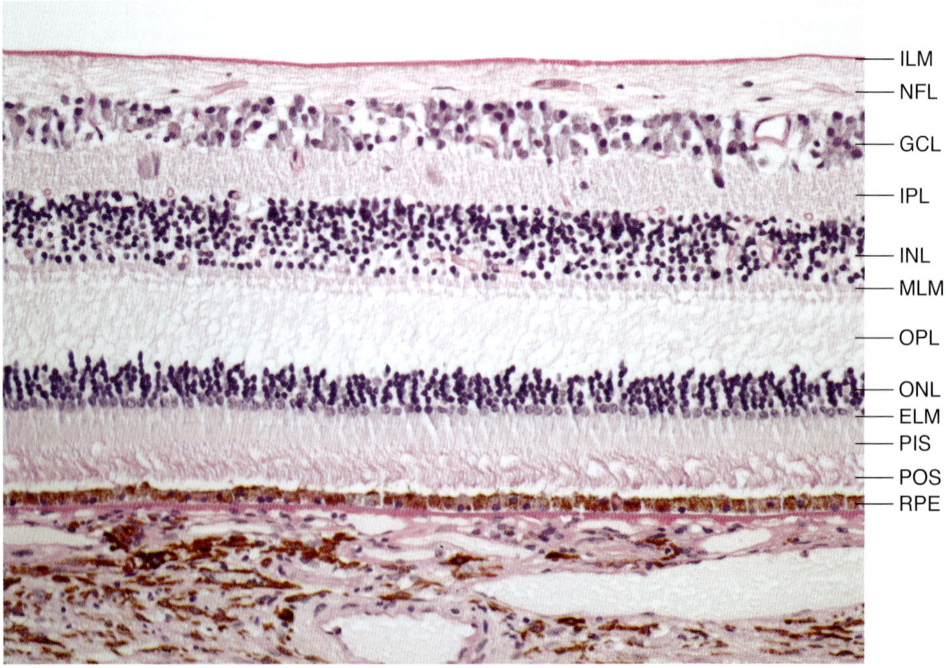

Figure 2-35 *(Continued)*

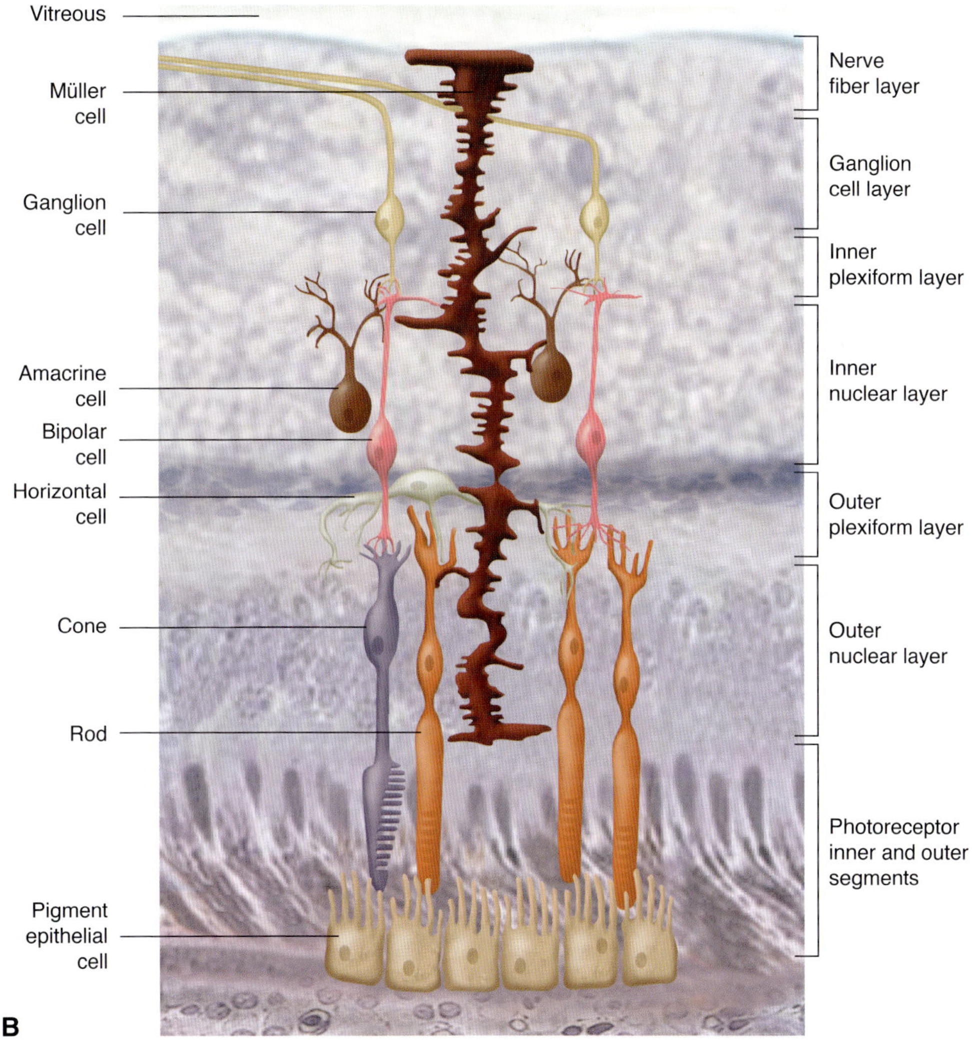

Figure 2-35 **A,** Normal retinal layers (periodic acid–Schiff [PAS] stain). From vitreous to choroid: ILM = internal limiting membrane; NFL = nerve fiber layer; GCL = ganglion cell layer; IPL = inner plexiform layer; INL = inner nuclear layer; MLM = middle limiting membrane; OPL = outer plexiform layer; ONL = outer nuclear layer; ELM = external limiting membrane; PIS = photoreceptor inner segment; POS = photoreceptor outer segment; RPE = retinal pigment epithelium. **B,** Cell types of the retina. *(Part A courtesy of Robert H. Rosa, Jr, MD. Part B illustration by Paul Schiffmacher; revised by Cyndie C.H. Wooley.)*

and horseradish peroxidase (Fig 2-36). A basal lamina covers the outer surface of the endothelium and is surrounded by pericytes, or mural cells, which suppress endothelial proliferation and, along with glial cells, contribute to the inner blood–retina barrier (Fig 2-37).

Müller cells and other glial elements are generally attached to the basal lamina of retinal blood vessels. Retinal blood vessels lack an internal elastic lamina and the continuous

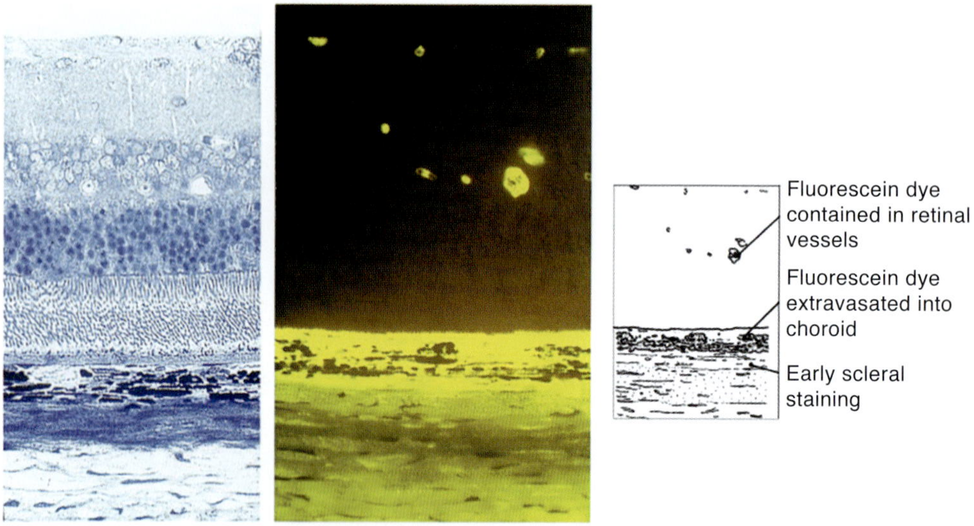

Figure 2-36 Blood–retina barriers. The inner blood–retina barrier is created by intercellular junctions between endothelial cells of the nonfenestrated retinal vessels. The outer blood–retina barrier consists of tight junctions between adjacent RPE cells. *Left:* Normal histologic section of rat retina. *Right:* Section of rat retina following injection of fluorescein. Note the containment of dye within the retinal vessels and the diffuse staining of the choroid by leakage of fluorescein from the fenestrated choriocapillaris. Further extravasation into the outer retina is blocked by the RPE. *(Reproduced with permission from Spalton D, Hitchings R, Hunter P.* Atlas of Clinical Ophthalmology. *3rd ed. Oxford: Elsevier/Mosby; 2005:409.)*

layer of smooth muscle cells found in other vessels in the body. In the absence of the latter, there is no autonomic regulation of the retinal vessels.

The retina possesses a dual circulation in which the inner retina is supplied by branches of the central retinal artery, and the outer retina is supplied by the choroid (see Fig 2-32). Retinal arterioles give rise to the superficial capillary plexus and the deep capillary plexus, which supply the ganglion cell layer and inner nuclear layer, respectively (Fig 2-38). The retinal vascular supply is discussed in detail in BCSC Section 12, *Retina and Vitreous.* The outer nuclear layer and remaining layers of the outer retina are perfused by the choroid. The outer plexiform layer represents a watershed zone in regard to perfusion. Perfusion by the 2 circulations can vary with the location in or thickness of the retina, as well as with light exposure. In approximately 18%–32% of eyes, a cilioretinal artery, derived from the posterior ciliary circulation, also supplies the macula.

Retinal vessels exhibit several characteristics. In contrast to choroidal vessels, retinal vessels demonstrate dichotomous branching. Also, retinal vessels do not normally cross the horizontal raphe. The occurrence of such suggests the presence of anastomoses, which can often be found in the temporal macula following retinal vein occlusions. Further, retinal arteries do not intersect with other arteries; similarly, retinal veins do not intersect with other veins. At arteriovenous crossings, the 2 vessels share a common sheath, which often represents the site of branch retinal vein occlusions.

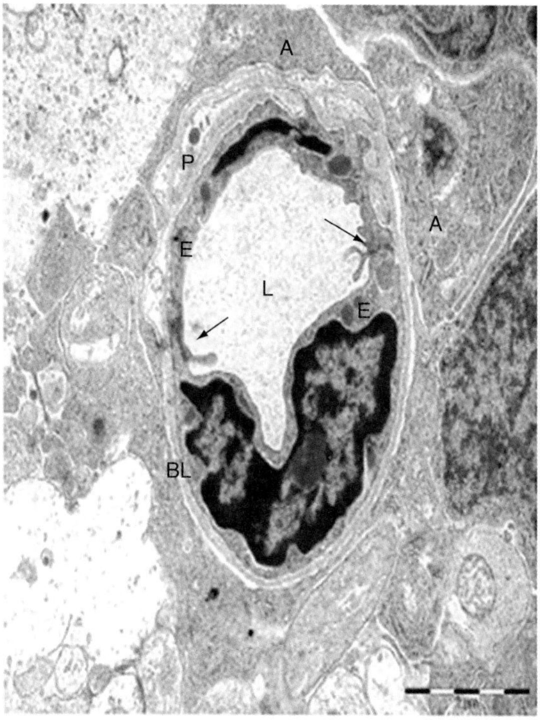

Figure 2-37 Inner blood–retina barrier. Electron micrograph of a retinal capillary in the inner nuclear layer. The inner blood–retina barrier consists of intercellular endothelial junctions (tight, adherens, and gap), pericytes, and contributions from glial cells (Müller cells, astrocytes). A = astrocyte; BL = basal lamina; E = endothelial cell; L = lumen; P = pericyte. Arrows = intercellular junctional complexes. *(Modified with permission from Klaassen I, Van Noorden CJ, Schlingemann RO. Molecular basis of the inner blood-retinal barrier and its breakdown in diabetic macular edema and other pathological conditions.* Prog Retin Eye Res. *2013;34:19–48, Fig 3.)*

Stratification of the neurosensory retina

The neurosensory retina can be divided into several layers (Fig 2-39; see also Fig 2-35). The photoreceptor outer segments represent the outermost layer and interact with the apical processes of the RPE. A potential space exists between this outermost layer of the neurosensory retina and the RPE and is the plane of separation in retinal detachment. The roof of the subsensory space is demarcated by the *external limiting membrane (ELM),* which separates the photoceptor nucleus from its inner and outer segments (see Fig 2-33). The ELM is not a true membrane and is formed by the attachment sites of adjacent photoreceptors and Müller cells. It is highly permeable, allowing the passage of oxygen and macromolecules from the choroid into the outer retina.

Photoreceptor nuclei are found in the *outer nuclear layer (ONL).* The *outer plexiform layer (OPL)* is composed of synapses between the photoreceptors and bipolar cells. Horizontal-cell fibers descend into this region and regulate synaptic transmission. The OPL also accommodates the oblique axons of the rods and cones as they radiate from the foveal center. Because it contains more fibers, the OPL is thicker in the perifoveal region

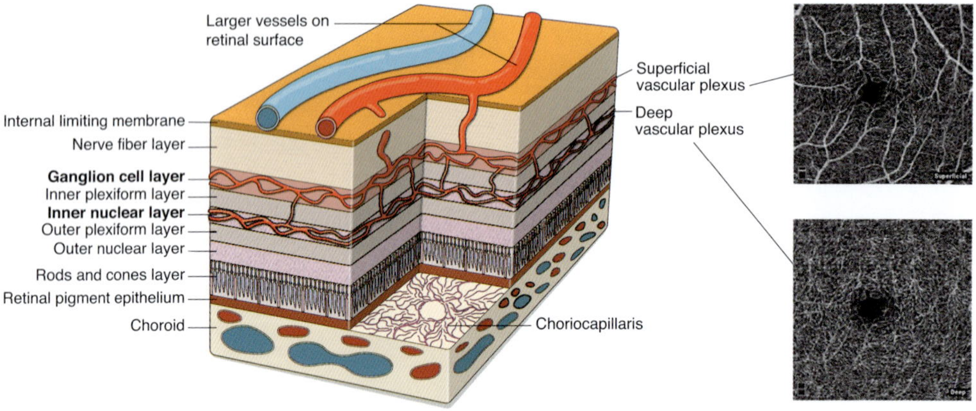

Figure 2-38 OCT angiograms *(right)* demonstrate the superficial vascular plexus and the deep vascular plexus, which arise from retinal arterioles. The schematic *(left)* shows the retinal layers supplied by these plexuses. *(Angiograms courtesy of Vikram S. Brar, MD. Schematic by Mark Miller.)*

(see Fig 2-39). The radial fibers in this portion of the OPL are known as the *Henle fiber layer.* At the edge of the foveola, the Henle layer lies almost parallel to the internal limiting membrane, resulting in petaloid or star-shaped patterns when these extracellular spaces are filled with fluid or exudate (Fig 2-40).

Like the ELM, the *middle limiting membrane (MLM)* is not a true membrane but is rather a junctional system in the inner third of the OPL, where synaptic and desmosomal connections occur between photoreceptor inner fibers and processes of bipolar cells. It is sometimes apparent on OCT as a linear density. Retinal blood vessels ordinarily do not extend beyond this point.

The *inner nuclear layer (INL)* contains nuclei of bipolar, Müller, horizontal, and amacrine cells. The *inner plexiform layer (IPL)* consists of axons of the bipolar and amacrine cells and dendrites of the ganglion cells and their synapses. Amacrine cells, like the horizontal cells of the OPL, probably play an inhibitory role in synaptic transmission. The *ganglion cell layer (GCL)* is made up of the cell bodies of the ganglion cells that lie near the inner surface of the retina. The *nerve fiber layer (NFL)* is formed by axons of the ganglion cells. Normally, these axons do not become myelinated until after they pass through the lamina cribrosa of the optic nerve.

Like the ELM and MLM, the *internal limiting membrane (ILM)* is not a true membrane. It is formed by the footplates of the Müller cells and attachments to the basal lamina. The basal lamina of the retina is smooth on the vitreal side but appears undulatory on the retinal side, where it follows the contour of the Müller cells. The thickness of the basal lamina varies. The ILM is the point of contact of the retina and the cortical vitreous, the vitreoretinal interface.

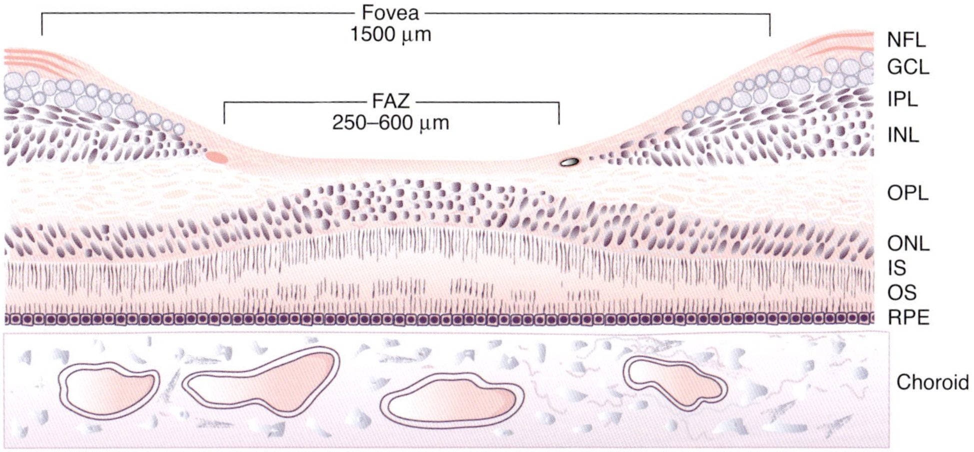

Figure 2-39 Schematic section through the fovea. FAZ = foveal avascular zone; GCL = ganglion cell layer; INL = inner nuclear layer; IPL = inner plexiform layer; IS = inner segment of the photoreceptor; NFL = nerve fiber layer; ONL = outer nuclear layer; OPL = outer plexiform layer (Henle fiber layer); OS = outer segment of the photoreceptors; RPE = retinal pigment epithelium. *(Illustration by Sylvia Barker.)*

Overall, cells and their processes in the retina are oriented perpendicular to the plane of the RPE in the middle and outer layers but parallel to the retinal surface in the inner layers. For this reason, deposits of blood or exudates tend to form round blots in the outer layers (where small capillaries are found) and linear or flame-shaped patterns in the NFL.

Drexler W, Morgner U, Ghanta RK, Kärtner FX, Schuman JS, Fujimoto JG. Ultrahigh-resolution ophthalmic optical coherence tomography. *Nat Med.* 2001;7(4): 502–507.

Topography of the Retina

There is considerable variation in retinal thickness (Figs 2-41, 2-42). The retina is thickest in the papillomacular bundle near the optic nerve (0.23 mm) and thinnest in the foveola (0.10 mm) and ora serrata (0.11 mm).

Macula

Clinically, retina specialists tend to regard the macula, which is 5–6 mm in diameter, as the area between the temporal vascular arcades. Histologically, it is the region with more than 1 layer of ganglion cell nuclei (Fig 2-43; see also Figs 2-32, 2-39, 2-40). See BCSC Section 12, *Retina and Vitreous,* for further detail.

The name *macula lutea* (which means *yellow spot*) derives from the yellow color of the central retina in dissected cadaver eyes or in eyes with retinal detachment involving the macula. This color is due to the presence of carotenoid pigments, located primarily

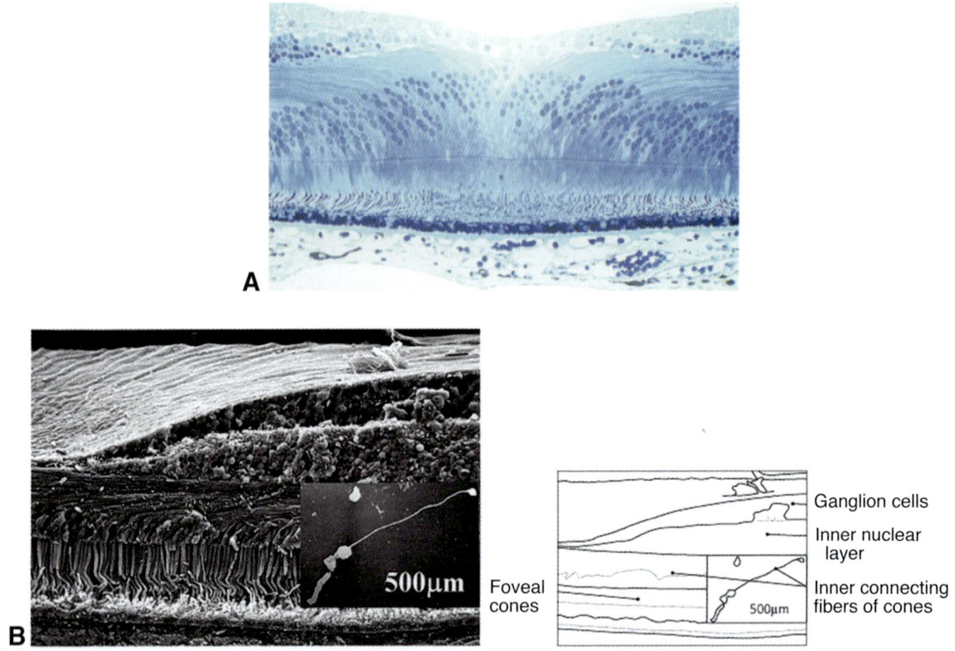

Figure 2-40 Henle fiber layer. **A,** Histologic section through the fovea. Note that only the outer nuclear layer and photoreceptors are present centrally. Oblique photoreceptor axons extend to the outer plexiform layer. These radial fibers are known as the *Henle fiber layer.* **B,** Electron micrograph showing the Henle fiber layer. *(Reproduced with permission from Spalton D, Hitchings R, Hunter P.* Atlas of Clinical Ophthalmology. *3rd ed. Oxford: Elsevier/Mosby; 2005:405–406.)*

in the Henle fiber layer. Two major pigments—zeaxanthin and lutein—have been identified whose proportions vary with their distance from the fovea. In the central area (0.25 mm from the fovea), the lutein-to-zeaxanthin ratio is 1:2.4, and in the periphery (2.2–8.7 mm from the fovea), the ratio is greater than 2:1. This variation in pigment ratio corresponds to the rod-to-cone ratio. Lutein is more concentrated in rod-dense areas of the retina; zeaxanthin is more concentrated in cone-dense areas.

Fovea

The *fovea* is a specialized portion of the macula that appears as a central retinal depression. At approximately 1.5 mm in diameter, it is comparable in size to the optic nerve head (see Fig 2-39). Its margins are clinically inexact, but in younger eyes, the fovea is evident ophthalmoscopically as an elliptical light reflex that arises from the slope of the thickened ILM of the retina. From this point inward, the basal lamina rapidly decreases in thickness as it dives down the slopes of the fovea toward the depths of the foveola, where it is barely visible, even by electron microscopy.

The *foveola* is a central depression in the floor of the fovea, located approximately 4.0 mm temporal and 0.8 mm inferior to the center of the optic nerve head. It is approximately 0.35 mm in diameter and 0.10 mm thick at its center. The borders of the foveola

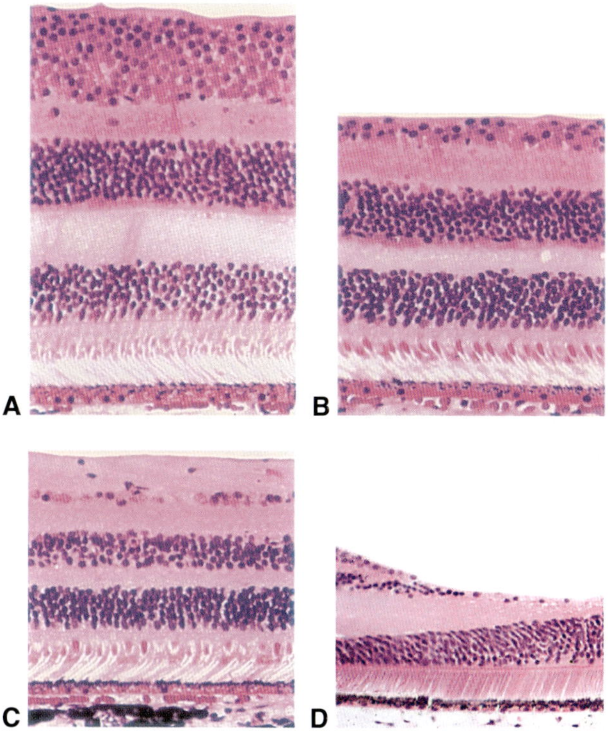

Figure 2-41 Regional differences in the thickness of retinal layers. **A,** Papillomacular bundle, which has the thickest ganglion cell layer. **B,** Macula with 2-cell-thick ganglion cell layer. **C,** Peripheral retina with single-cell ganglion cell layer and thinner inner and outer nuclear layers. **D,** Fovea, in which only the outer nuclear layer and photoreceptors are present. *(All parts courtesy of Thomas A. Weingeist, PhD, MD.)*

merge imperceptibly with the fovea. The nuclei of the photoreceptor cells in the region of the foveola bow forward toward the ILM to form the fovea externa (see Fig 2-40). Usually, only photoreceptors, Müller cells, and other glial cells are present in this area.

The photoreceptor layer of the foveola is composed entirely of cones, whose dense packing accounts for the high visual acuity and color vision for which this small area is responsible. The foveal cones are shaped like rods but possess all the cytologic characteristics of extramacular cones. The outer segments are oriented parallel to the visual axis and perpendicular to the plane of the RPE. In contrast, the peripheral photoreceptor cell outer segments are tilted toward the entrance pupil.

The location of the *foveal avascular zone (FAZ),* or capillary-free zone (Fig 2-44; see also Fig 2-39), is approximately the same as that of the foveola. Its appearance in fundus fluorescein angiograms varies greatly. The diameter of the FAZ ranges from 250 to 600 μm or greater; often, a truly avascular, or capillary-free, zone cannot be identified. This area of the retina is entirely perfused by the choriocapillaris and can be severely affected when retinal detachment involves the FAZ. Around the fovea is the *parafovea,* which is 0.5 mm wide and is where the GCL, the INL, and the OPL are thickest.

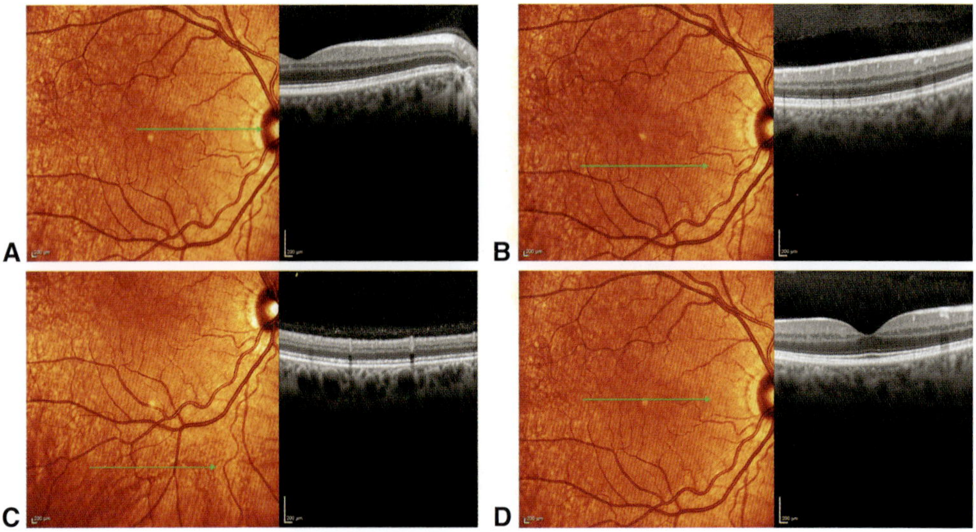

Figure 2-42 OCT images demonstrating the regional differences in retinal layer thickness that are described in Figure 2-41. **A,** Papillomacular bundle. **B,** Macula. **C,** Peripheral retina. **D,** Fovea. *(Courtesy of Vikram S. Brar, MD.)*

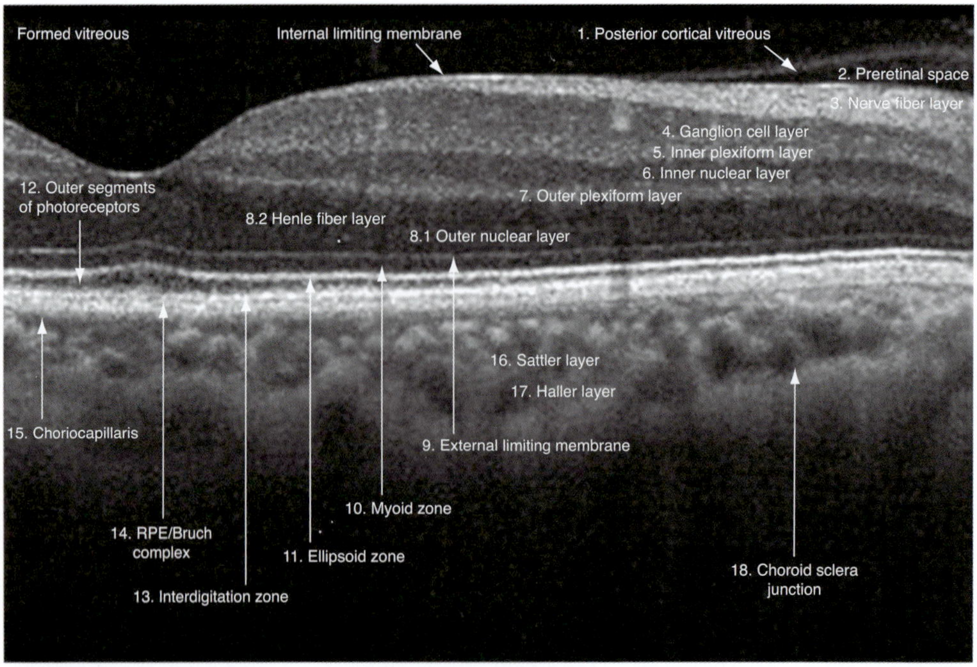

Figure 2-43 OCT image through the fovea. International consensus on segmentation of the normal retina on spectral-domain OCT. *(From Staurenghi G, Sadda S, Chakravarthy U, Spaide RF; International Nomenclature for Optical Coherence Tomography (IN•OCT) Panel. Proposed lexicon for anatomic landmarks in normal posterior segment spectral-domain optical coherence tomography: the IN•OCT consensus.* Ophthalmology. *2014;121(8):1572–1578.)*

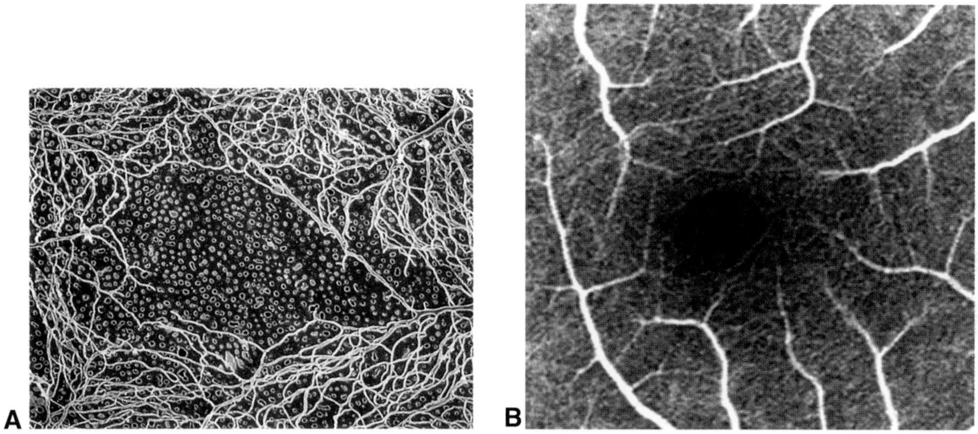

Figure 2-44 Foveal avascular zone. **A,** Scanning electron micrograph of a retinal vascular cast at the fovea, showing the foveal avascular zone (FAZ) and underlying choriocapillaris, the sole source of oxygen to the retina at this location. **B,** Fluorescein angiogram of the FAZ, obtained during the peak venous phase. Fluorescence from the choriocapillaris is blocked by the RPE. *(Part B courtesy of Vikram S. Brar, MD.)*

Surrounding this zone is the most peripheral region of the macula, the 1.5-mm-wide *perifovea.*

Orth DH, Fine BS, Fagman W, Quirk TC. Clarification of foveomacular nomenclature and grid for quantitation of macular disorders. *Trans Sect Ophthalmol Am Acad Ophthalmol Otolaryngol.* 1977;83(3 Pt 1):OP506–514.

Retinal Pigment Epithelium

The retinal pigment epithelium (RPE) develops from the outer layer of the optic cup and consists of a monolayer of hexagonal cells that extends anteriorly from the optic nerve head to the ora serrata, where it merges with the pigmented epithelium of the ciliary body (Fig 2-45). Its structure is deceptively simple considering its many functions:

- vitamin A metabolism
- maintenance of the outer blood–ocular barrier
- phagocytosis of the photoreceptor outer segments
- absorption of light (reduction of scatter)
- formation of the basal lamina of the Bruch membrane
- production of the mucopolysaccharide matrix surrounding the outer segments
- maintenance of retinal adhesion
- active transport of materials into and out of the RPE

Like other epithelial and endothelial cells, RPE cells are polarized. The basal aspect is intricately folded and provides a large surface of attachment to the thin basal lamina that forms the inner layer of the Bruch membrane. The apices have multiple villous processes that envelop and engage with the photoreceptor outer segments

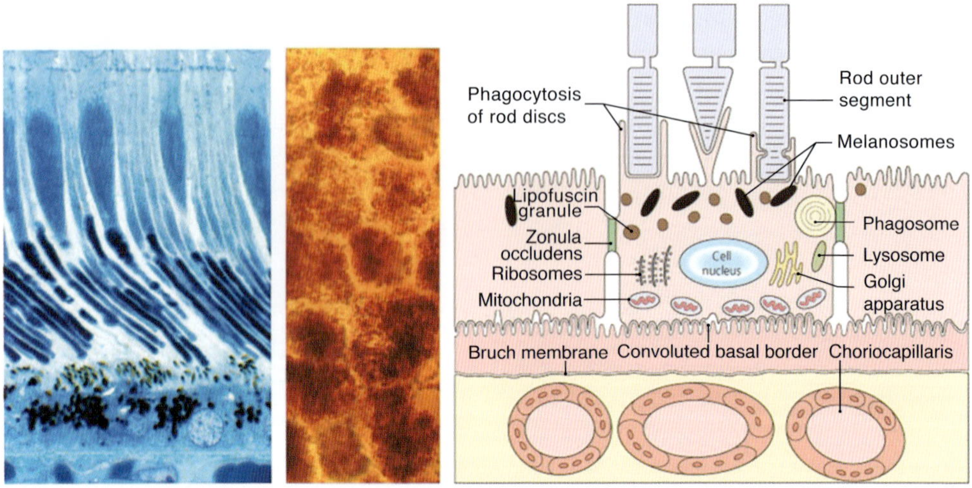

Figure 2-45 RPE. *Left:* Rod and cone outer segments interact with apical processes of the RPE. Note the pigment granules in the apical aspect of the RPE. *Center:* Flat preparation of RPE cells. Note the hexagonal shape and melanin granules. *Right:* Tight junctions between RPE cells act as a barrier to diffusion of solutes from the choriocapillaris and constitute the outer blood–retina barrier. Note the phagosome containing digested photoreceptor discs. Numerous mitochondria, which are required for this highly metabolic tissue, are also depicted. *(Modified with permission from Spalton D, Hitchings R, Hunter P.* Atlas of Clinical Ophthalmology. *3rd ed. Oxford: Elsevier/Mosby; 2005:401.)*

(see Fig 2-45). Separation of the RPE from the neurosensory retina is called *retinal detachment.*

Contiguous RPE cells are firmly attached by a series of lateral junctional complexes. The *zonulae occludentes* and *zonulae adherentes* not only provide structural stability but also play an important role in maintaining the outer blood–ocular barrier (see Fig 2-45). The zonula occludens is the junction at which adjacent plasma membranes are fused, forming a circular band or belt around the surface of adjacent cells. A small intercellular space is present between zonulae adherentes.

RPE cell diameter varies from 10–14 μm in the macula to 60 μm in the periphery. In addition, compared with RPE cells in the periphery, RPE cells in the fovea are taller and thinner, contain more melanosomes, and have larger melanosomes. These characteristics account in part for the decreased transmission of choroidal fluorescence observed during fundus fluorescein angiography. The eye of a fetus or infant contains between 4 and 6 million RPE cells. Although the surface area of the eye increases appreciably with age, the increase in the number of RPE cells is relatively small. No mitotic figures are apparent within the RPE of the normal adult eye.

The cytoplasm of the RPE cells contains multiple round and ovoid pigment granules *(melanosomes)* (see Fig 2-45). These organelles develop in situ during formation of the optic cup and first appear as nonmelanized premelanosomes. Their development contrasts sharply with that of the pigment granules in uveal melanocytes, which are derived from the neural crest and later migrate into the uvea.

Lipofuscin granules probably arise from the discs of photoreceptor outer segments and represent residual bodies from phagosomal activity. This so-called wear-and-tear pigment is less electron dense than are the melanosomes, and its concentration increases gradually with age. Clinically, these lipofuscin granules are responsible for the signal observed with fundus autofluorescence.

RPE cells also possess phagocytic function; they continually ingest the disc membranes shed by the outer segments of photoreceptor cells, enclosing them within *phagosomes.* Several stages of disintegration are evident at any given time. In some species, shedding and degradation of the membranes of rod and cone outer segments follow a diurnal rhythm synchronized with daily fluctuations of environmental light.

The cytoplasm of the RPE cell contains numerous mitochondria (which are involved in aerobic metabolism), rough-surfaced endoplasmic reticulum, a Golgi apparatus, and a large round nucleus (see Fig 2-45).

CLINICAL PEARL

Throughout life, incompletely digested residual bodies, lipofuscin, phagosomes, and other material are excreted beneath the basal lamina of the RPE. These contribute to the formation of *drusen,* which are accumulations of this extracellular material. Drusen can vary in size and are commonly classified by their ophthalmoscopic appearance as hard or soft. They are typically located between the basement membrane of RPE cells and the inner collagenous zone of Bruch membrane. Large soft drusen are associated with intermediate-stage age-related macular degeneration.

Bruch Membrane

The Bruch membrane is a PAS-positive lamina resulting from the fusion of the basal laminae of the RPE and the choriocapillaris of the choroid (Fig 2-46). It extends from the margin of the optic nerve head to the ora serrata. Ultrastructurally, the Bruch membrane consists of 5 elements:

- basal lamina of the RPE
- inner collagenous zone
- relatively thick, porous band of elastic fibers
- outer collagenous zone
- basal lamina of the choriocapillaris

It is highly permeable to small molecules such as fluorescein. Defects in the membrane may develop in myopia, pseudoxanthoma elasticum, trauma, or inflammatory conditions and may, in turn, lead to the development of choroidal neovascularization. With age, debris accumulates in and thickens the Bruch membrane.

Ora Serrata

The ora serrata separates the retina from the pars plana (Fig 2-47). Its distance from the Schwalbe line is between 5.75 mm nasally and 6.50 mm temporally. In myopia, this distance is greater; in hyperopia, it is shorter. Externally, the ora serrata lies beneath the spiral of Tillaux (see Chapter 1, Fig 1-16).

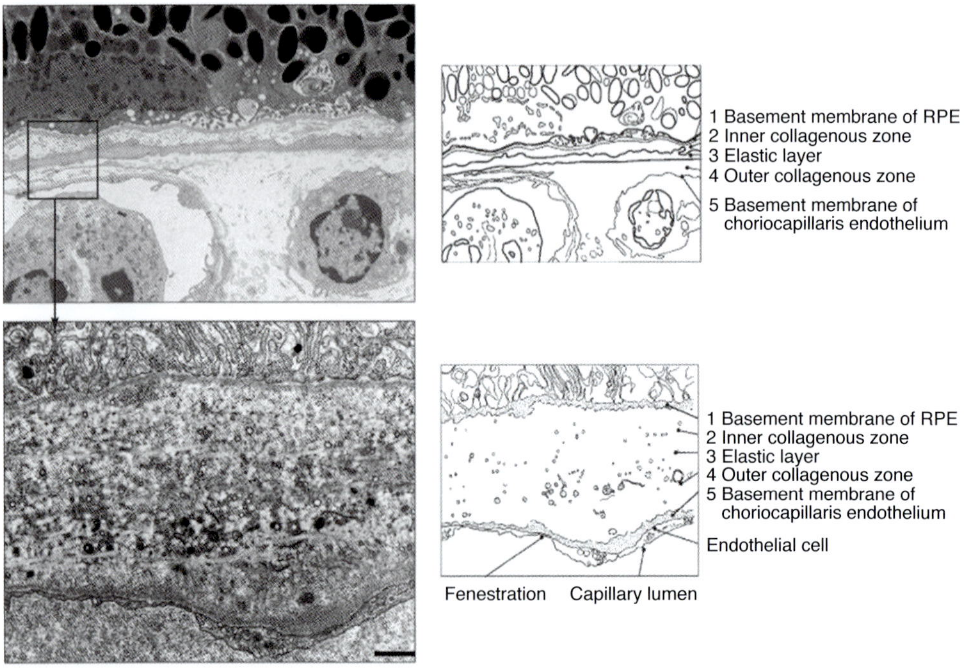

Figure 2-46 Electron micrograph demonstrating the layers of the Bruch membrane. In the upper panel, note the melanin granules in the RPE. In the lower panel, numerous infoldings of the basal surface of the RPE are evident. *(Reproduced with permission from Spalton D, Hitchings R, Hunter P.* Atlas of Clinical Ophthalmology. *3rd ed. Oxford: Elsevier/Mosby; 2005:400.)*

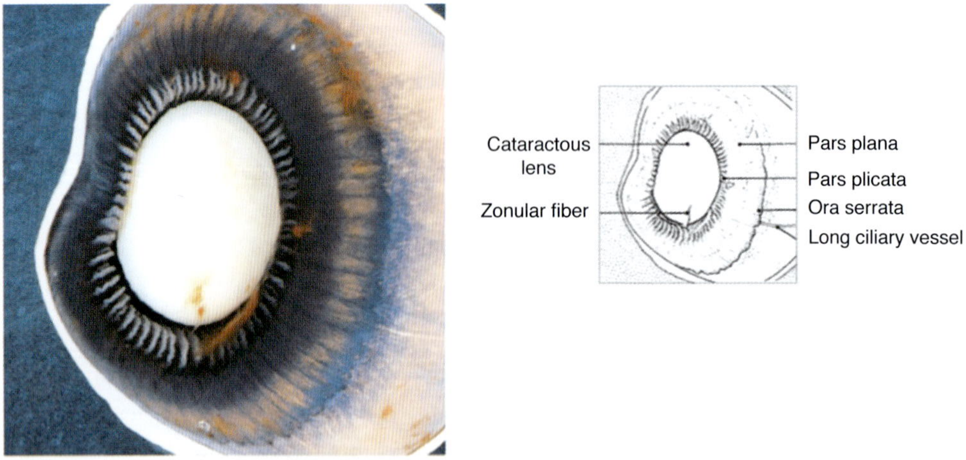

Figure 2-47 Gross photograph of the ora serrata. The pars plana and pars plicata are also shown. *(Reproduced with permission from Spalton D, Hitchings R, Hunter P.* Atlas of Clinical Ophthalmology. *3rd ed. Oxford: Elsevier/Mosby; 2005:259.)*

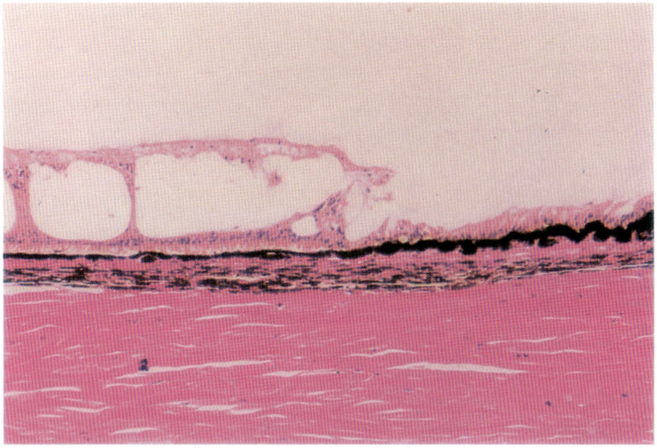

Figure 2-48 Ora serrata. Note the malformed appearance of the peripheral retina and the cystic changes at the junction between the pars plana and the retina (hematoxylin-eosin stain ×32). *(Courtesy of Thomas A. Weingeist, PhD, MD.)*

At the ora serrata, the diameter of the eye is 20 mm and the circumference is 63 mm; at the equator, the diameter is 24 mm and the circumference is 75 mm. Topographically, the margin of the ora serrata is relatively smooth temporally and serrated nasally. Retinal blood vessels end in loops before reaching the ora serrata.

The ora serrata is in a watershed zone between the anterior and posterior vascular systems, which may in part explain why peripheral retinal degeneration is relatively common. The peripheral retina in the region of the ora serrata is markedly attenuated. The photoreceptors are malformed, and the overlying retina frequently appears cystic in paraffin sections (Blessig-Iwanoff cysts; Fig 2-48).

Vitreous

The vitreous cavity occupies four-fifths of the volume of the globe. The transparent vitreous humor is important to the metabolism of the intraocular tissues because it provides a route for metabolites used by the lens, ciliary body, and retina. Its volume is close to 4.0 mL. Although it has a gel-like structure, the vitreous is 99% water. Its viscosity, however, is approximately twice that of water, mainly because of the presence of the mucopolysaccharide hyaluronic acid (Fig 2-49).

At the ultrastructural level, fine collagen fibrils (chiefly type II) and cells have been identified in the vitreous. The origin and function of these cells, termed *hyalocytes,* are unknown, but they probably represent modified histiocytes, glial cells, or fibroblasts. The fibrils at the vitreous base merge with the basal lamina of the nonpigmented epithelium of the pars plana and, posteriorly, with the ILM of the retina, the vitreoretinal interface.

The vitreous adheres to the retina peripherally at the vitreous base (Fig 2-50), which extends from 2.0 mm anterior to the ora serrata to approximately 4.0 mm posterior to it.

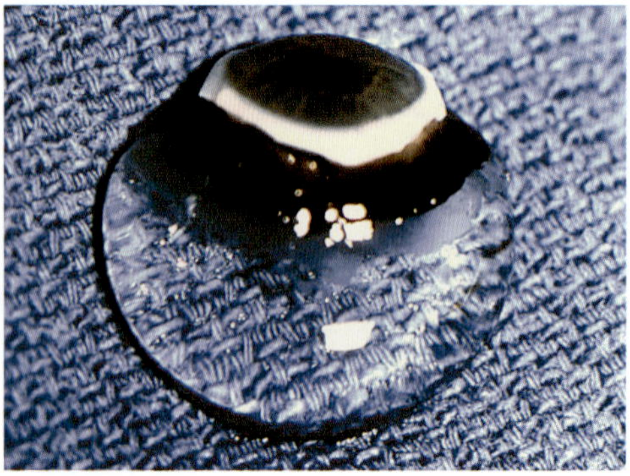

Figure 2-49 Vitreous. Gross photograph of the vitreous with the sclera, choroid, and retina removed from the eye of a 9-month-old child. *(Modified from Sebag J. Posterior vitreous detachment.* Ophthalmology. *2018;125(9):Fig 1.)*

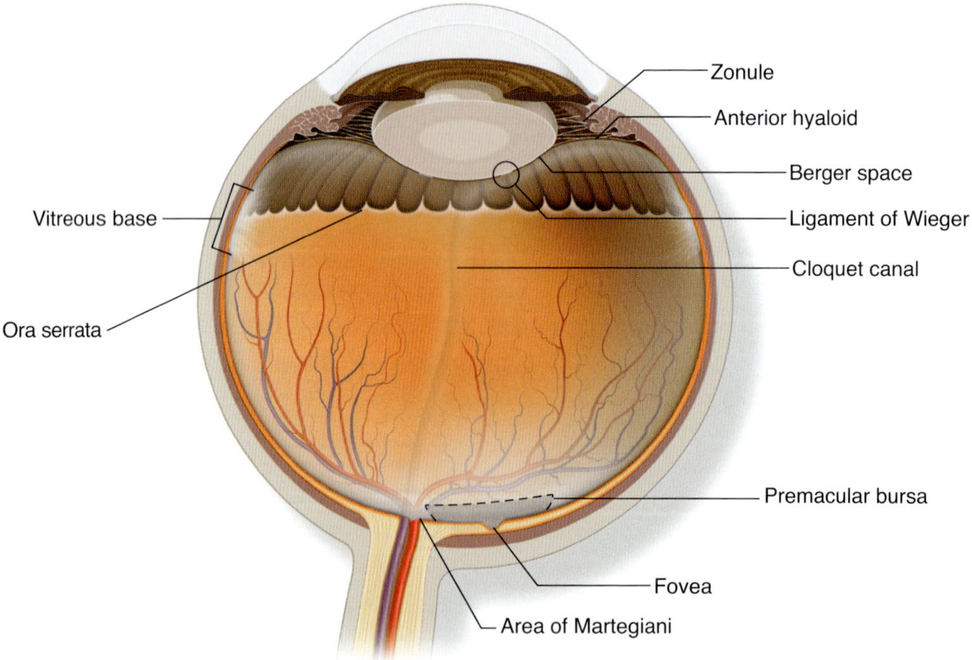

Figure 2-50 Vitreous. The vitreous is most firmly attached to the retina at the vitreous base, which straddles the ora serrata. Additional adhesions exist at the posterior lens capsule (hyaloideocapsular ligament; also known as *ligament of Weiger*), along the retinal vessels, at the perimacular region, and at the optic nerve margin. A prominent area of liquefaction of the premacular vitreous gel is called the *premacular bursa*, or *precortical vitreous pocket*. *(Illustration by Mark M. Miller.)*

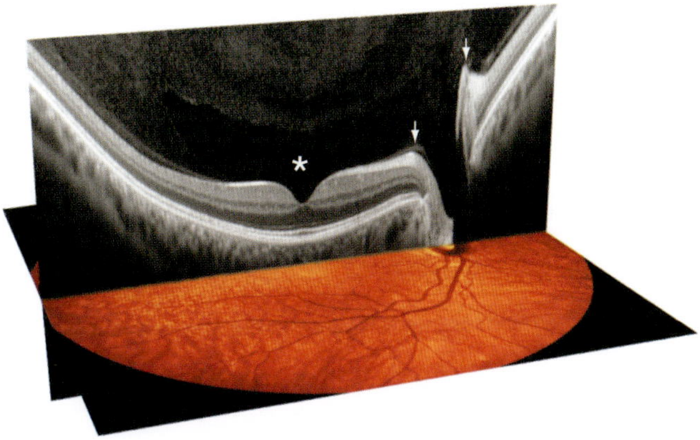

Figure 2-51 Posterior vitreous attachments. OCT image of the fovea and overlying vitreous. Note the adhesion of the vitreous at the margins of the optic nerve *(arrows)* and fovea (perimacular), with overlying premacular bursa *(*)*. *(Courtesy of Vikram S. Brar, MD.)*

Additional attachments exist at the optic nerve head margin, at the perimacular region surrounding the fovea, along the retinal vessels, and at the periphery of the posterior lens capsule (Fig 2-51). See Chapter 11 for further discussion of the vitreous.

Lund-Andersen H, Sander B. The vitreous. In: Levin LA, Nilsson SFE, Ver Hoeve J, Wu SM. *Adler's Physiology of the Eye.* 11th ed. Philadelphia: Elsevier/Saunders; 2011:164–181.

CHAPTER 3

Cranial Nerves: Central and Peripheral Connections

Highlights

- Cranial nerve (CN) II—Macular projections constitute 80%–90% of the total volume of the optic nerve. Nasal fibers, carrying input from the temporal visual field, cross at the optic chiasm whereas temporal fibers do not.
- CN III—CN III subnuclei supply their respective ipsilateral extraocular muscles. Exceptions are the subnucleus for the superior rectus muscle, which innervates the contralateral superior rectus; and the single, central levator palpebrae subnucleus, which supplies both levator muscles.
- CN IV fascicles completely decussate after leaving the nucleus, thus innervating the contralateral superior oblique muscle. CN IV has the longest intracranial course and is the only CN to exit dorsally from the brainstem.
- CN V, the largest of the CNs, provides sensation to the face and eye, as well as other structures of the head.
- CN VI is susceptible to injury from increased intracranial pressure.
- CN VII provides the efferent limb of the tear reflex.

Cranial nerves I–VI are depicted in Figure 3-1 in relation to the bony canals and arteries at the base of the skull. In Figure 3-2, the nerves are shown in relation to the brainstem, cavernous sinus, and orbit. For further study, see BCSC Section 5, *Neuro-Ophthalmology,* which describes these nerves as they apply to specific clinical entities.

Olfactory Nerve (First Cranial Nerve)

The olfactory nerve (CN I) originates from small olfactory receptors in the mucous membrane of the nose. Unmyelinated CN I fibers pass from these receptors in the nasal cavity through the cribriform plate of the ethmoid bone and enter the ventral surface of the olfactory bulb, where they form the nerve.

The olfactory tract runs posteriorly from the bulb beneath the frontal lobe of the brain in a groove (or sulcus) and lateral to the gyrus rectus (Fig 3-3). The gyrus rectus forms the anterolateral border of the suprasellar cistern. Meningiomas arising from the arachnoid cells in this area can cause important ophthalmic signs and symptoms associated with loss of olfaction.

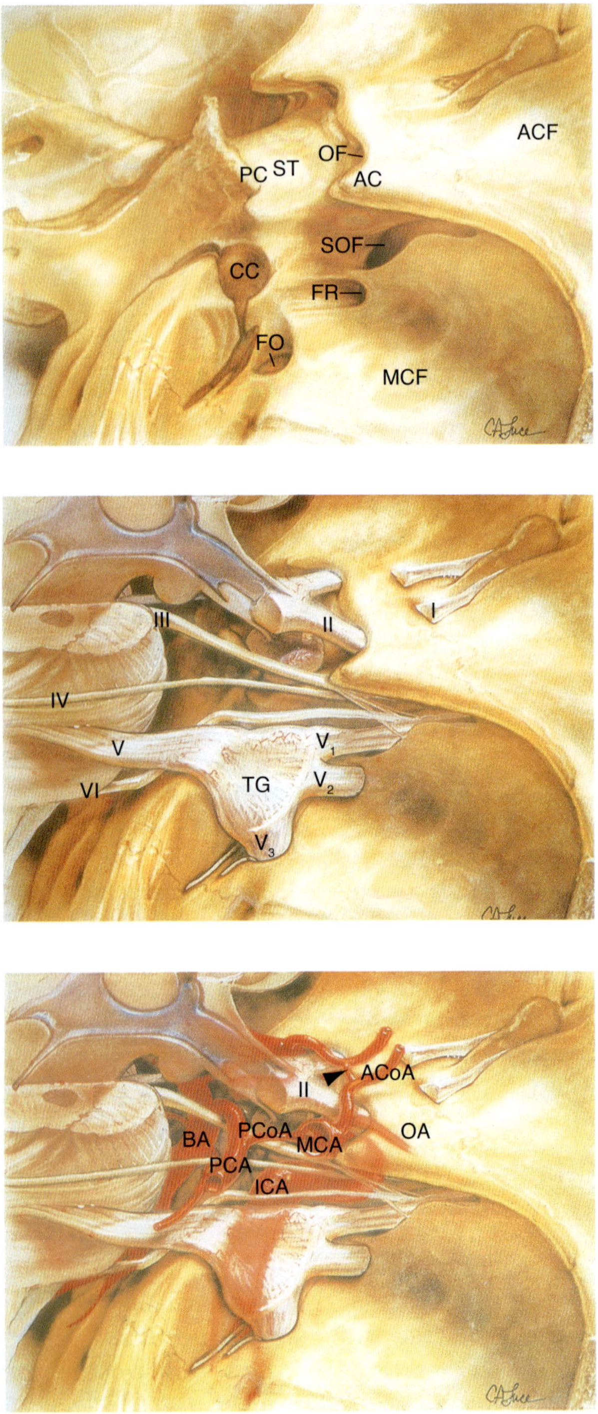

Figure 3-1 View from the right parietal bone looking downward into the skull base. Various anatomical relationships are shown at the base of the skull. The orbits are located to the right, out of the picture (the roof of the orbits is just visible). The floor of the right middle cranial fossa is in the lower part. **A,** The relationship between the bony canals is shown. AC = anterior clinoid; ACF = anterior cranial fossa; CC = carotid canal; FO = foramen ovale; FR = foramen rotundum; MCF = middle cranial fossa; OF = optic foramen; PC = posterior clinoid; SOF = superior orbital fissure; ST = sella turcica. **B,** The relationship between the cranial nerves (with trigeminal ganglion) is depicted. I = olfactory nerve; II = optic nerve; III = oculomotor nerve; IV = trochlear nerve; V = trigeminal nerve, with ophthalmic (V_1), maxillary (V_2), and mandibular (V_3) divisions; VI = abducens nerve; TG = trigeminal ganglion. **C,** The relationship between the arteries is demonstrated. ACoA (and *arrowhead*) = anterior communicating artery; BA = basilar artery; ICA = internal carotid artery; MCA = middle cerebral artery; OA = ophthalmic artery; PCA = posterior cerebral artery; PCoA = posterior communicating artery; II = optic nerve. *(Reproduced with permission from Zide BM, Jelks GW, eds.* Surgical Anatomy of the Orbit. *New York: Raven; 1985.)*

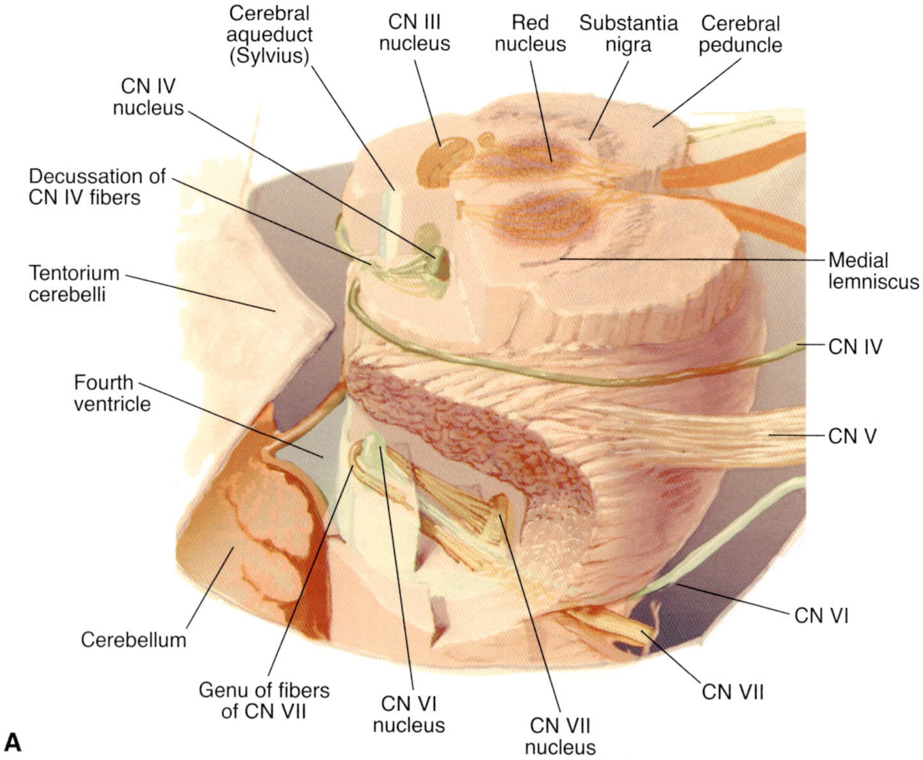

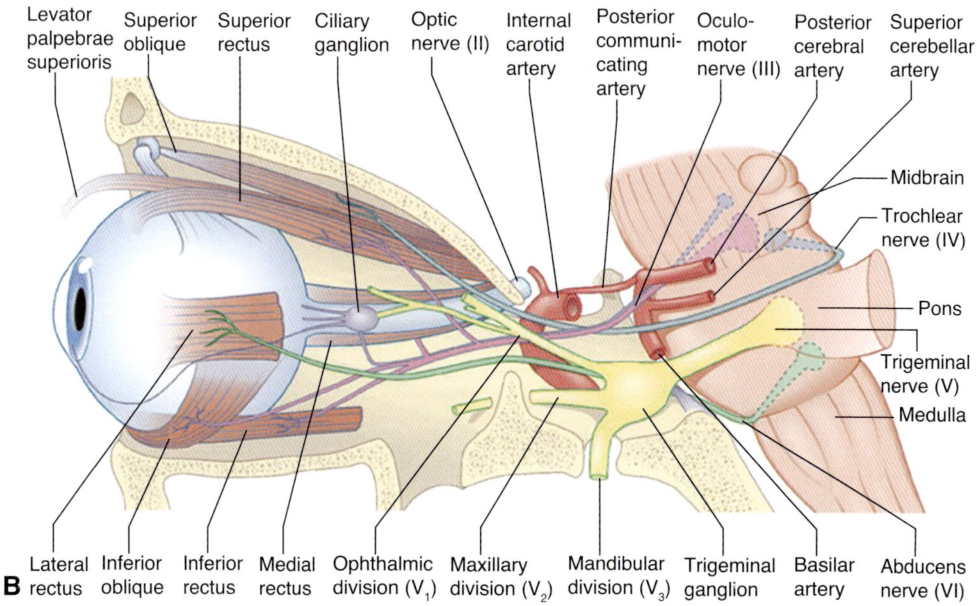

Figure 3-2 **A,** Intra-axial course of the ocular motor nerves at the level of the midbrain *(above)* and pons *(below)*. Note the relationship to the surrounding cerebellum and cranial nerves (CNs) V and VII. **B,** Schematic of CNs II–VI from the brainstem to the orbit. *(Part A illustration by Craig A. Luce. Part B modified with permission from Friedman NJ, Kaiser PK, Trattler WB.* Review of Ophthalmology. *3rd ed. Edinburgh: Elsevier; 2018:63.)*

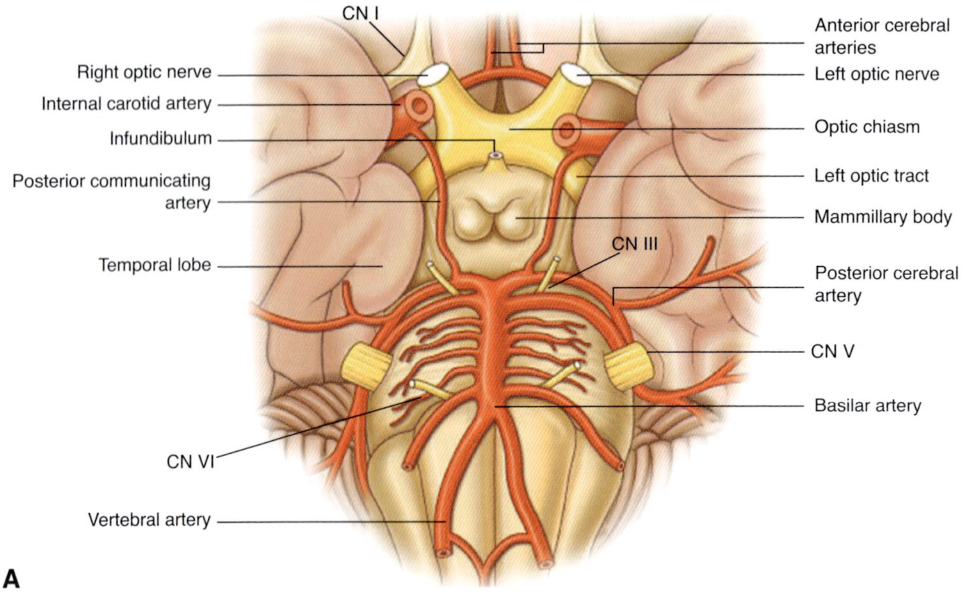

A

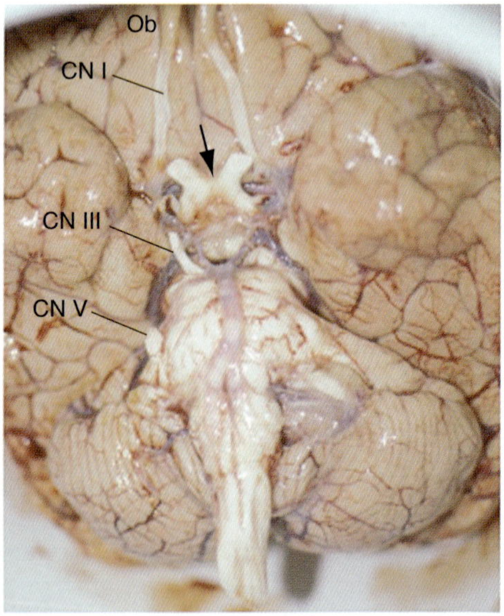

B

Figure 3-3 **A,** Schematic of the optic chiasm and brainstem. **B,** Photograph of the optic chiasm *(arrow)* in a human brain. CN I = olfactory nerve; CN III = oculomotor nerve; CN V = trigeminal nerve; CN VI = abducens nerve; Ob = olfactory bulb. *(Modified with permission from Liu GT, Volpe NJ, Galetta SL.* Neuro-Ophthalmology: Diagnosis and Management. *2nd ed. New York: Elsevier; 2010:238.)*

Optic Nerve (Second Cranial Nerve)

The optic nerve (CN II) consists of more than 1 million axons that originate in the ganglion cell layer of the retina and extend toward the lateral geniculate nucleus. The optic nerve begins anatomically at the optic nerve head (ONH) but physiologically and functionally within the ganglion cell layer that covers the entire retina and continues to the optic chiasm. It may be divided into the following 4 topographic areas (Fig 3-4, Table 3-1):

- intraocular region (ONH, consisting of the superficial nerve fiber layer [NFL], prelaminar area, laminar area, and retrolaminar area)
- intraorbital region (located within the muscle cone)
- intracanalicular region (located within the optic canal)
- intracranial region (ending at the optic chiasm)

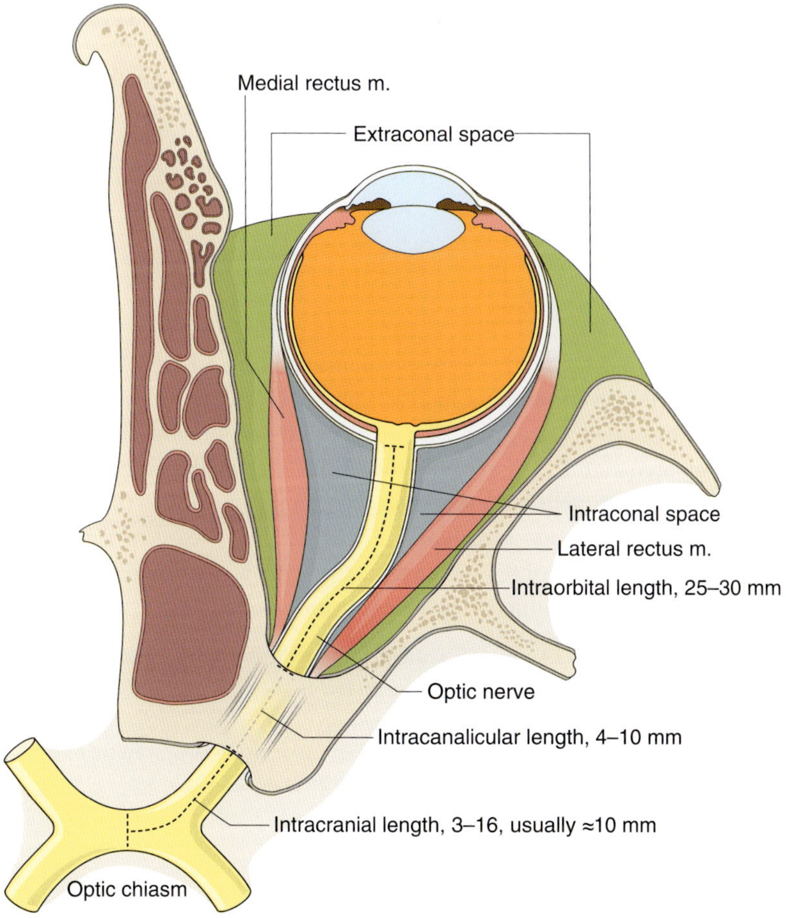

Figure 3-4 The optic nerve. Schematic of the 4 segments of the optic nerve. The intraconal *(blue)* and extraconal *(green)* spaces are also depicted. m. = muscle. *(Illustration by Mark Miller.)*

Table 3-1 Regional Differences in the Optic Nerve

Segment	Length, mm	Diameter, mm	Blood Supply
Intraocular	1		Varies by segment
Optic disc		1.76 (horizontal) 1.92 (vertical)	Branches of posterior ciliary arteries
Prelaminar			Short posterior ciliary arteries Recurrent choroidal arteries (debated) Cilioretinal arteries, if present
Laminar			Branches of arterial circle of Zinn-Haller, which arises from the para-optic branches of the short posterior ciliary arteries
Retrolaminar		3	Primary: Pial vessels and short posterior ciliary vessels Secondary: CRA and recurrent choroidal arteries
Intraorbital	25–30	3–4	
Distal			Intraneural branches of CRA
Proximal			Pial vessels and branches of ophthalmic artery
Intracanalicular	≈4–10		Branches of ophthalmic artery
Intracranial	3–16, usually ≈10	4–7	Branches of ophthalmic artery, anterior cerebral artery, and superior hypophysial artery

CRA = central retinal artery.
See also Figure 3-4.

The optic nerve originates directly from the diencephalon and, developmentally, is part of the brain and central nervous system. Its fibers are surrounded not by Schwann cells but by myelin produced by oligodendrocytes. The intraorbital portion is approximately 25–30 mm long, which is greater than the distance between the back of the globe and the optic canal (18 mm). For this reason, when the eye is in the primary position, the optic nerve runs a sinuous course. Axial proptosis secondary to thyroid eye disease or a retrobulbar tumor will first lead to straightening of the intraorbital optic nerve. Further elongation can lead to stretching of the optic nerve, which may cause chronic nerve injury and optic neuropathy.

Cascone P, Rinna C, Reale G, Calvani F, Iannetti G. Compression and stretching in Graves orbitopathy: emergency orbital decompression techniques. *J Craniofac Surg.* 2012;23(5): 1430–1433.

Soni CR, Johnson LN. Visual neuropraxia and progressive vision loss from thyroid-associated stretch optic neuropathy. *Eur J Ophthalmol.* 2010;20(2):429–436.

Intraocular Region

The ONH is the principal site of many congenital and acquired ocular diseases. Its anterior surface is visible ophthalmoscopically as the *optic disc,* an oval structure whose size reflects some ethnic and racial variance. The size of the ONH varies widely, averaging

1.76 mm horizontally and 1.92 mm vertically. The central depression, or *cup,* is located slightly temporal to the geometric center of the nerve head and represents an axon-free region. Results of studies have found that the cup maintains its size or enlarges throughout life. The main branches of the central retinal artery (CRA) and the central retinal vein (CRV) pass through the center of the cup.

The ONH can be divided into 4 topographic areas (Fig 3-5):

- superficial NFL
- prelaminar area
- laminar area
- retrolaminar area

These are discussed in the following sections. *Note:* The term *optic disc* has been used interchangeably in the literature to refer to the superficial NFL and the prelaminar area, or to the entire ONH. This book uses the term *optic nerve head* to refer to all 4 parts.

Garway-Heath DF, Wollstein G, Hitchings RA. Aging changes of the optic nerve head in relation to open angle glaucoma. *Br J Ophthalmol.* 1997;81(10):840–845.

Jonas JB, Gusek GC, Naumann GO. Optic disc, cup and neuroretinal rim size, configuration and correlations in normal eyes. *Invest Ophthalmol Vis Sci.* 1988;29(7):1151–1158.

Superficial nerve fiber layer

As the unmyelinated ganglion cell axons enter the nerve head, they retain their retinotopic organization, with fibers from the upper retina superiorly and those from the lower retina inferiorly. Fibers from the temporal retina are lateral; those from the nasal side are medial. Macular fibers, which constitute approximately one-third of the nerve, occupy the immediate temporal aspect of the ONH. All other temporal fibers with origins distal to the macula are laterally displaced above or below the macular fibers (Fig 3-6).

Prelaminar area

The ganglion cell axons that enter the nerve head are supported by a "wicker basket" of astrocytic glial cells and are segregated into bundles, or *fascicles,* that pass through the lamina cribrosa (see Fig 3-5). These astrocytes invest the optic nerve and form continuous circular tubes that enclose groups of nerve fibers throughout their intraocular and intraorbital course, separating them from connective tissue elements at all sites. At the edge of the nerve head, the Müller cells that make up the internal limiting membrane (ILM) are replaced by astrocytes. Astrocytes constitute 10% of the nerve head volume and form a membrane that not only covers the surface of the nerve head but is continuous with the ILM of the retina.

The pigment epithelium may be exposed at the temporal margin of the ONH to form a narrow, pigmented crescent. When the pigment epithelium and choroid fail to reach the temporal margin, crescents of partial or absent pigmentation may be noted. The relationship between the choroid and the prelaminar portion of the optic nerve partly accounts for the staining of the ONH normally observed in late phases of fluorescein fundus angiography. The ONH vessels do not leak, but the choroidal capillaries are freely permeable to fluorescein, which can therefore diffuse into the adjacent optic nerve layers.

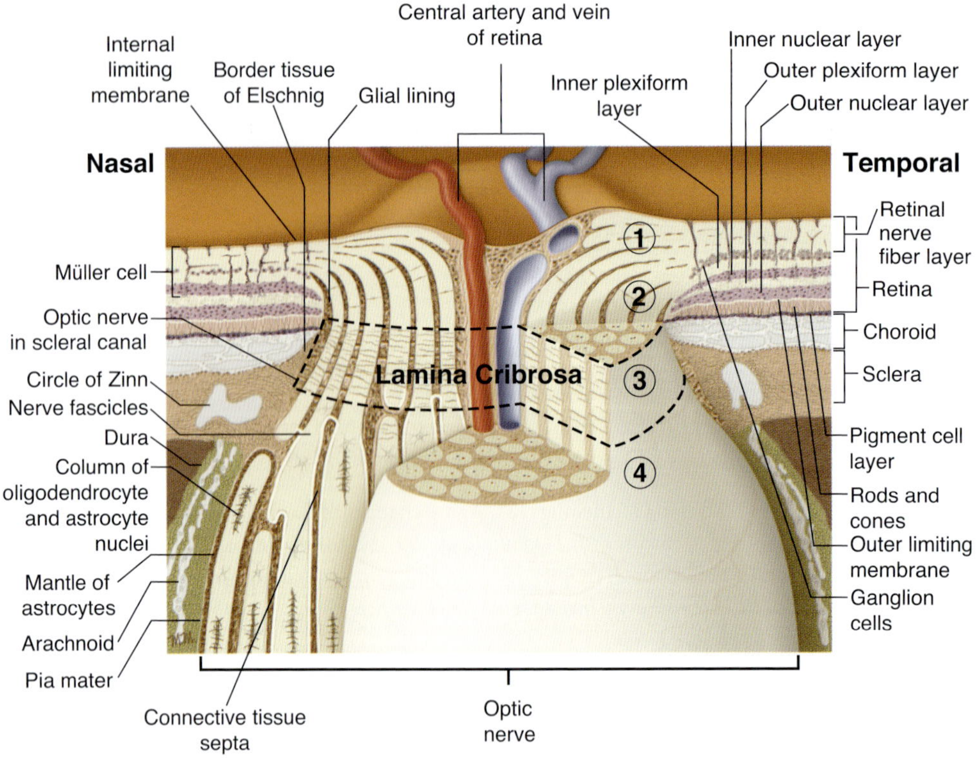

Figure 3-5 Schematic representation of the optic nerve head (ONH). The temporal retina has a thicker layer of ganglion cells, representing the increased ganglion cell concentration found in the macula. Müller glia traverse the neural retina to provide both structural and functional support. Where the retina terminates at the ONH edge, the Müller cells are continuous with the astrocytes, forming the internal limiting membrane. The border tissue of Elschnig is the dense connective tissue that joins the sclera with the Bruch membrane, enclosing the choroid and forming the scleral ring that defines the margin of the ONH. At the posterior termination of the choroid on the temporal side, the border tissue of Elschnig lies between the astrocytes surrounding the optic nerve canal and the stroma of the choroid. On the nasal side, the choroidal stroma is directly adjacent to the astrocytes surrounding the nerve. This collection of astrocytes surrounding the canal is known as the *border tissue,* which is continuous with a similar glial lining at the termination of the retina. The nerve fibers of the retina are segregated into approximately 1000 fascicles by astrocytes. On reaching the lamina cribrosa *(upper dashed line),* the nerve fascicles and their surrounding astrocytes are separated from each other by connective tissue. The lamina cribrosa is an extension of scleral collagen and elastic fibers through the nerve. The external choroid also sends some connective tissue to the anterior part of the lamina. At the external part of the lamina cribrosa *(lower dashed line),* the nerve fibers become myelinated, and columns of oligodendrocytes and a few astrocytes are present within the nerve fascicles. The bundles continue to be separated by connective tissue septa (derived from pia mater and known as *septal tissue*) all the way to the chiasm. A mantle of astrocytes, continuous anteriorly with the border tissue, surrounds the nerve along its orbital course. The dura, arachnoid, and pia mater are shown. The nerve fibers are myelinated. Within the bundles, the cell bodies of astrocytes and oligodendrocytes form a column of nuclei. The central retinal vessels are surrounded by a perivascular connective tissue throughout its course in the nerve. This connective tissue, known as the *central supporting connective tissue strand,* blends with the connective tissue of the lamina cribrosa. 1 = superficial nerve fiber layer; 2 = prelaminar area; 3 = laminar area; 4 = retrolaminar area. *(Illustration by Mark Miller.)*

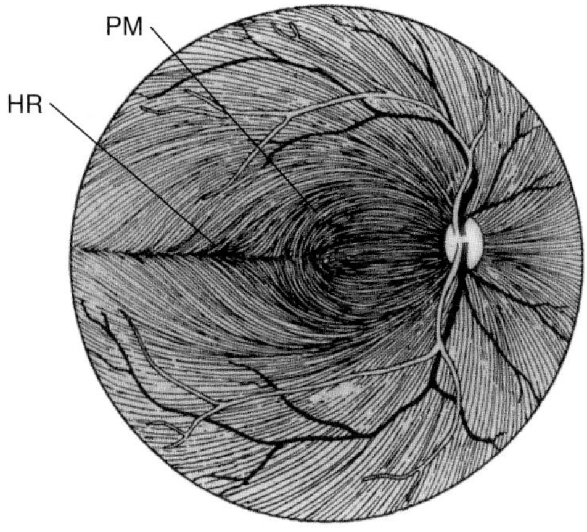

Figure 3-6 The pattern of the nerve fiber layer of axons from retinal ganglion cells to the ONH. Temporal axons originate above and below the horizontal raphe (HR) and take an arching course to the ONH. Axons arising from ganglion cells in the nasal macula project directly to the ONH as the papillomacular bundle (PM). *(Reproduced from Kline LB, Foroozan R, eds.* Optic Nerve Disorders. *2nd ed. Ophthalmology Monographs 10. New York: Oxford University Press, in cooperation with the American Academy of Ophthalmology; 2007:5.)*

Laminar area

The *lamina cribrosa* comprises approximately 10 connective tissue plates, which are integrated with the sclera and whose pores transmit the unmyelinated axon bundles of the retinal ganglion cells before they exit as the optic nerve. The openings are wider superiorly than inferiorly, which may imply less protection from the mechanical effects of pressure in glaucoma. The lamina contains type I and type III collagens, abundant elastin, laminin, and fibronectin. Astrocytes surround the axon bundles, and small blood vessels are present.

The lamina cribrosa serves the following 3 functions:

- scaffold for the optic nerve axons
- point of fixation for the CRA and CRV
- reinforcement of the posterior segment of the globe

Optical coherence tomography and scanning laser ophthalmoscopy are being used to facilitate anatomical study of the lamina cribrosa in pathologic states such as glaucoma and retinal vascular disease.

Retrolaminar area

As a result of myelination of the nerve fibers and the presence of oligodendroglia and the surrounding meningeal sheaths (internal, arachnoid, and external) (see Fig 3-5), the diameter of the optic nerve increases to 3 mm behind the lamina cribrosa. The retrolaminar nerve transitions to the intraorbital part of the optic nerve, to the apex of the orbit. The axoplasm of the neurons contains neurofilaments, microtubules, mitochondria, and smooth endoplasmic reticulum.

Intraorbital Region

Annulus of Zinn

The intraorbital part of the optic nerve lies within the muscle cone. Before passing into the optic canal, the nerve is surrounded by the annulus of Zinn, which is formed by the origins of the rectus muscles. The superior and medial rectus muscles partially share a connective tissue sheath with the optic nerve. This connection may partly explain why patients with retrobulbar neuritis report symptoms of pain on eye movement.

Meningeal sheaths

The *internal sheath,* the innermost meningeal sheath of the optic nerve, is continuous with the pia mater and arachnoid mater, which cover the brain and spinal cord (Fig 3-7). It is a vascular connective tissue coat, covered with meningothelial cells, that sends numerous septa into the optic nerve, dividing its axons into bundles. (The meningothelial cells can give rise to optic nerve sheath meningioma.) The septa continue throughout the intraorbital and intracanalicular regions of the nerve and end just before the chiasm. They contain collagen, elastic tissue, fibroblasts, nerves, and small arterioles and venules. The septa provide mechanical support for the nerve bundles and nutrition to the axons and glial cells. A mantle of astrocytic glial cells prevents the pia and septa from having direct contact with nerve axons.

The *arachnoid sheath,* which is composed of collagenous tissue and small amounts of elastic tissue, lines the dural sheath and is connected to the internal sheath across the subarachnoid space by vascular trabeculae. The subarachnoid space ends anteriorly at the level of the lamina cribrosa. Posteriorly, it is usually continuous with the subarachnoid space of the brain.

Because the central retinal vessels cross this space, a rise in intracranial pressure (ICP) can compress the retinal vein and raise the venous pressure within the retina above the intraocular pressure. This situation causes intraocular venous dilatation and the loss of spontaneous venous pulsation (SVP) at the nerve head. The presence of SVP indicates normal ICP. However, some individuals have normal ICP and absent SVP. Thus, the loss of previously documented SVP is more indicative of elevated ICP.

The *external,* or *dural, sheath* of the optic nerve is the thick outermost meningeal sheath and is continuous with the dura mater in the brain. It is 0.3–0.5 mm thick and consists of dense bundles of collagen and elastic tissue that fuse anteriorly with the outer layers of the sclera.

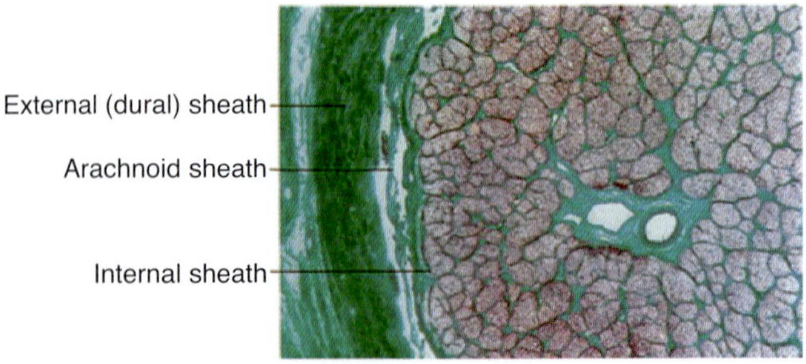

Figure 3-7 Meningeal sheaths. The dural sheath, which is the outer layer, is composed of collagenous connective tissue. The arachnoid sheath, the middle layer, is made up of fine collagenous fibers arranged in a loose meshwork. The internal sheath, the innermost layer, is made up of fine collagenous and elastic fibers and is highly vascularized. Elements from both the arachnoid and the internal sheaths are continuous with the optic nerve septa (Masson trichrome stain, ×64). *(Courtesy of Thomas A. Weingeist, PhD, MD.)*

The meninges of the optic nerve are supplied by sensory nerve fibers, which account in part for the pain experienced by patients with retrobulbar neuritis or other inflammatory optic nerve diseases.

Intracanalicular Region

The optic nerve and surrounding arachnoid sheath are tethered to the periosteum of the bony canal in the intracanalicular region. In blunt trauma, particularly over the eyebrow, the force of injury can be transmitted to the intracanalicular region, causing shearing and interruption of the blood supply to the nerve in this area. Such nerve damage is called *indirect traumatic optic neuropathy.* In addition, optic nerve edema in this area can lead to a compartment syndrome, further compromising the function of the optic nerve within the confined space of the optic canal.

Intracranial Region

After passing through the optic canals, the 2 optic nerves lie superior to the ophthalmic arteries and superior and medial to the *internal carotid arteries* (*ICAs;* see Fig 3-3). The anterior cerebral arteries cross over the optic nerves and are connected by the anterior communicating artery, which completes the anterior portion of the circle of Willis. The optic nerves then pass posteriorly over the cavernous sinus to join in the optic chiasm.

Visual Pathway

The visual pathway begins in the retina; impulses from the photoreceptors are transmitted to the optic chiasm via the optic nerve of each eye. Within the chiasm, the retinal fibers segregate into the right and left optic tracts. Each optic tract carries information for its respective field of vision. For example, the right optic tract consists of fibers from the ipsilateral temporal retina and the contralateral nasal retina. The corresponding hemifields represent the left half of the visual field for each eye. The optic tracts, whose cell bodies lie in the ganglion cell layer of the retina, go on to synapse at the lateral geniculate nucleus. The subsequent fibers further divide as they travel to the primary visual cortex (known variously as *V1, striate cortex,* or *Brodmann area 17*), where they terminate; the most inferior of the fibers (subserving the superior visual field) take one path and the more superior fibers (subserving the inferior visual field) follow a different one (Fig 3-8). Lesions at different locations along the visual pathway produce characteristic visual field defects that help localize the site of damage. Structures of the visual pathway are described further in the following sections and in BCSC Section 5, *Neuro-Ophthalmology.*

Optic chiasm

The optic chiasm makes up part of the anterior inferior floor of the third ventricle. It is surrounded by pia and arachnoid mater and is richly vascularized. The chiasm is approximately 12 mm wide, 8 mm long in the anteroposterior direction, and 4 mm thick.

The extramacular fibers from the inferonasal retina cross anteriorly in the chiasm at the "Wilbrand knee" before passing into the optic tract. Extramacular superonasal fibers cross directly to the opposite tract. Extramacular temporal fibers pursue a direct course through

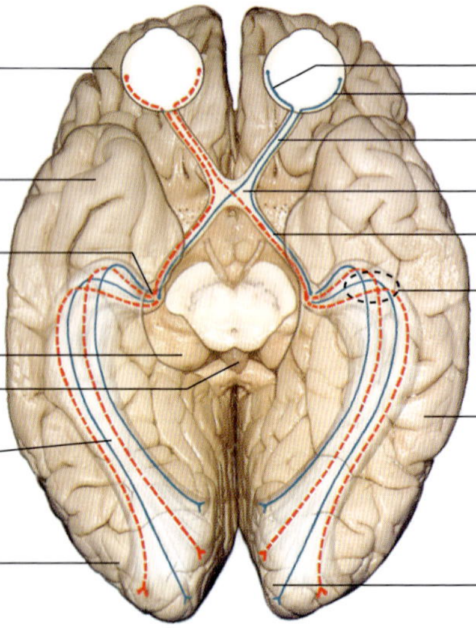

Figure 3-8 The visual pathways. *(Illustration by Dave Peace.)*

the chiasm to the optic tract as a bundle of uncrossed fibers. The macular projections are located centrally in the optic nerve and constitute 80%–90% of the total volume of the optic nerve and the chiasmal fibers. Nasal macular fibers cross in the posterior part of the chiasm. Approximately 53% of the optic nerve fibers are crossed, and 47% are uncrossed.

Optic tract

Each optic tract is made up of fibers from the ipsilateral temporal retina and the contralateral nasal retina. Fibers (both crossed and uncrossed) from the upper retinal projections travel medially in the optic tract; lower projections move laterally. The macular fibers are dorsolateral within the optic tracts.

Lateral geniculate nucleus

The lateral geniculate nucleus (LGN) is the synaptic zone for the higher visual projections. It is a mushroom-shaped structure in the posterior thalamus that receives approximately 70% of the optic tract fibers within its 6 alternating layers of gray and white matter (the other 30% of the fibers go to the pupillary nucleus). Layers 1, 4, and 6 of the LGN contain axons from the contralateral optic nerve. Layers 2, 3, and 5 arise from the ipsilateral optic nerve. The 6 layers, numbered consecutively from inferior to superior, give rise to the optic radiations (Fig 3-9).

Optic radiations

The optic radiations connect the LGN with the visual cortex of the occipital lobe. From the LGN, inferior fibers (which subserve the superior visual field) travel anteriorly, then laterally and posteriorly, looping around the temporal horn of the lateral ventricles in the temporal lobe (Meyer loop). Superior fibers (which subserve the inferior visual field) travel posteriorly through the parietal lobe (Fig 3-10).

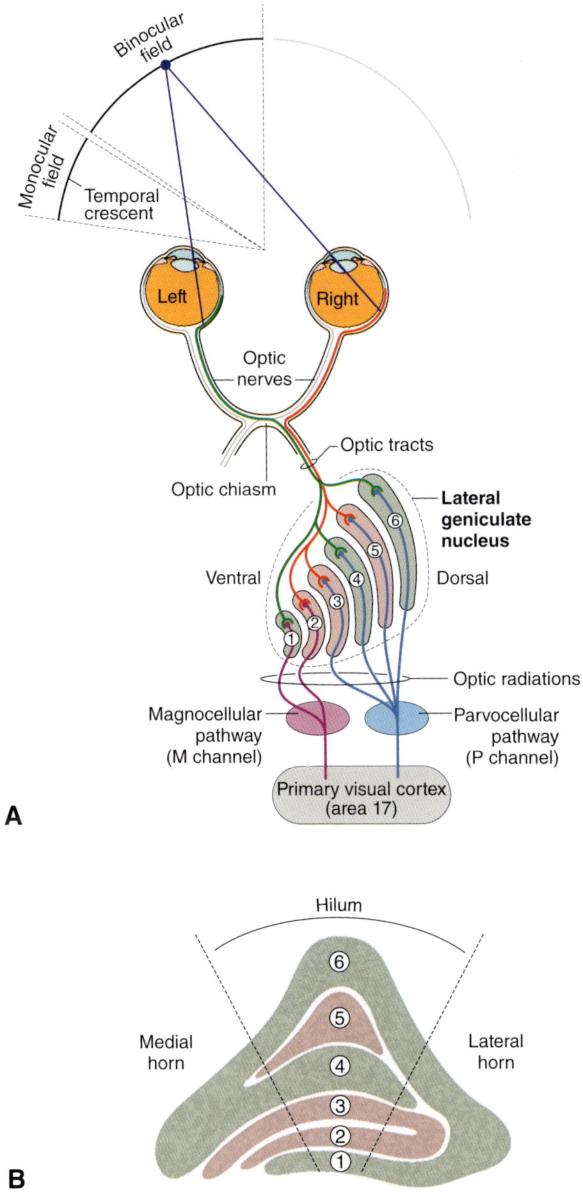

Figure 3-9 Lateral geniculate nucleus (LGN). **A,** The LGN receives the fibers of the corresponding optic tract. Layers 1, 4, and 6 receive input from the crossed fibers of the optic tract; layers 2, 3, and 5 receive input from the uncrossed fibers. Layers 1 and 2 represent the magnocellular pathways, which are concerned with detection of movement. The remaining 4 layers represent the parvocellular pathways, which are responsible for color vision and visual acuity. **B,** The hilum represents central (macular) vision and is perfused by the posterior choroidal artery, the medial horn represents inferior vision, and the lateral horn represents superior vision. These areas are perfused by the anterior choroidal artery. *(Redrawn with permission from Liu GT, Volpe NJ, Galetta SL.* Neuro-Ophthalmology: Diagnosis and Management. *2nd ed. New York: Elsevier; 2010:299–300. Illustration by Mark Miller.)*

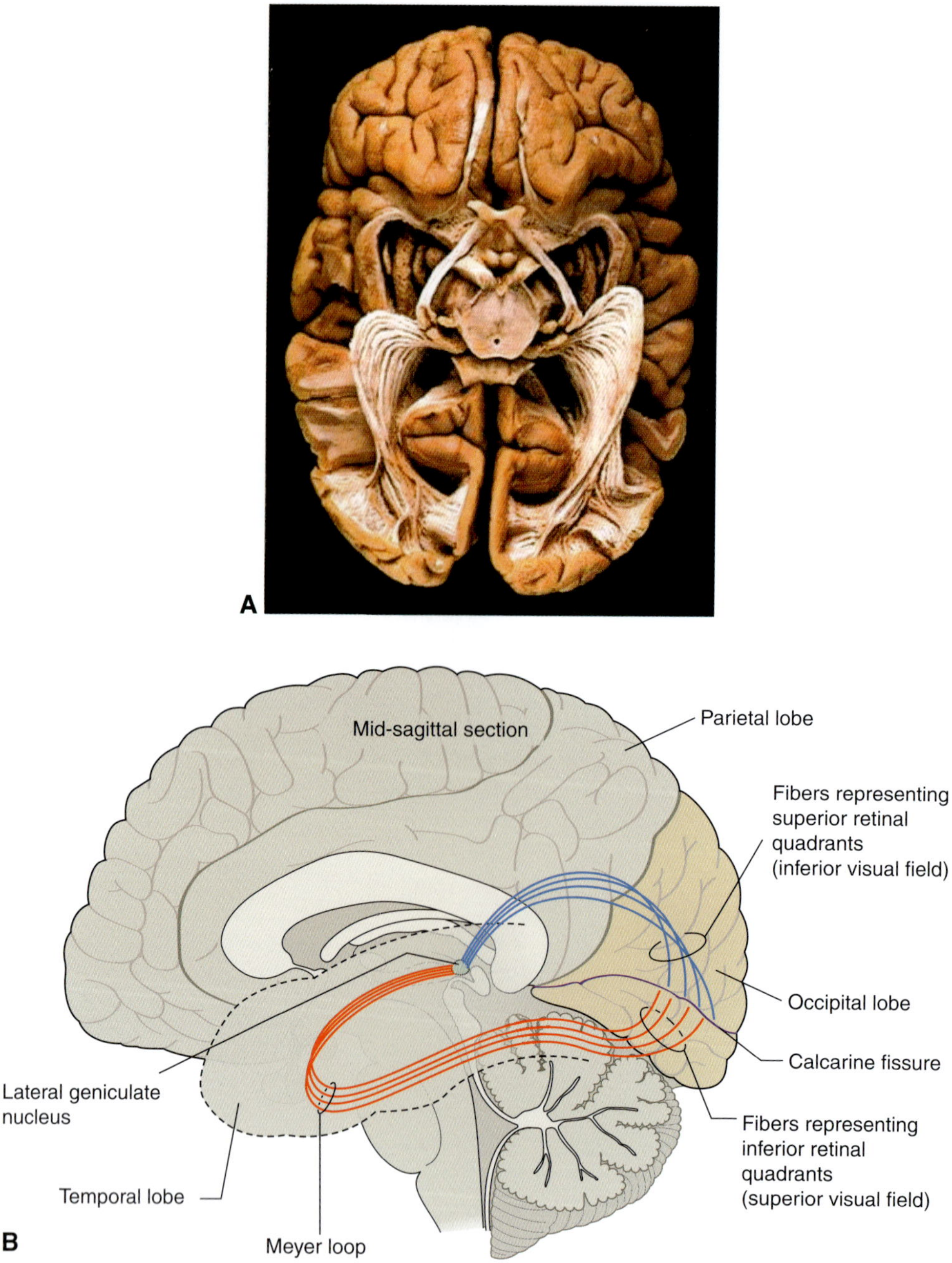

Figure 3-10 Optic radiations. **A,** Axial view of the brain demonstrating the optic chiasm, optic tract, and optic radiations, which connect the LGN to the occipital lobe. **B,** Schematic of the optic radiations, sagittal view. The lower radiations (subserving the superior visual field) course anteriorly before looping posteriorly in the temporal lobe. The upper radiations course dorsally in the parietal lobe to terminate in the occipital lobe above the calcarine fissure. *(Part A reproduced with permission from Sherbondy AJ, Dougherty RF, Napel S, Wandell BA. Identifying the human optic radiation using diffusion imaging and fiber tractography.* J Vis. *2008;8(10):12.1–11, Figure 1. Part B redrawn with permission from University of Texas at Dallas. Illustration by Mark Miller.)*

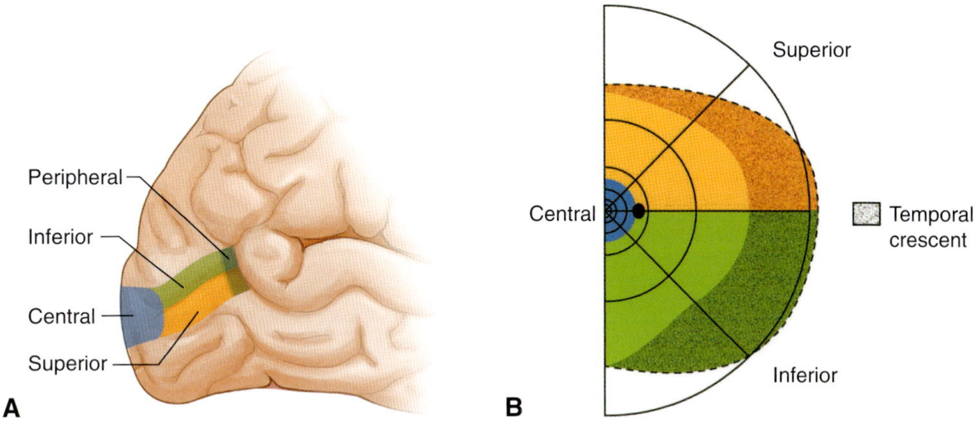

Figure 3-11 Primary visual cortex and corresponding visual field representation. **A,** Left occipital cortex showing the location of the striate cortex within the calcarine fissure. *Blue* represents the macula (central visual field); *green* represents the inferior visual field; and *orange* represents the superior visual field. The most peripheral fibers are represented by the stippled colors. **B,** Right visual hemifield, plotted with kinetic perimetry, corresponds to the regions of the striate cortex in part **A.** The stippled area corresponds to the monocular temporal crescent, which is mapped in the most anterior 8%, approximately, of the striate cortex. *(Illustrations by Christine Gralapp.)*

Primary visual cortex

The primary visual cortex, the thinnest area of the human cerebral cortex, has 6 cellular layers and occupies the superior and inferior lips of the calcarine fissure (also called *calcarine sulcus*) on the posterior and medial surfaces of the occipital lobes. Macular function is extremely well represented in the visual cortex and occupies the most posterior position at the tip of the occipital lobe. The most anterior portion of the calcarine fissure is occupied by contralateral nasal retinal fibers only (Fig 3-11).

Trobe JD. *The Neurology of Vision.* New York: Oxford University Press; 2001:1–42.

Blood Supply of the Optic Nerve and Visual Pathway

The blood supply of the optic nerve varies from one segment of the nerve to another. Although the blood supply can vary widely, a multitude of studies have revealed a basic pattern (Fig 3-12). See Table 3-1, which summarizes the blood supply of the optic nerve. The blood supply of the visual pathway is summarized in Table 3-2 and depicted in Figure 3-13. The following sections discuss the vascular supply of the intraocular and intraorbital segments in greater detail.

Intraocular region

The ophthalmic artery lies inferior to the optic nerve. The CRA and, usually, 2 long posterior ciliary arteries branch off from the ophthalmic artery after it enters the muscle cone at the annulus of Zinn.

The lumen of the CRA is surrounded by nonfenestrated endothelial cells with typical zonulae occludens that are similar to those in retinal blood vessels. The CRA, however,

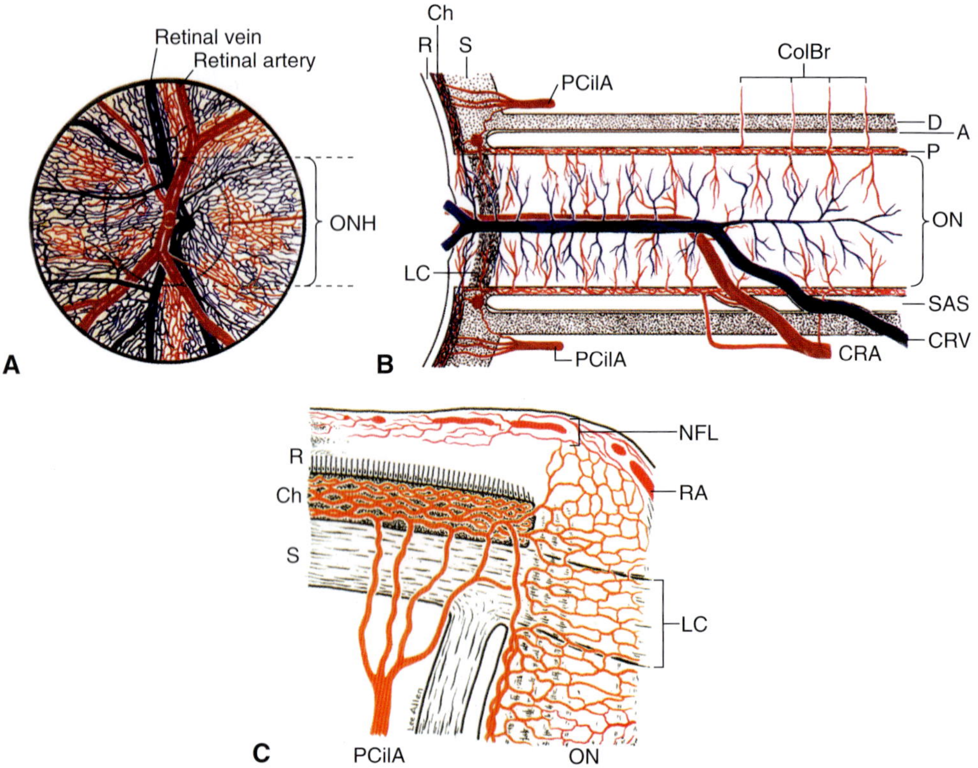

Figure 3-12 Schematic representation of the vascular supply to the optic nerve and ONH. Intraocular view **(A),** lateral view **(B),** and sagittal view **(C)** of the ONH. Short posterior ciliary arteries supply centripetal capillary beds of the anterior ONH. The central retinal artery (CRA) contribution is restricted to nerve fiber layer capillaries and capillaries of the anterior intraorbital optic nerve. Capillary beds at all levels drain into the central retinal vein (CRV). A = arachnoid; Ch = choroid; ColBr = collateral branches; D = dura; LC = lamina cribrosa; NFL = superficial nerve fiber layer of the ONH; ON = optic nerve; P = pia; PCilA = posterior ciliary artery; R = retina; RA = retinal arteriole; S = sclera; SAS = subarachnoid space. *(Part C reproduced with permission from Hayreh SS. The blood supply of the optic nerve head and the evaluation of it—myth and reality.* Prog Retin Eye Res. *2001;20(5):563–593.)*

differs from retinal arterioles in that it contains a fenestrated internal elastic lamina and an outer layer of smooth muscle cells surrounded by a thin basement membrane. The retinal arterioles have no internal elastic lamina, and they lose their smooth muscle cells shortly after entering the retina. The CRV consists of endothelial cells, a thin basal lamina, and a thick collagenous adventitia.

The lamina cribrosa is supplied by branches of the arterial circle of *Zinn-Haller* (Fig 3-14). This circle arises from the para-optic branches of the short posterior ciliary arteries and is usually embedded in the sclera around the nerve head. It is often incomplete and may be divided into superior and inferior halves. Involvement of the inferior half is the likely cause of altitudinal (superior or inferior hemifield) visual field defects following an episode of nonarteritic anterior ischemic optic neuropathy.

Of note, the posterior ciliary arteries are terminal arteries, and the area where the respective capillary beds from each artery meet is termed the *watershed zone.* When

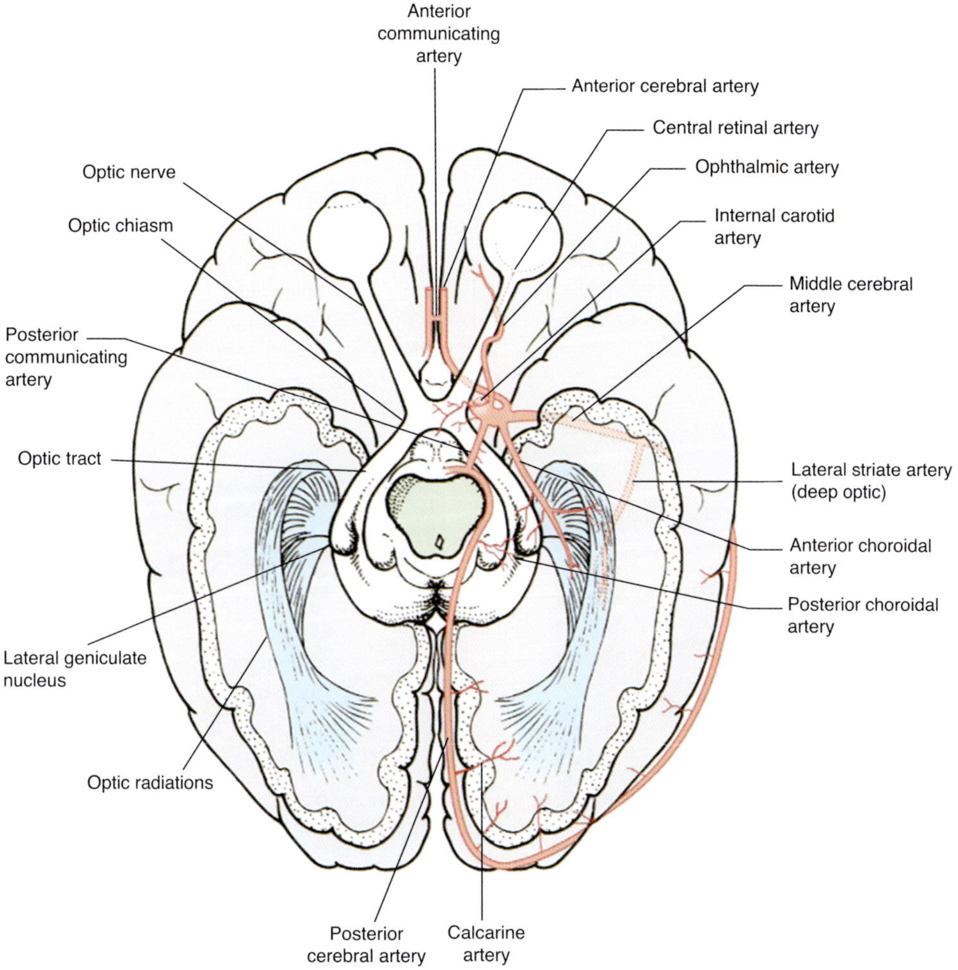

Figure 3-13 Vascular supply of the optic nerve and visual pathway. *(Modified with permission from Forrester JV, Dick AD, McMenamin PG, Roberts F, Pearlman E.* The Eye: Basic Sciences in Practice. *4th ed. Edinburgh: Elsevier; 2016:98.)*

perfusion pressure drops, the tissue lying within this area is the most vulnerable to ischemia. Consequences can be significant when the entire ONH or a part of it lies within the watershed zone.

Tan NY, Koh V, Girard MJ, Cheng CY. Imaging of the lamina cribrosa and its role in glaucoma: a review. *Clin Exp Ophthalmol.* 2018;46(2):177–188.

Intraorbital region

The intraorbital region of the optic nerve is supplied proximally by the pial vascular network and by neighboring branches of the ophthalmic artery. Distally, it is supplied by intraneural branches of the CRA. Most anteriorly, it is supplied by short posterior ciliary arteries and infrequently by peripapillary choroidal arteries.

Table 3-2 Blood Supply of the Visual Pathway

Structure	Blood Supply
Optic chiasm	Branches of anterior cerebral a., superior hypophysial a., internal carotid a., posterior communicating a., and posterior cerebral a.
Optic tract	Branches of posterior communicating a. and anterior choroidal a.
Lateral geniculate nucleus	Branches of anterior and posterior choroidal a.
Optic radiations	Anterior: Anterior choroidal a.
	Posterior: Lateral striate a. (middle cerebral a.) and branches of posterior cerebral a.
Primary visual cortex	Calcarine a. (primarily derived from the posterior cerebral a.) and sometimes branches of the middle cerebral a.

a. = artery.

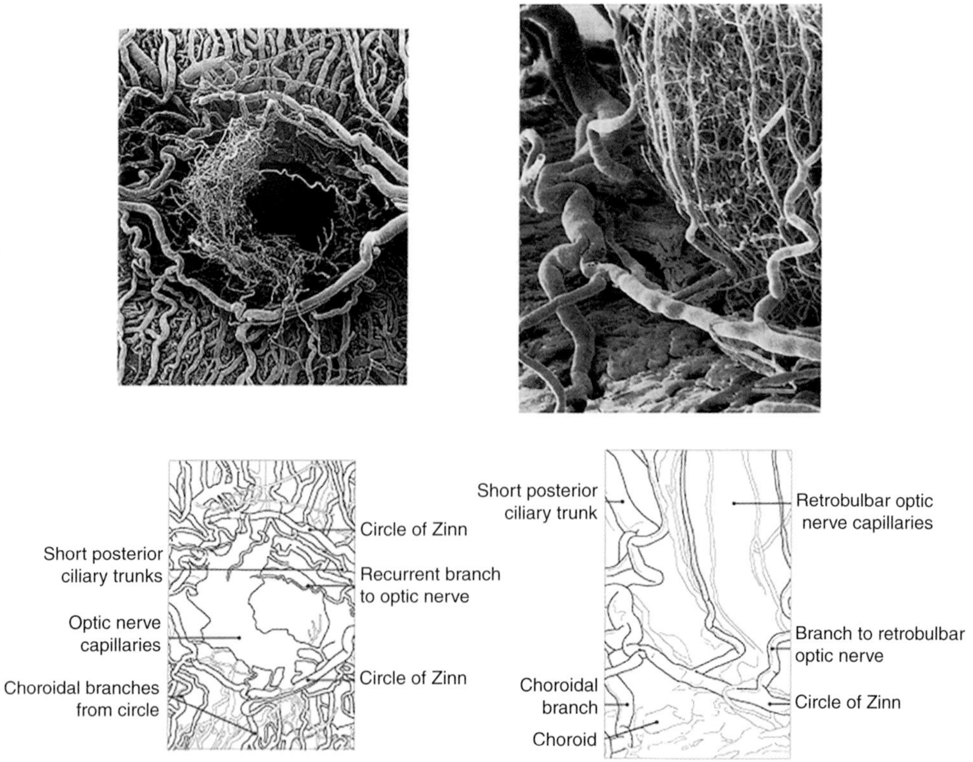

Figure 3-14 Circle of Zinn-Haller. Electron microscopy of the retrolaminar vascular circle *(left)*. Branches from the circle to the optic nerve *(right)*. *(Reproduced with permission from Spalton D, Hitchings R, Hunter P.* Atlas of Clinical Ophthalmology. *3rd ed. New York: Elsevier/Mosby; 2005:563.)*

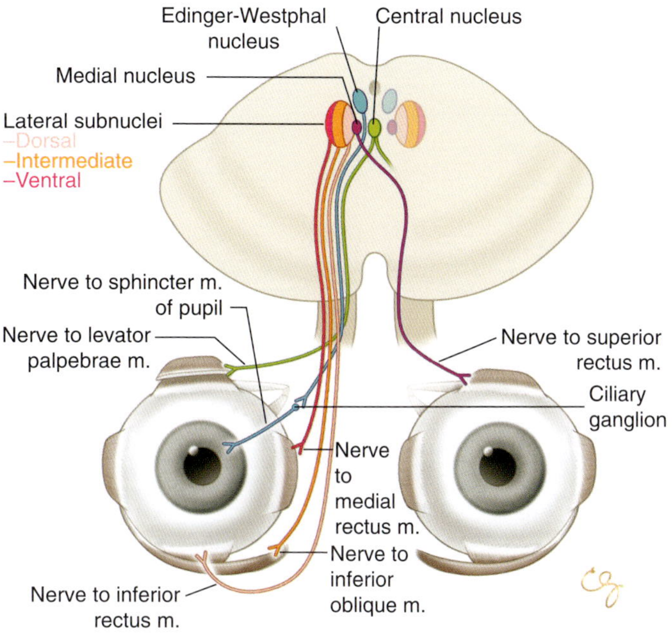

Figure 3-15 Oculomotor nucleus complex. Note that all extraocular muscles served by CN III are innervated by their respective ipsilateral nuclei except the superior rectus muscle. Parasympathetic fibers traveling to the pupillary sphincter muscle synapse in the ciliary ganglion in the orbit. m. = muscle. *(Illustration by Christine Gralapp.)*

Oculomotor Nerve (Third Cranial Nerve)

Although the oculomotor nerve (CN III) contains only 24,000 fibers, it supplies all the extraocular muscles except the superior oblique and the lateral rectus, which are innervated by the trochlear nerve and abducens nerve, respectively. It also provides parasympathetic cholinergic innervation to the pupillary sphincter and the ciliary muscle.

CN III arises from a complex group of cells in the rostral midbrain, or *mesencephalon,* at the level of the superior colliculus. This nuclear complex lies ventral to the periaqueductal gray matter, is immediately rostral to the CN IV nuclear complex, and is bounded inferolaterally by the medial longitudinal fasciculus.

The CN III nucleus consists of several distinct, large motor cell subnuclei, each of which subserves the extraocular muscle it innervates (Fig 3-15). The subnuclei innervate the following:

- ipsilateral inferior rectus muscle
- ipsilateral inferior oblique muscle
- ipsilateral medial rectus muscle
- contralateral superior rectus muscle

Except for a single central, caudal subnucleus that serves both levator palpebrae superioris muscles, the cell groups are paired. Notably, the shared innervation of both levator muscles is an example of Hering's law of equal innervation.

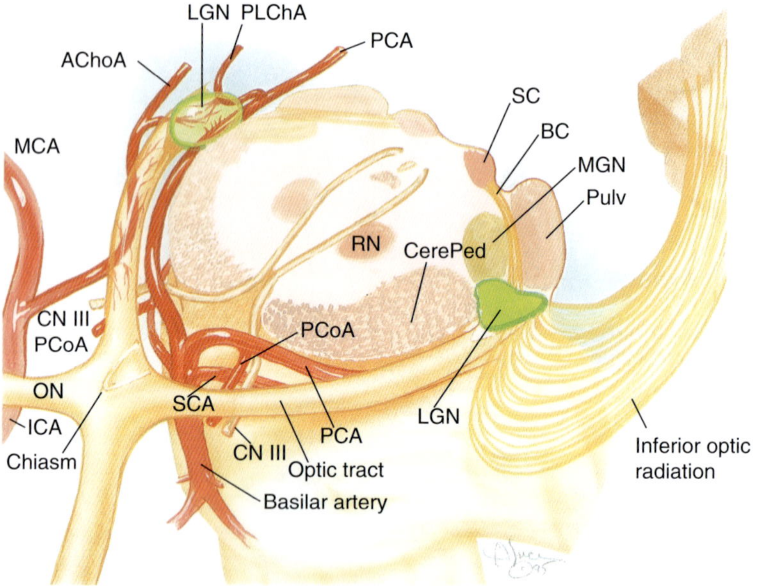

Figure 3-16 Relationship of the lateral geniculate nucleus (LGN) to nearby structures and its blood supply. AChoA = anterior choroidal artery; BC = brachium conjunctivum; CerePed = cerebral peduncles; ICA = internal carotid artery; MCA = middle cerebral artery; MGN = medial geniculate nucleus; ON = optic nerve; PCA = posterior cerebral artery; PCoA = posterior communicating artery; PLChA = posterior lateral choroidal artery; Pulv = pulvinar; RN = red nucleus; SC = superior colliculus; SCA = superior cerebellar artery. *(Illustration by Craig A. Luce.)*

CLINICAL PEARL

Hering's law of equal innervation. The paired levator palpebrae superioris muscles receive equal innervation from the single central nucleus of CN III. In cases of unilateral ptosis, both muscles receive increased stimulation to compensate for the single ptotic eyelid. When the ptotic lid is elevated manually, the increased stimulation is released to both eyelids and the contralateral lid becomes relatively more ptotic.

Fibers from the dorsal subnucleus to the superior rectus uniquely cross, or *decussate,* in the caudal aspect of the nucleus and therefore supply the contralateral superior rectus muscles. The Edinger-Westphal nucleus is rostral in location. It provides the parasympathetic preganglionic efferent innervation to the ciliary muscle and pupillary sphincter. The most ventral subnuclei supply the medial rectus muscles. A subnucleus for ocular convergence has been described but is not consistently found in primates.

The fascicular portion of CN III travels ventrally from the nuclear complex, through the red nucleus, between the medial aspects of the cerebral peduncles, and through the corticospinal fibers (see Fig 3-2). It exits in the interpeduncular space. In the subarachnoid space, CN III passes below the posterior cerebral artery (PCA) and above the superior cerebellar artery, the 2 major branches of the basilar artery (Fig 3-16). The nerve

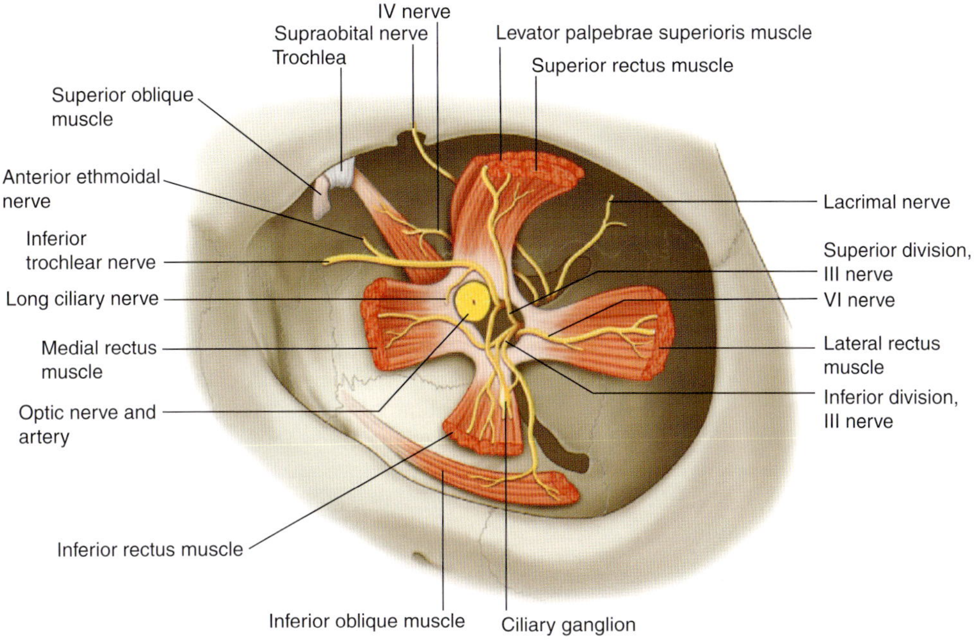

Figure 3-17 Anterior view of the left orbital apex showing the distribution of the nerves as they enter through the superior orbital fissure and optic canal. This view also shows the annulus of Zinn, the fibrous ring formed by the origin of the 4 rectus muscles. *(Reproduced with permission from Levin LA, Nilsson SFE, Ver Hoeve J, Wu SM.* Adler's Physiology of the Eye. *11th ed. Philadelphia: Elsevier/Saunders; 2011:187.)*

travels forward in the interpeduncular cistern lateral to the posterior communicating artery (PCoA) and penetrates the arachnoid between the free and attached borders of the tentorium cerebelli. About 20% of patients with PCoA aneurysms have isolated oculomotor nerve palsy on presentation, and about 80% of aneurysms occurring with CN III palsy were located in the PCoA—usually at the junction of the PCoA and the ICA.

The oculomotor nerve pierces the dura mater on the lateral side of the posterior clinoid process (see Fig 3-24), initially traversing the roof of the cavernous sinus (see Fig 3-25). It runs along the lateral wall of the cavernous sinus and above CN IV and enters the orbit through the superior orbital fissure (see Fig 3-1).

CN III usually separates into superior and inferior divisions after passing through the annulus of Zinn in the orbit (Fig 3-17). Alternatively, it may divide within the anterior cavernous sinus. The nerve maintains a topographic organization even in the midbrain, so lesions almost anywhere along its course may cause a divisional nerve palsy.

The superior division of CN III innervates the superior rectus and levator palpebrae superioris muscles. The larger inferior division splits into 3 branches to supply the medial rectus, inferior rectus, and inferior oblique muscles.

The parasympathetic fibers wind around the periphery of the nerve, enter the inferior division, and course through the branch that supplies the inferior oblique muscle. They join the ciliary ganglion, where they synapse with the postganglionic fibers, which emerge as many short ciliary nerves. These nerves pierce the sclera and travel through the choroid to innervate the pupillary sphincter and the ciliary muscle. The superficial location of these fibers makes them more vulnerable to compression, such as from an aneurysm, than to ischemia.

Golshani K, Ferrell A, Zomorodi A, Smith TP, Britz GW. A review of the management of posterior communicating artery aneurysms in the modern era. *Surg Neurol Int.* 2010;1:88.

Trobe JD. Searching for brain aneurysm in third cranial nerve palsy. *J Neuro-Ophthalmol.* 2009;29(3):171–173.

CLINICAL PEARL

A pupil-sparing oculomotor nerve palsy, even in the context of systemic vascular disease, is not a perfect indicator of the absence of an enlarging aneurysm. A number of neuro-ophthalmologists therefore recommend emergency imaging (by computed tomography/computed tomography angiography or magnetic resonance imaging/magnetic resonance angiography) for any patient with new-onset CN III palsy with incomplete ptosis.

Pathways for the Pupil Reflexes

Light reflex

The light reflex (also called *pupillary light reflex, pupillary reflex*) consists of a simultaneous and equal constriction of the pupils in response to illumination of one eye or the other (Fig 3-18). Of note, when the preganglionic parasympathetic fibers leave each Edinger-Westphal nucleus, they run on the superficial surface of the oculomotor nerve (CN III) as it leaves the brainstem, then spiral downward to lie medially in the nerve at the level of the petroclinoid ligament and inferiorly in the inferior division of CN III as it enters the orbit. These fibers synapse in the ciliary ganglion (Fig 3-19) and give rise to postganglionic myelinated short ciliary nerves, approximately 3%–5% of which are pupillomotor. The rest are designated for the ciliary muscle and are concerned with the near reflex.

Near reflex

The near reflex (also called *near synkinesis, near triad*), is a synkinesis that occurs when attention is changed from distance to near (see Fig 3-18). This reflex includes the triad of accommodation, pupil constriction, and convergence. The convergence reflex is initiated in the occipital association cortex, from which impulses descend along corticofugal pathways to relay in pretectal and possibly tegmental areas. From these relays, fibers pass to the Edinger-Westphal nuclei and both motor nuclei of the medial rectus muscles. Fibers for the near reflex approach the pretectal nucleus from the ventral aspect; thus, compressive dorsal lesions of the optic tectum spare the near pupil reflex relative to the light reflex (light–near dissociation). Efferent fibers for accommodation follow the same general pathway as do those for the light reflex, but their final distribution (via the short ciliary nerves) is to the ciliary muscle.

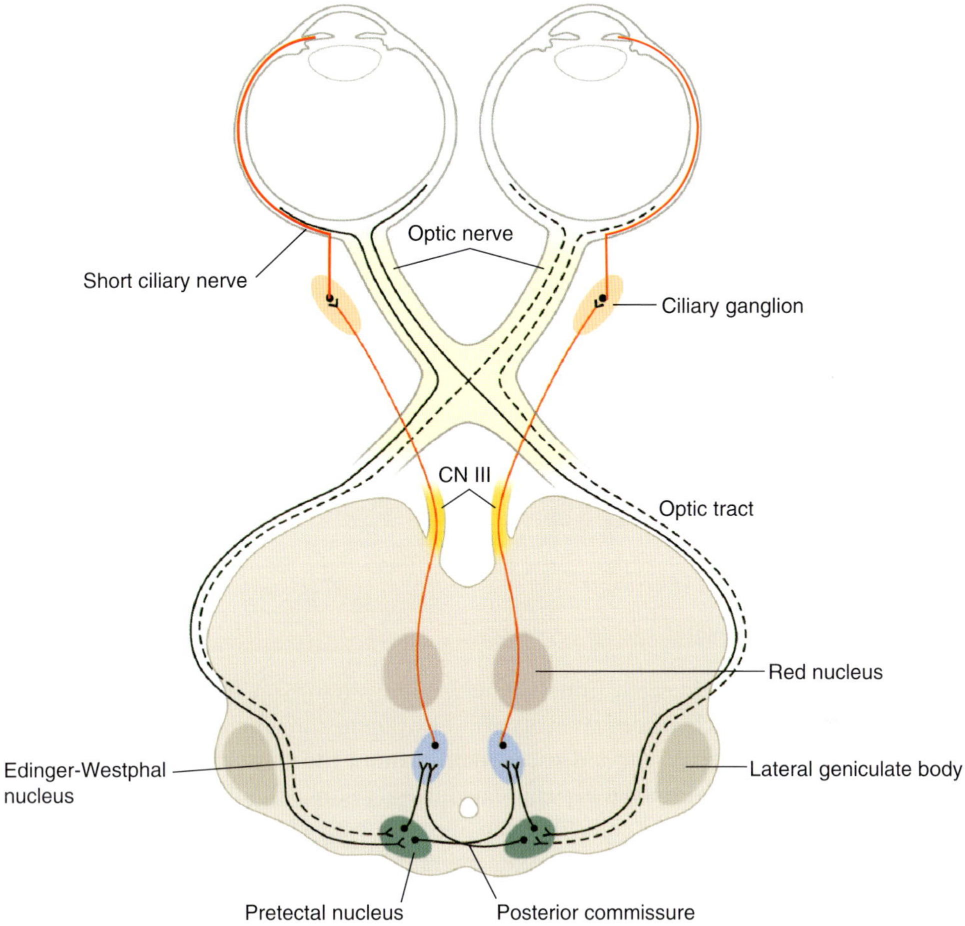

Figure 3-18 Pathway of the pupillary reflexes. *Light reflex (pupillary light reflex):* Light from each eye passes via electrical signals through the optic nerve, and nasal fibers decussate in the optic chiasm, providing signals in both optic tracts. The pupillary fibers exit the optic tract posteriorly, reaching the pretectal nuclei at the level of the superior colliculus in the midbrain. Efferent fibers project to the ipsilateral and contralateral Edinger-Westphal nuclei. Preganglionic parasympathetic fibers leave each Edinger-Westphal nucleus and run on the superficial surface of the oculomotor nerve as it leaves the brainstem. The fibers follow the inferior division of CN III as it enters the orbit, synapsing in the ciliary ganglion. Postganglionic myelinated short ciliary nerves (3%–5% of which are pupillomotor) then innervate the iris and the ciliary muscle. *Near reflex:* Fibers for the near reflex follow a similar efferent course, inducing miosis, but they also act at the ciliary muscle to induce accommodation. *(Illustration by Christine Gralapp.)*

Trochlear Nerve (Fourth Cranial Nerve)

The trochlear nerve (CN IV) contains the fewest nerve fibers (approximately 3400) of any CN but has the longest intracranial course (75 mm). The nerve nucleus is located in the caudal midbrain at the level of the inferior colliculus near the periaqueductal gray matter, ventral to the aqueduct of Sylvius. It is continuous with the caudal end of the CN III

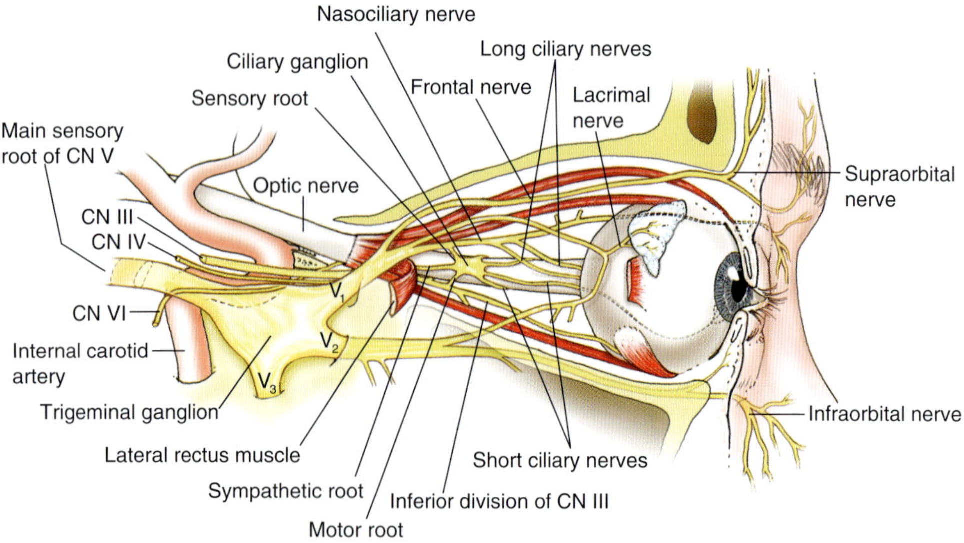

Figure 3-19 Schematic of the lateral orbit demonstrating the ciliary ganglion and CNs II–VI. *(Illustration by Dave Peace.)*

nucleus and differs histologically from that nucleus only in the smaller size of its cells. Like the CN III nucleus, it is bounded ventrolaterally by the medial longitudinal fasciculus.

The fascicles of CN IV curve dorsocaudally around the periaqueductal gray matter and completely decussate in the superior medullary velum. The nerves exit the brainstem just beneath the inferior colliculus (see Figs 3-1, 3-2). CN IV is the only CN that is completely decussated (the superior rectus subnuclei of CN III project contralaterally; however, the CN III fascicles themselves do not decussate once they leave the nuclear complex), and CN IV is the only CN to exit the dorsal surface of the brainstem (see Figs 3-2, 3-22). As it curves around the brainstem in the ambient cistern, CN IV runs beneath the free edge of the tentorium, passes between the posterior cerebral and superior cerebellar arteries (like CN III, but more laterally), and then pierces the dura mater to enter the cavernous sinus (see Fig 3-24).

CN IV travels beneath CN III and above the ophthalmic division of CN V in the lateral wall of the cavernous sinus (see Fig 3-25). It enters the orbit through the superior orbital fissure outside the annulus of Zinn and runs superiorly to innervate the superior oblique muscle. Because of its location outside the muscle cone, CN IV is usually not affected by injection of retrobulbar anesthetics (see Fig 3-17).

Trigeminal Nerve (Fifth Cranial Nerve)

The trigeminal nerve (CN V), the largest CN, possesses both sensory and motor divisions. The sensory portion serves the greater part of the scalp and the forehead, face, eyelids, eyes, lacrimal glands, extraocular muscles, ears, dura mater, and tongue. The motor portion innervates the muscles of mastication through branches of the mandibular division.

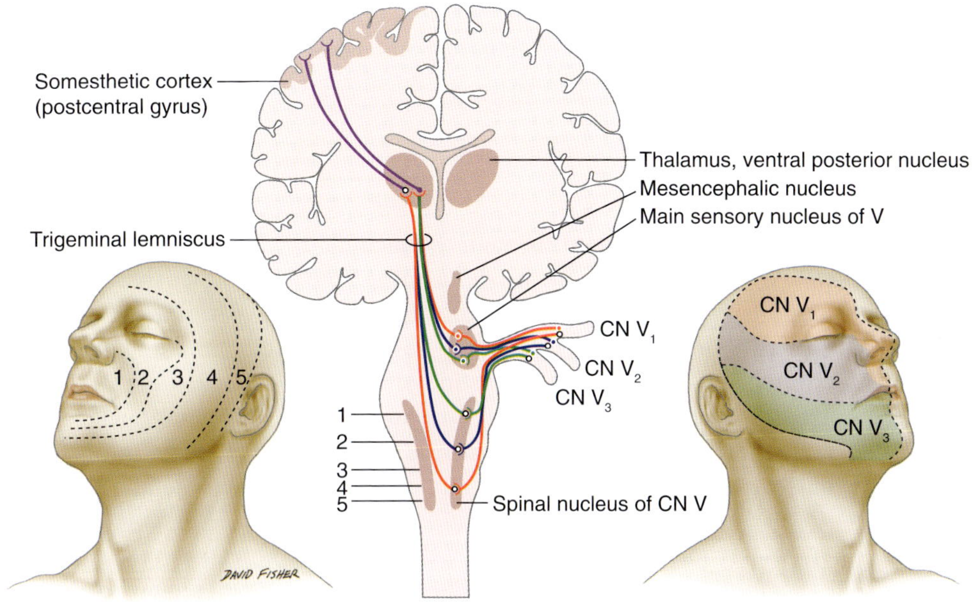

Figure 3-20 Diagram of the central pathways and peripheral innervation of CN V. The numbers 1–5 indicate the locations of dermatomes on the face and their corresponding representation in the brainstem. *(Illustration by David Fisher; used with permission from Kline LB.* Neuro-Ophthalmology Review Manual. *6th ed. Thorofare, NJ: Slack; 2008:174.)*

The CN V nuclear complex extends from the midbrain, through the pons and medulla, to the upper cervical segments, often as caudal as the C4 vertebra. It consists of the following 4 nuclei, listed from rostral to caudal:

- mesencephalic nucleus
- main sensory nucleus
- spinal nucleus and tract
- motor nucleus

Important interconnections exist between the different subdivisions of the CN V sensory nuclei and the reticular formation (Fig 3-20).

Mesencephalic Nucleus

The mesencephalic nucleus mediates *proprioception* and *deep sensation* from the masticatory, facial, and extraocular muscles. The nucleus extends inferiorly into the posterior pons as far as the main sensory nucleus.

Main Sensory Nucleus

The main sensory nucleus lies in the pons, lateral to the motor nucleus. It is continuous with the mesencephalic nucleus (above) and with the spinal nucleus (below). The main sensory nucleus receives its input from ascending branches of the sensory root, and it serves *light touch* from the skin and mucous membranes. The sensory root of CN V, upon entering the pons, divides into an ascending tract and a descending tract. The ascending tract terminates in the main sensory nucleus, and the descending tract ends in the spinal nucleus.

Spinal Nucleus and Tract

The spinal nucleus and tract extend through the medulla to C4. The nucleus receives *pain* and *temperature* afferents from the descending spinal tract, which also carries cutaneous components of CN VII, CN IX, and CN X that serve sensations from the ear and external auditory meatus. The sensory fibers from the ophthalmic division of CN V (V_1) terminate in the most ventral portion of the spinal nucleus and tract. Fibers from the maxillary division (V_2) end in the midportion of the spinal nucleus (in a ventral–dorsal plane). The fibers from the mandibular division (V_3) end in the dorsal parts of the nucleus (the 3 divisions of CN V are discussed in greater detail later in the chapter).

The cutaneous territory of each of the CN V divisions is represented in the spinal nucleus and tract in a rostral–caudal direction. Fibers from the perioral region are thought to terminate most rostrally in the nucleus; fibers from the peripheral face and scalp end in the caudal portion. The zone between them, the midfacial region, is projected onto the central portion of the nucleus. This “onionskin” pattern of cutaneous sensation (see Fig 3-20) has been revealed by clinical studies of patients with damage to the spinal nucleus and tract.

> **CLINICAL PEARL**
>
> Damage to the trigeminal sensory nucleus at the level of the brainstem causes bilateral sensory loss in concentric areas of the face, with the sensory area surrounding the mouth in the center. If a patient verifies this distribution of sensory loss, the lesion is in the brainstem. Conversely, sensory loss that follows the peripheral distribution of the trigeminal sensory divisions (ophthalmic, maxillary, and mandibular) indicates that the lesion lies in the divisions of CN V (V_1, V_2, V_3) and is a fascicular lesion.

Axons from the main sensory and spinal nuclei, as well as portions of the mesencephalic nucleus, relay sensory information to higher sensory areas of the brain. The axons cross the midline in the pons and ascend to the thalamus along the ventral and dorsal trigeminothalamic tracts. They terminate in the nerve cells of the ventral posteromedial nucleus of the thalamus. These cells, in turn, send axons through the internal capsule to the postcentral gyrus of the cerebral cortex.

The afferent limb of the oculocardiac reflex is mediated by the trigeminal nerve. It is connected to the efferent limb, which is mediated by the parasympathetic neurons of the vagus nerve, via short internuncial fibers to the reticular formation.

Meuwly C, Golanov E, Chowdhury T, Erne P, Schaller B. Trigeminal cardiac reflex: new thinking model about the definition based on a literature review. *Medicine (Baltimore)*. 2015;94(5):e484.

Motor Nucleus

The motor nucleus is located in the pons, medial to the main sensory nucleus. It receives fibers from both cerebral hemispheres, the reticular formation, the red nucleus, the tectum, the medial longitudinal fasciculus, and the mesencephalic nucleus. The motor nucleus gives rise to the axons that form the motor root, which supplies the muscles of mastication (pterygoid, masseter, and temporalis), the tensor tympani muscle, the tensor veli palatini muscle, the mylohyoid muscle, and the anterior belly of the digastric muscle.

Intracranial Pathway of Cranial Nerve V

The intracranial segment of the trigeminal nerve emerges from the upper lateral portion of the ventral pons, passes over the petrous apex (the crest of the petrous part of temporal bone), forms the *trigeminal ganglion,* and then divides into 3 branches (see Figs 3-1, 3-2). The trigeminal ganglion, also called the *gasserian* or *semilunar ganglion,* contains the cell bodies of origin of all CN V sensory axons. The crescent-shaped ganglion occupies a recess in the dura mater posterolateral to the cavernous sinus. This recess, called the *Meckel cave,* is near the apex of the petrous part of the temporal bone in the middle cranial fossa. Medially, the trigeminal ganglion is close to the ICA and the posterior cavernous sinus.

Divisions of Cranial Nerve V

The 3 divisions of CN V are the ophthalmic (V_1), the maxillary (V_2), and the mandibular (V_3).

Ophthalmic division (CN V_1)

The ophthalmic division enters the cavernous sinus lateral to the ICA and courses beneath CN III and CN IV (see Figs 3-24, 3-25). Within the sinus, it gives off a tentorial–dural branch, which innervates the cerebral vessels, dura mater of the anterior fossa, cavernous sinus, sphenoid wing, petrous apex, Meckel cave, tentorium cerebelli, falx cerebri, and dural venous sinuses. CN V_1 passes into the orbit through the superior orbital fissure and divides into 3 branches: frontal, lacrimal, and nasociliary (see Fig 3-17).

Frontal nerve The frontal nerve (see Fig 3-19) divides into the supraorbital and supratrochlear nerves, which provide sensation to the medial portion of the upper eyelid and the conjunctiva, forehead, scalp, frontal sinuses, and side of the nose. The supratrochlear nerve exits the orbit 17 mm from midline, whereas the supraorbital nerve exits at 27 mm from midline, through either a notch or a true foramen.

Lacrimal nerve The lacrimal nerve innervates the lacrimal gland and the neighboring conjunctiva and skin. The lacrimal gland receives its parasympathetic supply from the retro-orbital plexus (discussed later, in the section Facial Nerve [Seventh Cranial Nerve]). Occasionally, the lacrimal nerve exits the orbit via a lacrimal foramen to supply the lateral forehead. Otherwise, that area is supplied by branches of the supraorbital nerve.

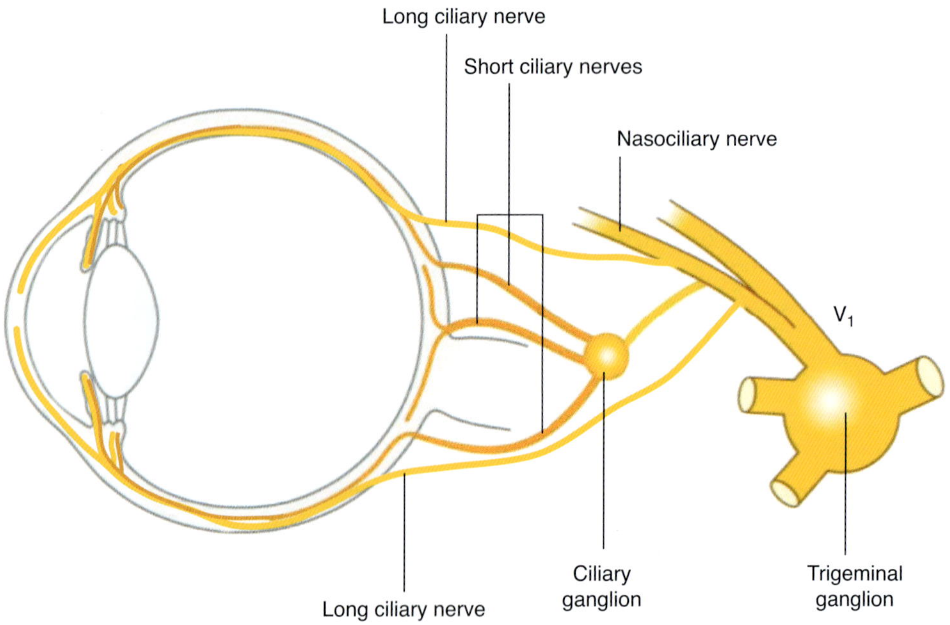

Figure 3-21 Divisions of the nasociliary nerve. The nasaociliary nerve is a branch of V_1, the ophthalmic division of CN V. The posterior ciliary nerves supply sensation to the globe. The paired long ciliary nerves innervate the anterior structures; the short ciliary nerves, posterior structures. The short posterior ciliary nerves also carry sympathetic and parasympathetic fibers to the iris dilator and sphincter muscles, respectively. In addition, they carry parasympathetic fibers to the ciliary muscle, where they induce accommodation. *(Modified with permission from Levin LA, Nilsson SFE, Ver Hoeve J, Wu SM.* Adler's Physiology of the Eye. *11th ed. Philadelphia: Elsevier/Saunders; 2011:91.)*

Nasociliary nerve Branches from the nasociliary nerve supply sensation to the middle and inferior turbinates, septum, lateral nasal wall, and tip of the nose. The infratrochlear branch serves the lacrimal drainage system, the conjunctiva, and the skin of the medial canthal region. The ciliary nerves (short and long) carry sensory fibers from the ciliary body, the iris, and the cornea. The short ciliary nerves also carry the sympathetic and parasympathetic fibers from the ciliary ganglion to the iris dilator and sphincter, respectively, and the parasympathetic fibers to the ciliary muscle (Fig 3-21). The sensory short ciliary fibers pass through the ciliary ganglion to join, along with the long ciliary fibers, the nasociliary nerve. Thus, the short ciliary nerves carry sensory (V_1), sympathetic, and parasympathetic fibers (see Fig 3-19).

Maxillary division (CN V_2)

The maxillary division leaves the trigeminal ganglion to exit the skull through the foramen rotundum, which lies below the superior orbital fissure (see Fig 3-1). CN V_2 courses through the pterygopalatine fossa into the inferior orbital fissure and then passes through the infraorbital canal as the infraorbital nerve. After exiting the infraorbital foramen, CN V_2 divides into an inferior palpebral branch, a nasal branch, and a superior labial branch, supplying the lower eyelid, the side of the nose, and the upper lip, respectively. The teeth, maxillary sinus, roof of the mouth, and soft palate are also innervated by branches of the maxillary division. These branches can be damaged after fractures of the orbital floor.

Mandibular division (CN V_3)

The mandibular division contains sensory and motor fibers. It is the only division of CN V that contains motor fibers. It exits the skull through the foramen ovale (see Fig 3-1) and provides motor input for the masticatory muscles. Sensation is supplied to the mucosa and skin of the mandible, lower lip, tongue, external ear, and tympanum.

Standring S, ed. *Gray's Anatomy: The Anatomical Basis of Clinical Practice.* 41st ed. Edinburgh: Elsevier Limited; 2016.

Abducens Nerve (Sixth Cranial Nerve)

The nucleus of the abducens nerve (CN VI) is situated in the floor of the fourth ventricle, beneath the facial colliculus in the caudal pons. The medial longitudinal fasciculus lies medial to the CN VI nucleus. The fascicular portion of CN VI runs ventrally through the paramedian pontine reticular formation and the pyramidal tract and leaves the brainstem in the pontomedullary junction (see Figs 3-1, 3-2).

CN VI then takes a vertical course along the ventral face of the pons and is crossed by the anterior inferior cerebellar artery. It continues through the subarachnoid space along the surface of the clivus to perforate the dura mater below the petrous apex, approximately 2 cm below the posterior clinoid process (see Fig 3-24). It then passes intradurally through or around the inferior petrosal sinus and beneath the petroclinoid (Gruber) ligament through the Dorello canal, after which it becomes extradural and enters the cavernous sinus. This long route (especially along the surface of the clivus and beneath the petroclinoid ligament) is responsible for this nerve's susceptibility to stretch injury leading to paresis in the context of increased intracranial pressure. In the cavernous sinus, CN VI runs below and lateral to the ICA and may transiently carry sympathetic fibers from the carotid plexus (see Fig 3-25). It passes through the superior orbital fissure within the annulus of Zinn to enter the medial surface of the lateral rectus muscle, which it innervates.

Facial Nerve (Seventh Cranial Nerve)

The facial nerve (CN VII) is a complex, mixed sensory and motor nerve. The motor root contains special visceral efferent fibers that innervate the muscles of facial expression. The sensory root conveys the sense of taste from the anterior two-thirds of the tongue and sensation from the external auditory meatus and the retroauricular skin. It also provides preganglionic parasympathetic innervation by way of the sphenopalatine and submandibular ganglia to the lacrimal, submaxillary, and sublingual glands.

The motor nucleus of CN VII is a cigar-shaped column 4 mm long, located in the caudal third of the pons. It is ventrolateral to the CN VI nucleus, ventromedial to the spinal nucleus of CN V, and dorsal to the superior olive (Fig 3-22; see also Fig 3-2A). The signal for facial movement starts in the primary motor cortex in the precentral gyrus.

The dorsal motor subnucleus controls the upper half of the face and receives corticobulbar input from *both* cerebral hemispheres, whereas the lateral subnucleus controls the lower half of the face and receives corticobulbar input from the *contralateral* cerebral hemisphere.

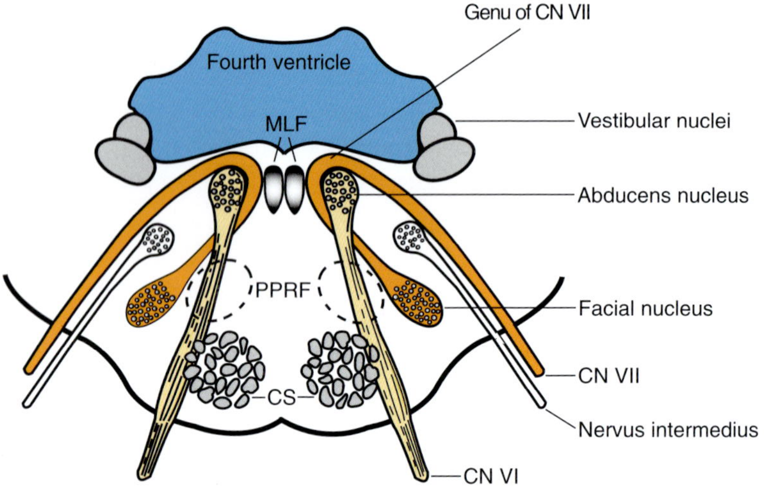

Figure 3-22 Cross section of the pons at the level of CN VI (abducens nerve) nucleus. CS = corticospinal tract; MLF = medial longitudinal fasciculus; PPRF = pontine paramedian reticular formation. *(Illustration by Sylvia Barker.)*

Therefore, pathology involving the CN VII nucleus would affect only the contralateral lower face; peripheral CN VII pathology causes an ipsilateral hemifacial palsy.

The facial nerve has several important anatomical relationships with adjacent structures. Fibers from the motor nucleus course dorsomedially to approach the floor of the fourth ventricle and then ascend immediately dorsal to the CN VI nucleus. At the rostral end of the CN VI nucleus, the main facial motor fibers arch over its dorsal surface (forming the internal genu of CN VII) and then pass ventrolaterally between the spinal nucleus of CN V and the CN VII nucleus to exit the brainstem at the pontomedullary junction. The bulge formed by the CN VII genu in the floor of the fourth ventricle is the *facial colliculus* (see Figs 3-2A, 3-22).

CNs VII and VIII (the acoustic nerve) pass together through the lateral pontine cistern in the cerebellopontine angle and enter the internal auditory meatus in a common meningeal sheath.

The main branch of CN VII exits the stylomastoid foramen just behind the styloid process at the base of the mastoid. It then passes through the superficial and deep lobes of the parotid gland and divides into the superior temporofacial branch (which further divides into the temporal, zygomatic, and buccal subbranches) and the cervicofacial branch. Commonly, the temporal branch supplies the upper half of the orbicularis oculi muscle, and the zygomatic branch supplies the lower half, although the inferior orbicularis is sometimes innervated by the buccal branch. The frontalis, corrugator supercilii, and pyramidalis muscles are usually innervated by the temporal branch.

The temporal (or frontal) branch of the facial nerve crosses the zygomatic arch superficially at the junction of the anterior one-third and posterior two-thirds of the arch. It then enters the more superficial layer of the temporoparietal fascia while staying below the *superficial musculoaponeurotic system (SMAS)*. A good approximation of the course of the nerve across the zygomatic arch follows the point at which a line between the tragus and the lateral eyelid commissure is bisected by a line that begins at the earlobe. The nerve can be injured in the context of perizygomatic or temple surgical approaches, such as Tenzel or Mustardé semicircular flap reconstruction of the eyelid, temporal artery biopsy, and cosmetic forehead and midface surgery.

Tear Reflex Pathway

Reflex lacrimation is controlled by afferents from the sensory nuclei of CN V. The tear reflex arc is shown in Figure 3-23. The efferent preganglionic parasympathetic fibers pass peripherally as part of the nervus intermedius and divide into 2 groups near the external genu of CN VII. The lacrimal group of fibers passes to the pterygopalatine ganglion in the greater superficial petrosal nerve. The salivatory group of fibers projects through the chorda tympani nerve to the submandibular ganglion to innervate the submandibular and sublingual salivary glands.

The greater superficial petrosal nerve extends forward on the anterior surface of the petrous part of temporal bone to join the deep petrosal nerve (sympathetic fibers) and form the nerve of the pterygoid canal (vidian nerve). This nerve enters the pterygopalatine fossa; joins the pterygopalatine ganglion; and gives rise to unmyelinated postganglionic fibers that innervate the globe, lacrimal gland, glands of the palate, and nose. The parasympathetic fibers destined for the orbit enter it via the superior orbital fissure, along with branches of the ophthalmic nerve (CN V_1). Here, they are joined by sympathetic fibers from the carotid plexus and form a retro-orbital plexus of nerves, whose rami oculares supply orbital vessels or enter the globe to supply the choroid and anterior segment structures. Some of these fibers enter the globe directly; others enter via connections with the short ciliary nerves. The rami oculares also supply the lacrimal gland.

Emotional lacrimation is mediated by parasympathetic efferent fibers originating in the superior salivatory nucleus and the lacrimal nucleus in the caudal pons, both of which lie posterolateral to the motor nucleus. The lacrimal nucleus receives input from the hypothalamus, mediating emotional tearing; there is also supranuclear input from the cortex and the limbic system.

The Cerebral Vascular System

The CNs can be affected by the surrounding cerebrovascular system, which includes both arterial and venous components. CN palsies can be harbingers of life-threatening conditions. Thus, it is imperative to understand the CNs' anatomical relationships with adjacent structures. For further discussion of the cerebral vasculature and the various resultant syndromes of the CNs, see BCSC Section 5, *Neuro-Ophthalmology*.

Cavernous Sinus

The cavernous sinus is an interconnected series of venous channels located just posterior to the orbital apex and lateral to the sphenoid sinus and pituitary fossa. The following structures are located within the venous cavity:

- the ICA, surrounded by the sympathetic carotid plexus
- CNs III, IV, and VI
- the ophthalmic and maxillary divisions of CN V

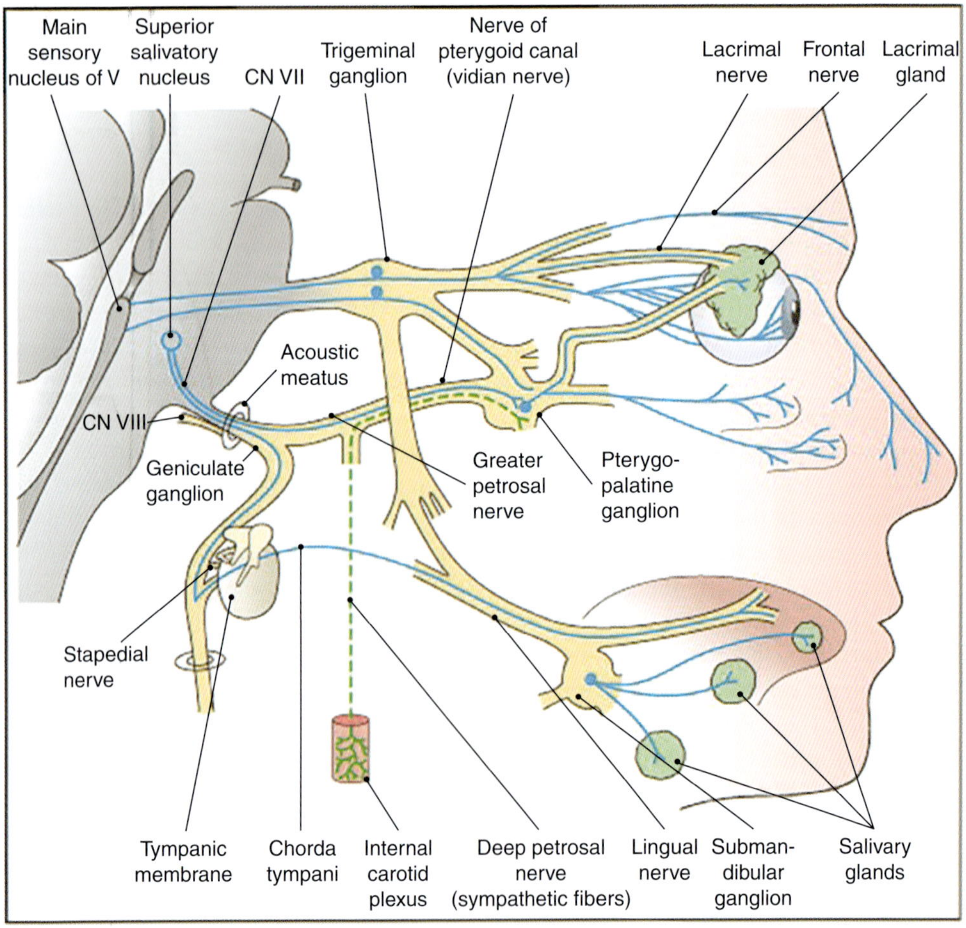

Figure 3-23 Lacrimal reflex arc (after Kurihashi). The afferent pathway is provided by the first and second divisions of CN V. The efferent pathway proceeds from the lacrimal nucleus (close to the superior salivatory nucleus) via CN VII (nervus intermedius), through the geniculate ganglion, the greater superficial petrosal nerve, and the nerve of the pterygoid canal (vidian nerve) (where it is joined by sympathetic fibers from the deep petrosal nerve). The fibers then pass to the pterygopalatine ganglion, where they synapse with postganglionic fibers. These fibers reach the lacrimal gland directly, via the retro-orbital plexus of nerves (particularly CN V_1). The fibers carry cholinergic and vasoactive intestinal polypeptide (VIP)-ergic fibers to the gland. *(Modified with permission from Spalton D, Hitchings R, Hunter P.* Atlas of Clinical Ophthalmology. *3rd ed. New York: Elsevier/Mosby; 2005:642.)*

Figure 3-24 shows the entry of CNs III–VI into the cavernous sinus from the midbrain. Figure 3-25 depicts the relative location of these structures in different parts of the cavernous sinus.

Other Venous Sinuses

Other venous sinuses include the superior sagittal, transverse, straight, sigmoid, and petrosal sinuses. The various components of the venous system are depicted in Figure 3-26.

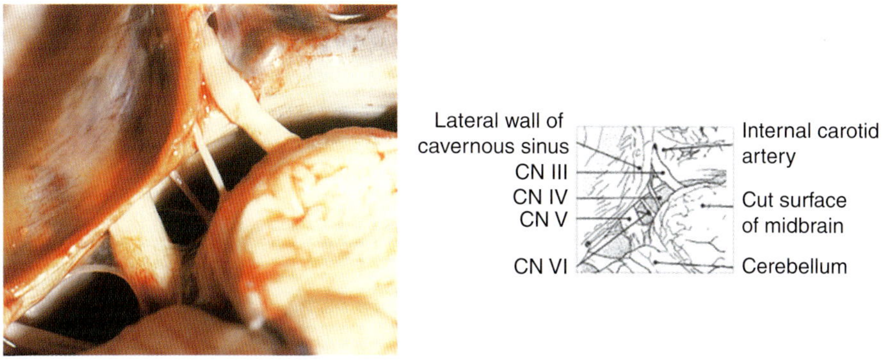

Figure 3-24 CNs III–VI exit the midbrain and enter the cavernous sinus. *(Reproduced with permission from Spalton D, Hitchings R, Hunter P.* Atlas of Clinical Ophthalmology. *3rd ed. New York: Elsevier/Mosby; 2005:642.)*

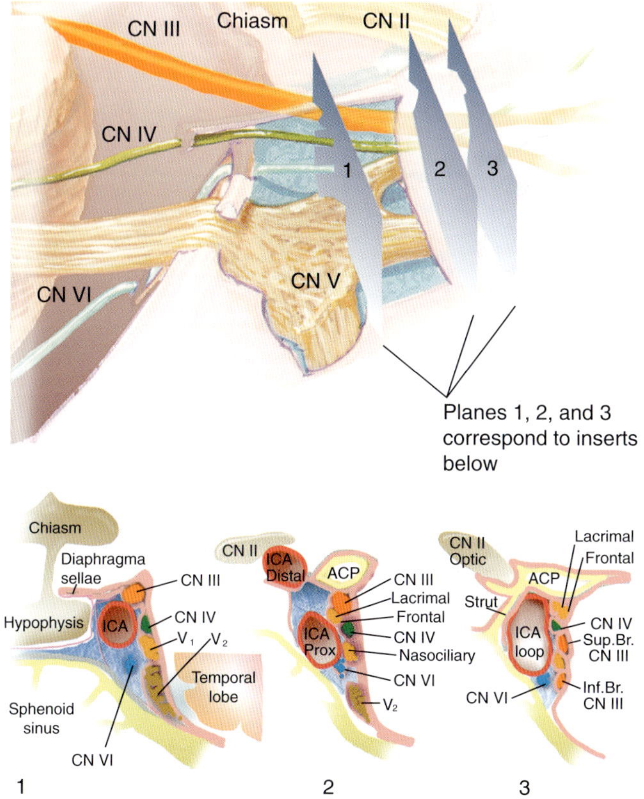

Figure 3-25 Intracavernous course of the ocular motor nerves. CNs III and IV run in the lateral wall of the cavernous sinus along with CN V_1 and CN V_2. CN VI runs in close approximation to the carotid artery within the cavernous sinus itself. As the nerves course toward the anterior aspect of the cavernous sinus and the superior orbital fissure, the ophthalmic division of CN V (CN V_1) divides into 3 branches: the lacrimal, frontal, and nasociliary nerves. ACP = anterior clinoid process; ICA = internal carotid artery; Inf. Br. = inferior branch; Prox = proximal; Sup. Br. = superior branch. *(Illustrations by Craig A. Luce.)*

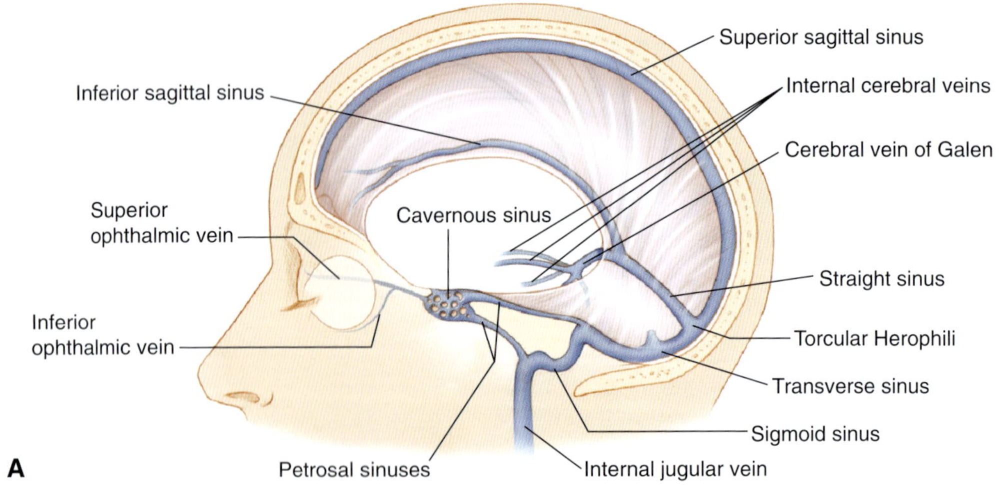

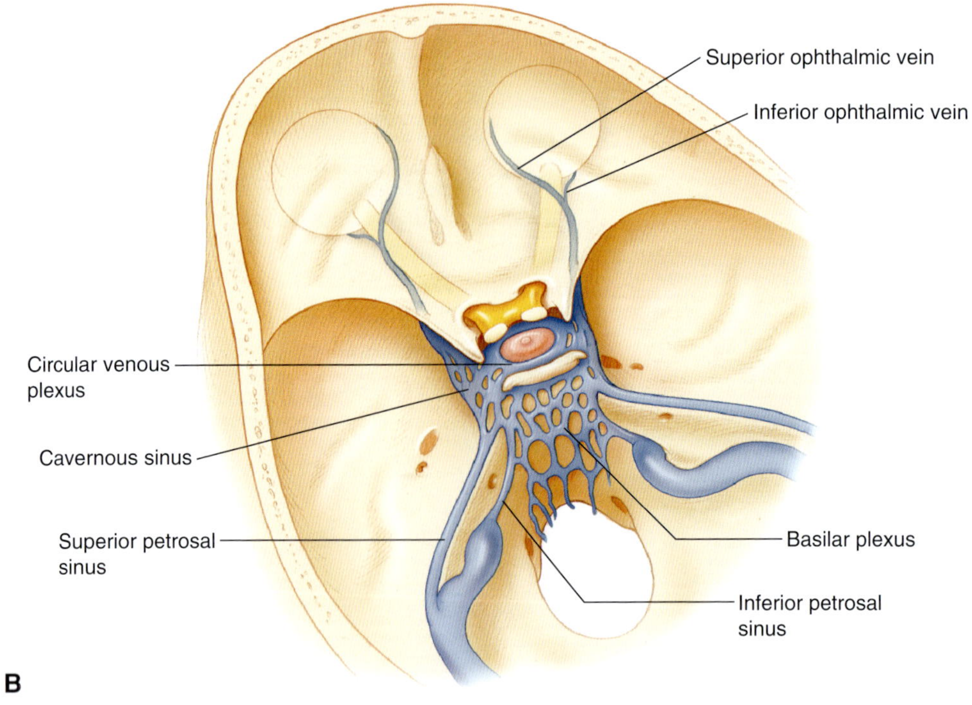

Figure 3-26 **A,** Cerebral venous sinus system. **B,** Drainage of the cavernous sinus. *(Illustrations by Christine Gralapp.)*

Thrombosis in any portion of the venous sinuses can lead to increased venous pressure and may cause intracranial hypertension with secondary CN VI palsy and papilledema.

Circle of Willis

The major arteries supplying the brain are the right and left ICAs (which distribute blood primarily to the rostral portion of the brain, anterior circulation) and the right and left

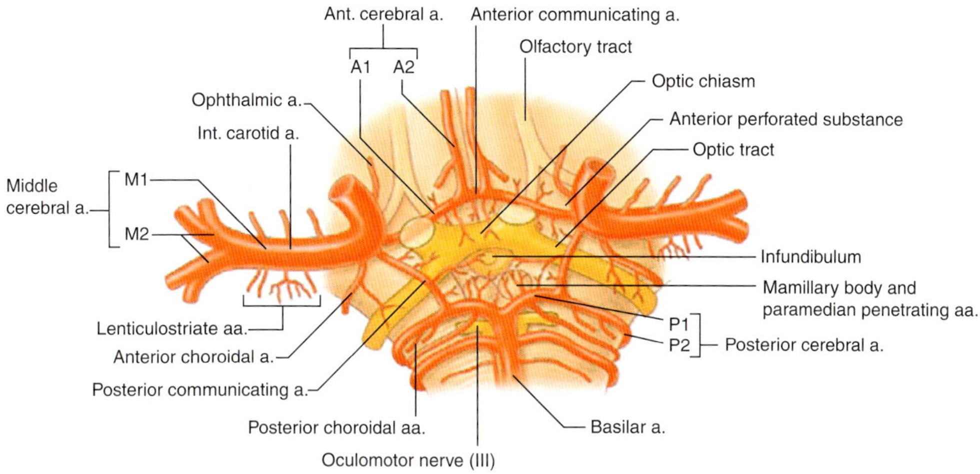

Figure 3-27 The circle of Willis represents an anastomosis of the anterior, middle, and posterior cerebral arteries. Branches from these vessels supply the distal segment of the intracranial optic nerves, optic chiasm, and optic tract. a. = artery; aa. = arteries; Ant. = anterior; Int. = internal. *(Modified with permission from Liu GT, Volpe NJ, Galetta SL.* Neuro-Ophthalmology: Diagnosis and Management. *2nd ed. New York: Elsevier; 2010:295.)*

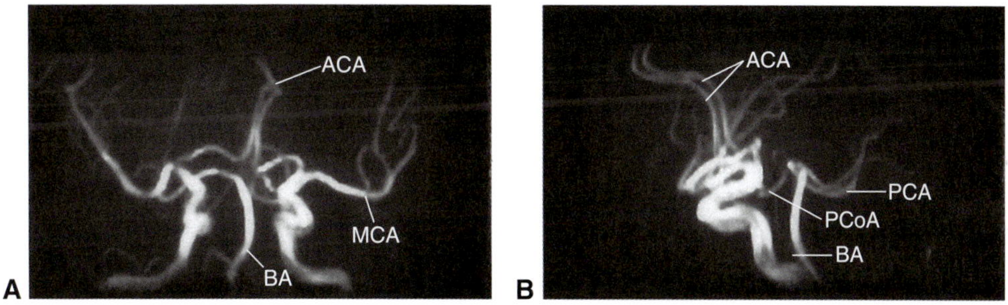

Figure 3-28 **A,** Magnetic resonance angiogram showing the circle of Willis in an anteroposterior view. **B,** An oblique view from the same patient. ACA = anterior cerebral artery; BA = basilar artery; MCA = middle cerebral artery; PCA = posterior cerebral artery; PCoA = posterior communicating artery. *(Courtesy of T. Talli, MD, and W. Yuh, MD.)*

vertebral arteries (which join to form the basilar artery, posterior circulation). The basilar artery distributes blood primarily to the brainstem and the posterior portion of the brain. These arteries interconnect at the base of the brain at the circle of Willis, also called the *cerebral arterial circle* (Figs 3-27, 3-28; see also Figs 3-3, 3-16). These interconnections (anastomoses) help distribute blood to all regions of the brain, even when a portion of the system becomes occluded. CN III, in particular, can be affected by vascular lesions within this region.

PART II

Embryology

CHAPTER 4

Ocular Development

This chapter includes related videos, which can be accessed by scanning the QR codes provided in the text or going to www.aao.org/bcscvideo_section02.

Highlights

- The eye develops from 2 germ layers, the ectoderm and the mesoderm.
- Most of the eye forms from different types of ectoderm: surface ectoderm, neuroectoderm, and neural crest cells.
- The eye is formed by a series of genetic cascades; alteration of these cascades results in ocular malformations such as microphthalmia and coloboma.

General Principles

Embryogenesis can be thought of as a series of steps that build on one another; each step creates a ripple effect on all subsequent steps. The steps are regulated by genetic programs that are activated in specific cell types and in a specific order. These genetic programs consist of cascades of genes that are expressed in response to external cues. Often, the same genes participate in different cascades and play different roles in different contexts.

For example, gene products that activate transcription in a particular program may repress transcription in the context of another program, depending on the position of the program within the overall developmental cascade. The cascades are regulated by diffusible ligands (growth factors and hormones) that create overlapping zones of concentration gradients that allow cells to triangulate their position within the developing embryo and determine which program to activate. Misactivation of genetic cascades, whether the result of gene mutations, oocyte abnormalities, or exposure to teratogens, causes embryologic abnormalities that, in the most severe cases, are embryonic lethal or, in less severe cases, give rise to congenital abnormalities.

During gastrulation (development from a single-layered blastula to a multilayered gastrula), 3 germ layers form in all animal embryos: ectoderm (superficial layer of cells), mesoderm (middle layer), and endoderm (inner layer) (Figs 4-1, 4-2). In addition, vertebrate embryos have an ectomesenchymal cell population that arises from neuroectoderm at the dorsal edge of the neural tube. These cells, known as *neural crest cells,* are transient migratory stem cells that can form tissues with ectodermal and mesodermal

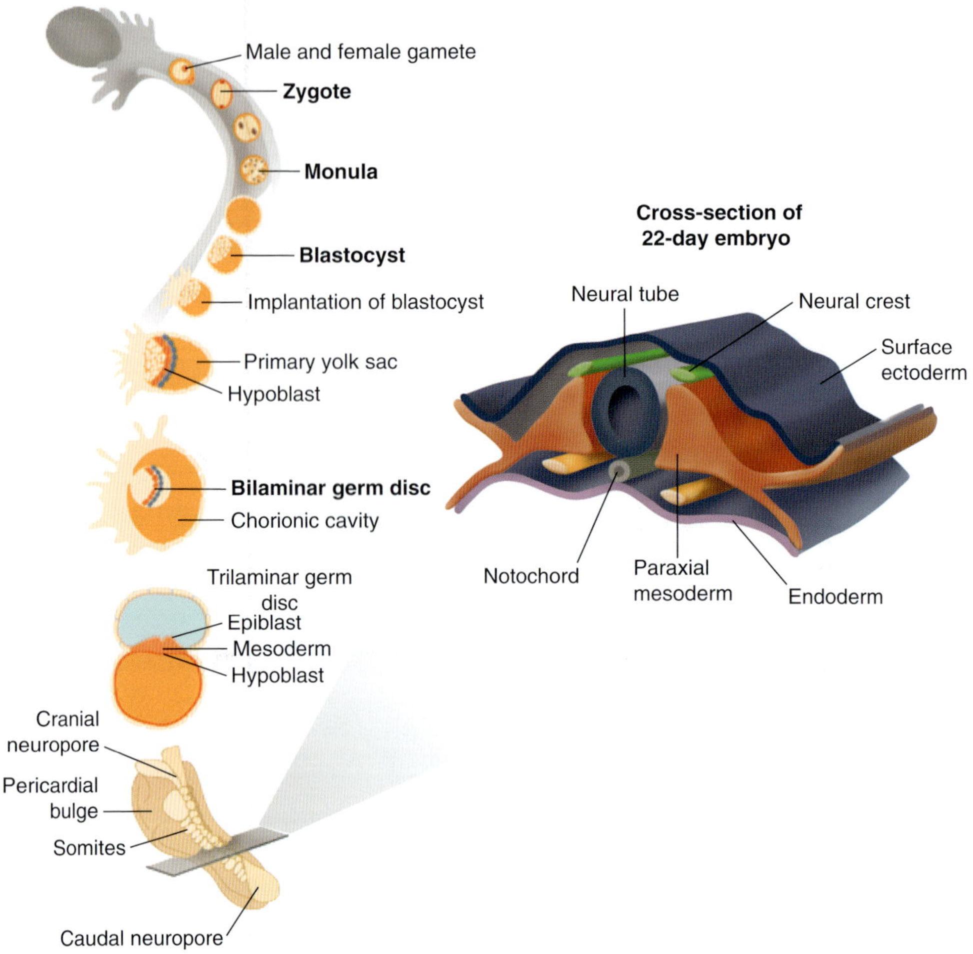

Figure 4-1 Early stages of embryonic development. The cross section demonstrates the neural tube and underlying notochord with adjacent neural crest cells *(green)* and mesoderm *(red)*. There is overlying surface ectoderm and underlying endoderm. The optic sulci develop within the neuropore at day 22. *(Illustration by Paul Schiffmacher. Adapted from Forrester JV, Dick AD, McMenamin PG, Roberts F, Pearlman E.* The Eye: Basic Sciences in Practice. *4th ed. Edinburgh: Elsevier; 2016, eFig 2-1.)*

characteristics (Fig 4-3). There are several types of neural crest cells, depending on their location and subsequent contributions. Ocular structures are derived from cranial neural crest cells, which are referred to as *neural crest cells* in this chapter.

The eye and orbital tissues develop from ectoderm, mesoderm, and neural crest cells, with the neural crest cells making a particularly large contribution. In addition, neural crest cells make key contributions to facial, dental, and cranial structures (Fig 4-4). For this reason, syndromes that arise from neural crest maldevelopment (eg, Goldenhar syndrome) often involve the eye as well as facial, dental, and calvarial abnormalities.

Following gastrulation, the ectoderm separates into surface ectoderm and neuroectoderm. Each makes a key contribution to development of the eye (Fig 4-5, Table 4-1).

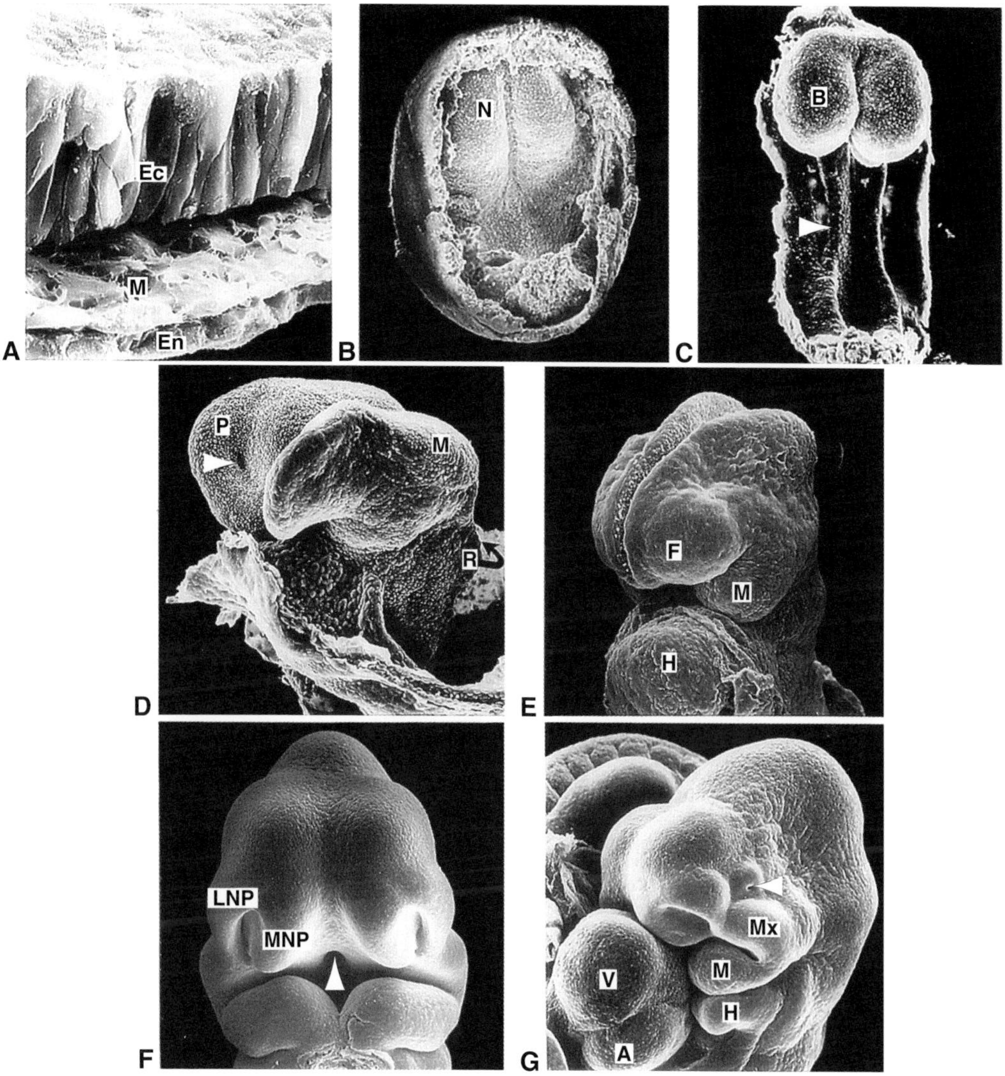

Figure 4-2 Scanning electron micrographs of normal craniofacial development. **A:** A parasagittal section through the cranial aspect of a gastrulation-stage mouse embryo. The cells of the 3 germ layers—ectoderm (**Ec**), mesoderm (**M**), and endoderm (**En**)—have distinct morphologies. **B:** The developing neural plate (**N**) is apparent in a dorsal view of this presomite mouse embryo. **C:** Neural folds *(arrowhead)* can be observed in the developing spinal cord region. The lateral aspects of the brain (**B**) region have not yet begun to elevate in this mouse embryo in the head-fold stage. **D:** Three regions of the brain can be distinguished at this 6-somite stage: prosencephalon (**P**), mesencephalon (**M**), and rhombencephalon (**R**, *curved arrow*). Optic sulci *(arrowhead)* are visible as evaginations from the prosencephalon. **E:** The neural tube has not yet fused in this 12-somite embryo. The stomodeum, or primitive oral cavity, is bordered by the frontonasal prominence (**F**), the first visceral arch (mandibular arch, **M**), and the developing heart (**H**). **F:** Medial and lateral nasal prominences (**MNP, LNP**) surround olfactory pits in this 36-somite mouse embryo. The Rathke pouch *(arrowhead)* can be distinguished in the roof of the stomodeum. **G:** In this lateral view of a 36-somite mouse embryo, the first and second (hyoid, **H**) visceral arches are apparent. The region of the first arch consists of maxillary (**Mx**) and mandibular (**M**) components. Note the presence of the eye with its invaginating lens *(arrowhead)*. Atrial (**A**) and ventricular (**V**) heart chambers can be distinguished. *(Reproduced from Sulik KK, Johnston MC. Embryonic origin of holoprosencephaly: interrelationship of the developing brain and face.* Scan Electron Microsc. *1982;(Pt 1):311.)*

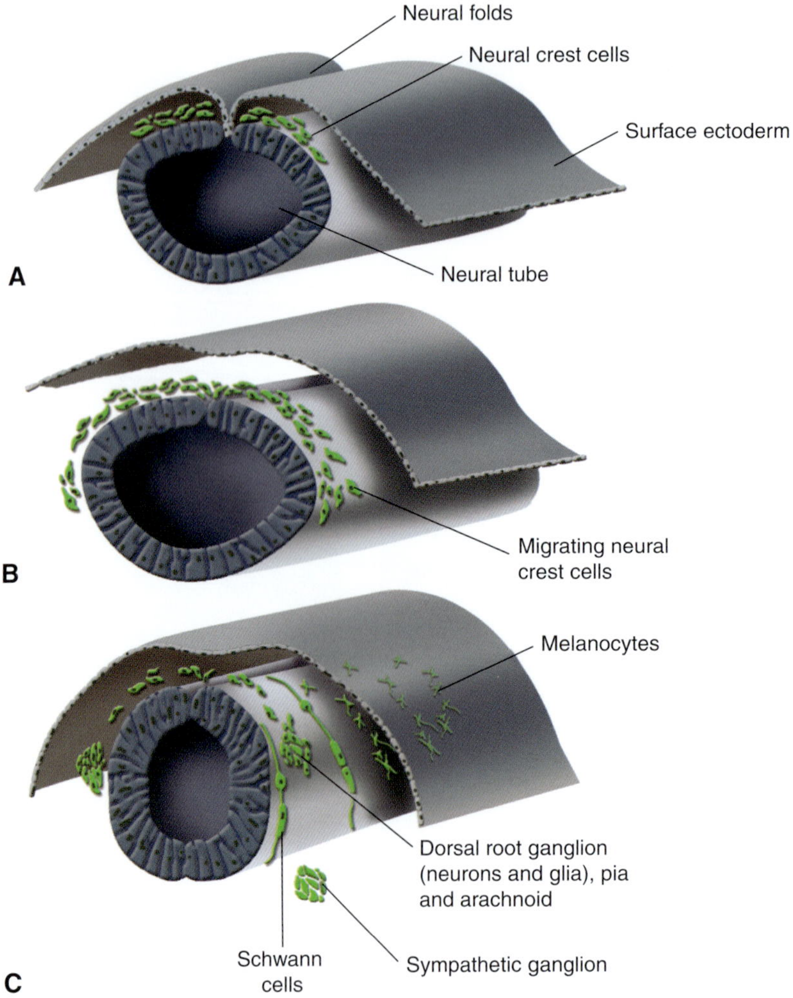

Figure 4-3 Migration of neural crest cells. **A,** Origin of neural crest cells from the junction of surface ectoderm and neuroectoderm *(light blue)* at the dorsal edge of the neural tube. **B,** Lateral/ventral migration. **C,** Differentiation of neural crest cells; note the development of melanocytes, dorsal root ganglia (including sensory ganglia of cranial nerve V), and autonomic ganglia. *(Illustration by Paul Schiffmacher. Adapted from Forrester JV, Dick AD, McMenamin PG, Roberts F, Pearlman E.* The Eye: Basic Sciences in Practice. *4th ed. Edinburgh: Elsevier; 2016, eFig 2-2.)*

Billon N, Iannarelli P, Monteiro MC, et al. The generation of adipocytes by the neural crest. *Development.* 2007;134(12):2283–2292.

Foster CS, Sainz de la Maza M, Tauber J. *The Sclera.* New York: Springer Science + Business Media LLC; 2012.

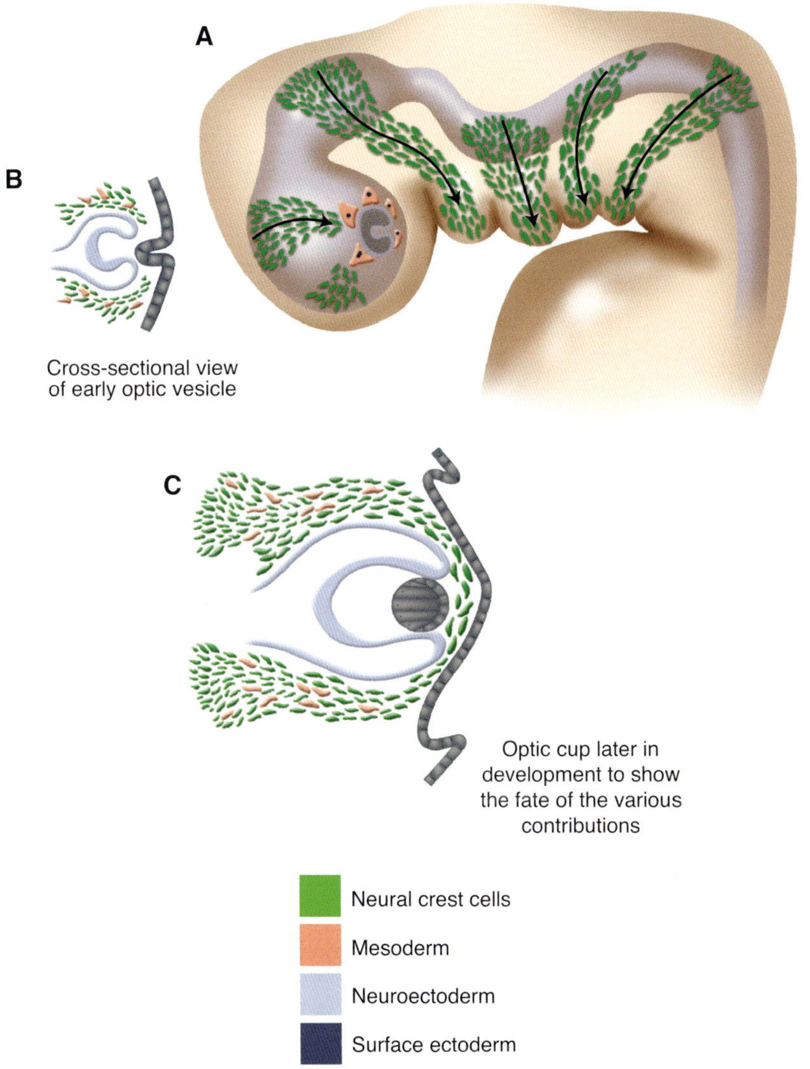

Figure 4-4 Migration of neural crest cells. **A,** Lateral and ventral migration of neural crest cells that will contribute to the development of the face and eye. In the head, neural crest cells contribute to tissues initially thought to be of mesodermal origin only. This does not occur in the trunk. Note the optic vesicle at the rostral ventral aspect. **B,** Cross section of the optic vesicle with invagination of the neuroectoderm (which will contribute to the retina, retinal pigment epithelium, optic nerve) and overlying surface ectoderm (contributes to lens). **C,** The neural crest cells and mesoderm surrounding the neuroectoderm will contribute to the sclera, cornea, and uvea (melanocytes), among numerous other ocular structures. *(Illustration by Paul Schiffmacher. Adapted from Forrester JV, Dick AD, McMenamin PG, Roberts F, Pearlman E.* The Eye: Basic Sciences in Practice. *4th ed. Edinburgh: Elsevier; 2016:113.)*

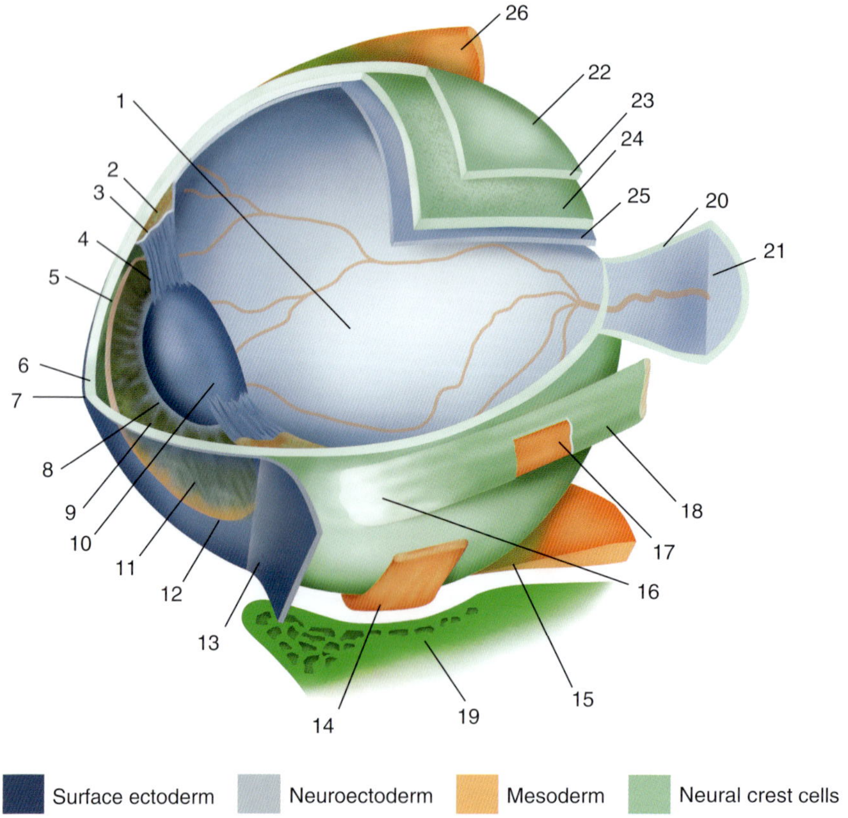

Figure 4-5 Embryologic origin of the ocular tissues. 1, Vitreous body; 2, ciliary muscle; 3, ciliary body epithelium; 4, zonular fibers; 5, corneal endothelium; 6, corneal stroma; 7, corneal epithelium; 8, iris sphincter; 9, iris dilator; 10, lens; 11, iris stroma; 12, trabecular meshwork; 13, conjunctiva; 14, inferior oblique muscle; 15, inferior rectus muscle; 16, medial rectus tendon; 17, medial rectus muscle; 18, medial rectus muscle sheath; 19, inferior orbital bones; 20, optic nerve sheath; 21, optic nerve; 22, bulbar sheath; 23, sclera; 24, choroid; 25, neurosensory retina and retinal pigment epithelium; 26, superior rectus muscle. *(Developed by Evan Silverstein, MD, and Vikram S. Brar, MD. Illustration by Cyndie C. H. Wooley; original art by Paul Schiffmacher.)*

Eye Development

Figure 4-6 and Table 4-2 outline the timeline of ocular development. Video 4-1 presents an animation of ocular embryology.

VIDEO 4-1 Ocular embryology.
Animation developed by Evan Silverstein, MD.
Access all Section 2 videos at www.aao.org/bcscvideo_section02.

At 22 days, the optic primordium appears in neural folds. Two optic pits, derived from neuroectoderm, develop on either side of the midline and eventually form the *optic vesicles.* The narrow neck of these vesicles directly connects the optic vesicle and the developing forebrain. Once the optic vesicle touches the inner aspect of the surface ectoderm, the vesicle

Table 4-1 Derivatives of Embryonic Tissues

Ectoderm
- *Neuroectoderm*
  - Ciliary body epithelium (nonpigmented and pigmented)
  - Iris epithelium (nonpigmented and pigmented)
  - Iris sphincter and dilator muscles
  - Neurosensory retina
  - Optic nerve, axons, and glia
  - Retinal pigment epithelium
  - Vitreous
- *Neural crest cells*
  - Bones: midline and inferior orbital bones; parts of orbital roof and lateral rim
  - Cartilage
  - Choroid/iris stroma (also see Mesoderm)
  - Ciliary ganglion
  - Connective tissue of orbit
  - Corneal stroma and endothelium
  - Extraocular muscle sheaths and tendons
  - Orbital fat (also see Mesoderm)
  - Melanocytes (uveal and epithelial)
  - Meningeal sheaths of the optic nerve
  - Schwann cells of ciliary nerves
  - Sclera, except temporal sclera (also see Mesoderm)
  - Trabecular meshwork
  - Vitreous (also see Mesoderm)
  - Vasculature: muscle and connective tissue sheaths of ocular and orbital vessels
- *Surface ectoderm*
  - Corneal epithelium
  - Conjunctival epithelium
  - Epithelium, glands, cilia of skin of eyelids, and caruncle
  - Lacrimal drainage system
  - Lacrimal gland (also from neural crest)
  - Lens
  - Vitreous

Mesoderm
- Choroid
- Ciliary body
- Extraocular muscle fibers
- Fat (also see Neural crest cells)
- Iris stroma
- Temporal sclera (also see Neural crest cells)
- Vascular endothelium
- Vitreous (also see Neural crest cells)

invaginates to form a bilayered optic cup. (Note that the embryologic optic cup is not the same as the anatomical optic cup of the optic nerve head.) The inner layer forms the neural retina, and the outer layer forms the retinal pigment epithelium (RPE) (see Fig 4-6D).

As the optic cup forms, 2 processes take place. First, the surface ectoderm begins to invaginate to form the lens. Second, the area between the cup and the surface ectoderm fills with a combination of mesodermal and neural crest–derived cells—the ectomesenchyme that will form much of the anterior segment of the eye (see Fig 4-6E). In the area surrounding the posterior aspect of the optic cup, the same group of cells will give rise to the hyaloid vessels, choroid, and sclera (see Fig 4-6C–E).

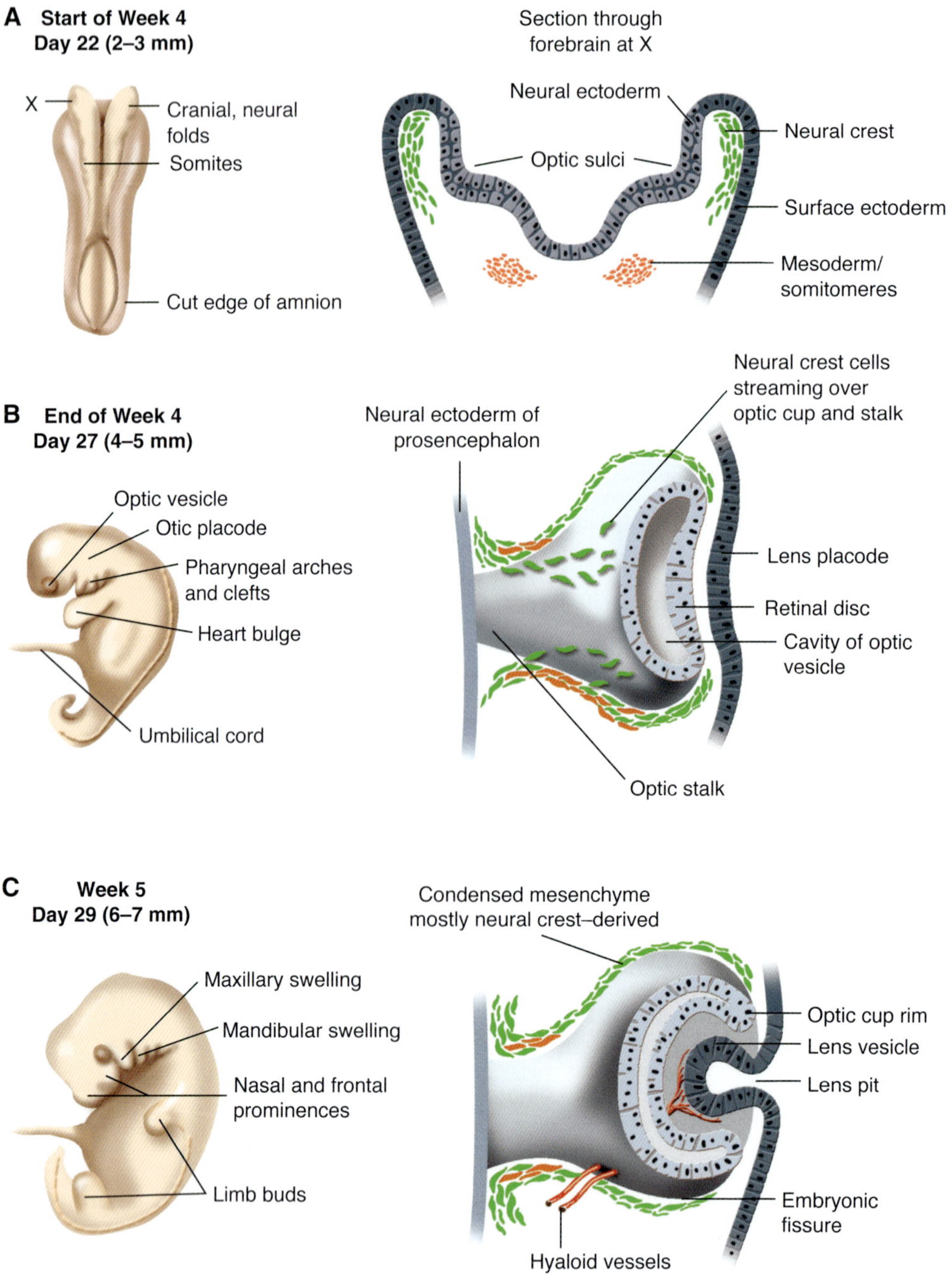

Figure 4-6 Embryonic development of the eye. The contributions of the surface ectoderm, neuroectoderm, neural crest cells, and mesoderm are shown. RPE = retinal pigment epithelium. *(Illustration by Paul Schiffmacher. Adapted from Forrester JV, Dick AD, McMenamin PG, Roberts F, Pearlman E.* The Eye: Basic Sciences in Practice. *4th ed. Edinburgh: Elsevier; 2016:104–105.)*

(Continued)

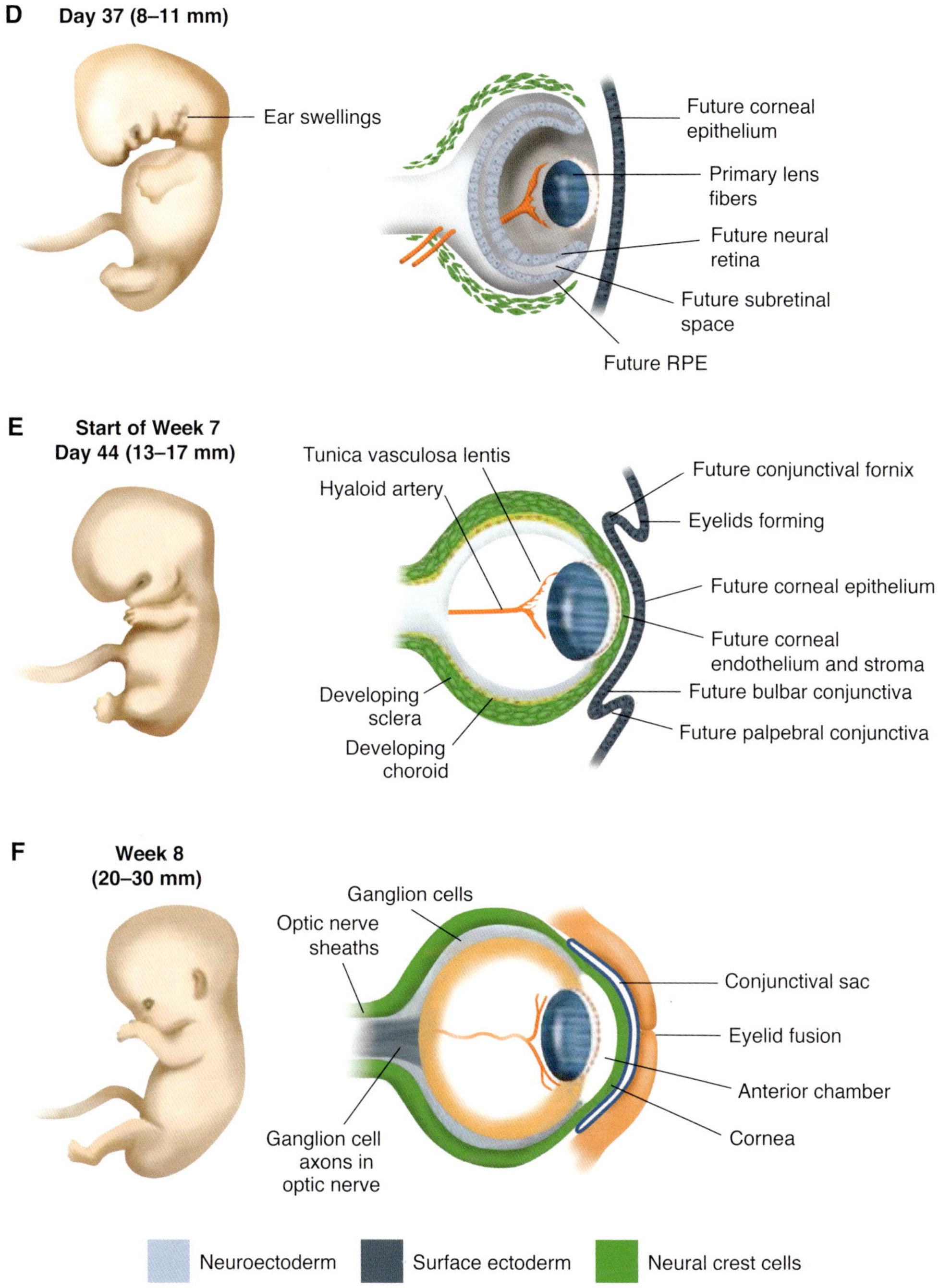

Figure 4-6 *(continued)*

Table 4-2 Chronology of Embryonic and Fetal Development of the Eye

22 days	Optic primordium appears in neural folds (1.5–3.0 mm).
25 days	Optic vesicle evaginates. Neural crest cells migrate to surround vesicle.
27 days	Vesicle induces lens placode.
4–5 weeks	Eyelid folds appear.
Second month	Invagination of optic and lens vesicles occurs. Hyaloid artery enters the eye via the embryonic fissure. Closure of embryonic fissure begins. Pigment granules appear in retinal pigment epithelium. Primordia of lateral rectus and superior oblique muscles grow anteriorly. Eyelid folds meet and fuse. Retinal differentiation begins with nuclear and marginal zones. Migration of retinal cells begins. Neural crest cells of corneal endothelium migrate centrally. Corneal stroma follows. Cavity of lens vesicle is obliterated. Secondary vitreous surrounds hyaloid system. Choroidal vasculature develops. Axons from ganglion cells migrate to optic nerve. Glial lamina cribrosa forms. Bruch membrane appears.
Third month	Precursors of rods and cones differentiate. Anterior rim of optic vesicle grows forward, and ciliary body starts to develop. Sclera condenses. Vortex veins pierce sclera.
Fourth month	Retinal vessels grow into nerve fiber layer near optic disc. Folds of ciliary processes appear. Iris sphincter develops. Descemet membrane forms. Schlemm canal appears. Hyaloid system starts to regress. Glands and cilia develop.
Fifth month	Photoreceptors develop inner segments. Choroidal vessels form layers. Iris stroma is vascularized. Eyelids begin to separate.
Sixth month	Ganglion cells thicken in macula. Recurrent arterial branches join the choroidal vessels. Dilator muscle of iris forms.
Seventh month	Outer segments of photoreceptors differentiate. Central fovea starts to thin. Fibrous lamina cribrosa forms. Choroidal melanocytes produce pigment. Circular muscle forms in ciliary body.
Eighth month	Anterior chamber angle completes formation. Hyaloid system disappears.
Ninth month	Retinal vessels reach the periphery. Myelination of fibers of optic nerve is complete to lamina cribrosa. Pupillary membrane disappears.

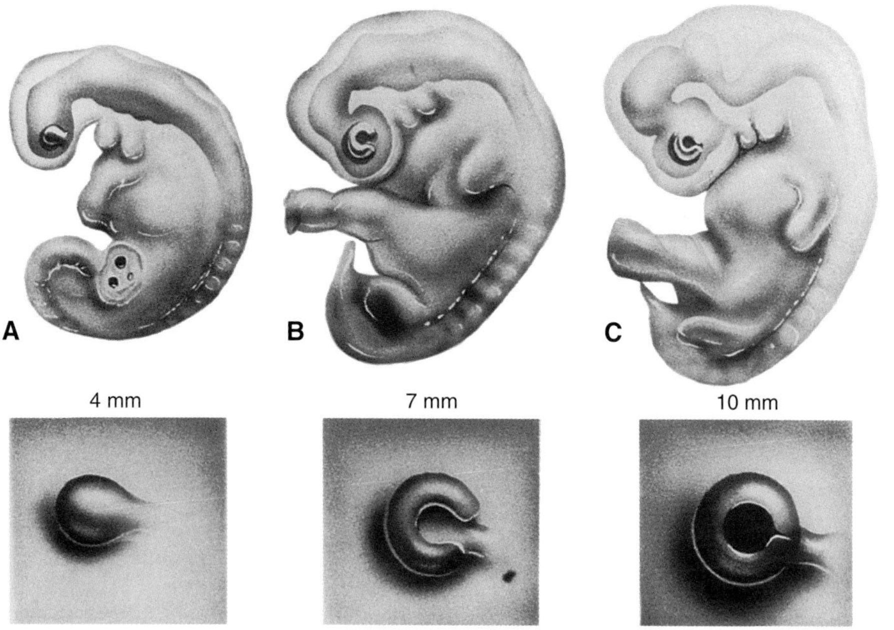

Figure 4-7 Ocular and somatic development. **A,** Flexion of the neural tube and ballooning of the optic vesicle. **B,** Upper-limb buds appear as the optic cup and embryonic fissure emerge. **C,** Completion of the optic cup with closure of the fissure. Convolutions appear in the brain, and leg buds appear. Measurements show the size of the embryo. *Bottom:* Optic vesicle; optic cup with open embryonic fissure; cup with fissure closing.

The invagination of the optic cup occurs asymmetrically (Fig 4-7), with a ventral fissure that facilitates entry of mesodermal and neural crest cells. The fissure closes at its center first and then "zips" both anteriorly and posteriorly. Failure of fissure closure leads to a coloboma. Anterior colobomas are the most common (they cause iris and occasionally anterior scleral defects); central colobomas are the least common; and posterior colobomas occur with a frequency somewhere in between (they give rise to optic nerve head, retinal, and choroidal defects). The location of fissure closure correlates with the inferonasal quadrant, which is where colobomas are clinically found. See BCSC Section 6, *Pediatric Ophthalmology and Strabismus,* for further discussion of congenital and developmental disorders.

The following sections discuss development of individual ocular structures.

Lens

Lens formation begins with proliferation of surface ectoderm cells to form a lens plate, followed by inward invagination of the plate to form a lens pit. As the pit deepens, it closes anteriorly and detaches to form the lens vesicle (see Fig 4-6C). The remaining cells at the surface form the corneal epithelium (see Fig 4-6D). Invading neural crest cells form the corneal stroma and endothelium, along with other anterior segment structures (see Fig 4-6E).

The lens vesicle is a single-layer structure composed of cuboidal cells surrounding a large lumen, and it sits within the optic cup. The anterior cells remain cuboidal and single

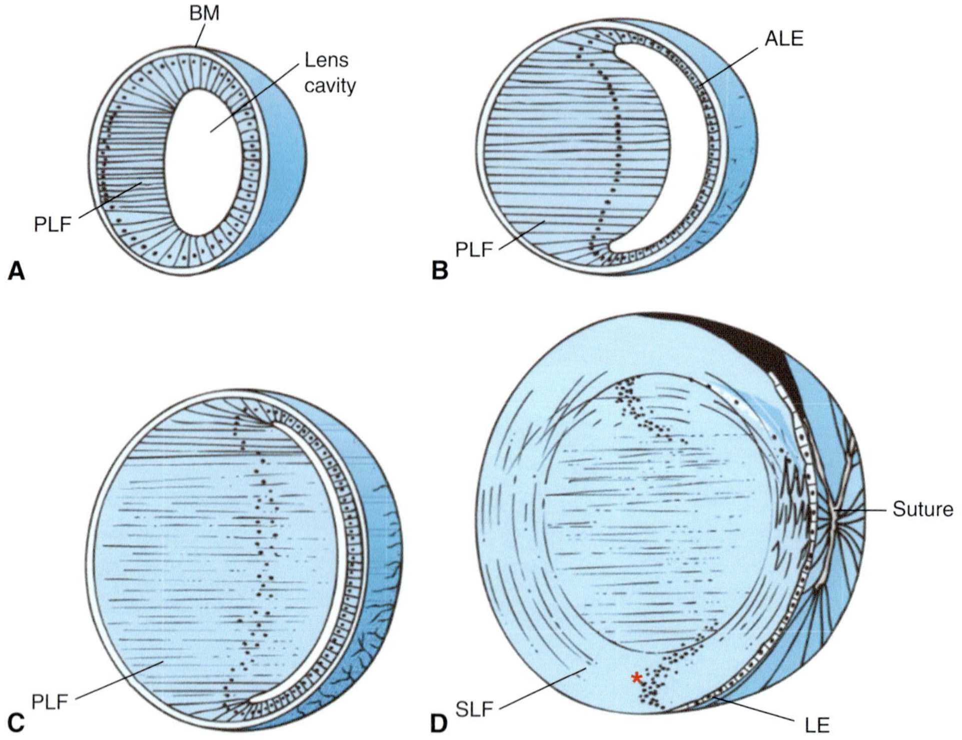

Figure 4-8 Lens formation. **A,** Lens vesicle. **B,** Anterior cells remain cuboidal, whereas the posterior cells elongate. **C,** The posterior cells eventually fill the lens vesicle, giving rise to the embryonic nucleus. **D,** The anterior cells give rise to the lens epithelium (LE). Note the lens bow region *(*)* extending from the epithelial cells, giving rise to the secondary lens fibers (SLF). ALE = anterior lens epithelium; BM = basement membrane; PLF = primary lens fibers. *(Modified with permission from Forrester JV, Dick AD, McMenamin PG, Roberts F, Pearlman E.* The Eye: Basic Sciences in Practice. *4th ed. Edinburgh: Elsevier; 2016:121–123.)*

layered throughout life, but the rest of the lens epithelium cells become elongated, and their proliferation fills the optic vesicle. These cells form the primary lens fibers that eventually form the embryonal nucleus. The remaining outer cells create a true basement membrane known as the *lens capsule* (Fig 4-8).

Development of the lens vesicle is supported by a branching network of vessels, derived from the hyaloid artery, known as the *tunica vasculosa lentis*. Failure of this tissue to regress can lead to conditions ranging from pupillary membranes that are seen on routine slit-lamp examination, to a malformation called *persistent fetal vasculature* (also called *persistent hyperplastic primary vitreous*), which can be associated with lenticular opacity and abnormal development of the eye.

The lens is a unique structure in that its basement membrane surrounds its cellular component. The lens capsule is transparent, thickest at its equator, and thinnest posteriorly. It is composed of type IV collagen and glycosaminoglycans (also known as *GAGs*). The elasticity of the lens capsule is key to facilitating changes in lens shape to achieve accommodation. The anterior lens (cuboidal) epithelium continues to form new lens fibers throughout life (see Fig 4-8D), leading to the lenticular thickening observed with age. The zonular fibers of the lens form as part of the tertiary vitreous, with mostly mesodermal and ectodermal contributions.

Posterior Segment

Retina

The neural retina develops from the invagination of the inner aspect of the optic cup, and the RPE develops from the outer layer. The apposed surfaces of these 2 layers are ciliated. The inner-layer cilia go on to form photoreceptors, while the outer-layer cilia regress. Although the physical space between these layers eventually closes, it remains a potential space; retinal detachments occur when fluid accumulates, due to various etiologies, within this space.

Neural (inner) retinal development is driven by overlapping cascades of genetic programs; several "master" switches help determine lineages and drive cell fate, such as Nrl (neural retina leucine zipper), a transcription factor of the Maf subfamily that serves as an intrinsic regulator of rod photoreceptor development. Retinal development occurs concentrically, beginning in the center of the optic cup and extending peripherally. Lamination of the neural retina occurs at approximately 8–12 weeks of gestation with the formation of inner and outer neuroblastic layers. Ganglion cells appear to be the first to differentiate; early in the second trimester, they proliferate rapidly (Fig 4-9). The internal and external limiting membranes form when cells cease to proliferate and begin to differentiate.

Retinal vasculature develops from remnants of the hyaloid artery; this artery is retained within the optic nerve and eventually becomes the central retinal artery (Fig 4-10). Endothelial cells organize posteriorly, with vessel development following the same concentric pattern as retinal development (this is the basis for zones I–III [location of involvement] in the classification of retinopathy of prematurity).

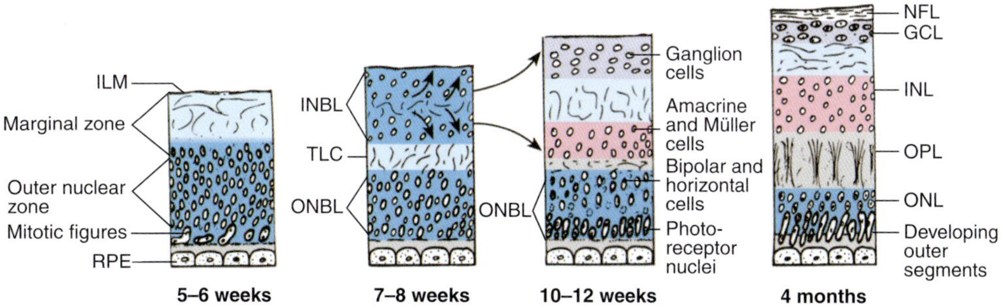

Figure 4-9 Development of the neural retina. The inner neuroblastic layer (INBL) gives rise to ganglion, Müller, and amacrine cells. The outer neuroblastic layer (ONBL) gives rise to bipolar and horizontal cells. Later, the cell bodies and outer segments of the photoreceptors develop. GCL = ganglion cell layer; ILM = internal limiting membrane; INL = inner nuclear layer; NFL = nerve fiber layer; ONL = outer nuclear layer; OPL = outer plexiform layer; RPE = retinal pigment epithelium; TLC = transient layer of Chievitz. *(Reproduced with permission from Forrester JV, Dick AD, McMenamin PG, Roberts F, Pearlman E.* The Eye: Basic Sciences in Practice. *4th ed. Edinburgh: Elsevier; 2016:115.)*

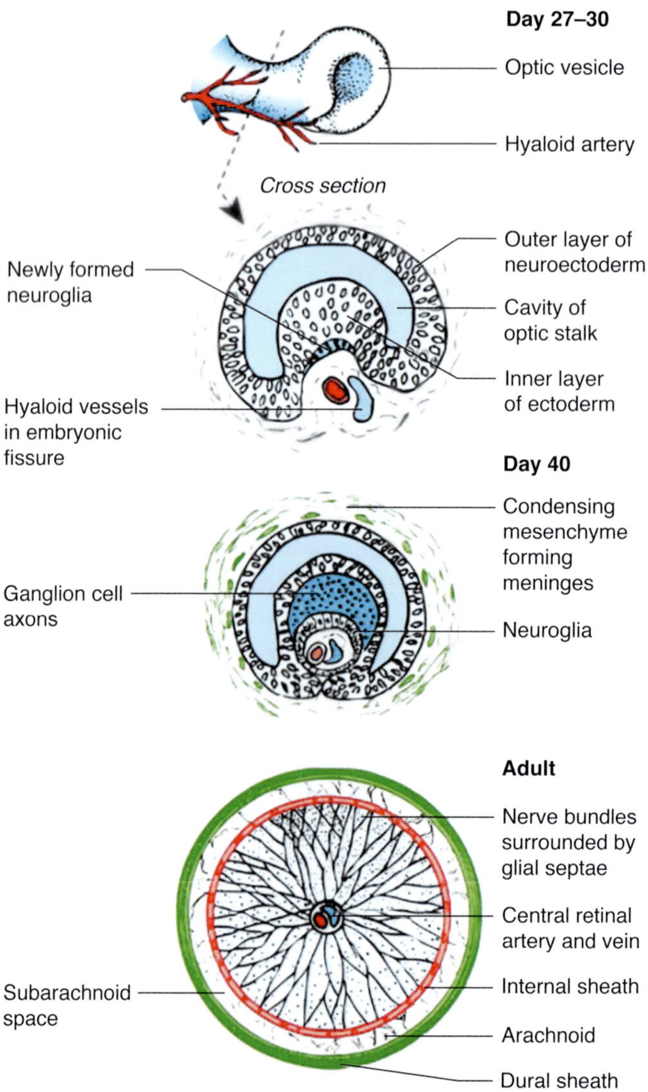

Figure 4-10 Development of the optic nerve. The hyaloid artery enters the eye via the embryonic fissure. As the fissure closes, the artery is retained within the optic nerve stalk and becomes the central retinal artery. Condensation of the surrounding neural crest cells and mesoderm form the optic nerve sheath and pial vessels. The developing ganglion cells grow toward the optic nerve stalk along the inner layer of ectoderm. The outer layer will form the lamina cribrosa. Astroglia generate the septae around the nerve bundles. These cells later give rise to oligodendrocytes, which myelinate the postlaminar axons of the retinal ganglion cells. *(Modified with permission from Forrester JV, Dick AD, McMenamin PG, Roberts F, Pearlman E.* The Eye: Basic Sciences in Practice. *4th ed. Edinburgh: Elsevier; 2016:117.)*

Retinal pigment epithelium

The RPE forms from proliferating pseudostratified columnar epithelial cells that create lateral tight junctions and deposit a basement membrane, which later becomes the inner layer of the Bruch membrane. The RPE is the only pigmented tissue in the body that is *not* derived from neural crest cells, although these cells are located at the anterior-most edge of the neural crest, suggesting shared origins.

Optic nerve

The optic nerve develops from the optic stalk, the narrow stalk that connects the optic vesicle with the forebrain (see Fig 4-6B, C). The optic stalk is highly active in regulating cell migration into and around the developing eye, mostly through release of ligands and expression of growth factor receptors. It initially forms from neuroectodermal cells surrounded by neural crest cells. In the sixth week of gestation, neuroectodermal cells begin to vacuolate and degenerate, providing space for axons from the ganglion cells of the inner retina (see Fig 4-10). The surrounding neural crest cells form meninges, whereas neuroectodermal cells form surrounding oligodendrocytes (to form myelin sheaths). Peripheral nerves, including most cranial nerves, are surrounded by myelin supplied by Schwann cells. The exception is the optic nerve, which is surrounded by oligodendrocytes. This difference is an important reason for the optic nerve's susceptibility to neuritis.

Vitreous

The vitreous is probably formed from both mesodermal and ectodermal components: Neural crest cells of the inner optic cup probably contribute the connective fibers of the vitreous. The hyaloid vasculature develops from mesodermally derived cells (Fig 4-11; see also Fig 4-6C, D, and Fig 4-10). The primary vitreous, the earliest vitreous in the embryo, forms a central conical structure that contains the hyaloid vasculature (Fig 4-12) and is surrounded by secondary vitreous. The secondary vitreous forms from hyalocytes as the primary vitreous begins to regress, eventually (by the sixth fetal month) enveloping the regressed primary vitreous. Between months 4 and 6, the zonular fibers of the lens develop from tertiary vitreous and are distinct from the primary and secondary vitreous. Remnants of the primary vitreous include the Cloquet canal and its anterior extension, the hyaloideocapsular ligament (also known as *ligament of Weiger*).

Uvea

The uvea (also called *uveal tract*)—comprising the ciliary body, iris, and choroid—develops from a combination of mesoderm and neural crest cells. The corresponding epithelial layers of the ciliary body and iris are derived from the neuroectoderm and are not considered part of the uvea, the pigmented vascular layer of the eye. The uvea obtains its dark color from neural crest–derived melanocytes residing within it. Its blood vessels and ciliary muscles are derived from the mesoderm.

Ciliary body and iris

At the anterior aspect of the optic cup, the surrounding mesoderm proliferates, pushing the neuroectoderm inward and centrally between the corneal endothelium and the anterior lens surface, giving rise to the ciliary body and iris epithelium (Fig 4-13).

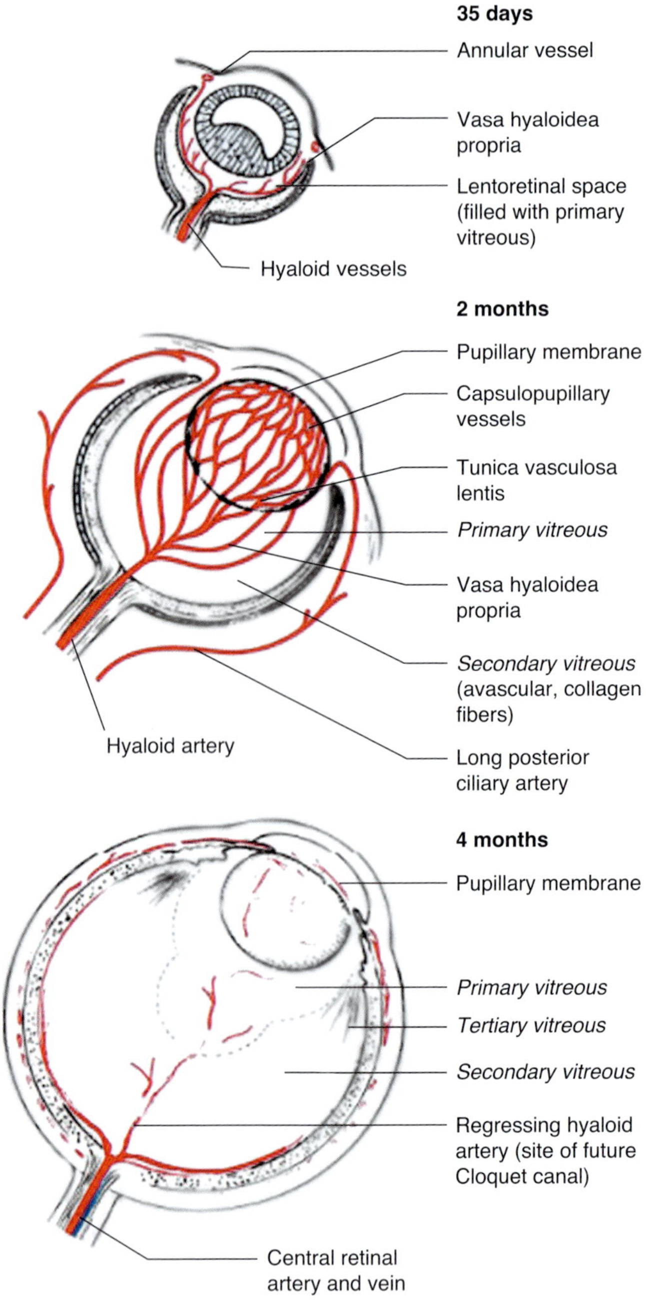

Figure 4-11 Development of the vitreous. The mesoderm gives rise to the hyaloid artery, which is contained within the primary vitreous. This vascular system supplies the tunica vasculosa lentis. The secondary vitreous forms from hyalocytes as the primary vitreous regresses. The zonular fibers develop from the tertiary vitreous. *(Modified with permission from Forrester JV, Dick AD, McMenamin PG, Roberts F, Pearlman E.* The Eye: Basic Sciences in Practice. *4th ed. Edinburgh: Elsevier; 2016:123.)*

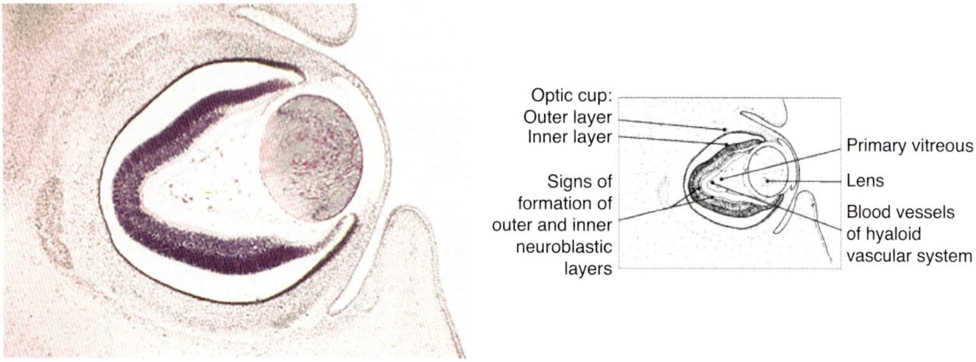

Figure 4-12 Illustration and corresponding histologic image showing the relationship between the optic cup, primary vitreous, and lens. The ciliary body and iris are absent. Note the cornea and eyelids developing from surface ectoderm. *(Reproduced with permission from Spalton D, Hitchings R, Hunter P.* Atlas of Clinical Ophthalmology. *3rd ed. New York: Elsevier/Mosby; 2005:398.)*

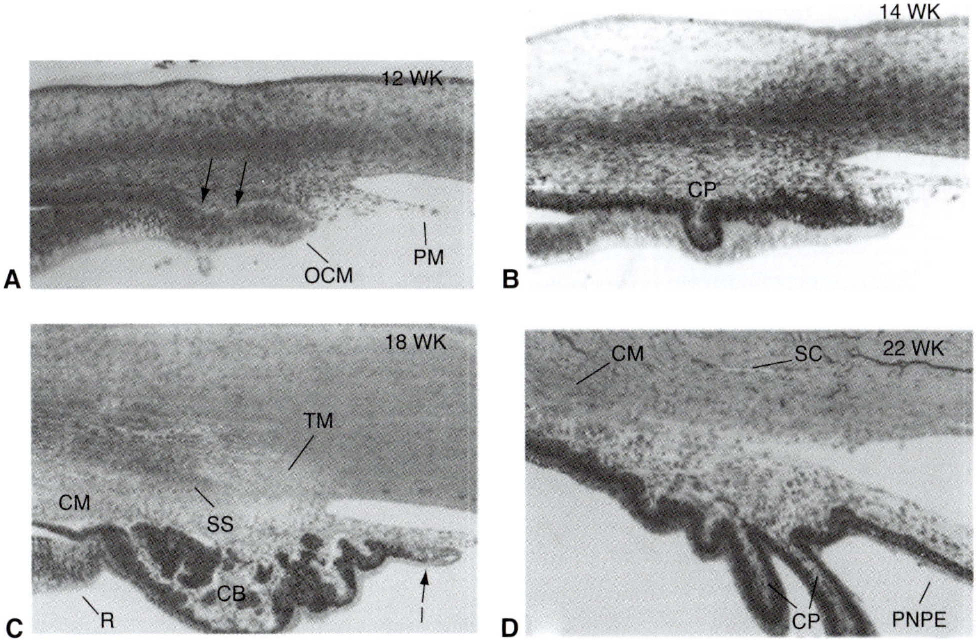

Figure 4-13 Development of the iris and ciliary body in a human fetal eye from 12 to 22 weeks. **A,** *Arrows* indicate proliferating vascular mesoderm behind the neuroectoderm at the optic cup margin (OCM). **B,** Continued growth of the mesoderm, with infolding of the neuroectoderm and development of a ciliary process (CP). Note the inner pigmented and outer nonpigmented layers of the ciliary epithelium. **C,** Anteriorly, the neuroectoderm forms the epithelial layers of the iris (I). At this stage, the angle recess is present, with developing trabecular meshwork (TM) and ciliary muscle (CM) and intervening scleral spur (SS). **D,** Developing CPs and iris. Note that the posterior nonpigmented epithelium of the iris (PNPE) is continuous with the nonpigmented ciliary epithelium. The PNPE will acquire pigment as the iris develops. CB = ciliary body; PM = pupillary membrane; R = retina; SC = Schlemm canal. *(Modified with permission from Forrester JV, Dick AD, McMenamin PG, Roberts F, Pearlman E.* The Eye: Basic Sciences in Practice. *4th ed. Edinburgh: Elsevier; 2016:125.)*

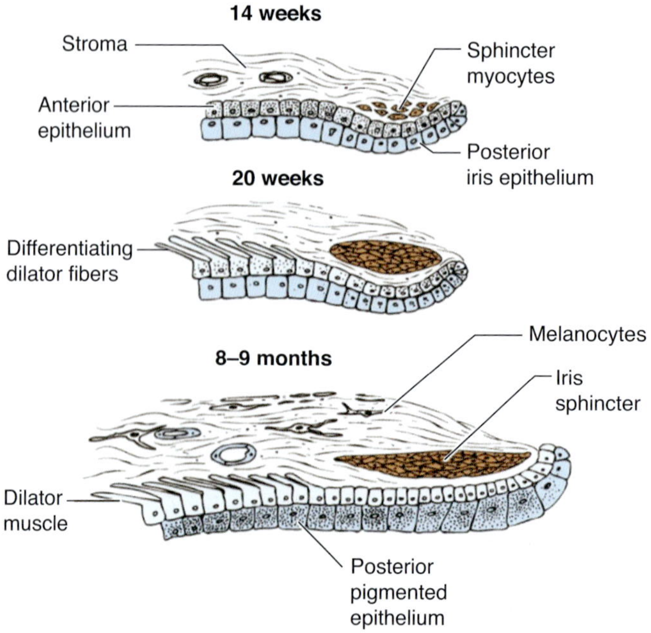

Figure 4-14 Development of the iris. The iris sphincter and dilator muscles are derived from neuroectoderm. The dilator muscle arises directly from the anterior iris epithelium. *(Modified with permission from Forrester JV, Dick AD, McMenamin PG, Roberts F, Pearlman E.* The Eye: Basic Sciences in Practice. *4th ed. Edinburgh: Elsevier; 2016:126.)*

The mesodermal proliferation results in formation of the ciliary muscle and leads to infolding of the neuroectoderm. These folds give rise to the ciliary processes, which are lined by 2 layers of epithelium: an inner pigmented layer and an outer nonpigmented layer. The outer nonpigmented layer of the ciliary body is continuous with the retina posteriorly and the nonpigmented posterior epithelium of the iris anteriorly. The latter acquires pigment over the course of development, starting at the pupil margin and progressing radially to the iris root, leading to the posterior iris pigment epithelium found in the adult eye. Pigmentation does not occur in the anterior epithelial layer of the iris.

Anteriorly, the neuroectoderm incorporates surrounding mesenchymal elements from the tunica vasculosa lentis. The subsequent anterior component, of mesodermal origin, gives rise to the iris stroma and vasculature. Posteriorly, the neuroectoderm continues as the epithelial layers of the iris and gives rise to the sphincter and dilator muscles. The dilator muscles are a direct extension of the anterior iris epithelium (Fig 4-14).

Choroid

Condensation of neural crest cells and mesoderm surrounding the optic cup produces the choroid on the inner aspect of the cup and the sclera and cornea on its outer aspect (see Fig 4-6D, E). A layer of small blood vessels, the *choriocapillaris,* forms first and is fenestrated. This is followed by development of an outer layer of larger vessels, which gives rise to the vortex veins and branches of the posterior ciliary circulation. Subsequently, a middle layer of arterioles forms between the choriocapillaris and the outer layer of larger vessels. Melanocytes develop in the choroid later in gestation.

Cornea, Anterior Chamber, and Sclera

Cornea and anterior chamber

The surface ectoderm closes over the lens pit and gives rise to the corneal epithelium (see Fig 4-6D). This is followed by 3 successive waves of migration of neural crest–derived ectomesenchymal cells (Figs 4-15, 4-16; see also Fig 4-6E). The first wave gives rise to the corneal endothelium, passing between the surface ectoderm and the anterior lens vesicle. The second wave passes between the endothelium and epithelium to give rise to the keratocytes of the corneal stroma. The third wave, consisting of cells of neural crest and mesodermal origin, contributes to iris development. The corneal endothelial cells meet with developing iris, forming the angle recess. The trabecular meshwork and the Schlemm canal develop from mesenchymal cells posterior to the recess. The endothelial cells that line the canal and collector channels are derived from adjacent capillaries, which will eventually form the episcleral venous plexus. The resultant aqueous vein receives aqueous humor and delivers it to the venous circulation (see Chapter 2, Figs 2-17, 2-18). The trabecular beams undergo further maturation and stratification to form the layered trabecular meshwork. Alteration in this process has been implicated in the development of congenital glaucoma and anterior chamber dysgenesis. The scleral spur forms between the trabecular meshwork and the ciliary muscle as the anterior chamber angle develops (see Fig 4-13C, D).

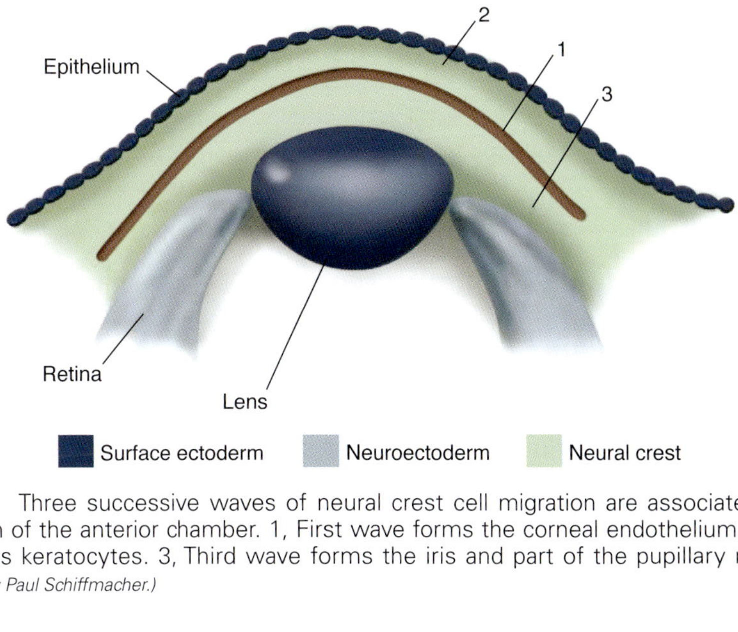

Figure 4-15 Three successive waves of neural crest cell migration are associated with differentiation of the anterior chamber. 1, First wave forms the corneal endothelium. 2, Second wave forms keratocytes. 3, Third wave forms the iris and part of the pupillary membrane. *(Illustration by Paul Schiffmacher.)*

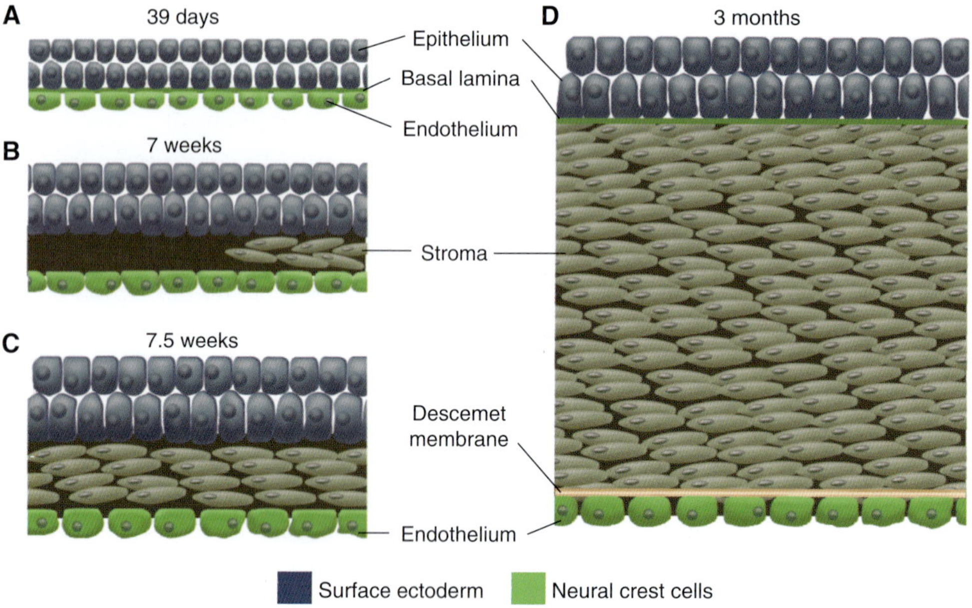

Figure 4-16 Development of the cornea in the central region. **A,** At day 39, 2-layered epithelium rests on the basal lamina and is separated from the endothelium (single layer) by a narrow acellular space. **B,** At week 7, neural crest–derived ectomesenchymal cells from the periphery migrate into the space between the epithelium and the endothelium. **C,** Mesenchymal cells (future keratocytes) are arranged in 4–5 incomplete layers by 7½ weeks of gestation; a few collagen fibrils are present among the cells. **D,** By 3 months, the epithelium has 2–3 layers of cells, and the stroma has approximately 25–30 layers of keratocytes that are arranged more regularly in the posterior half. Thin, uneven Descemet membrane lies between the most posterior keratocytes and the single layer of endothelium. *(Illustration by Cyndie C. H. Wooley.)*

Sclera

The sclera is formed from mesodermal (temporal sclera) and neural crest–derived ectomesenchymal elements. The sclera joins the developing cornea near the equator of the eye but continues to develop and expand to surround the developing optic cup. The scleral spur and Tenon capsule form later, at the time of extraocular muscle insertion.

Development of the Extraocular Muscles, Adnexa, and Orbit

Extraocular Muscles

The extraocular muscles (EOMs) form from paraxial and prechordal mesoderm, following cues from the developing eye as well as from surrounding neural crest–derived mesenchyme. Indeed, the interactions among the optic cup, mesoderm, and neural crest cells are crucial to the proper development and organization of the EOMs. If the optic cup fails to form and the eye vesicle turns into a cyst (microphthalmia spectrum), the EOMs often develop anomalously, an outcome that is likely because signals from the optic cup are necessary for proper migration of neural crest cells into the eye and surrounding tissues, and subsequent signals from these neural crest–derived cells are required for proper development and organization of the EOMs. Interestingly, eyeless blind cave fish have embryonic eyes, likely because the developing eyes serve as important organizers of facial and head development (possibly through the morphogenic actions of retinoic acid).

Congenital cranial dysinnervation disorders involving the EOMs include Duane retraction syndrome, Marcus Gunn jaw-winking syndrome, Möbius syndrome, and congenital fibrosis of the extraocular muscles (see BCSC Section 6, *Pediatric Ophthalmology and Strabismus*). Genetic studies have identified mutations in genes for neuron biology and axon guidance (eg, *KIF21A, PHOX2A, TUBB3*) that cause these EOM syndromes.

By extrapolation, congenital ptosis and other congenital EOM disorders probably result from delays in muscle innervation. Current models suggest that as the muscle mesenchyme and associated nerve jointly develop, a delay in innervation of the muscle mesenchyme can cause premature differentiation of that mesenchyme into connective tissue (ie, fibrosis). The extent of delay may correlate with the severity of fibrosis (eg, severity of the congenital ptosis and levator muscle dysfunction). Furthermore, the delay in, or absence of, innervation may provide a window for inappropriate innervation by another cranial nerve, such as trigeminal innervation of the levator muscle (Marcus Gunn jaw-winking syndrome) or oculomotor innervation of the lateral rectus muscle (Duane retraction syndrome).

Bohnsack BL, Gallina D, Thompson H, et al. Development of extraocular muscles requires early signals from periocular neural crest and the developing eye. *Arch Ophthalmol.* 2011;129(8):1030–1041.

Engle EC. Human genetic disorders of axon guidance. *Cold Spring Harb Perspect Biol.* 2010;2(3):a001784.

Adnexa

The upper eyelid first develops at 4–5 weeks of gestation as a proliferation of surface ectoderm in the region of the future outer canthus. During the second month, both the upper and lower eyelids become discernible as undifferentiated skinfolds that surround mesenchyme of neural crest origin (see Figs 4-6E, F and 4-12). Later, mesodermal mesenchyme infiltrates the eyelids and differentiates into the palpebral musculature. The eyelid folds grow toward each other as well as laterally. Starting near the inner canthus, the margins of the folds fuse between weeks 8 and 10 of gestation. As the folds adhere to each other, development of the cilia and glands begins. The orbicularis muscle condenses in the fold in week 12. The eyelid adhesions begin to gradually break down late in the fifth month (Fig 4-17), coincident with the secretion of sebum from the sebaceous glands and cornification of the surface epithelium.

The lacrimal gland begins to develop between the sixth and seventh weeks of gestation. Solid cords of epithelial cells proliferate from the basal cell layer of the conjunctiva in the temporal region of the fornix. Neural crest–derived mesenchymal cells aggregate at the tips of the cords and differentiate into acini. At approximately 3 months, ducts of the gland form by vacuolation of the cord cells and the development of lumina. Lacrimal gland (reflex) tear production does not begin until 20 or more days after birth. Therefore, newborn infants cry without tears.

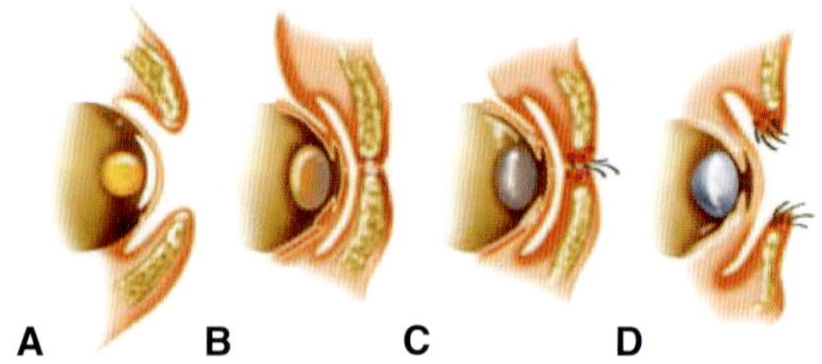

Figure 4-17 Development of the eyelids. **A,** During the seventh week, the upper and lower eyelid folds grow over the developing eye. **B,** Eyelid folds fuse during weeks 8 to 10; fusion starts along the nasal margin. **C,** Subsequently, cilia and glandular structures develop. **D,** From the fifth to seventh months, the eyelids gradually separate. *(Illustration by Paul Schiffmacher.)*

Orbit

Orbital development involves key contributions from ectodermal, mesodermal, and neural crest–derived elements. By the fourth week of gestation, the frontonasal and maxillary processes of neural crest cells occupy the space that surrounds the optic cups. The bones, cartilage, fat, and connective tissues of the orbit develop from these cells. All bones of the orbit are membranous except the sphenoid, which is initially cartilaginous. Ossification begins during the third month of gestation, and fusion occurs between the sixth and seventh months.

Genetic Cascades and Morphogenic Gradients

The embryonic genome is not transcribed until the stage of midblastula transition, which takes place several hours after fertilization. Instead, maternal messenger RNA (mRNA) is found in the oocyte, providing the initial genetic instruction set to the fertilized egg. Once embryonic transcription begins, it follows a set of predefined genetic programs.

Homeobox Gene Program

The blueprint for the embryonic program involves the homeobox genes *(HOX)*. These genes are so named because they contain a distinctive and highly conserved segment of DNA, approximately 180 base pairs long, that encodes a conserved 60–amino acid sequence constituting the homeodomain. The homeodomain provides a protein with specific DNA-binding capabilities.

The function of *HOX* genes as master regulators arises from the ability of these genes to regulate expression of downstream genes through homeodomain binding to DNA promoter sequences, wherein they act as switches of gene transcription. Each set of switches drives a particular cell fate, and transcriptional cascades of these switches lead to the development of different tissues and organs.

As expected, specific *HOX* genes are crucial for development of the eye (Fig 4-18). The paired box 6 gene, *PAX6,* in particular, appears to be a master switch for eye development. The PAX6 transcription factor is expressed in a band in the anterior neural plate, very early in the primordial eye field, and ectopic expression of *PAX6* can lead to ectopic eyes

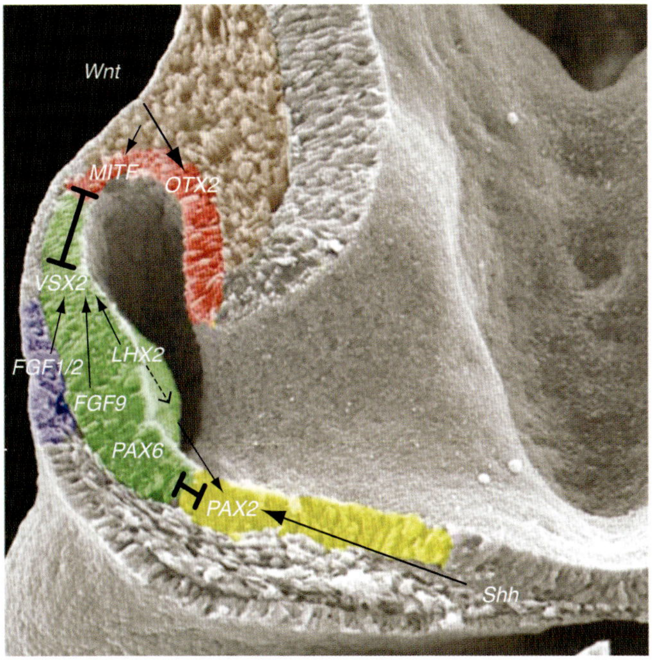

Figure 4-18 Scanning electron micrograph of an optic vesicle (dorsal is at top of image; optic stalk cavity to the left). The section is color coded to indicate the homeobox genes and diffusible extracellular factors expressed in a particular location that predetermine tissue development. Red = retinal pigment epithelium; green = retina; blue = lens; yellow = optic stalk. FGF = fibroblast growth factor; *LHX2* = LIM homeobox 2 gene; *MITF* = microphthalmia-associated transcription factor; *OTX2* = orthodenticle homeobox 2 gene; *PAX2* = paired box 2 gene; *PAX6* = paired box 6 gene; Shh = sonic hedgehog; *VSX2* = visual system homeobox 2 gene; Wnt = Wnt transcription factor. *(Modified with permission from Forrester JV, Dick AD, McMenamin PG, Roberts F, Pearlman E.* The Eye: Basic Sciences in Practice. *4th ed. Edinburgh: Elsevier; 2016:110.)*

and aniridia, Peters anomaly, coloboma, and microphthalmia. The following *HOX* genes also play key roles in development of the eye, and mutations in these genes have been reported in patients with the conditions given within parentheses: paired box 2, *PAX2* (renal coloboma syndrome), retina and anterior neural fold homeobox gene, *RAX* (eg, microphthalmia), and paired like homeodomain 2, *PITX2* (eg, Peters anomaly, Axenfeld-Rieger syndrome).

Shaham O, Menuchin Y, Farhy C, Ashery-Padan R. Pax6: a multi-level regulator of ocular development. *Prog Retin Eye Res.* 2012;31(5):351–376.

Growth Factors, Diffusible Ligands, and Morphogens

Gene-expression cascades are clearly crucial for eye development, just as they are for development of most organs. However, to respond to cues in real time, cells in the developing eye require additional signals. These signals take the form of diffusible extracellular factors (termed *morphogens*) that are active in the earliest stages of embryonic development (see Fig 4-18).

The most important of these factors include retinoic acid (RA), Wnt, fibroblast growth factors (FGFs), the hedgehog family members Shh and Ihh, and insulin-like growth factor (IGF). These factors fall into 2 broad groups: Group 1 ligands interact with intracellular receptors that directly regulate gene expression (eg, RA). Group 2 ligands interact with cell-surface receptors that initiate an intracellular signaling cascade (eg, Wnt, FGF), often involving protein phosphorylation cascades, to eventually affect gene expression and intracellular remodeling (eg, cytoskeleton), cell motility, protein trafficking, and other processes. Defects in Wnt signaling cause familial exudative vitreoretinopathy (incomplete vascularization of the peripheral retina), leading to vitreous bleeding, tractional retinal detachments, and severe visual impairment.

Cells respond differently to ligands depending on ligand concentration in the context of a concentration gradient (also termed *morphogenic gradient*). In many cases, cells and tissues that have multiple potential fates utilize these diffusible ligands to activate a particular fate. For example, FGF signaling in the optic vesicle regulates expression of the basic helix-loop-helix transcription factor MITF (microphthalmia-associated transcription factor) in the optic cup, which in turn regulates the balance between development of neural retina and pigment epithelium. The interested reader is referred to several excellent reviews on the topic of eye development and diffusible ligands in embryogenesis.

Kish PE, Bohnsack BL, Gallina D, Kasprick DS, Kahana A. The eye as an organizer of craniofacial development. *Genesis.* 2011;49(4):222–230.

Rogers KW, Schier AF. Morphogen gradients: from generation to interpretation. *Annu Rev Cell Dev Biol.* 2011;27:377–407.

Sadler TW. *Langman's Medical Embryology.* 13th ed. Philadelphia: Lippincott Williams & Wilkins; 2014.

Tabata T. Genetics of morphogen gradients. *Nat Rev Genet.* 2001;2(8):620–630.

Future Directions

The embryologic study of how a single cell (zygote) gives rise to a multitude of cell and tissue types led to the field of stem cell biology. The first successful culture of human embryonic stem cell (hESC) lines derived from spare in vitro fertilization blastocysts was reported in 1998. Stem cells range from totipotent to pluripotent to multipotent as they become more limited in their potential to form the entire range of cell and tissue types.

The strict definition of *stem cells* refers to cells that have the ability to self-renew via asymmetric cell division; the more colloquial and common definition refers to multipotent but lineage-restricted progenitor cells (eg, limbal stem cells). Although stem cell research has generally depended on the study of hESCs, the advent of induced pluripotent stem cell (iPSC) technology has allowed stem cells to be grown from a small sample of adult somatic cells, such as skin cells, and provided a more easily accessible and less politically charged model for the study of pluripotency. Stem cell models have been extremely useful in the study of organogenesis, tissue differentiation, and associated genetic cascades.

A breakthrough in ophthalmic research was reported in 2012 by Nakano and colleagues, who demonstrated the ability to generate 3-dimensional neural retina from hESCs, called *retinal organoids,* entirely in vitro. As they grow, retinal organoids follow the steps of normal embryonic development, including invagination of the optic vesicle and formation of the optic cup, in giving rise to complex, stratified retinal tissue opposed by retinal pigment epithelium (Video 4-2). This has allowed researchers to study human retinal development and disease outside the organism using simple retinal networks that function like a developing human retina. Human retinal organoids have already been used successfully to model retinal diseases and conditions affecting the retina, such as microphthalmia, Best vitelliform macular dystrophy, gyrate atrophy, Leber congenital amaurosis, and retinitis pigmentosa. Future therapies employing regenerative transplantation approaches, however, are more likely to utilize lineage-restricted progenitor cells so as to increase the likelihood of proper regeneration of function while reducing the risk of cancer.

VIDEO 4-2 Invagination of hESC-derived neural retina.
Used with permission from Nakano T, Ando S, Takata N, et al. Self-formation of optic cups and storable stratified neural retina from human ESCs. Cell Stem Cell. *2012;10(6):771–785.*

Eiraku M, Takata N, Ishibashi H, et al. Self-organizing optic-cup morphogenesis in three-dimensional culture. *Nature.* 2011;472:51–56.

Forrester JV, Dick AD, McMenamin PG, Roberts F, Pearlman E. Embryology and early development of the eye and adnexa. In: *The Eye, Basic Sciences in Practice.* 4th ed. New York: Elsevier; 2016:103–129.

Gage PJ, Zacharias AL. Signaling "cross-talk" is integrated by transcription factors in the development of the anterior segment in the eye. *Dev Dyn.* 2009;238(9):2149–2162.

Graw J. The genetic and molecular basis of congenital eye defects. *Nat Rev Genet.* 2003; 4(11):876–888.

Swaroop A, Kim D, Forrest D. Transcriptional regulation of photoreceptor development and homeostasis in the mammalian retina. *Nat Rev Neurosci.* 2010;11(8):563–576.

PART III
Genetics

Introduction

Genetics is the study of heredity and the variations in inherited characteristics and diseases. Although genetics is a relatively new science compared with such disciplines as anatomy and physiology, its significance in the overall understanding of human life cannot be overstated. Genetic knowledge can enhance our understanding of the processes of cellular function, embryology, and development, as well as our concepts of disease. Many researchers think that as much as 90% of medical disease either has a major genetic component or involves genetic factors that may significantly influence the disease.

The discovery of previously unknown genes, such as the *homeobox genes* (eg, the *HOX* and *PAX* gene families)—which regulate, guide, and coordinate early embryologic development and differentiation—has opened new areas of understanding of physiology at the cellular or tissue level. (These genes, also called *homeotic selector genes,* are discussed in Part II, Embryology, as well.) Another example is the identification of the genes that appear to be transcribed as initiating events in the process of *apoptosis,* or programmed cell death, which itself appears crucial for normal embryogenesis as well as for degenerative diseases and cancers.

Genetic disorders affect about 5% of live-born infants in the United States. Approximately 50% of childhood blindness has a genetic cause. Some 20,000–25,000 human genes involving about 180,000 exons are known. In 10%–15% of known genetic diseases, clinical findings are limited to the eye; a similar percentage includes systemic disorders with ocular manifestations.

Terminology

Familiarity with the vocabulary of genetics and molecular biology will greatly enhance the reader's understanding of the following 2 chapters on molecular and clinical genetics. The reader is thus encouraged to review the genetics glossary in the appendix of this book, which includes many key genetics terms, as well as to consult online resources, 2 examples of which follow.

National Cancer Institute Dictionary of Genetics Terms. https://www.cancer.gov/publications/dictionaries/genetics-dictionary

National Human Genome Research Institute Talking Glossary of Genetic Terms. https://www.genome.gov/genetics-glossary/

CHAPTER 5

Molecular Genetics

Highlights

- Cell division occurs via a complex process known as the *cell cycle.* The function of tumor suppressor genes is to regulate this cycle. Mutations to these genes result in numerous conditions with ophthalmic manifestations, examples of which are neurocutaneous disorders (phakomatoses) and retinoblastoma.
- Approximately 99% of DNA does not code for proteins and may be involved in regulation of gene expression. The term *epigenetics* refers to the study of heritable processes that alter gene expression without changing the DNA sequence.
- Transcription factors determine the rate of messenger RNA production from DNA. The family of *PAX* genes encodes for transcription factors, mutations of which are involved in the development of numerous ophthalmic conditions.
- Alternate splicing allows different isoforms of a particular protein to be expressed. Vascular endothelial growth factor and its receptors have various isoforms due to this mechanism.
- Mitochondrial DNA (mtDNA) is passed on to children from their mothers. Many diseases with ophthalmic manifestations occur because of mutations in mtDNA, including chronic progressive external ophthalmoplegia and Leber hereditary optic neuropathy.
- New gene therapies such as AAV (adeno-associated virus) vector gene therapy and the CRISPR-Cas9 system have the potential to treat many previously untreatable eye diseases.

The Cell Cycle

The cell cycle is the series of events that take place in a cell leading to its duplication and division (Fig 5-1). The 4 distinct phases are

- G_1 (growth, preparation for DNA synthesis)
- S (DNA synthesis/chromosome replication)
- G_2 (growth, preparation for mitosis)
- M (mitosis and cytokinesis)

The M phase consists of 2 processes: *mitosis,* in which the cell's chromosomes are divided between the 2 sister cells, followed by *cytokinesis,* in which the cell's cytoplasm divides in

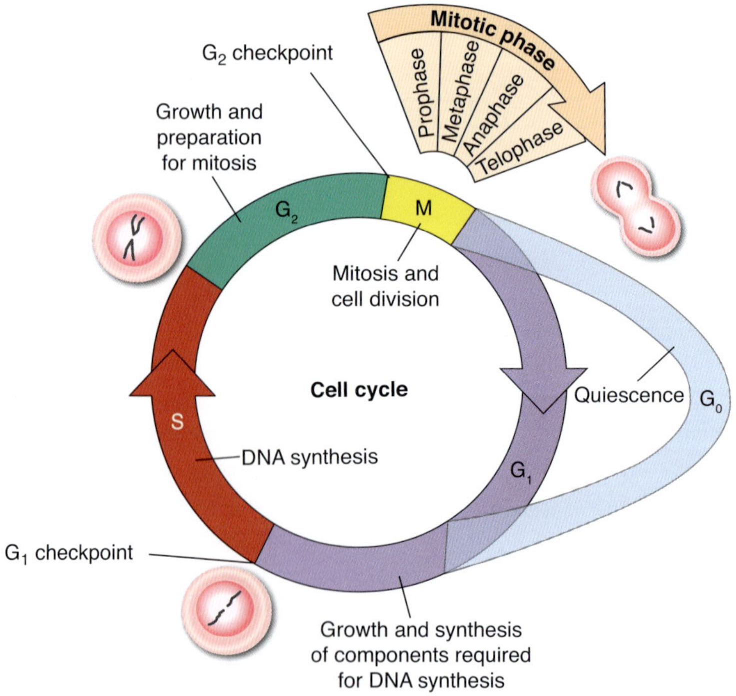

Figure 5-1 In the cell cycle, the progression from DNA synthesis (S) to mitosis (M) includes phases before (G_1) and after (G_2) the replication of DNA. Upon receiving signals to differentiate, cells leave the cycle and enter the final stage of cell differentiation, or terminal differentiation. Regulation of the cycle occurs at numerous checkpoints, before the cell progresses from one phase to another. Under certain circumstances, cells may return to quiescence (G_0) or enter the pathway to programmed cell death (apoptosis).

half and forms distinct cells. Cells that have temporarily stopped dividing are said to have entered a state of quiescence called the *G_0 phase.* The M phase can be subdivided into several distinct, sequential phases:

- *prophase* (chromatin is condensed into chromosomes)
- *metaphase* (chromosomes align in the middle of the cell)
- *anaphase* (chromosomes split and migrate to opposite poles of the cell)
- *telophase* (2 daughter nuclei form at the poles of the cell)

Mitosis refers to somatic cell division, whereas meiosis refers to replication of germ cells.

Meiosis

Meiosis is a specialized type of cell division necessary for sexual reproduction in eukaryotes because the cells produced by meiosis are ova and sperm. It consists of 2 successive cell divisions, meiosis I and meiosis II. Unlike in mitosis, in meiosis the chromosomes undergo a recombination that shuffles the genes from each parent, producing a different genetic combination in each gamete. The outcome of meiosis is 4 genetically unique haploid cells, whereas the outcome of mitosis is 2 genetically identical diploid cells.

Interphase consists of the G_1 and S phases (there is no G_2 phase in meiosis) and is followed by meiosis I and then meiosis II. Meiosis I and II are each divided into prophase, metaphase, anaphase, and telophase stages, as in the mitotic cell cycle. In the G_1 phase, each of the chromosomes consists of a single (very long) molecule of DNA. At this stage in humans, the cells contain 46 chromosomes, the same number as in somatic cells. During S phase, the chromosomes duplicate, so that each of the 46 chromosomes becomes a complex of 2 identical sister chromatids.

During meiosis I, homologous chromosomes (a matched pair, 1 derived from each parent) separate into 2 cells. The entire haploid content of each chromosome is contained in each of the resulting daughter cells; the first meiotic division thus reduces the ploidy of the original cell by half.

During meiosis II, each chromosome's sister strands (the chromatids) are decoupled, and the individual chromatids are segregated into haploid daughter cells. The 2 cells resulting from meiosis I divide during meiosis II, creating 4 haploid daughter cells.

Chromosomal *crossing over* is the exchange of genetic material between homologous chromosomes that results in recombinant chromosomes. It occurs during prophase of the first meiotic division (prophase I), usually when matching regions on matching chromosomes break and then reconnect to the other chromosome. Although the same genes appear in the same order, the alleles are different. It is theoretically possible to have any combination of parental alleles in an offspring. This theory of *independent assortment* of alleles is fundamental to genetic inheritance. However, the chances of recombination are greater the farther apart 2 genes are from each other. The genetic distance is described in centimorgans (cM; named for Thomas Hunt Morgan, who described crossing over), and a distance of 1 cM between genes represents a 1% chance of their crossing over in 1 meiosis.

Genetic *linkage* describes the tendency of genes to be inherited together as a result of their proximity on the same chromosome. *Linkage disequilibrium* occurs when combinations of alleles are present in a population more or less frequently than would be expected based on their distances apart from each other. This concept is applied in searches for a gene that may cause a particular disease.

Although crossovers typically occur between homologous regions of matching chromosomes, a mismatch or unbalanced recombination may occur. This rare event can be a local duplication or deletion of genes on 1 chromosome, a translocation of part of 1 chromosome onto a different one, or an inversion of a part of the chromosome.

Cell Cycle Regulation

In the cell cycle, transition from one phase to the next is regulated at checkpoints (see Fig 5-1). Important checkpoints occur at the following:

- G_1: transition from G_1 to S
- G_2: transition from G_2 to M

Checkpoints allow monitoring of the cell to verify the successful, error-free completion of the previous phase. At the G_1 checkpoint, cell size and the availability of nutrients and growth factors are assessed, and the cell is checked for DNA damage. After completion of this checkpoint, the cell is committed to proceeding with cell division; otherwise, it enters the quiescent G_0 phase. Before the cycle progresses to the M phase, further inspection of the DNA occurs at the G_2 checkpoint. If damaged DNA is detected at either checkpoint, it may be repaired, or programmed cell death (see the section Apoptosis) may be initiated.

Checkpoint regulation occurs via a family of proteins known as *cyclins* and *cyclin-dependent kinases (CDKs).* At the G_1 checkpoint, CDK phosphorylation of proteins of the retinoblastoma (Rb) family facilitates downstream transcription in preparation for S phase. Tumor suppressor genes like the Rb family often have a role in regulation of the cell cycle, dysregulation of which can lead to cancer (see the section "Tumor suppressor genes").

Sun A, Bagella L, Tutton S, Romano G, Giordano A. From G0 to S phase: a view of the roles played by the retinoblastoma (Rb) family members in the Rb-E2F pathway. *J Cell Biochem.* 2007;102(6):1400–1404.

Gene Structure

Composed of DNA, *genes* are the molecular units of heredity and are located primarily in the cell nucleus, where they are assembled into *chromosomes* of varying sizes. Paired chromosomes are numbered from largest (1) to smallest (22), and there are 2 additional sex chromosomes (XY or XX). The 4 bases present in DNA—adenine (A), cytosine (C), guanine (G), and thymine (T)—are combined into a double-helix structure that allows replication, transcription, and translation. The genetic structure (Fig 5-2) can be likened to the sections of an encyclopedia, with genes the chapters, *exons* the sentences, *trinucleotides* the words, and *nucleotides* the letters.

Mitochondria, the site of oxidative phosphorylation, are the power plants of the cell. The mitochondria are a vestige of a symbiotic relationship between 2 primitive unicellular organisms that merged to form eukaryotic organisms (most animals and plants). The fact that mitochondria still contain their own DNA is a reminder of their independent origin. Each mitochondrion contains 2–10 copies of a very short, circular segment containing 13 protein-coding genes involved in oxidative phosphorylation. Because mitochondria contain several segments of DNA and each cell contains several mitochondria, there may be variation of the mitochondrial DNA (mtDNA) within a cell and between cells of the same person, a state known as *heteroplasmy.* Humans acquire mitochondria from the ovum, and thus mtDNA follows maternal line inheritance.

Chromosomal DNA replication and RNA synthesis (transcription) occur within the nucleus. Messenger RNA (mRNA) is transported to ribosomes in the cytoplasm, where translation to the amino acid sequences of proteins occurs. Following the mRNA molecule's initiation codon (start sequence) is the structural *open reading frame (ORF),* which is composed of *exons* (sequences that code for amino acids that will be present in the final protein) and *introns* (sequences that are spliced out during the processing of mRNA). Following the last exon is the *3′ untranslated region (3′ UTR).* The function of this region is partly regulatory.

The development of introns in higher organisms may have had evolutionary benefits. The compartmentalization of coding segments into exons may have permitted more rapid evolution of proteins by allowing for alternative processing of precursor RNA (alternative

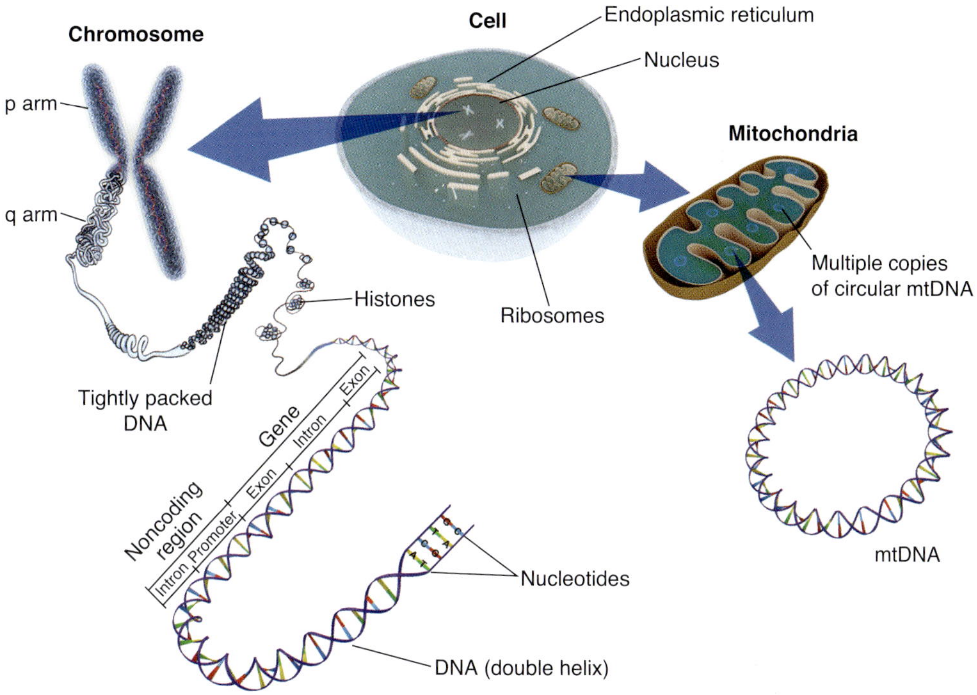

Figure 5-2 Structures of the cell showing the location of DNA within chromosomes and mitochondria. The basic double helix of nucleotides is divided into noncoding regions, including introns and promoter regions, and coding exons, which form genes. The figure shows a noncoding intron between 2 exons. The intron is spliced out before the segment is translated. This modification occurs following transcription, though before messenger RNA (mRNA) is finalized.

splicing) and for rearrangements of exons during gene duplication (exon shuffling). Some introns contain complete, separate genes, and some of these may cause disease or influence the expression of other genes. Expansion of unstable repeats within introns can cause abnormal splicing and result in genetic disease. Small insertions and deletions are very common and referred to as *indels.*

Noncoding DNA

The majority of DNA—approximately 99% of the base sequences in human DNA—does not code for proteins. Noncoding DNA is composed of highly repetitive sequences, some of which include *satellites, microsatellites, short interspersed elements (SINEs),* and *long interspersed elements (LINEs).* The 300-base-pair (bp) *Alu* sequence, named after the restriction enzyme used to identify it, is the repetitive DNA that appears most frequently. Noncoding DNA comprises introns, promoters, and other regions within chromosomes and mitochondria and is involved in regulating gene expression and exon splicing.

RNA transcribed from noncoding DNA may directly influence the transcription of other sequences and participate in normal genome repair and regulation. Some of the repetitive sequences of nontranscribed DNA form *telomeric DNA,* which is essential for the correct formation and maintenance of chromosomes. Loss of telomeric DNA correlates with cell senescence. Defects in telomeric DNA maintenance have been proposed to be associated with carcinogenesis.

Gene Transcription and Translation: The Central Dogma of Genetics

The central dogma of gene transcription and translation is that the DNA code is transcribed as mRNA code and then translated as amino acid code of the resulting protein (Fig 5-3). The trinucleotides that correspond with amino acids have some redundancy in the system, so that a nucleotide change may not necessarily result in a change in amino acid. The coding region of DNA is composed of exons, several of which are spliced together to make the full coding sequence of RNA. Although the central dogma specifies that DNA determines RNA sequence and that RNA determines amino acid sequence, there are feedback and regulatory mechanisms of gene expression that are both genetically and environmentally determined. These mechanisms, such as methylation and histone

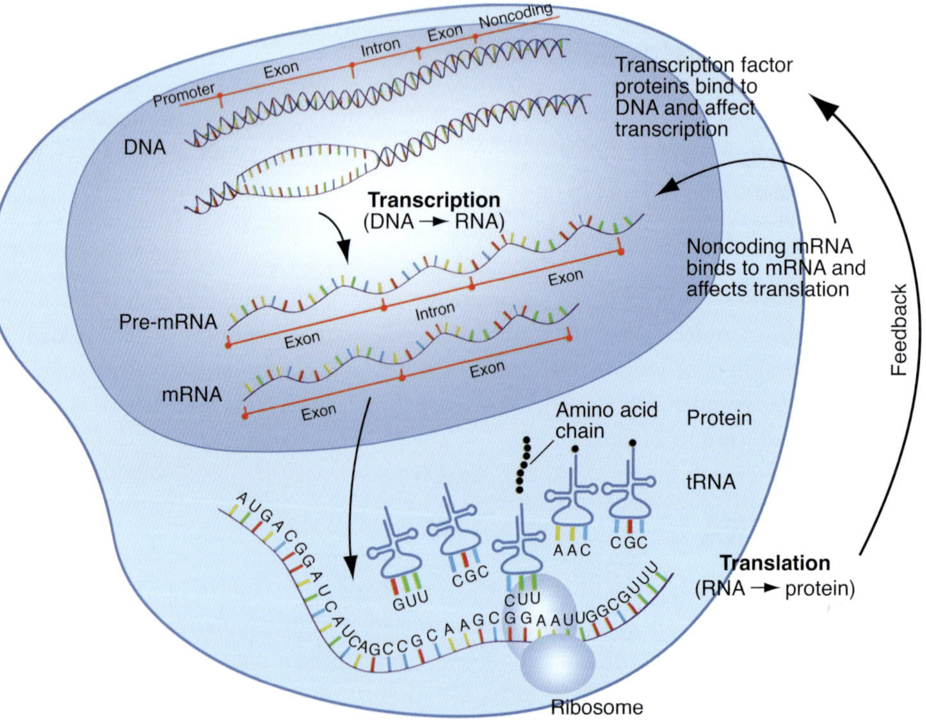

Figure 5-3 The central dogma of genetics, as represented schematically, is that DNA sequence codes are transcribed to the mRNA sequence, and then the mRNA transcription is translated into the amino acid sequence of the coded protein. However, proteins in the form of transcription factors and complementary short RNA sequences can modify translation and transcription. These proteins are being investigated as potential forms of therapy.

formation, can silence gene expression. In addition, small segments of RNA can block mRNA. The study of the influence of these regulatory mechanisms in gene and disease expression is known as *epigenetics.*

Genes control cellular activity through 2 processes:

1. transcription *(expression),* in which DNA molecules give rise to RNA molecules, followed by translation in most cases
2. *translation,* in which RNA directs the synthesis of proteins. Translation occurs in ribosomes, where mRNA induces transfer RNA (tRNA)–mediated recruitment of amino acids to "build" a protein. A more in-depth description of translation is beyond the scope of this chapter.

Transcription factors are proteins that bind to specific DNA sequences and thus control the flow (or transcription) of genetic information from DNA to mRNA. Transcription factors perform this function by promoting or repressing the recruitment of RNA polymerase to specific genes.

Approximately 10% of genes in the human genome code for transcription factors. They contain one or more DNA-binding domains, which attach to specific sequences of DNA adjacent to the genes that they regulate. There are numerous families of these genes, including the homeobox and paired box genes. *PAX6* acts as a master control gene for the development of the eye, an example of the key role of transcription factors in embryogenesis.

Many ophthalmic diseases result from transcription-factor mutations. *PAX2* mutations cause colobomas of the optic nerve and renal hypoplasia. *PAX3* mutations cause Waardenburg syndrome with dystopia canthorum (types WS1 and WS3). *PAX6* mutations are the basis of virtually all cases of aniridia, occasional cases of Peters anomaly, and several other rarer phenotypes, specifically autosomal dominant keratitis and dominant foveal hypoplasia.

Fitzpatrick DR, van Heyningen V. Developmental eye disorders. *Curr Opin Genet Dev.* 2005;15(3):348–353.

Intron Excision

Messenger RNA undergoes excision of the introns by a highly organized process called *splicing,* which leaves the mRNA composed of only exons, or coding segments. The exons can then undergo translation in the ribosomes. Splicing takes place in specialized structures called *spliceosomes,* which are composed of RNA and proteins. Errors of splicing can lead to genetic disease. Approximately 15% of point mutations that cause human disease do so by generating splicing errors that result in aberrations such as exon skipping, intron retention, or use of a cryptic splice site. For example, mutations in proteins that are vital in splicing can cause retinitis pigmentosa (RP).

Alternative Splicing and Isoforms

Alternative splicing is the creation of multiple pre-mRNA sequences from the same gene by the action of different promoters. These promoters cause certain exons to be skipped during transcription of the gene. The protein products of alternative splicing are often called *isoforms.* The promoters are usually tissue specific, so different tissues express different isoforms. The gene for dystrophin is an example of alternative splicing: full-length dystrophin is the major isoform expressed in muscle; shorter isoforms predominate in the retina, peripheral nerve, and central nervous system.

Another example of alternative splicing's relevance underlies the basis of the cornea's avascularity. Vascular endothelial growth factor (VEGF) receptor 1 is a key blood vessel receptor that binds and transduces a signal from the primary mediator of angiogenesis, VEGF. In the cornea, high levels of an alternatively spliced isoform, soluble VEGF receptor 1 (sVEGFR-1), are expressed. As this isoform is soluble, it is present in the extracellular matrix and serves as an endogenous VEGF trap or decoy receptor. Without it, there are increased levels of free VEGF, and the cornea becomes vulnerable to vascular invasion.

Ambati BK, Nozaki M, Singh N, et al. Corneal avascularity is due to soluble VEGF receptor-1. *Nature.* 2006;443(7114):993–997.

Methylation

Regions of DNA that are undergoing transcription lack 5-methyl cytosine residues, which normally account for 1%–5% of total DNA. Evidence suggests a close correlation between methylation and gene inactivation. Regulation of DNA methylation may be responsible for imprinting control. Methylation may account for variation in phenotypic expression of some diseases.

Hjelmeland LM. Dark matters in AMD genetics: epigenetics and stochasticity. *Invest Ophthalmol Vis Sci.* 2011;52(3):1622–1631.

X-Inactivation

The random permanent inactivation of 1 of the 2 X chromosomes in the female, resulting in the lack of expression of the majority of genes on that chromosome, is a significant event during early development of the human embryo. The time of X-inactivation is not precisely known but is thought to vary over a period of several cell divisions during the blastocyst–gastrula transition. X-inactivation is also known as *lyonization,* after its discoverer, Mary Lyon. Lyonization affects the severity of the phenotype of several X-linked retinal conditions, such as RP and incontinentia pigmenti.

Imprinting

Genomic imprinting is a heritable yet reversible process by which a gene is modified, depending on which parent provides it. The mechanism is unclear but appears to operate at the chromatin organization level and involves heterochromatization and methylation of CpG (cytosine-phosphate-guanine) sites. Examples of genes that can be imprinted include the Wilms tumor–suppressor gene and the human *SNRPN* (small nuclear ribonucleoprotein polypeptide N) gene.

Prader-Willi and Angelman syndromes are examples of diseases resulting from abnormalities of imprinting. Approximately 70%–80% of patients with Prader-Willi syndrome harbor a deletion of the paternally derived 15q11–q13, resulting in the loss of this region's normal contribution from the paternal line. About 70%–80% of patients with Angelman syndrome also have a deletion of 15q11–q13, but from the maternally derived chromosome, resulting in loss of the maternal contribution. Chromosome 15 uniparental disomy, wherein both copies of chromosome 15 are inherited from the same parent, can also cause each syndrome. The 2 chromosomes 15 in uniparental disomy are maternal in Prader-Willi syndrome and paternal in Angelman syndrome. The *SNRPN* gene maps to 15q11–q13 but appears to be expressed only from the paternally inherited allele.

DNA Damage and Repair

DNA is constantly sustaining damage from mutagens such as ultraviolet (UV) light, chemicals, and spontaneous deamination. Each cell loses 10,000 bases per day from spontaneous DNA breakdown related to normal body temperature alone. In the absence of repair, these mutations would accumulate and result in tumor formation. Damaged DNA is estimated to cause approximately 80%–90% of cancers in humans.

Repair

Damaged DNA sites are repaired chiefly by 2 mechanisms: *excision repair* and *mismatch repair.* The processes of replication, transcription, mismatch repair, excision repair, and gene expression are closely coordinated by cross-acting systems. Enzymes that cut or patch segments of DNA during crossing over at meiosis are also involved in DNA repair. Molecules that unwind double-stranded DNA (called *helicases*) are involved in replication, transcription, and DNA excision repair.

The tumor protein P53, also called TP53 or p53, appears to play an extremely important role as the "guardian of the genome" by preventing cells from proliferating if their DNA is irreparably damaged. Levels of p53 increase after UV or ionizing radiation exposure. The p53 gene inhibits DNA replication directly and binds with 1 of the RNA polymerase transcription factors, TFIIH. If the degree of damage is slight, increased production of p53 induces reversible cell arrest until DNA repair can take place. If DNA damage is too great or irreversible, p53 production is massively increased and apoptosis occurs, probably through stimulation of the expression of the *BAX* gene, whose product promotes apoptosis. Loss of p53 causes cells to fail to arrest in response to DNA damage, and these cells do not enter apoptosis. Thus, mutations of p53 predispose to tumorigenesis.

The gene mutated in ataxia-telangiectasia (Louis-Bar syndrome), a protein kinase called *ATM,* also appears to be integrally involved in DNA repair, possibly by informing the cell of radiation damage. The *ATM* gene product associates with synaptonemal complexes, promotes chromosomal synapsis, and is required for meiosis. Individuals with ataxia-telangiectasia have a threefold greater risk of cancer.

Xeroderma pigmentosum is a severe condition in which the functions of enzymes that repair UV-damaged DNA are crippled. Patients with this condition typically have diffuse pigmented anomalies on their sun-exposed skin and are at high risk for basal cell and squamous cell carcinoma, as well as melanoma. Ocular surface cancers (squamous cell carcinoma and melanoma) can also develop in affected patients.

Lim R, Sethi M, Morley AMS. Ophthalmic manifestations of xeroderma pigmentosum: a perspective from the United Kingdom. *Ophthalmology*. 2017;124(11):1652–1661.

Apoptosis

Apoptosis is a Greek word describing leaves dropping from trees. (*Ptosis,* drooping of the upper eyelid, comes from the same root.) Apoptosis is the process of programmed cell death that occurs in multicellular organisms, in contrast to necrosis, a form of traumatic cell death that results from acute cellular injury. Biochemical events in apoptosis result in characteristic cell changes and cell death. Morphological changes include cell shrinkage, nuclear fragmentation, chromatin condensation, and chromosomal DNA fragmentation. Several key events in apoptosis focus on the mitochondria, including the release of caspase activators, changes in electron transport, loss of mitochondrial transmembrane potential, altered cellular reduction-oxidation (redox) reactions, and activation of pro- and anti-apoptotic Bcl-2 family proteins.

Apoptosis is crucial in the developing human embryo; scaffolding cells such as those involved in eyelid opening are removed by epidermal apoptosis. In later life, excessive apoptosis causes atrophy, such as occurs in RP or glaucoma, whereas insufficient apoptosis results in uncontrolled cell proliferation, such as occurs in cancers, including retinoblastoma.

Mutations and Disease

Mutations Versus Polymorphisms

Mutations are changes in DNA that can lead to disease, whereas polymorphisms are variations in DNA that were previously thought to rarely cause disease. The difference is not always easy to determine. In general, mutations change amino acid sequence or, more dramatically, lead to a shortening or nonproduction of the protein encoded by the gene. Polymorphisms tend not to cause a change in the amino acid sequence (because of the built-in redundancy in the DNA code) or a change from one amino acid to a similar amino acid. However, some synonymous changes, though not changes in amino acid sequence, could affect splicing. Many of the disease-associated single nucleotide polymorphisms (SNPs) identified in genome-wide association studies (GWAS) are found in the noncoding regions of the genome.

Mutations

Mutations can involve a change in a single base pair; simple deletion or insertion of DNA material; or more complex rearrangements such as inversions, duplications, or translocations. Deletion, insertion, or duplication of any number of base pairs in other than groups of 3 creates a frameshift in the entire DNA sequence downstream, resulting in the eventual formation of a stop codon and truncation of the message.

Mutations that result in no active gene product being produced are called *null mutations.* Null mutations include missense or nonsense mutations that (1) produce either a stop codon directly or a frameshift with creation of a premature stop codon downstream or (2) cause an alteration at the acceptor splice junction site, resulting in the loss of exons or inappropriate incorporation of introns into the spliced mRNA.

Mutations can also lead to a gain of function that may be beneficial (leading to evolution) or detrimental (leading to disease). An example of a beneficial gain in function is the emergence, among bacteria, of antibiotic resistance. An example of a detrimental gain of function is a receptor protein that binds too tightly with its target protein, creating loss of normal physiologic function. Most autosomal dominant disorders are of this type.

Single base-pair mutations may code for the same amino acid or a tolerable change in the amino acid sequence, leading to harmless polymorphisms or DNA variations that are in turn inherited. These are called *conserved base-pair mutations.*

Polymorphisms

A polymorphism is any variation in DNA sequence that occurs, by convention, at a frequency of greater than 1% in the normal population. Key polymorphisms associated with disease include those in the region of the *CFH* gene in age-related macular degeneration and the *LOXL1* gene in pseudoexfoliation syndrome. Many polymorphisms are silent and simply linked to the disease mutation, but some may influence disease.

Cancer Genes

Cancer can result from any of a number of genetic mechanisms, including the activation of oncogenes and the loss of tumor suppressor genes. The product of proto-oncogenes is often involved in signal transduction of external messages to the intracellular machinery that governs normal cell growth and differentiation. As such, the DNA sequences of proto-oncogenes are highly conserved in nature between such different organisms as humans and yeast. Proto-oncogenes can be activated to oncogenes by loss or disruption of normal gene regulation.

Oncogenes

Oncogenes were first detected in retroviruses, which had acquired them from their host in order to take control of cell growth. These oncogenes are often identified by names that refer to the viral source, as for example, *ras* (*ra*t *s*arcoma virus). They are known to be activated not only in virus-induced malignancies but in common nonviral cancers in humans. Oncogenes behave the same way that autosomal dominant traits behave, and only 1 mutant allele is needed for tumor formation, presumably by a dominant-negative effect on regulation of signal transduction.

Tumor suppressor genes

Tumor suppressor genes, also called *antioncogenes,* are genes that must be present in 1 functional copy to prevent uncontrolled cell proliferation. Although some may represent genes whose products participate in checkpoints for the cell cycle, a characteristic of tumor suppressor genes is the diversity of their normal functions. Examples of tumor suppressor genes include the genes for retinoblastoma, Wilms tumor, neurofibromatosis types 1 and 2, tuberous sclerosis, ataxia-telangiectasia, and von Hippel–Lindau disease. All of these examples (except ataxia-telangiectasia) behave as autosomal dominant traits, but the mechanism of tumor formation for tumor suppressor genes is very different from that for oncogenes. If 1 allele is already defective because of a hereditary mutation, the other allele must also be lost for tumor formation to occur (also known as the *2-hit hypothesis*). This loss of the second allele is termed *loss of heterozygosity,* and it can occur from a second mutation, gene deletion, chromosomal loss, or mitotic recombination.

Mitochondrial Disease

A significant number of disorders associated with the eye or visual system involve mitochondrial deletions and mutations. Mitochondrial diseases should be considered whenever the inheritance pattern of a trait suggests maternal transmission. Although the inheritance pattern might superficially resemble that of an X-linked trait, maternal transmission differs in that all of the offspring of affected females—both daughters and sons—can inherit the trait, but only the daughters can pass it on.

The phenotype and severity of mitochondrial disease appear to depend on the nature of the mutation, the presence or degree of heteroplasmy (coexistence of more than 1 species of mitochondrial DNA [mtDNA]—ie, wild type and mutant), and the oxidative needs of the tissues involved. Spontaneous deletions and mutations of mtDNA accumulate with age, and the effect of this accumulation is to decrease the efficiency and function of the electron transport system, reducing the availability of adenosine triphosphate (ATP). When energy production becomes insufficient to maintain the function of cells or tissue, disease occurs. There appears to be an important interaction between age and tissue threshold of oxidative phosphorylation and the expression of inherited mutations of mtDNA.

With each cell division, the number of mutant mtDNA copies that are partitioned to a given daughter cell is random, unlike in mendelian inheritance. After a number of cell divisions, some cells, purely by chance, receive more normal or more mutant copies of mtDNA, resulting in a drift toward homoplasmy in subsequent cell lines. This process is called *replicative segregation.* With mtDNA deletions, preferential replication of the smaller deleted molecules causes an increase of the deleted copy over time. The trend toward homoplasmy helps explain why disease worsens with age and why organ systems not previously involved in multisystem mitochondrial disease become involved.

Causes of mitochondrial diseases can be categorized as follows:

- large rearrangements of mtDNA (deletions or insertions), such as chronic progressive external ophthalmoplegia (CPEO), Kearns-Sayre syndrome, and Pearson marrow-pancreas syndrome
- mutations of mtDNA-encoded ribosomal RNA (rRNA), such as occur in maternally inherited sensorineural deafness and aminoglycoside-induced deafness
- mutations of mtDNA-encoded tRNA, such as occur in the syndromes of MELAS (*m*itochondrial *e*ncephalomyopathy, *l*actic *a*cidosis, and *s*trokelike episodes),

MERRF (*m*yoclonic *e*pilepsy with *r*agged *r*ed *f*ibers), MIDD (*m*aternally *i*nherited *d*iabetes and *d*eafness), and (in about 30% of cases) CPEO
- missense and nonsense mutations, such as are present in Leber hereditary optic neuropathy; and neuropathy, ataxia, and RP

Chronic Progressive External Ophthalmoplegia

CPEO is a disorder involving progressive ptosis and paralysis of eye muscles associated with a ragged red myopathy, usually as a result of deletion of a portion of the mitochondrial genome. Patients with CPEO commonly have pigmentary retinopathy that does not create significant visual disability. Infrequently, they may have more marked retinal or other system involvement, the so-called *CPEO-plus syndromes.* In Kearns-Sayre syndrome, CPEO is associated with heart block and severe RP with marked visual impairment. Pearson marrow-pancreas syndrome results from a large deletion of mtDNA and presents in younger patients with an entirely different phenotype involving sideroblastic anemia and pancreatic exocrine dysfunction. However, in patients afflicted during their later years, Pearson marrow-pancreas syndrome can present with a phenotype resembling that of Kearns-Sayre syndrome.

Roughly 50% of patients with CPEO have demonstrable mtDNA deletions, whereas virtually all patients with Kearns-Sayre syndrome have large deletions. Of patients with CPEO who do not harbor demonstrable mtDNA deletions, up to 30% may have a point mutation at nucleotide position 3243, the same mutation in the tRNA for leucine that in other individuals is associated with MELAS syndrome. For all syndromes associated with deletions, such as Kearns-Sayre and CPEO, detection of the deletion usually requires study of the muscle tissue.

MELAS and MIDD

Two different disorders—mitochondrial encephalomyopathy, lactic acidosis, and stroke-like episodes (MELAS) and maternally inherited diabetes and deafness (MIDD; also called *type 2 diabetes mellitus with deafness*)—are associated with an mtDNA point mutation (A-to-G change at nucleotide position 3243), which affects an mtDNA-encoded tRNA. Macular retinal pigment epithelial atrophy and this mutation have been described in patients with MELAS.

Isashiki Y, Nakagawa M, Ohba N, et al. Retinal manifestations in mitochondrial diseases associated with mitochondrial DNA mutation. *Acta Ophthalmol Scand.* 1998;76(1):6–13.

Yu-Wai-Man P, Griffiths PG, Hudson G, Chinnery PF. Inherited mitochondrial optic neuropathies. *J Med Genet.* 2009;46(3):145–158.

Leber Hereditary Optic Neuropathy

The most important ophthalmic disease of mitochondria is Leber hereditary optic neuropathy (LHON), which is more prevalent in males than in females but does not fit a classic X-linked pattern of transmission. The trait is not transmitted to the offspring of affected males, but virtually every daughter and son of a female patient with LHON inherits the trait. In approximately 50% of cases, LHON development is correlated with a single base change (G to A at nucleotide position 11778 in the *ND-4* gene) in human mtDNA involved in the synthesis of NADH dehydrogenase. In addition to optic atrophy, patients can exhibit peripapillary microangiopathy. LHON can also occur from other so-called primary mutations at nucleotide positions 3460 of *ND-1* and 14484 of *ND-6,* as well as several other rare mutations. At least 12 secondary mutations have been associated with LHON, often when multiple mutations are present in an individual's mitochondria. Some authors think that these secondary mutations cause disease by additive detrimental effects on the electron transport system of oxidative phosphorylation. Most of these secondary mutations appear in the general population, and debate persists on whether each mutation alone is truly pathogenic.

The likelihood of improvement of visual acuity over time appears to differ among patients with the separate mutations associated with LHON. Mutation at nucleotide position 11778 is associated with the least likelihood of recovery, and mutation at nucleotide position 14484 is associated with the greatest likelihood.

Neuropathy, Ataxia, and Retinitis Pigmentosa

Neuropathy, ataxia, and retinitis pigmentosa (NARP) is associated with a single base-pair mutation at nucleotide position 8993 in the *ATPase-6* gene. The NARP phenotype occurs when the percentage of mutant mtDNA is less than 80%, whereas the same mutation present at much higher proportions (greater than 95%) can cause Leigh syndrome, a severe neurodegenerative disease of infancy and early childhood. The 8993 mutation is demonstrable in fibroblasts and lymphoblasts.

The Search for Genes in Specific Diseases

A variety of methods have been used to assign individual genes to specific chromosomes, to link individual genes to one another, and to link diseases to specific genes.

Polymerase Chain Reaction

Polymerase chain reaction (PCR) is a technique used in molecular biology to amplify a single copy or a few copies of a segment of DNA or RNA by several orders of magnitude, generating thousands to millions of copies of a particular DNA sequence. PCR is a common and indispensable technique used in clinical and research laboratories for a broad variety of applications. Clinically, PCR has been utilized in establishing the etiology of ocular infections. For example, PCR performed on ocular fluids can detect numerous members of the herpes virus family.

PCR methods rely on thermal cycling, which involves exposing the reactants to repeated cycles of heating and cooling, permitting different temperature-dependent reactions of DNA melting and enzyme-driven DNA replication. Primers (short DNA fragments) containing sequences complementary to the target region, along with a DNA polymerase (usually Taq polymerase), enable selective and repeated amplification. As PCR progresses, the

DNA generated is itself used as a template for replication, setting in motion a chain reaction in which the original DNA template is exponentially amplified.

Sugita S, Ogawa M, Shimizu N, et al. Use of a comprehensive polymerase chain reaction system for diagnosis of ocular infectious diseases. *Ophthalmology.* 2013;120(9):1761–1768.

Genetic Markers

Occasionally in cytogenetic studies, a genetic marker such as a large deletion or translocation (eg, 11p13 in aniridia) may be visible. Other markers used to identify the location of genes include blood groups (eg, as in Duffy blood group and Coppock cataract); restriction fragment length polymorphisms (RFLPs; eg, as in RP); microsatellites of variable number of tandem repeats (VNTRs); and most recently SNPs, as used in many GWAS. Cytogenetic tests are conducted on white blood cells, whereas the other genetic markers test DNA that is extracted most commonly from peripheral blood or saliva.

If a specific chromosomal structure is abnormal or even normally variant, its transmission through a family with a hereditary disease, as mapped by a pedigree, may support the assumption that the mutant gene and the variant chromosome are comigrating. Thus, the mutant gene is likely to be physically located on the variant chromosome—that is, the gene is a cytogenetic marker for the disease.

Gene Dosage

If a portion of a chromosome containing a specific gene is deleted, the amount of the gene product will be determined only by the remaining homologue. For example, people with an interstitial deletion of part of the long arm of chromosome 13 may have serum levels of esterase D that are 50% of normal. When several such individuals were also found to have retinoblastoma, it was suggested that both the esterase and the retinoblastoma genes are located in the missing segment. In contrast to the reduced activity caused by a deletion, a duplication may produce 150% of normal activity of a given gene product, as a result of either a chromosomal trisomy or a triplication of a specific chromosomal segment. Gene dosage appears to be a mechanism of disease in anterior segment dysgenesis, caused by duplication or deletion of the *FOXC1* gene; both 50% and 150% of the transcription factor lead to this dysgenesis.

Linkage and Disease Association

Even if no information is known about the nature or function of a gene for a disease, linkage studies may be able to localize the gene to a given chromosome or a specific marker. In 1937, Bell and Haldane recognized the first linkage between 2 diseases on a human chromosome: congenital color vision deficiency and hemophilia on the X chromosome. Subsequent investigations have led to the chromosomal mapping of a large number of different human ocular diseases.

Gene assignments

Every chromosome has numerous defined genes. The Human Genome Project identified and mapped approximately 20,000–25,000 genes. In addition, the database Online

Mendelian Inheritance in Man, OMIM (https://omim.org), lists information on all known mendelian disorders. Human gene mapping has 2 major applications. The first is identification of the gene for a specific genetic disease by its linkage to a known marker. For example, suppose gene A causes a hereditary disease and gene B is a known enzyme or polymorphic marker closely linked to A. Even though no biochemical test exists for A, a tight linkage to B would allow a reasonable probability of identifying the disease for prenatal diagnosis and sometimes for carrier detection. The second impact of mapping is as an aid to understanding the cause of the phenotypic malformations in specific chromosomal diseases. For example, the phenotype of Down syndrome may result from triplication of only the distal long arm of chromosome 21 through a chromosome rearrangement rather than trisomy of the entire chromosome.

It is possible to detect linkage by observing the frequency with which a polymorphic marker is inherited with a disease trait. The physical distance represented by 1 cM corresponds to approximately 1 million bp (1000 kb) and to a 1% chance that recombination will result from a single meiosis (a 0.01 recombination fraction). When a genetic marker is sufficiently close to a disease gene, both are rarely separated by meiotic recombination. The frequency of this separation by chromosomal exchange at meiosis is termed the *recombination frequency*. To be linked, markers should be no more than about 20 cM apart. For perspective, the average chromosome contains about 150 cM, and there are approximately 3300 cM in the entire human genome, which corresponds to 3×10^9 bp.

When determining linkage between a gene and a marker, geneticists compare different models by calculating likelihood ratios. When the likelihood ratio is 1000:1 that the odds of one model are greater than those of another, the first is accepted over the second. The base 10 logarithm of the likelihood ratio (*LOD score; l*ogarithm of *od*ds score) is usually reported. An LOD score of 1–2 is of potential interest in terms of linkage; 2–3 is suggestive; and greater than 3 is generally considered proof of linkage. Although an LOD score of 3 gives a probability ratio of 1000:1 in favor of linkage versus independent assortment, this score does not indicate a type I error as low as 0.001 but, in fact, indicates an error that is close to 0.05, the standard significance level used in statistics. (BCSC Section 1, *Update on General Medicine,* explains these concepts in depth.)

Candidate Gene Approaches

Candidate gene screening

The process of candidate gene screening involves screening for mutations of genes that are abundantly expressed within a tissue and are either important for function or specifically expressed only in that tissue. Sometimes, the candidate gene is one that recapitulates the human disease in transgenic animals. Examples of candidate gene screening discoveries include the findings of mutations of peripherin/*RDS* in autosomal dominant RP and macular dystrophies and the finding of mutations of the rod cyclic guanosine monophosphate (cGMP) β-subunit of rod phosphodiesterase and the cGMP–gated cation channel in autosomal recessive RP.

Positional candidate gene screening

Whenever linkage studies localize a gene to a given chromosomal region, genes already known to reside in the same region become candidate genes for that disease. Following are some examples of disease localization that resulted from linkage to a given region, which in turn led to finding the disease-causing gene by screening for mutations of genes in the region: autosomal dominant RP from rhodopsin mutations (3q); Sorsby fundus dystrophy from *TIMP3* mutations (22q); and Oguchi disease from point deletions within the arrestin gene (2q).

Mutation Screening

Direct Sequencing

The development of techniques for rapid sequencing of DNA was one of the most significant advances in molecular genetics. Currently, it costs far less to sequence a stretch of DNA than to sequence and characterize the amino acid peptide that the DNA produces.

Although other mutation screening techniques exist, sequencing of DNA is the surest and most direct. Sequencing of complementary DNA (cDNA) derived from mRNA provides a quick look at the reading frames (exons) of the gene, whereas sequencing of genomic DNA is more time-consuming because of the presence of introns between the exons. The intron–exon boundaries must be known and multiple PCR assays set up in order to screen not only the exons and their splice junction sites but also upstream and downstream regions that may be important for gene activation and regulation.

DNA sequencing techniques currently in use include the enzymatic (or Sanger sequencing) method, which can be automated (Fig 5-4), and next-generation sequencing (NGS), also known as *massively parallel sequencing.* NGS offers the ability to sequence the entire genome of an individual. Some NGS methods use as probes allele-specific oligonucleotides that are constructed to employ hybridization to recognize a specific DNA sequence in order to detect a specific point mutation (Fig 5-5).

Early methods of mutation detection included Sanger sequencing using radioactive and later fluorescent probes; the single-stranded conformational polymorphism (SSCP) technique; denaturing gradient gel electrophoresis (DGGE); and the use of RFLPs.

Whole-exome sequencing will identify many potential mutations; however, identification of true disease-causing mutations will require considerable bioinformatic information.

Zhang J, Chiodini R, Badr A, Zhang G. The impact of next-generation sequencing on genomics. *J Genet Genomics.* 2011;38(3):95–109.

Genome-Wide Association Studies

Although karyotyping and linkage analysis can still be used to identify disease-associated genes, most research is now centered on GWAS and NGS. The *International HapMap Project,* which followed the creation of the human gene map, compared the DNA sequence of 1184 reference individuals from 11 global populations (creating a catalog called

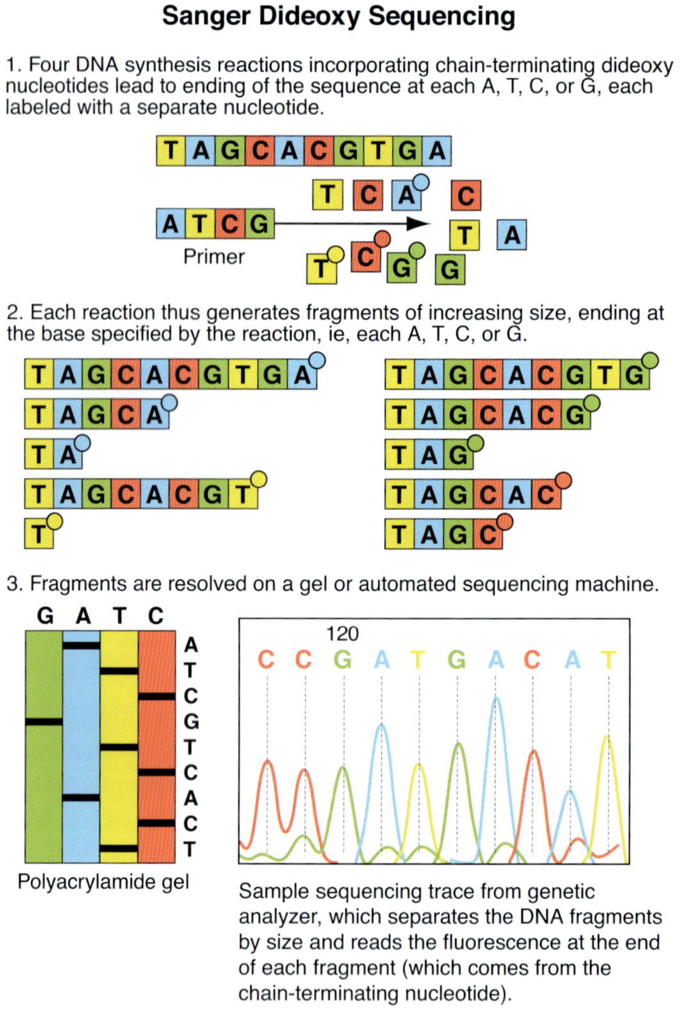

Figure 5-4 Schematic representation of the original Sanger dideoxy chain-termination sequencing method. The results produced are shown in step 3: DNA fragments resolved on a polyacrylamide gel and a sequencing trace from a modern automated sequencing machine. *(Original figure from Oxbridge Biotech Roundtable; redrawn by Mark Miller.)*

the *HapMap*) to identify regions of variation between individuals and racial groups. By using the HapMap to study individuals from a similar population, genetics researchers find that many people will share a series of SNPs or a haplotype. Thus, it is possible to test only one or a few SNPs but to infer a large number of adjacent SNPs by imputation. Chip or bead platforms enable the investigation of 100,000 to millions of SNPs across the genome, forming the basis of a GWAS.

Results of a GWAS are usually presented in a *Manhattan plot,* so named because it brings to mind the New York City skyline. In a Manhattan plot, the chromosomes are arranged in order along the x-axis, and the *P* value (as –log P) of the association of the

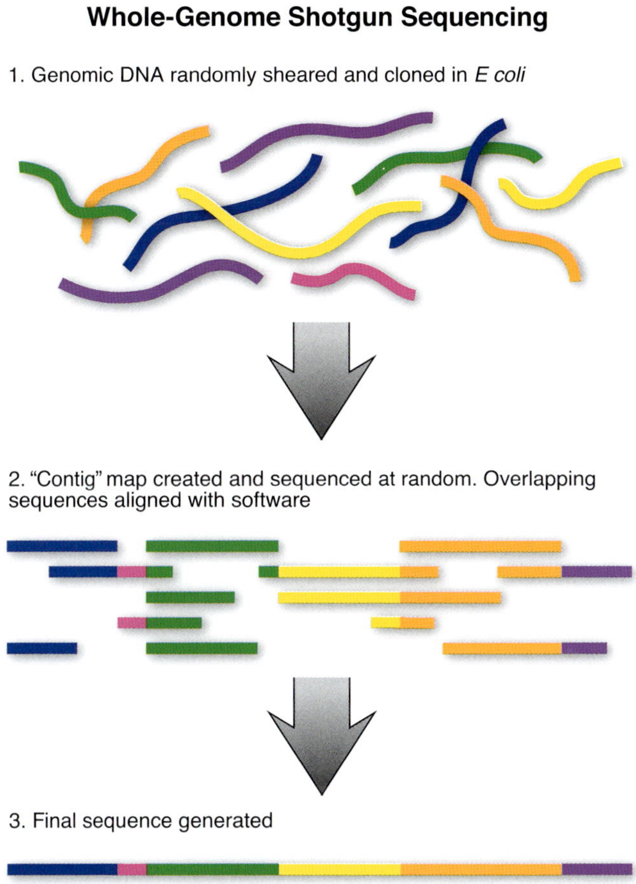

Figure 5-5 Schematic summary of the whole-genome shotgun sequencing method of next-generation sequencing (NGS). At a basic level, all NGS technologies use the same principle: fragment the DNA, add primers/adapters, amplify, and sequence. In whole-genome shotgun sequencing, a DNA sample is randomly broken into numerous small fragments that are then sequenced using the chain-termination method. Multiple overlapping DNA fragments produced from numerous repetitions of this process are then assembled into a single continuous sequence on a computer program. *(Original figure from Oxbridge Biotech Roundtable; redrawn by Mark Miller.)*

disease or trait with the particular SNP at that chromosomal location is given on the y-axis. Figure 5-6 shows a Manhattan plot for glaucoma. A significant gene association (threshold $\approx 5 \times 10^{-8}$) will often have multiple adjacent SNPs at high levels of significance, and thus a column of points will rise on the plot. It is rare that the SNPs themselves are the disease-causing mutations. Usually they are linked in the haplotype to the mutation, which is why researchers will then use fine-mapping of the region by looking at a large number of SNPs in the nearby region.

Combining numerous studies, usually of multiple ethnic groups, in meta-analyses allows for identification of additional associated gene regions. Figure 5-7 shows how GWAS meta-analyses combine data from individual GWAS. Figure 5-8 shows the meta-analysis

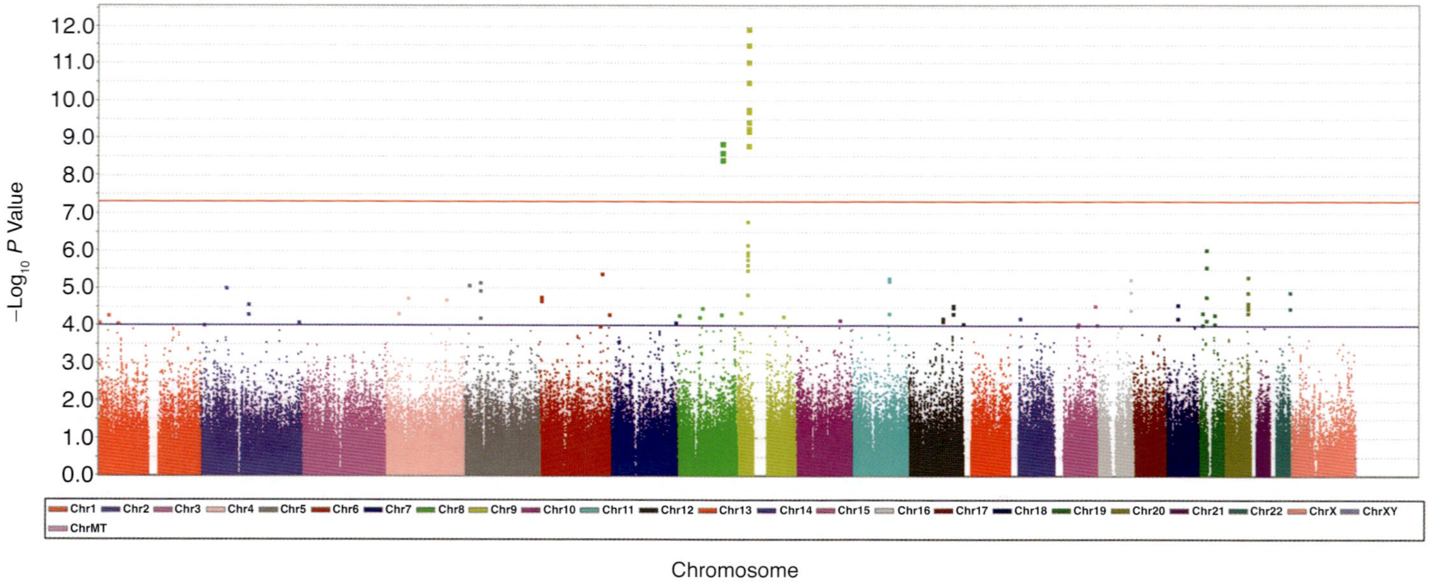

Figure 5-6 Manhattan plot for glaucoma, identifying the *CDKN2BAS* region at 9p21 and the *SIX1/SIX6* region at 14q23. *(Reproduced with permission from Wiggs JL, Yaspan BL, Hauser MA, et al. Common variants at 9p21 and 8q22 are associated with increased susceptibility to optic nerve degeneration in glaucoma.* PLoS Genet. *2012;8(4):e1002654.)*

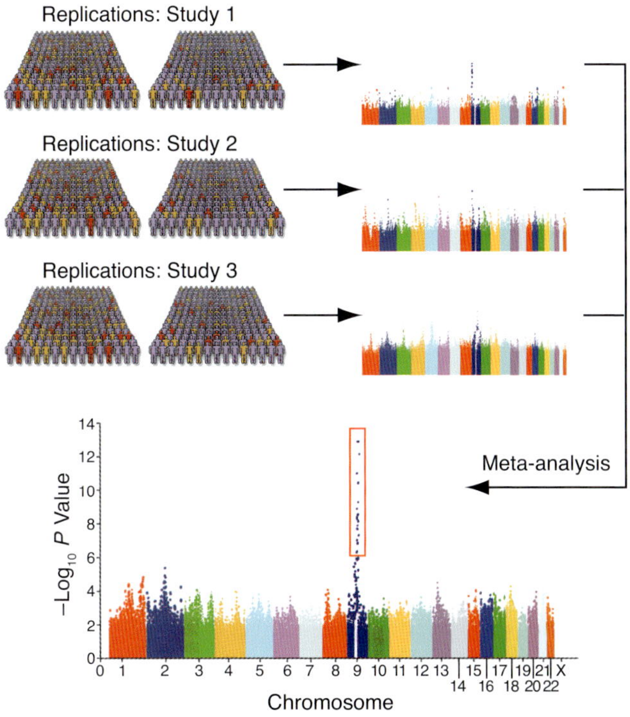

Figure 5-7 Meta-analysis of Manhattan plots. *(Reproduced with permission from Manolio TA. Genomewide association studies and assessment of the risk of disease.* N Engl J Med. *2010;363(2):166–176.)*

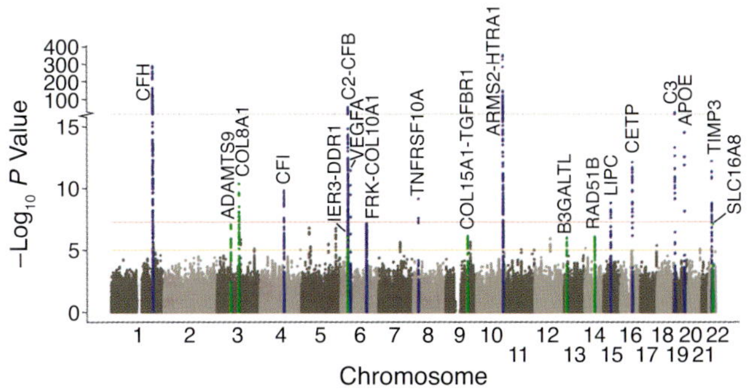

Figure 5-8 Manhattan plot for age-related macular degeneration meta-analysis identifying numerous associated genes. *(Reproduced with permission from Fritsche LG, Chen W, Schu M, et al. Seven new loci associated with age-related macular degeneration.* Nat Genet. *2013;45(4):433–439.)*

of GWAS for age-related macular degeneration (AMD), with 19 loci now identified. The effect size for all of these genes is usually small, but cumulatively they account for approximately 40% of AMD heritability.

Comparison of GWAS from different ethnic groups can help clarify whether the SNP itself is disease causing or just linked to the true disease-causing mutation(s). An example is the *LOXL1* gene, which is associated with pseudoexfoliation. One SNP was associated with disease in the Caucasian population, but disease was associated with the alternate SNP in the Japanese population (Fig 5-9A). Thus, it is unlikely that this SNP is actually disease causing but more likely that different SNPs are associated with the true disease-causing mutation in East Asian and White, or Caucasian-derived, populations. In contrast, another SNP had equivalent association in both populations (Fig 5-9B).

For a catalog of GWAS including ophthalmic studies, see the European Molecular Biology Laboratory–European Bioinformatics Institute (EMBL-EBI) catalog at http://www.ebi.ac.uk/gwas/.

Determining Whether Genetic Change Is a Pathogenic Mutation

If a patient is to be considered for a gene-based therapy, it is important for the clinician to understand how bioinformatics weights the likelihood that a genetic change is a pathogenic mutation. With the huge amount of genetic information provided by whole-exome sequencing, whole-genome sequencing, and genome arrays used in GWAS, many variants of unknown significance have been identified. Numerous types of evidence are used to distinguish a benign polymorphism from a pathogenic mutation. These include population data on the frequency of a variant in cases and controls; segregation data in pedigrees; computational and predictive data, which include SIFT (sorting intolerant from tolerant) and PolyPhen (polymorphism phenotyping); and functional data from cell and animal models (Table 5-1).

Stone EM, Andorf JL, Whitmore SS, et al. Clinically focused molecular investigation of 1000 consecutive families with inherited retinal disease. *Ophthalmology*. 2017;124(9):1314–1331.

Gene Therapy

Gene therapy holds much promise, but the field remains in its infancy. The potential for cure is not matched by either technology or understanding. Key challenges remain in characterizing mutations of genes for major diseases, understanding the pathogenic relevance of identified genes, and developing proper delivery systems for curative gene constructs (the main long-term gene therapy vehicle—viruses—is currently limited by the size of the gene, inflammatory effects, and the risk of oncogenesis).

Replacement of Absent Gene Product in X-Linked and Recessive Diseases

For genetic diseases in which the mutant allele produces either no message or an ineffective gene product (called a *null allele*), correction of the disorder may be possible by simple replacement of the gene in the deficient cells or tissues. It is theoretically possible to transfer normal genes into human cells that harbor either null or mutant genes not producing a stable, translated product. Vectors used to carry the genetic material into the cells include adenoviruses, retroviruses (especially adeno-associated viruses [AAVs]), and plasmid–liposome complexes. AAV vector gene therapy has been successful in curing

Study or Subgroup	XFG Events	XFG Total	XFS Events	XFS Total	Weight	Odds Ratio M-H, Fixed, 95% CI
1.1.1 Caucasian						
Aragon-Martin US+European	225	264	156	188	13.6%	1.18 [0.71, 1.97]
Fan mostly American	237	282	93	116	10.6%	1.30 [0.75, 2.27]
Lemmela Finnish	126	152	82	100	8.5%	1.06 [0.55, 2.06]
Pasutto Germany	522	622	321	408	31.5%	1.41 [1.03, 1.95]
Pasutto Italian	212	260	128	152	15.1%	0.83 [0.48, 1.42]
Thorleifsson Iceland	124	150	83	106	8.5%	1.32 [0.71, 2.47]
Subtotal (95% CI)		**1730**		**1070**	**87.8%**	**1.22 [1.00, 1.49]**
Total events	1446		863			
Heterogeneity: Chi² = 3.12, df = 5 (P = 0.68); I² = 0%						
Test for overall effect: Z = 1.97 (P = 0.05)						
1.1.2 Japanese						
Fuse Japanese	3	72	1	40	0.6%	1.70 [0.17, 16.86]
Hayashi Japanese	0	54	1	64	0.7%	0.39 [0.02, 9.73]
Ozaki Japanese	8	212	14	206	6.9%	0.54 [0.22, 1.31]
Tanito Japanese	7	166	7	118	4.0%	0.70 [0.24, 2.05]
Subtotal (95% CI)		**504**		**428**	**12.2%**	**0.64 [0.34, 1.21]**
Total events	18		23			
Heterogeneity: Chi² = 0.96, df = 3 (P = 0.81); I² = 0%						
Test for overall effect: Z = 1.38 (P = 0.17)						
Total (95% CI)		**2234**		**1498**	**100.0%**	**1.15 [0.95, 1.39]**
Total events	1464		886			
Heterogeneity: Chi² = 7.67, df = 9 (P = 0.57); I² = 0%						
Test for overall effect: Z = 1.45 (P = 0.15)						
Test for subgroup differences: Not applicable						

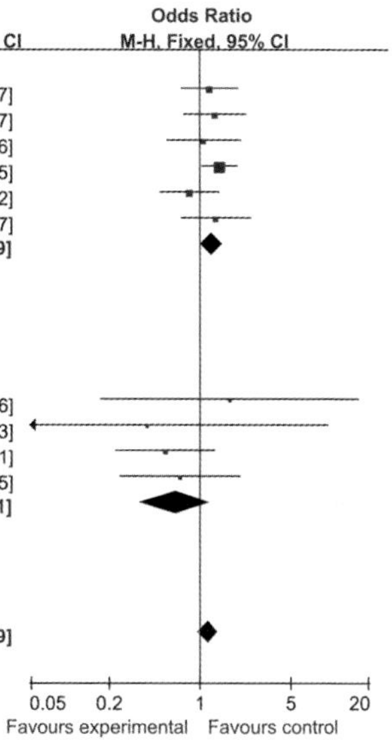

A

Study or Subgroup	XFG Events	XFG Total	XFS Events	XFS Total	Weight	Odds Ratio M-H, Fixed, 95% CI
1.2.1 Caucasian						
Aragon-Martin US+European	199	264	135	186	16.3%	1.16 [0.75, 1.77]
Fan mostly American	218	286	86	114	12.2%	1.04 [0.63, 1.73]
Lemmela Finnish	120	162	85	118	10.6%	1.11 [0.65, 1.89]
Pasutto Germany	476	618	294	406	34.1%	1.28 [0.96, 1.70]
Pasutto Italian	211	264	116	146	12.5%	1.03 [0.62, 1.70]
Thorleifsson Iceland	113	150	78	106	9.4%	1.10 [0.62, 1.94]
Yang Utah (US)	83	98	20	26	2.0%	1.66 [0.57, 4.82]
Subtotal (95% CI)		**1842**		**1102**	**97.2%**	**1.17 [0.98, 1.39]**
Total events	1420		814			
Heterogeneity: Chi² = 1.31, df = 6 (P = 0.97); I² = 0%						
Test for overall effect: Z = 1.75 (P = 0.08)						
1.2.2 Japanese						
Fuse Japanese	2	72	0	40	0.3%	2.87 [0.13, 61.31]
Ozaki Japanese	2	212	5	206	2.1%	0.38 [0.07, 2.00]
Tanito Japanese	1	166	1	118	0.5%	0.71 [0.04, 11.45]
Subtotal (95% CI)		**450**		**364**	**2.8%**	**0.66 [0.21, 2.16]**
Total events	5		6			
Heterogeneity: Chi² = 1.31, df = 2 (P = 0.52); I² = 0%						
Test for overall effect: Z = 0.68 (P = 0.50)						
Total (95% CI)		**2292**		**1466**	**100.0%**	**1.15 [0.97, 1.37]**
Total events	1425		820			
Heterogeneity: Chi² = 3.50, df = 9 (P = 0.94); I² = 0%						
Test for overall effect: Z = 1.62 (P = 0.10)						
Test for subgroup differences: Not applicable						

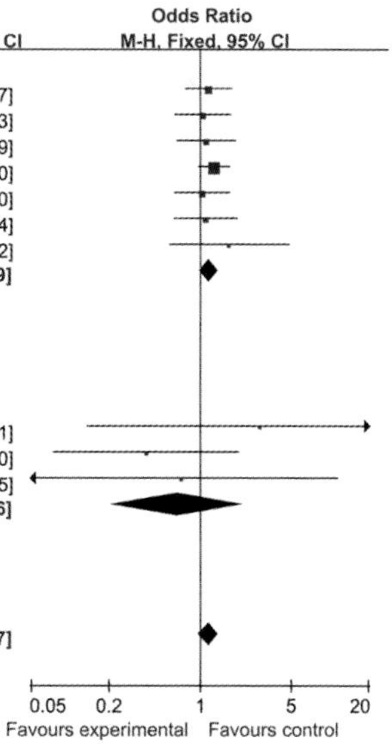

B

Figure 5-9 Forest plots *(at right)* of meta-analyses for single nucleotide polymorphisms (SNPs) near *LOX1* in pseudoexfoliation syndrome (XFS) and pseudoexfoliation glaucoma (XFG). A forest plot is a graphical display designed to illustrate the relative strength of effects found in different quantitative scientific studies that address the same question; essentially, it graphically represents a meta-analysis of the results. **A,** Meta-analysis of the association of SNP rs1048661 with a combined group of XFS and XFG cases. Subgroup meta-analysis indicated that the odds ratios (ORs) of SNP rs1048661 G allele are reversed in Caucasian and Japanese populations. **B,** Meta-analysis of the association of SNP rs3825942 with a combined group of XFS and XFG cases. Subgroup meta-analysis indicated that the ORs of SNP rs3825942 G allele are consistent in Caucasian and Japanese populations. Square = study-specific OR, with the size of the square proportional to the weight of the study; horizontal line = 95% confidence interval (CI); diamond = summary OR with its corresponding 95% CI. *(Reproduced with permission from Chen H, Chen LJ, Zhang M, et al. Ethnicity-based subgroup meta-analysis of the association of* LOXL1 *polymorphisms with glaucoma.* Mol Vis. *2010;16:167–177.)*

Table 5-1 Does a Change in a Gene Really Cause Disease?

	Strong Evidence That a DNA Change Is Benign	Moderate Evidence That a DNA Change Is Pathogenic	Strong Evidence That a DNA Change Is Pathogenic
Population data	eg, Frequency of the DNA change is too high in controls	eg, DNA change is absent in population databases	eg, Frequency of the DNA change in affected cases is statistically increased over that in controls
Segregation data	eg, No segregation of DNA change with disease in families	eg, Odds of DNA change and disease occurring together are >1 in 16 in a family	eg, Odds of DNA change and disease occurring together are >1 in 32 in a family
Computational and predictive data	eg, Evidence that a DNA change is silent or that there is no change to gene product	eg, DNA change affects gene product, such as missense mutation or protein truncation	eg, DNA change produces an amino acid change that is established as pathogenic or as a null mutation
Functional data; cell or animal models	eg, Well-established functional data show no deleterious effect	eg, Mutation hot spot in well-studied functional domain	eg, Well-established functional studies show a deleterious effect

Note: Bioinformaticians in genetics laboratories use multiple types of data (population, segregation, computational, and functional) to help determine the likelihood of DNA change being a pathogenic mutation. Often, data are incomplete in some domains. The more information there is supporting pathogenicity, the more confident the clinician can be in applying the results of genetic testing to patient management in areas such as predictive DNA testing or gene therapy. Genetic testing for inherited retinal disease is now more than 75% sensitive in detecting the causative mutation.

many disorders in animal models, such as the *RPE65* gene mutation that causes RP in the Briard dog.

Human gene therapy trials with *RPE65* suggested no major early adverse effects and some improvement in visual function. In 2017, the US Food and Drug Administration approved the use of voretigene neparvovec-rzyl (AAV2-hRPE65v2) in patients with confirmed biallelic *RPE65*-mediated retinal dystrophy (ie, Leber congenital amaurosis [LCA] and RP). The current cost of treating both eyes is $850,000. Also, mutations in *RPE65* account for only a small percentage of LCA (see Chapter 6, Fig 6-4); thus, this therapy is not suitable for all patients with LCA. Studies in younger subjects (<3 years) are also under way, and several other retinal dystrophy genes are under investigation for human gene therapy trials.

Carvalho LS, Vandenberghe LH. Promising and delivering gene therapies for vision loss. *Vision Res.* 2015;111(Pt B):124–133.

Russell S, Bennett J, Wellman JA, et al. Efficacy and safety of voretigene neparvovec (AAV2-hRPE65v2) in patients with RPE65-mediated inherited retinal dystrophy: a randomised, controlled, open-label, phase 3 trial. *Lancet.* 2017;390(10097):849–860.

Strategies for Dominant Diseases

Dominant diseases are caused by production of a gene product that is either insufficient *(haploid insufficiency)* or conducive to disease *(dominant-negative effect)*. Theoretically, haploid insufficiency should be treatable by gene replacement therapy as outlined in the previous section for X-linked and recessive diseases. For dominant disorders produced by defective developmental genes, this correction would have to occur in early fetal development.

Disorders resulting from a dominant-negative effect require a different approach. Thus, strategies for treatment of dominant disease differ, depending on whether a functional gene product is produced. Some genes code for RNA molecules that can bind to mRNA from another gene and block the other molecule's ability to be translated. Greater understanding of these genes may enable the creation of either drugs or new gene-encoded RNA molecules that can block the translation of mRNA for defective alleles, thus allowing only the normal allele to be expressed.

Another approach is the use of oligonucleotide or antisense DNA that are designed to bind with mRNA from mutant alleles, stopping the mRNA from being translated by ribosomes (Fig 5-10). Although many problems need to be resolved for such therapy to be effective, this approach holds promise for autosomal dominant disorders in which disease is caused by expression of the mutant gene product.

The use of ribozymes, RNA molecules that have the ability to cleave certain RNA molecules, provides another approach. A third method utilizes *short interfering RNA (siRNA)*, also known as *small interference RNA*, to bind to mRNA and lead to the eventual

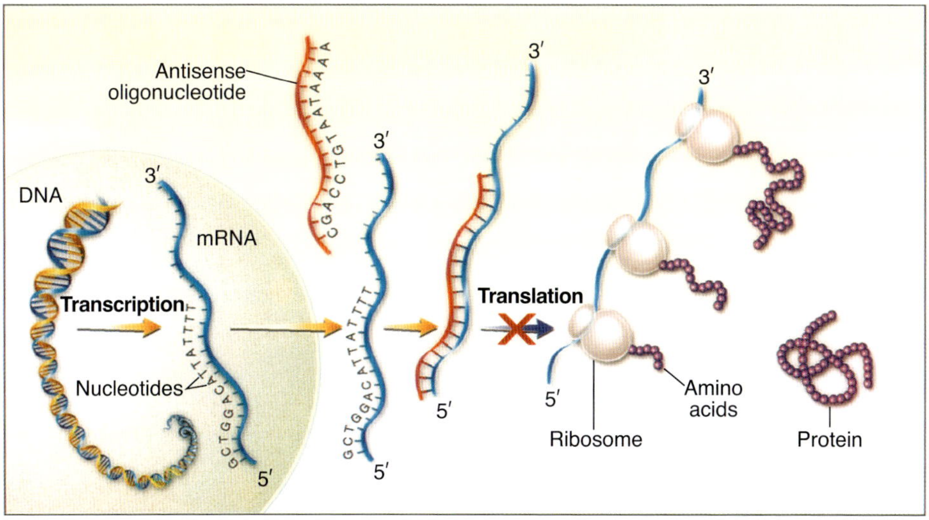

Figure 5-10 Blockade of translation by antisense oligonucleotides. Normal gene transcription of DNA into mRNA is followed by translation of mRNA into protein. Antisense oligonucleotides complementary to a portion of mRNA bind mRNA, preventing translation—either by the steric effect of the binding process itself or (possibly) by inducing degradation of the mRNA by RNase. *(Reproduced with permission from Askari FK, McDonnell WM. Antisense-oligonucleotide therapy.* N Engl J Med. *1996;334(5):316–318.)*

degradation of specific mRNA molecules. The use of siRNA molecules as potential therapeutic agents has become increasingly popular, and this approach has proven to be a powerful means by which to study the function of novel gene products. However, one challenge with siRNA therapy is achieving intracellular delivery. Another challenge is cell-surface TLR3 receptor stimulation, which can induce immune or antiangiogenic processes as a generic class property.

A new form of genome editing known as *CRISPR–Cas9* (clustered, regularly interspaced, short palindromic repeats–CRISPR-associated protein 9) has been used to correct point mutations in the DNA sequence of cells. Combining the technology of CRISPR–Cas9 with that of induced pluripotent stem cells (iPSCs) could potentially allow a scenario in which a skin biopsy is performed on a patient with an inherited retinal disease, skin cells are induced to produce pluripotent stem cells, and the causative mutation is edited out with CRISPR–Cas9. The cells could then be grown into the appropriate retinal cell line and implanted in the diseased eye. Before clinical trials commence, this personalized therapy, which would be costly, must still overcome issues with immunity and the risk of tumor development.

Burnight ER, Gupta M, Wiley LA, et al. Using CRISPR-Cas9 to generate gene-corrected autologous iPSCs for the treatment of inherited retinal degeneration. *Mol Ther*. 2017; 25(9):1999–2013.

Hung SSC, McCaughey T, Swann O, Pébay A, Hewitt AW. Genome engineering in ophthalmology: application of CRISPR/Cas to the treatment of eye disease. *Prog Retin Eye Res*. 2016;53:1–20.

CHAPTER 6

Clinical Genetics

Highlights

- Obtaining a family history and recognizing patterns of inheritance are important for accurate diagnosis and management of hereditary eye diseases.
- Although it is important to know whether genes are X-linked, mitochondrial, or autosomal, there is little clinical value in knowing autosomal assignments (1–22), which can be found easily with online databases such as OMIM (Online Mendelian Inheritance in Man).
- Chromosomal abnormalities may be evident with cytogenetics. Two important ones for ophthalmologists involve the *RB1* gene on chromosome arm 13q and the *PAX6* gene on chromosome arm 11p, defects in which result in retinoblastoma and aniridia, respectively.
- The phakomatoses are mostly due to recessive oncogenes, with loss of genes causing germline or somatic tumors in a pattern similar to that in retinoblastoma.
- Carriers of genetic conditions should be examined for clinical signs of those conditions.
- Appropriate referral for genetic counseling and genetic testing is important in most mendelian diseases.
- Currently, American Academy of Ophthalmology (AAO) guidelines do not recommend genetic testing for common eye diseases such as age-related macular degeneration (AMD) and primary open-angle glaucoma (POAG) outside the research setting.

Introduction

> The most valuable tool in clinical genetics is the question: "Does anyone else in the family have . . . ?"

At present, a positive family history carries greater specificity and sensitivity than most laboratory genetic tests. Even with all the DNA mutations currently known for diseases, the vast majority of mutations remains to be identified, and the full hand of genetic cards dealt to each person is not known. Genetics is important in every ophthalmic consultation, from those involving rare inborn errors of metabolism or congenital malformations to common eye diseases, such as myopia, glaucoma, cataract, and age-related macular degeneration (AMD). Even susceptibility to infection and trauma can be genetic. An understanding of the genetic basis of a disease may be particularly useful for arriving at a correct diagnosis when another family member has a similar disease. In addition, it is important for clinicians to recognize that a patient presenting with a particular eye problem may be at increased risk for an unrelated disease, such as glaucoma, because of an affected parent.

The ophthalmologist has an important obligation to patients with genetic eye diseases—either to provide genetic counseling or to arrange for referral to a geneticist or genetic counselor. Clinicians now have patients presenting with DNA test results for themselves or their families. The results may range from the identification of high-risk retinoblastoma gene mutations (which would significantly influence the management of at-risk children within the family) to genetic associations that are of no more value than iridology (genes have been associated with iris crypts and furrows). It is important to understand the clinical settings in which a genetic test is crucial, useful, or irrelevant to patient management. These distinctions will change in the future as new clinical trials define treatments based on genetic background.

When a patient presents with a DNA result for a disease for which no effective treatment based on such results is currently available, the clinician may be asked the following question: "What should we do about this?" The best answer is: "Participate in, or help fund, research so we can find out what the best treatments are." The US National Institutes of Health (NIH) website ClinicalTrials.gov is a good place to refer these patients.

The key recommendations of the AAO Task Force on Genetic Testing policy are given at the end of this chapter. When faced with the option of ordering genetic tests, clinicians should ask the same question they ask before ordering any tests: How will this change management? The best utilization of genetic testing comes from knowledge of the family history. An accurate family history might help an ophthalmologist save not only a patient's sight but also, in cases of retinoblastoma or Marfan syndrome, the patient's life.

Pedigree Analysis

Establishing a pedigree or drawing a family tree is the key to clinical genetics. The most useful strategy is to start with open questions, such as, *Are there any eye diseases in the family?* Then proceed further to more targeted questions, as in the case of potential Leber hereditary optic neuropathy (LHON): *Did any men on the maternal side of your family lose vision as a young adult?*

For patients with a family history, it is best to convert this information into a pedigree diagram—which can be a challenge in some electronic medical records. An initial, rough outline can be drawn on paper and the information can be entered into a simple or more sophisticated pedigree-drawing software program. The standard protocol for pedigree symbols is outlined in Figure 6-1.

Drawing one's own extended family tree is a useful exercise for the clinician. A basic pedigree should include parents, siblings, and children and should note those affected or unaffected by the disorder of interest. Often, specific inquiry of grandparents, uncles, aunts, and cousins can help clarify the inheritance pattern.

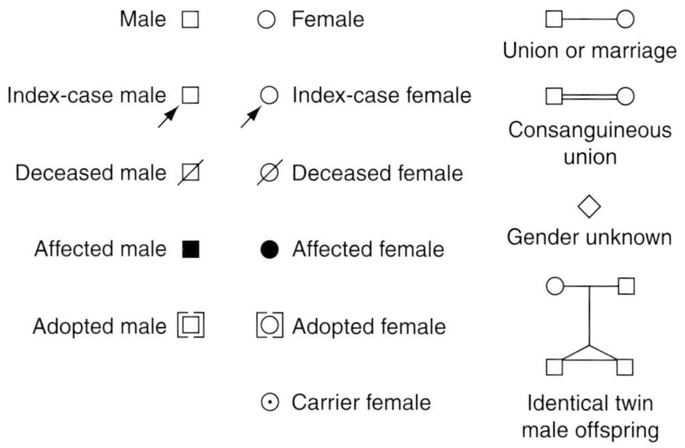

Figure 6-1 Symbols commonly used for pedigree analysis. *(Courtesy of David A. Mackey, MD.)*

The interviewer should always ascertain whether brothers and sisters are half siblings or full siblings. This procedure may not only limit the possible patterns of inheritance, but also identify other individuals at risk for the disorder under consideration. Information regarding parentage must be pursued aggressively (but always privately and confidentially). Although incest and nonpaternity are sensitive social issues, their occurrence is not rare. Therefore, when considering rare autosomal recessive diseases, the interviewer must ask specifically about consanguinity. Are the parents cousins? Are there common last names in the families of both parents? Were the parents born in the same area, or do they belong to known ethnic or religious isolates?

Age at death may be useful in specific situations and can be recorded near the appropriate symbols. In the case of a child with ectopia lentis and no family history of similar ocular disease, a clinician may find the identification of a relative who died from a dissecting thoracic aorta in his fourth decade of life very informative, leading to a tentative consideration of Marfan syndrome in the differential diagnosis. In another example, the clinician's casual observation of atypical tear-shaped congenital hypertrophy of the retinal pigment epithelium (CHRPE) in each eye (Fig 6-2) in a young adult may trigger remembrance that a parent had died at age 50 years from metastatic adenocarcinoma of the colon and a sibling from a brain tumor at age 10 years. Taken together, this information may lead to a diagnosis of Gardner syndrome and referral to a gastroenterologist for further diagnostic evaluation.

Taking a family history does not end with the initial consultation because it may be the first time a patient has heard of the disease. On discussing the new diagnosis with the family, the patient may discover additional family history. Clinicians should encourage patients to talk to their families, and then have patients update their family history at subsequent consultations. For more complicated genetic diseases, a genetic counselor will be able to assist patients with an extensive pedigree.

Bennett RL, French KS, Resta RG, Doyle DL. Standardized human pedigree nomenclature: update and assessment of the recommendations of the National Society of Genetic Counselors. *J Genet Couns.* 2008;17(5):424–433.

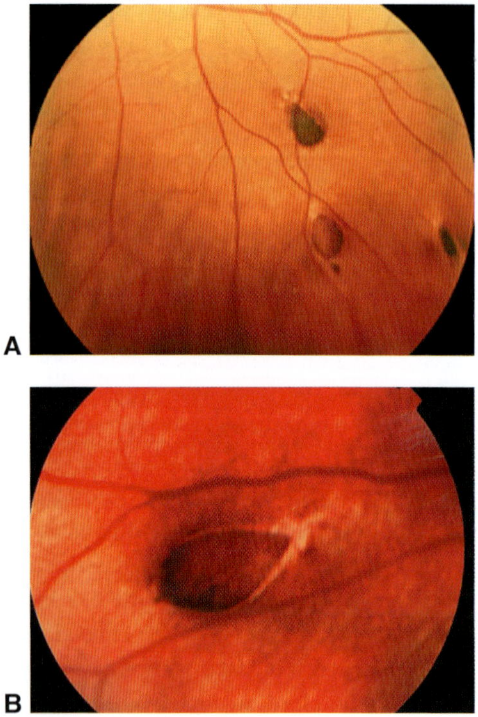

Figure 6-2 Atypical congenital hypertrophy of the retinal pigment epithelium (CHRPE) is found in 70%–80% of individuals with familial adenomatous polyposis (FAP). Patients with FAP and other tumors may have Gardner or Turcot syndrome, depending on the type and location of the tumor. Parts **A** and **B** demonstrate atypical tear-shaped CHRPE with depigmentation at 1 margin, usually the apex, which points toward the optic nerve. They can be multiple (as shown in part A) or solitary (as shown in part B). *(Reproduced with permission from Bowling B.* Kanski's Clinical Ophthalmology: A Systematic Approach. *8th ed. Oxford: Elsevier Limited; 2016:516.)*

Bennett RL, Steinhaus KA, Uhrich SB, et al. Recommendations for standardized human pedigree nomenclature. Pedigree Standardization Task Force of the National Society of Genetic Counselors. *Am J Hum Genet.* 1995;56(3):745–752.

Patterns of Inheritance

Many of the terms used in this section are defined in the Genetics Glossary in the appendix. See also the section Terminology: Hereditary, Genetic, Familial, Congenital later in this chapter.

Dominant Versus Recessive Inheritance

The terms *dominant* and *recessive* were first used by Gregor Mendel. In classical genetics, a dominant gene is always expressed with similar phenotype, whether the mutant gene is present in a homozygous or heterozygous state. Stated simply, a dominant gene mutation is expressed when present in only a single copy. A genetic disorder is called *recessive* if its expression is masked by a normal allele or, more precisely, if it is expressed only in the homozygote (or compound heterozygote) state when both alleles at a specific locus are mutant.

A *trait* is the consequence of the gene's action. It is the trait, or phenotypic expression of the gene at a clinical level, rather than the gene itself, that is dominant or recessive. A trait is recessive if its expression is suppressed by the presence of a normal gene (as in galactosemia) and dominant if it is apparently unaffected by a single copy of the normal allele (as in Marfan syndrome). If the alleles are different and yet are both manifested in the phenotype, they are said to be *codominant.* Examples of phenotypes with codominant inheritance patterns include the ABO blood types, HLA types, and hemoglobin variants (as involved in sickle cell disease).

As a result of epigenetic factors, a gene may have a greater or lesser effect on the individual or an organ, and therefore the trait may be more or less apparent. Thus, the designation of a trait as either dominant or recessive depends on the testing method used. Although classically a dominant gene has the same phenotype when the mutant allele is present in either the heterozygous or the homozygous state, most dominant medical diseases act more like codominant diseases, in which individuals who are homozygous for a mutant allele or who harbor 2 mutant alleles will have more severe expression than will those with only 1 mutant allele.

In experiments, the biochemical mechanisms of dominant hereditary diseases appear different from those of recessive disorders. Recessive traits usually result from enzyme deficiencies caused by mutations of the gene specifying the affected enzyme. The altered enzyme often can be shown to be structurally abnormal or unstable. Heterozygotes usually have approximately 50% of normal enzyme activity but are clinically unaffected, implying that half of the normal enzyme activity is compatible with near-normal function. If adequate biochemical testing can be performed and the specific enzyme isolated, the reduced enzyme activity can be quantified and the heterozygous genetic state inferred. Thus, clinically unaffected heterozygotes can be detected for such disorders as homocystinuria (decrease in cystathionine β-synthase), galactokinase deficiency (low blood galactokinase activity), classic galactosemia (galactose-1-phosphate uridyltransferase deficiency), gyrate atrophy of the choroid and retina (decreased ornithine aminotransferase), and Tay-Sachs disease (decreased hexosaminidase A). Table 6-1 outlines known enzyme disorders with ocular manifestations.

Rajappa M, Goyal A, Kaur J. Inherited metabolic disorders involving the eye: a clinicobiochemical perspective. *Eye* (London). 2010;24(4):507–518.

Autosomal Recessive Inheritance

An autosomal recessive disease is expressed fully only in the presence of a mutant gene at the same locus on both homologous chromosomes (ie, homozygosity for a mutant gene) or of 2 different mutant alleles at the same locus (compound heterozygosity). A single mutant allele is sufficient to cause a recessive disorder if the normal allele on the homologous chromosome is deleted. A recessive trait can remain latent through several generations until the chance mating of 2 heterozygotes for a mutant allele gives rise to an affected individual. The frequency of heterozygotes (carriers) for a given disorder will always be considerably greater than that of homozygotes. It is estimated that all human beings inherit numerous mutations for different recessive disorders for which they are heterozygotes.

Enzyme defects

Autosomal recessive diseases often result from defects in enzymatic proteins. Most of the so-called inborn errors of metabolism that result from enzyme defects are autosomal

Table 6-1 Known Enzyme Disorders and Corresponding Ocular Signs

Disorder	Defective Enzyme	Ocular Sign
Storage diseases		
Fabry disease	Ceramide trihexosidase (α-galactosidase A)	Corneal epithelial verticillate changes; aneurysmal dilation and tortuosity of retinal and conjunctival vessels
GM_1 gangliosidosis type I (generalized gangliosidosis)	β-Galactosidase-1	Macular cherry-red spot; optic atrophy; corneal clouding (mild)
GM_2 gangliosidosis type I (Tay-Sachs disease)	Hexosaminidase A	Macular cherry-red spot; optic atrophy
GM_2 gangliosidosis type II (Sandhoff disease)	Hexosaminidase A and B	Macular cherry-red spot
Krabbe disease (leukodystrophy)	Galactosylceramidase (or galactocerebrosidase)	Optic atrophy
Mannosidosis	α-Mannosidase	Lenticular opacities
Metachromatic leukodystrophy	Arylsulfatase A	Retinal discoloration, degeneration
Mucopolysaccharidosis IH (Hurler syndrome)	α-L-Iduronidase	Corneal opacity; pigmentary retinal degeneration
Mucopolysaccharidosis IS (Scheie syndrome)	α-L-Iduronidase	Corneal opacity; pigmentary retinal degeneration
Mucopolysaccharidosis II (Hunter syndrome)	Iduronate-2-sulfatase	Corneal opacity (mild type); older patients
Mucopolysaccharidosis III, type A (Sanfilippo syndrome)	Heparan *N*-sulfatase	Pigmentary retinal degeneration; optic atrophy
Metabolic disorders		
Albinism	Tyrosinase	Foveal hypoplasia; nystagmus; iris transillumination
Alkaptonuria	Homogentisic acid oxidase	Dark sclera
Crigler-Najjar syndrome	Bilirubin uridine diphosphate glucuronosyltransferase	Extraocular movement disorder
Ehlers-Danlos syndrome type VI	Lysyl hydroxylase	Microcornea, corneal ectasia; blue sclera; ectopia lentis; angioid streaks; retinal detachment
Familial dysautonomia (Riley-Day syndrome)	Dopamine-β-hydroxylase	Alacrima; corneal hypoesthesia; exodeviation; methacholine-induced miosis
Galactokinase deficiency	Galactokinase	Cataracts
Galactosemia	Galactose-1-phosphate uridyltransferase	Cataracts
Gyrate atrophy of the choroid and retina	Ornithine aminotransferase	Degeneration of the choroid and retina; cataracts; myopia
Homocystinuria	Cystathionine β-synthase	Dislocated lens
Hyperglycinemia	Glycine cell transport	Optic atrophy
Intermittent ataxia	Pyruvate decarboxylase	Nystagmus
Leigh necrotizing encephalopathy	Pyruvate carboxylase	Optic atrophy
Maple syrup urine disease	Branched-chain decarboxylase	Ophthalmoplegia; nystagmus
Niemann-Pick disease	Sphingomyelinase	Macular cherry-red spot
Refsum disease	Phytanoyl-CoA hydroxylase	Retinal degeneration
Sulfite oxidase deficiency	Sulfite oxidase	Ectopia lentis
Tyrosinemia type II	Tyrosine aminotransferase	Pseudodendritic keratitis

recessive traits, although a few are X-linked recessive disorders (eg, Lesch-Nyhan syndrome).

In some other disorders with genetic blocks in metabolism, the phenotypic consequences are related to the lack of a normal product distal to the block. One example is *albinism,* in which the metabolic block involves a step between the amino acid tyrosine and the formation of melanin. In still other inborn errors of metabolism, the phenotypic expression results from excessive production of a product through a normally alternative and minor metabolic pathway.

Carrier heterozygotes

The heterozygous carrier of a mutant gene may show minimal evidence of the gene defect in recessive conditions. However, dysfunction may be evident at a biochemical level. Thus, carrier heterozygotes have been detected by a variety of methods:

- identification of abnormal metabolites by electrophoresis (eg, galactokinase deficiency)
- hair bulb assay (eg, oculocutaneous albinism and Fabry disease)
- monitoring of enzyme activity in leukocytes (eg, galactose-1-phosphate uridyltransferase in galactosemia)
- skin culture for analysis of enzyme activity in fibroblasts (eg, ornithine aminotransferase deficiency in gyrate atrophy of the retina and choroid)
- assay of serum and tears (eg, hexosaminidase A in Tay-Sachs disease)

In contrast to the transmission of dominant traits, most reproduction resulting in transmission of recessive disorders involves phenotypically normal heterozygous parents. Among 4 offspring produced by parents carrying the same gene for an autosomal recessive disease, on average, 1 will be affected (homozygote), 2 will be carriers (heterozygotes), and 1 will be genetically and phenotypically unaffected. Thus, clinically unaffected heterozygous parents will produce offspring with a ratio of 1 clinically affected to 3 clinically normal. There is no predilection for either sex. In 2-child families, the patient with a recessive disease is frequently the only affected family member. For instance, approximately 40%–50% of patients with retinitis pigmentosa (RP) have no family history of the disorder. However, their age at onset, rate of progression, and other phenotypic characteristics are similar to those with defined recessive inheritance patterns.

> When a child is born with a recessive disorder, the genetic risk for each subsequent child of the same parents is 25%.

This concept has specific implications for genetic counseling. All offspring of an affected individual will be carriers; they are unlikely to be affected with the disorder unless their clinically unaffected parent is also by chance a carrier of the gene. The normal-appearing sibling of a child with a recessive disorder has a statistical risk of 2 chances in 3 of being a genetic carrier. As the genes for recessive diseases are identified, these individuals and their offspring will benefit from predictive DNA testing.

Consanguinity

The mating of close relatives can increase the probability that their children will inherit a homozygous genotype for recessive traits, particularly relatively rare ones. For example, the probability that the same allele is present in first cousins is 1 in 8. In the offspring of a first-cousin sexual union, 1 of every 16 genes is commonly present in a homozygous state. It follows that each offspring from a first-cousin union has a 1 in 16 chance of manifesting an autosomal recessive trait within a given family. Approximately 1% of all sexual unions may be consanguineous. A vigorous search for consanguinity between the parents should be made in any case of a rare recessive disease.

In contrast, the expression of common recessive genes is less influenced by inbreeding because most homozygous offspring are the progeny of unrelated parents. This pattern is usually the case with such frequent disorders as sickle cell disease and cystic fibrosis. The characteristics of autosomal recessive inheritance are summarized in Table 6-2.

Pseudodominance

Occasionally, an affected homozygote mates with a heterozygote. Of their offspring, 50% will be carriers and 50% will be affected homozygotes. Because this segregation pattern mimics that of dominant inheritance, it is called *pseudodominance.* Such matings are usually rare and are unlikely to affect more than 2 vertical generations.

Autosomal Dominant Inheritance

When an autosomal allele leads to a regular, clearly definable abnormality in the heterozygote, the trait is termed *dominant.* Autosomal dominant traits often represent defects in structural nonenzymatic proteins, such as in fibrillin in Marfan syndrome or collagen in Stickler syndrome. In addition, a dominant mode of inheritance has been observed for some malignant neoplastic syndromes, such as retinoblastoma, von Hippel–Lindau disease, tuberous sclerosis, and Gardner syndrome. Although the neoplasias in these diseases are inherited as autosomal dominant *traits,* the defect is recessive at the cellular level, with the tumors arising from loss of function of both alleles.

> Nearly all bearers of dominant disorders in the human population are heterozygotes.

In dominant inheritance, the heterozygote is clinically affected, and a single mutant gene interferes with normal function. Occasionally, depending on the frequency of the abnormal gene in the population and the phenotype, 2 carriers of the same abnormality produce children. Any offspring of 2 heterozygous parents has a 25% risk of being an affected homozygote.

It has been suggested that dominant diseases are caused by mutations affecting structural proteins, such as cell receptor growth factors (eg, *FGFR2* in Crouzon syndrome) or by functional deficits generated by abnormal polypeptide subunits (eg, unstable hemoglobins). The dominant disorders aniridia and Waardenburg syndrome result from

Table 6-2 Characteristics of Autosomal Recessive Inheritance

The mutant gene usually does not cause clinical disease (recessive) in the heterozygote.
Individuals inheriting both genes (homozygotes) of the defective type express the disorder.
Typically, the trait appears only in siblings, not in their parents or offspring or in other relatives.
The ratio of normal to affected in a sibship is 3:1. The larger the sibship, the more often will more than one child be affected.
The sexes are affected in equal proportions.
Parents of the affected person may be genetically related (consanguinity); the rarer the trait, the more likely.
Affected individuals have children who, though phenotypically normal, are carriers (heterozygotes) of the gene.

Table 6-3 Characteristics of Autosomal Dominant Inheritance With Complete Penetrance

The trait appears in 2 or more successive generations (vertical transmission).
Affected males and females are equally likely to transmit the trait to male and female offspring. Thus, male-to-male transmission occurs.
Each affected individual has an affected parent, unless the condition arose by new mutation in the given individual.
Males and females are affected in equal proportions.
Unaffected persons do not transmit the trait to their children.
The trait is expressed in the heterozygote but is more severe in the homozygote.
The age of fathers of isolated (new mutation) cases is usually advanced.
The more severely the trait interferes with survival and reproduction, the greater the proportion of isolated (new mutation) cases.
Variability in expression of the trait from generation to generation and between individuals in the same generation is expected.
Affected persons transmit the trait on average to 50% of their offspring.

loss of 1 of the 2 alleles for the developmental transcription factors PAX6 and PAX3, respectively.

In some instances, dominantly inherited traits are not clinically expressed. In other instances—such as in some families with autosomal dominant RP—pedigree analysis can sometimes show a defective gene in individuals who do not manifest any discernible clinical or functional impairment. This situation is called *incomplete penetrance* or *skipped generation.*

Conclusive evidence of autosomal dominant inheritance with complete penetrance requires demonstration of the disease in at least 3 successive generations. Transmission of the disorder from a male to his male offspring, with both sexes showing the typical disease, must also occur. The characteristics of autosomal dominant inheritance with complete (100%) penetrance are summarized in Table 6-3. In the usual clinical situation, any offspring of an affected heterozygote with a dominant disorder, regardless of sex, has a 1 in 2 chance of inheriting the mutant gene and thereby demonstrating some effect. The degree of variability in the expression of certain traits is usually more pronounced in autosomal dominantly inherited disorders than in other types of genetic disorders. Moreover, when a clinical disorder is inherited in more than one mendelian pattern, the dominantly inherited disorder is, in general, clinically less severe than the recessively inherited one.

Counseling for recurrence risk of autosomal dominant traits must involve a thorough examination of not only the affected person (who may have the full syndrome) but also the parents. If 1 parent is even mildly affected, the risk of additional genetically affected siblings rises to 50%. It is crucial that ophthalmologists not miss variable expressivity when they have the opportunity to examine the parents of their patient and other family members. In some ocular disorders, family members can inherit a gene for a dominant trait and not show clinically apparent manifestations. In these cases, electrophysiologic testing or genetic testing can be used to detect the impairment. For example, a relatively inexpensive genetic test can show which clinically normal family members carry the mutation for Best vitelliform macular dystrophy.

X-Linked Inheritance

A trait determined by genes on either of the sex chromosomes is properly termed *sex-linked.* This genetic pattern became widely known with the occurrence of hemophilia in European and Russian royal families.

The rules governing all modes of sex-linked inheritance can be derived logically by considering the chromosomal basis. Females have 2 X chromosomes, 1 of which will go to each ovum. Males have both an X and a Y chromosome. The male parent contributes his only X chromosome to all his daughters and his only Y chromosome to all his sons. Traits determined by genes carried on the Y chromosome are transmitted from a father to 100% of his sons. Among these Y chromosomal genes is the *testis-determining factor* (*TDF;* also called *sex-determining region Y,* or *SRY*). Genes controlling tooth size, stature, spermatogenesis, and hairy pinnae (hypertrichosis pinnae auris) are also on the Y chromosome. All other sex-linked traits or diseases are thought to result from genes on the X chromosome and are properly termed *X-linked.* Some X-linked conditions have considerable frequencies in human populations; congenital color vision defects such as protan and deutan anomalies were among the first human traits assigned to a specific chromosome.

The distinctive feature of X-linked inheritance, both dominant and recessive, is the absence of father-to-son transmission. Because the male X chromosome passes only to daughters, all daughters of an affected male will inherit the mutant gene.

X-linked recessive inheritance

A male has only 1 copy of any X-linked gene and therefore is said to be *hemizygous* for the gene, rather than homozygous or heterozygous. Because there is no normal gene to balance a mutant X-linked gene in the male, its resulting phenotype, whether dominant or recessive, will always be expressed. A female may be heterozygous or homozygous for a mutant X-linked gene. X-linked traits are commonly called *recessive* if they are caused by genes located on the X chromosome, as these genes express themselves fully only in the absence of the normal allele. Thus, males (with their single X chromosome) are predominantly affected. All their phenotypically healthy but heterozygous daughters are carriers. By contrast, each son of a heterozygous woman has an equal chance of being unaffected or hemizygously affected.

Table 6-4 Characteristics of X-Linked Recessive Inheritance

Usually only males are affected.
An affected male transmits the gene to all of his daughters (obligate carriers) and none of his sons.
All daughters of affected males, even those phenotypically normal, are carriers.
Affected males in a family either are brothers or are related to one another through carrier females (eg, maternal uncles).
If an affected male has children with a carrier female, on average 50% of their daughters will be homozygous and affected and 50% will be heterozygous and carriers.
Heterozygous females may rarely be affected (manifesting heterozygotes) because of lyonization.
Female carriers transmit the gene on average to 50% of their sons, who are affected, and to 50% of their daughters, who will be carriers.
There is no male-to-male transmission.

A female will be affected with an X-linked recessive trait under a limited number of circumstances:

- She is homozygous for the mutant gene by inheritance (ie, from an affected father and a heterozygous [or homozygous] mother).
- Her mother is heterozygous and her father contributes a new mutation.
- She has Turner syndrome, with only 1 X chromosome, or a partial deletion of 1 X chromosome and therefore is effectively hemizygous.
- She has a highly unusual skewing of inactivation of her normal X chromosome, as explained by the Lyon hypothesis (discussed in the section Lyonization later in this chapter).
- Her disorder is actually an autosomal genocopy of the X-linked condition.

Table 6-4 summarizes the characteristics of X-linked recessive inheritance. X-linked recessive inheritance should be considered when all affected individuals in a family are males, especially when they are related through historically unaffected women (eg, uncle and nephew, or multiple affected half brothers with different fathers). Many X-linked RP pedigrees have been mislabeled as autosomal dominant because of manifesting female carriers. The key feature of an X-linked pedigree is no male-to-male transmission.

X-linked dominant inheritance

X-linked dominant traits are caused by mutant genes expressed in a single dose and carried on the X chromosome. Thus, both heterozygous women and hemizygous men are clinically affected. Females are affected nearly twice as frequently as males. All daughters of males with the disease are affected. However, all sons of affected males are free of the trait unless their mothers are also affected. Because only children of affected males provide information in discriminating X-linked dominant from autosomal dominant disease, it may be impossible to distinguish these modes on genetic grounds when the pedigree is small or the available data are scarce. Some X-linked dominant disorders, such as incontinentia pigmenti (Bloch-Sulzberger syndrome), may prove lethal to the hemizygous male. The characteristics of X-linked dominant inheritance are summarized in Table 6-5.

Table 6-5 Characteristics of X-Linked Dominant Inheritance

Both males and females are affected, but the incidence of the trait is approximately twice as high in females as in males (or exclusively in females if the trait is lethal in the male).
An affected male transmits the trait to all of his daughters and to none of his sons.
Heterozygous affected females transmit the trait to both sexes with equal frequency.
The heterozygous female tends to be less severely affected than the hemizygous male.

X-linked disorders

Females with X-linked diseases have milder symptoms than males. Occasionally, males may be so severely affected that they die before the reproductive period, thus preventing transmission of the gene. Such is the case with Duchenne muscular dystrophy, in which most affected males die before their midteens. In other disorders, males are so severely affected that they die before birth, and only females survive. Families with such disorders would include only affected daughters, unaffected daughters, and normal sons at a ratio of 1:1:1. Incontinentia pigmenti is one such lethal genetic disorder. In affected females, an erythematous, vesicular skin eruption develops perinatally, which progresses to marbled, curvilinear pigmentation. The syndrome includes dental abnormalities, congenital or secondary cataracts, retinal neovascularization with tractional retinal detachment, and pseudogliomas.

Among the most severe X-linked dominant disorders with lethality for the hemizygous males is Aicardi syndrome. No verified birth of a male with this entity has ever been reported. Females have profound cognitive disabilities and delays; muscular hypotonia; blindness associated with a characteristic lacunar juxtapapillary chorioretinal dysplasia and optic disc anomalies; and central nervous system (CNS) abnormalities, the most common characteristic of which is agenesis of the corpus callosum. No recurrences have been reported among siblings, and parents can be reassured that the risk in subsequent children is minimal. All instances of the disease appear to arise from a new X-dominant lethal mutation, and affected females do not survive long enough to reproduce. The distal end of the short arm of the X chromosome appears to be the crucial area, because some patients with a deletion in this region have also been shown to have features of Aicardi syndrome.

Maternal Inheritance

When nearly all offspring of an affected woman appear to be at risk for inheriting and expressing a trait, and the daughters are at risk for passing on the trait to the next generation, the pattern of inheritance is called *maternal inheritance.* The disease stops with all-male offspring, whether affected or not. This form of inheritance is highly suggestive of a mitochondrial disorder. The structure and molecular aspects of the mitochondrial genome and a general discussion of mitochondrial disease are covered in Chapter 5.

Terminology: Hereditary, Genetic, Familial, Congenital

Hereditary indicates that a disease or trait under consideration results directly from an individual's particular genetic composition (or *genome*) and that it can be passed from one generation to another. *Genetic* denotes that the disorder is caused by a defect of genes, whether acquired or inherited. In some instances, such as mutations in genes related to ocular melanoma, the disease is clearly genetic, but it is not passed to subsequent generations and is therefore not hereditary. Thus, the terms *hereditary* and *genetic* are not synonymous but are sometimes used to convey similar concepts. Both hereditary and genetic disorders may be congenital or develop later in life.

A condition is *familial* if it occurs in more than one member of a family. It may, of course, be hereditary but need not be. A familial disorder can be caused by common exposure to infectious agents (eg, adenoviral conjunctivitis), excess food intake (eg, obesity), or environmental agents, such as cigarette smoke. Genetic factors, however, may contribute to the effects of exposure to these environmental factors and may cloud the picture.

The term *congenital* refers to characteristics present at birth. These characteristics may be hereditary or familial, or they may occur as an isolated event, often as the result of an infection (eg, rubella, toxoplasmosis, or cytomegalovirus) or a toxic agent (eg, as in thalidomide embryopathy or fetal alcohol syndrome). The presence of such characteristics *at birth* or shortly after (in the first weeks of life) is the defining factor. Pediatric ophthalmology literature has traditionally used the terms *congenital nystagmus, congenital esotropia, congenital glaucoma*, and *congenital cataract*; however, in many cases, these disorders are not present at birth and would be more accurately referred to as *infantile.*

Heritability refers to the proportion of phenotypic variation in a population that is attributable to genetic variation among individuals. Estimation of heritability aims to answer the "nature versus nurture" debate and to allow researchers to pursue genetic and/or environmental determinants of disease, although most cases involve a combination of the 2 determinants. Heritability studies compare the phenotypic similarity of genetically closely related individuals with that of less closely related individuals. The best example of this type of study is a comparison of the correlation of identical twins (monozygotic twins, who share 100% of their DNA sequence) with that of nonidentical twins (dizygotic twins, who share 50% of their DNA sequence). With both twins sharing the same age and similar intrauterine and early childhood environments, most of the variation is thought to be due to genetic factors. An example of a twin study concerning the highly heritable trait of central corneal thickness is shown in Figure 6-3.

A condition known to be genetic and hereditary (eg, RP) may appear in only 1 individual of a family. Such an individual is said to have a *simplex,* or *isolated,* form of a genetic disease. A genetically determined trait may be isolated in the pedigree for several reasons:

- The pedigree is small.
- The full expression of the disease has not been sought or has not manifested in other relatives.
- The disorder represents a new genetic mutation or chromosomal change.
- The disorder is recessive, and the investigation to determine whether the parents are carriers has been inadequate.
- There is nonpaternity.

Clinically similar disorders may be inherited in several different ways. For example, RP can occur from an autosomal dominant, autosomal recessive, X-linked recessive, or mitochondrial mutation. These various genetic forms represent distinct gene defects with

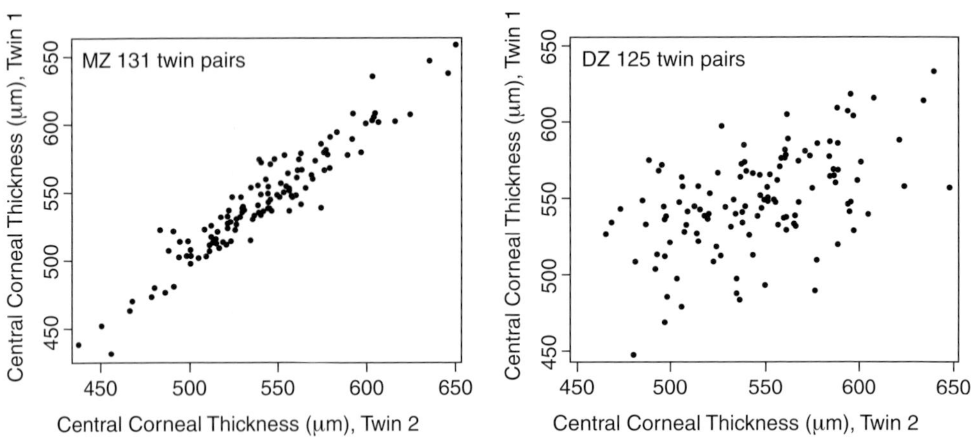

Figure 6-3 Comparison of correlation level for central corneal thickness in a set of monozygotic (MZ) twins with that of a set of dizygotic (DZ) twins. *Left,* Comparison for the MZ twins (correlation, 0.95). *Right,* Comparison for the DZ twins (correlation, 0.52). The difference in the correlation levels of the 2 sets of twins allows for calculation of the heritability of central corneal thickness, which in this example is 95%. *(Courtesy of David A. Mackey, MD.)*

different alterations in gene structure and various biochemical pathogeneses, each of which has similar clinical phenotypic expressions. Clarification of genetic heterogeneity is important, because only with the proper diagnosis and correct identification of the inheritance pattern can appropriate genetic counseling and prognosis be offered.

Some genetic disorders originally thought to be a single and unique entity are found, on close scrutiny, to be two or more fundamentally distinct entities. Further clarification of the inheritance pattern or biochemical analysis permits separation of initially similar disorders. Such has been the case for Marfan syndrome and homocystinuria. Patients with these disorders tend to be tall and thin, with long arms, legs, fingers, and toes; they also have ectopia lentis. However, the presence of dominant inheritance, aortic aneurysms, and valvular heart disease in Marfan syndrome distinguishes it from the recessive pattern and thromboembolic disease of homocystinuria.

Genetic heterogeneity is a general term that applies to the phenotypic similarity that may be produced by two or more fundamentally distinct genetic entities; this term implies that the genes are nonallelic. Leber congenital amaurosis, which has more than 14 causative genes, is a good example (Fig 6-4). Once the location on a chromosome is determined for a particular disease gene, and the gene's molecular structure is identified, most examples of genetic heterogeneity cease to be a problem for diagnosis or classification. However, clinical, allelic, and locus heterogeneity can remain perplexing issues. For example, mutations of the Norrie disease gene, *NDP,* usually result in the typical phenotype of pseudoglioma from exudative retinal detachments, but some *NDP* mutations have been associated with X-linked exudative vitreoretinopathy without any systemic associations.

Sanfilippo PG, Hewitt AW, Hammond CJ, Mackey DA. The heritability of ocular traits. *Surv Ophthalmol.* 2010;55(6):561–583.

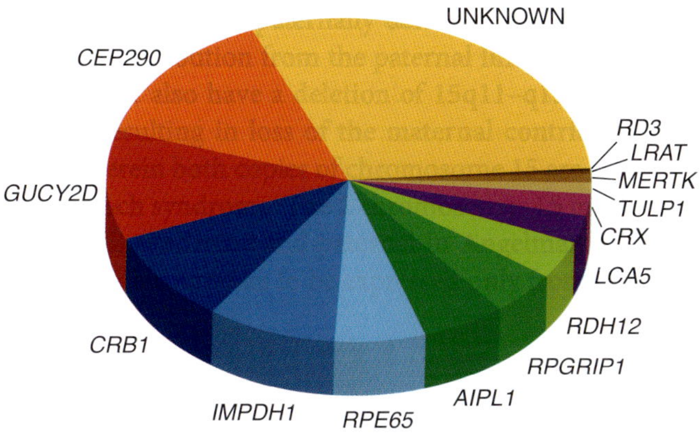

Figure 6-4 Prevalence of the 14 causative genes known in 2008 for cases of Leber congenital amaurosis (led by *CEP290* in approximately 15% of cases). Mutations for approximately 30% of cases remain to be identified. *(Reproduced with permission from den Hollander AI, Roepman R, Koenekoop RK, Cremers FP. Leber congenital amaurosis: genes, proteins and disease mechanisms.* Prog Retin Eye Res. *2008;27(4):391–419.)*

Genes and Chromosomes

The word *gene* comes from the Greek *genes* ("giving birth to") and is used as a term for individual units of hereditary information. Genes are the basic units of inheritance and include the sequence of nucleotides that codes for a single trait or a single polypeptide chain and its associated regulatory regions. Human genes vary substantially in size, from approximately 500 base pairs (bp) to more than 2 million bp. However, more than 98% of human genes range in size from less than 10 kilobase pairs (kb; 1 kb = 1000 bp) to 500 kb. Many are considerably larger than 50 kb. Whereas a single human cell contains enough DNA for 6 million genes, approximately 20,000–25,000 genes are found among the 23 pairs of known chromosomes. Although the remaining 95% of genetic material is likely to be involved in the regulation of gene expression, its precise function is largely unknown.

The relative sequence of the genes, which are arranged linearly along the chromosome, is called the *genetic map.* The physical position or region on a chromosome occupied by a single gene is known as a *locus.* The physical contiguity of various gene loci becomes the vehicle for close association of genes with one another *(linkage)* and their clustering in groups that characteristically move together or separately *(segregation)* from one generation to the next.

Each normal human somatic cell has 46 chromosomes composed of 23 pairs. Each member of a homologous pair carries matched, though not necessarily identical, genes in the same sequence. One member of each chromosome pair is inherited from the father, and the other from the mother. Each normal sperm or ovum contains 23 chromosomes, 1 representative from each pair; thus, each parent transmits half of his or her genetic information to each child. Of the 46 chromosomes, 44 are called *autosomes* because they provide information on somatic characteristics; the remaining 2 chromosomes are X and Y (see the section X-Linked Inheritance earlier in this chapter).

It is important to know whether genes are located on the X chromosome, mitochondrial DNA, or the autosomes; however, there is rarely any clinical value in knowing in which autosome (1–22) a gene is located. In the past, when only a few eye disease genes were known or just the location of a gene was known, clinicians often remembered the chromosomal locations. Now, with certain diseases, such as RP, there are numerous genes involved. Information on genes, including their chromosomal locations, can be readily found in electronic databases, such as OMIM (https://omim.org).

Alleles

The alternative forms of a particular gene at the same locus on each of an identical pair of chromosomes are called *alleles* (Greek for *reciprocals*). If both members of a pair of alleles for a given autosomal locus are identical (ie, the DNA sequence is the same), the individual is *homozygous* (a *homozygote*). If the allelic genes are distinct from each other (ie, the DNA sequence differs), the individual is *heterozygous* (a *heterozygote*). Different gene defects can cause dramatically different phenotypes and still be allelic. For example, sickle cell disease (SS hemoglobinopathy) caused by homozygosity of 1 mutant gene is substantially different from the phenotypic expression of SC hemoglobinopathy, yet the *Hb S* gene and the *Hb C* gene are allelic.

The term *polyallelism* refers to the many possible variants or mutations of a single gene. Mutant proteins that correspond to mutant alleles frequently possess slightly different biochemical properties. Among the mucopolysaccharidoses, for example, the enzyme α-L-iduronidase is defective in both Hurler and Scheie syndromes. Because these disorders stem from mutations of the same gene, they are abnormalities of the same enzyme and are, therefore, allelic. However, the clinical severity of these 2 disorders (age at onset; age at detection; and severity of affliction of skeleton, liver, spleen, and cornea) is entirely different, presumably because the function of the mutant enzyme is less altered by the Scheie syndrome mutation. Because the enzyme is a protein composed of hundreds of amino acids, a mutation resulting in a base substitution within a certain codon might cause a change in one or more amino acids in a portion of the enzyme remote from its active site, thus reducing its effect on the enzyme's function. However, the substitution of 1 amino acid at a crucial location in the enzyme's active site might abolish most or all of its enzymatic activity. Several examples of allelic disorders appear among the mucopolysaccharidoses.

The phenotype of the usual heterozygote is determined by 1 mutant allele and 1 "normal" allele. However, the genotype of a compound heterozygote comprises 2 different mutant alleles, each at the same locus. The genetic Hurler-Scheie compound heterozygote is biochemically proven and clinically manifests features intermediate between those in the homozygotes of the 2 alleles. Whenever detailed biochemical analysis is performed, the products of the 2 alleles manifest slightly different properties (eg, rates of enzyme activity or electrophoretic migration).

In contrast, and as noted earlier, some genetic disorders originally thought to be single and unique may, on close scrutiny, reveal two or more fundamentally distinct entities. Occasionally, this genetic heterogeneity is observed with diseases that are inherited in the same manner, such as tyrosinase-negative and tyrosinase-positive oculocutaneous albinism.

Because these 2 conditions are phenotypically similar and each is inherited as an autosomal recessive trait, it was formerly assumed that they were allelic. When a tyrosinase-negative person with albinism bears children with a tyrosinase-positive person with albinism, the offspring appear clinically normal. This observation excludes the possibility that these 2 conditions are allelic: each form of albinism occurs only when an offspring is homozygous for one of the genes causing the condition. Defects in separate gene loci (the tyrosinase gene and the *P* gene) are now known to cause oculocutaneous albinism. The offspring of individuals with phenotypically similar but genotypically different disorders are called *double heterozygotes* because they are heterozygous for each of the 2 loci.

Ashworth JL, Biswas S, Wraith E, Lloyd IC. Mucopolysaccharidoses and the eye. *Surv Ophthalmol.* 2006;51(1):1–17.

Fenzl CR, Teramoto K, Moshirfar M. Ocular manifestations and management recommendations of lysosomal storage disorders I: mucopolysaccharidoses. *Clin Ophthalmol.* 2015;9:1633–1644.

Mitosis

A cell may undergo 2 types of cell division: mitosis and meiosis. Mitosis gives rise to the multiple generations of genetically identical cells needed for the growth and maintenance of the organism. When mitosis is about to begin, the cell accurately duplicates all of its chromosomes. The replicated chromosomes then separate into 2 identical groups that migrate apart and eventually reach opposite sides of the cell. The cell and its contents then divide, forming 2 genetically identical daughter cells, each with the same diploid chromosome number and genetic information as the parent cell.

Meiosis

In contrast to mitosis, meiosis leads to the production of cells that have only 1 member of each chromosome pair (Fig 6-5). The specialized cells that arise from meiosis and participate in sexual reproduction are called *gametes.* The male gamete is a sperm, and the female gamete, an ovum. During meiosis, a modified sequence of divisions systematically reduces the number of chromosomes in each cell by one-half to the *haploid* number. Consequently, each gamete contains 23 chromosomes, 1 representative of each pair. This assortment occurs randomly, except that 1 representative of each pair of chromosomes is incorporated into each sperm or egg.

At conception, a sperm and an ovum unite, forming a *zygote,* a single cell that contains 46 chromosomes. Because both parents contribute equally to the genetic makeup of their offspring, new and often advantageous gene combinations may emerge.

Segregation

Two allelic genes, which occupy the same gene locus on 2 homologous chromosomes, separate with the division of the 2 chromosomes during meiosis, and each goes to a different gamete. Thus, the genes are said to *segregate,* a property limited to allelic genes, which cannot occur together in a single offspring of the bearer. For example, if a parent is a compound heterozygote for both hemoglobin S and hemoglobin C, which occupy the

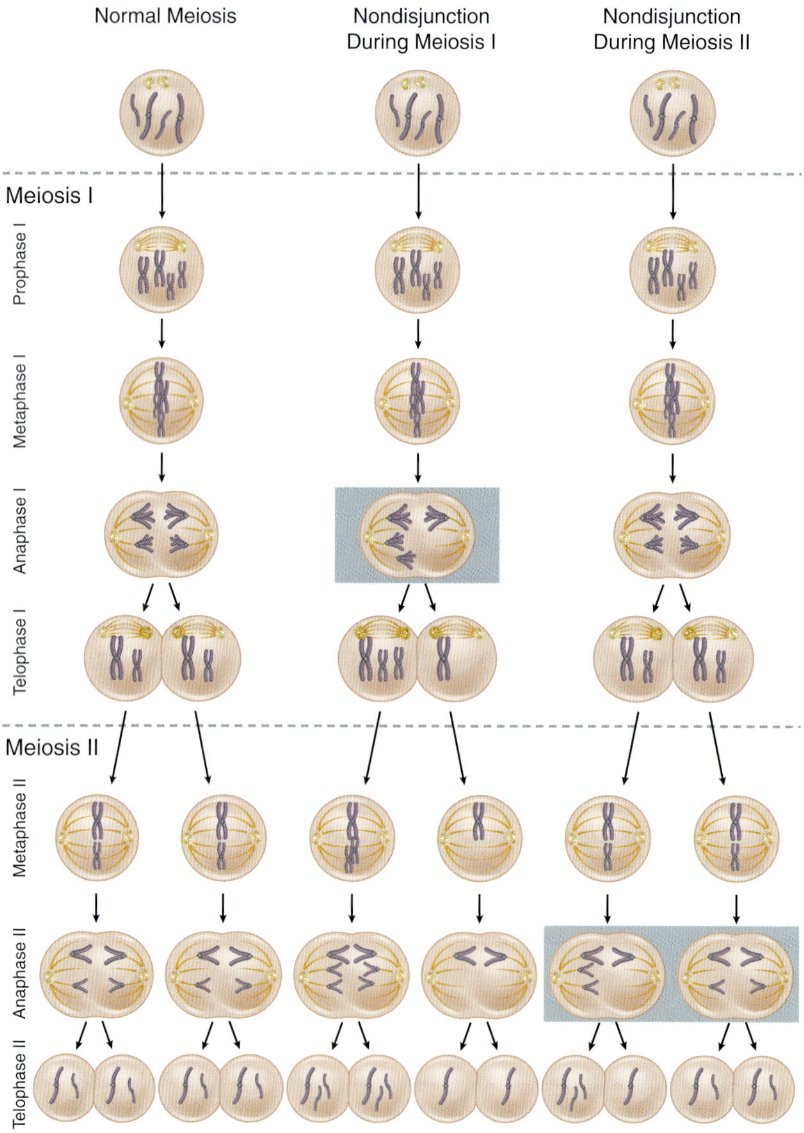

Figure 6-5 Normal meiosis and chromosomal nondisjunction *(blue boxes)* occurring at different phases of meiosis. *(Illustration by Cyndie C.H. Wooley.)*

same genetic locus on homologous chromosomes, then none of the offspring will inherit both hemoglobins from that parent; each will inherit either one or the other.

Independent Assortment

Genes on different *(nonhomologous)* chromosomes may or may not separate together during meiotic cell division. This random process, called *independent assortment,* states that nonallelic genes assort independently of one another. Because *crossing over* (exchange of chromosomal material between the members of a pair of homologous chromosomes) can occur in meiosis, 2 nonallelic genes originally on opposite members of the chromosomal pair may end up together on either of the 2 or may remain separated, depending on their original positions and on the sites of genetic interchange. Thus, the gametes of an individual with 2 nonallelic dominant traits, or *syntenic traits,* located on the same chromosome could produce 4 possible offspring. A child may inherit

- both traits, if the separate alleles remain on the same chromosome and the child inherits this chromosome
- neither trait, if the genes remain on 1 chromosome but the child inherits the opposite chromosome with neither allele
- only 1 of the 2 alleles, if crossing over occurred between the loci, and the child receives the chromosome with that particular allele

This scheme for nonallelic traits depends on the independent assortment of chromosomes in the first division of meiosis. Approximately 50 crossovers (1–3 per chromosome) occur during an average meiotic division.

Linkage

Linkage is the major exception or modification to the law of independent assortment. Genes located reasonably closely together on the same chromosome tend to be transmitted together, from generation to generation, more frequently than chance alone would allow for; therefore, they are said to be linked. The closer together the 2 loci are, the less likely they are to be affected by crossovers. Linear physical proximity along a chromosome cannot be considered an automatic guarantor of linkage, however. In fact, certain sites on each chromosome may be more vulnerable to homologous crossing over than others.

Mutations

Change in the structure or sequence of a gene is called a *mutation.* A mutation can occur randomly anywhere along the DNA sequence of a gene and may result when one nucleotide is substituted for another *(point mutation).* A mutation that occurs in a noncoding portion of the gene may or may not be of clinical consequence. Similarly, a mutation may structurally alter a protein but in a manner that does not notably compromise its function. A new mutation that compromises function may appear in a given gene as the gene is transmitted from parent to offspring.

More gross mutations may involve deletion, translocation, insertion, or internal duplication of a portion of the DNA. Some mutations cause either destruction of the offspring or sterility. Others are less harmful or are potentially beneficial and become established in subsequent generations. Mutations can occur spontaneously for reasons that are not understood. They may also be induced by exposure to a variety of environmental agents called *mutagens,* such as radiation, viruses, and certain chemicals.

Mutations may arise in somatic as well as germinal cells, but these are not transmitted to subsequent generations. Somatic mutations in humans are difficult to identify, although some account for the inception of certain forms of neoplasia (eg, retinoblastoma).

Polymorphisms

Many base changes have little or no deleterious effect on the organism. A *polymorphism* is defined as the occurrence of 2 or more alleles at a specific locus with a frequency greater than 1% each in a given population. Single nucleotide polymorphisms (SNPs) are important for gene mapping in genome-wide association studies (GWAS).

Genome, Genotype, Phenotype

The genome is the sum of the genetic material within a cell or an organism—thus, the total genetic endowment. By contrast, the genotype defines the genetic constitution, and thus biological capability, with regard to a specific locus (eg, individual blood groups or a specific single enzyme). Phenotype indicates the observable or manifest physical, physiologic, biochemical, or molecular characteristics of an individual, which are determined by the genotype but can be modified by the environment.

A clinical picture produced entirely by environmental factors that nevertheless closely resembles, or is even identical to, a phenotype is known as a *phenocopy.* Thus, for example, the pigmentary retinopathy of congenital rubella has occasionally been confused with a hereditary dystrophic disorder of the retina, RP. Similarly, amiodarone-induced changes in the corneal epithelium resemble those observed as cornea verticillata in the X-linked dystrophic disorder Fabry disease.

Single-Gene Disorders

Approximately 4500 different diseases are known to be caused by a defect in a single gene. As a group, these disorders are called *monogenic,* or *mendelian,* diseases. They most often show 1 of 3 patterns of inheritance: autosomal dominant, autosomal recessive, or X-linked. Disorders of mitochondrial DNA are inherited in a fourth manner, termed *maternal inheritance.*

Anticipation

Variability is an intrinsic property of human genetic disease that reflects the quantitative and qualitative differences in phenotype among individuals with the "same" mutant allele. Even within a single family with a genetic disease, each affected individual may manifest the disease to a different degree, with different features, or at a different age. For example, there is wide variation in both severity and age at detection of features of myotonic dystrophy (also called *Steinert disease*), which include motor myotonia, cataracts, gonadal atrophy, and presenile baldness. Even within a single family, the characteristic cataracts may begin to affect vision at any time from the second to the seventh decade of life.

Such variability of clinical manifestation led to the concept of *anticipation,* the phenomenon of apparently earlier and more severe onset of a disease in successive generations within a family. Before 1990, most geneticists thought that anticipation was not a biological phenomenon but rather an artifact of ascertainment. With the relatively recent discovery of triplet or trinucleotide tandem-repeat expansion diseases, anticipation has been shown to reflect the increased length of trinucleotide tandem repeats from one generation to the next. Anticipation occurs in autosomal dominant disorders. Myotonic dystrophy, fragile X syndrome, Huntington disease, and Kennedy disease (a form of spinobulbar muscular atrophy) are some of the diseases whose discovery contributed to the rejuvenation of the concept of anticipation.

Some human variability may result from the intrinsic differences in the genetic background of every human being. Other recognizable or presumptive influences on the variable intra- or interfamilial phenotype of the same gene include the following factors:

- sex influences or limitations
- maternal factors, such as intrauterine environment and even cytoplasmic (eg, mitochondrial) inheritance factors
- modifying loci
- genetic heterogeneity, including both isoalleles and genocopies
- gene alterations induced either by position effects with other genes or by somatic mutations
- epigenetic factors, methylation, and histone formation

Obviously, nongenetic factors (eg, diet, temperature, and drugs) may affect gene expression, either as phenocopies or through ecologic parameters.

Penetrance

The presence or absence of any effect of a gene is called *penetrance.* If a gene generates any evidence of phenotypic features, no matter how minimal, it is termed *penetrant.* If it is not expressed at any level of detection, it is termed *nonpenetrant.*

> Penetrance is an all-or-nothing concept, statistically representing the fraction of individuals carrying a given gene who manifest any evidence of the specific trait.

In families with an autosomal dominant mutant gene that has 100% penetrance of the phenotype, an average of 50% of the offspring will inherit the gene and show evidence of the disease.

Although penetrance has an exact statistical definition, its clinical ascertainment is affected by diagnostic awareness and the methods of physical examination. For example, many mild cases of Marfan syndrome would be missed without careful biomicroscopy of the fully dilated pupil and echocardiography of the heart valves and great vessels. Similarly, if the criteria for identification of the retinoblastoma gene include indirect ophthalmoscopy and scleral depression, some "nonpenetrant" parents or siblings in families with "dominantly inherited" retinoblastoma may be found to have a spontaneously involuted tumor, which clearly identifies them as bearers of the gene. In another example, some family members who have a gene for Best macular dystrophy will be identified not by clinical ophthalmoscopic examination but only by electro-oculographic testing. Therefore, in examining a potential bearer of a gene, the examiner must carefully search for any manifestations of the gene's effects in all susceptible tissues before dismissing someone as from a "skipped generation."

Expressivity

The presence of a defective gene does not necessarily imply a complete expression of every potential manifestation. The variety of ways and levels of severity in which a particular genetic trait manifests among different affected individuals is called *expressivity.* In neurofibromatosis (NF) 1, for example, an affected child may have only Lisch nodules of the iris and café-au-lait spots. The affected parent may also have extensive punctiform and pedunculated neurofibromas of the skin, plexiform neurofibroma, and optic nerve glioma.

> It is extremely rare that all affected members in the same family have uniform textbook presentations of the disorder.

Differences in the age at onset of clinical manifestations are one way that dominant disorders demonstrate expressivity. For example, in NF1, an affected individual may have the following sequence: only café-au-lait spots at birth, Lisch nodules that gradually increase in number and size at about age 5–10 years, punctiform neurofibromas of the skin in early adolescence, subareolar neurofibromas after puberty (females), and visual impairment from the effect of an optic glioma in the late teenaged years. Although all of these features are phenotypic components of the mutant gene, each feature has a characteristic age at onset and a natural history of growth and effect within the umbrella of the total disease. See the section "Genetics of the phakomatoses" for additional discussion of NF1.

Pleiotropism

Alteration within a single mutant gene may have consequences in various tissues in a given individual. The presentation of multiple phenotypic abnormalities in different organ systems produced by a single mutant gene is termed *pleiotropism.* For example:

- Marfan syndrome: Ectopia lentis occurs with arachnodactyly, aortic aneurysms, and long extremities.
- DIDMOAD (*d*iabetes *i*nsipidus, *d*iabetes *m*ellitus, *o*ptic *a*trophy, and neural *d*eafness) syndrome: Optic atrophy is found in association with juvenile diabetes mellitus, diabetes insipidus, and moderate perceptive hearing impairment.
- Alport syndrome: Neurosensory hearing loss can be associated with hereditary hematuric nephritis, lenticular changes (anterior lenticonus, spherophakia, cataracts), arcus juvenilis, and whitish-yellow retinal lesions.
- Bardet-Biedl syndrome: This is characterized by pigmentary retinopathy, obesity, genital hypoplasia, mental debility, and polydactyly.

In each of these disorders, a single mutant gene is responsible for dysfunction in multiple organ systems.

Chromosome Analysis

Cytogenetics is the branch of genetics concerned with the study of chromosomes and their properties. Chromosomal defects are changes in the chromosome number or structure that damage sensitive genetic functions and lead to developmental or reproductive disorders. These defects usually result from (1) a disruption of the mechanisms controlling chromosome movement during cell division; or (2) alterations of chromosome structure that lead to changes in the number or arrangement of genes or to abnormal chromosomal behavior.

Chromosomal abnormalities occur in approximately 1 of 200 term pregnancies and in 1%–2% of all pregnancies involving parents older than 35 years. About 7% of perinatal deaths and some 40%–50% of retrievable spontaneous abortuses have significant chromosomal aberrations. Virtually any change in chromosome number during early development profoundly affects the formation of tissues and organs and the viability of the entire organism. Most major chromosomal disorders are characterized by both developmental delay and cognitive disability, as well as a variety of somatic abnormalities.

Indications for and Types of Chromosome Analysis

Ophthalmologists should be aware of the value of learning the constitutional and tumor karyotypes for infants with retinoblastoma, especially if the tumor represents a new genetic mutation. Chromosome analysis (also called *karyotyping*) is also suggested in patients with isolated (nonfamilial) aniridia (which is often associated with Wilms tumor) and other systemic malformations.

A chromosomally abnormal state in a previous child warrants consideration of amniocentesis or chorionic villus sampling for prenatal diagnosis in subsequent pregnancies to avoid the risk of recurrence. An alternative is the use of preimplantation genetic diagnosis (discussed later in the chapter, under Reproductive Issues).

Karyotype

The systematic display of chromosomes from a single somatic cell is called a *karyotype*. Chromosome preparations are most commonly obtained from peripheral venous blood, although bone marrow, skin fibroblasts, and cells from amniotic fluid or chorionic villi are useful under specific circumstances. Chromosome analysis can be obtained directly from neoplastic tissues, as in retinoblastoma and Wilms tumor, for example.

Fluorescence in situ hybridization and chromosome arm painting

With the fluorescence in situ hybridization (FISH) technique, DNA fragments from genes of interest are first tagged with a fluorescent compound and then annealed or hybridized to chromosomes. In the process of chromosome arm painting, the regions of interest are stained to determine whether duplication, deletion, or rearrangement has occurred. Such fluorescent molecular probes can be used to detect and often quantify the presence of specific DNA sequences on a chromosome and can identify microscopic abnormalities that would be indiscernible by conventional cytogenetic methods.

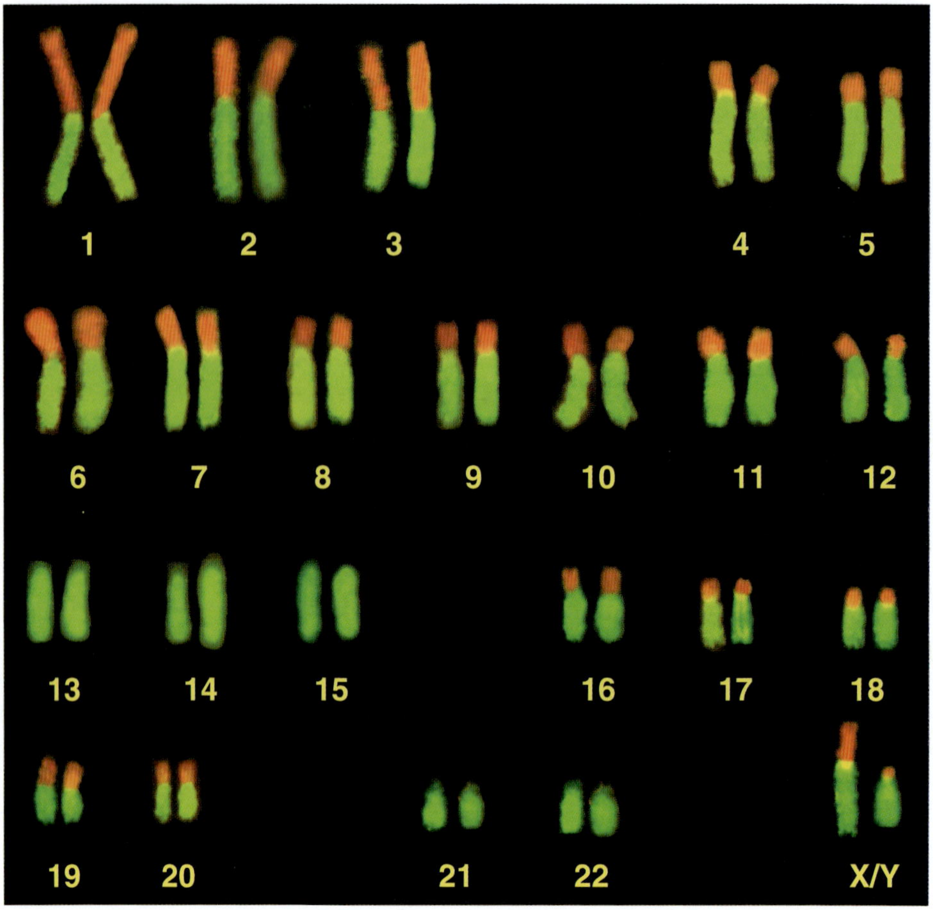

Figure 6-6 Composite karyotype of all human chromosomes hybridized with chromosome arm painting. Metaphase chromosomes were hybridized simultaneously with corresponding short-arm *(red)* and long-arm *(green)* painting probes, and a composite karyotype was generated. *(Reproduced with permission from Guan XY, Zhang H, Bittner M, Jiang Y, Meltzer P, Trent J. Chromosome arm painting probes.* Nat Genet. *1996;12(1):10–11.)*

Using microdissections of chromosomal regions and FISH, probes have been developed that label entire arms of chromosomes and each of the individual chromosomes (multicolor spectral karyotyping and combinatorial multifluor FISH). With 2-color FISH, both arms of each chromosome can be labeled simultaneously (Fig 6-6). These probes are valuable for detecting and understanding the mechanisms of complex chromosomal rearrangement.

Speicher MR, Gwyn Ballard S, Ward DC. Karyotyping human chromosomes by combinatorial multi-fluor FISH. *Nat Genet.* 1996;12(4):368–375.

Aneuploidy of Autosomes

Aneuploidy denotes an abnormal number of chromosomes in cells. The presence of 3 homologous chromosomes in a cell, rather than the normal pair, is termed *trisomy.*

Monosomy is the presence of only 1 member of any pair of autosomes or only 1 sex chromosome. The absence of a single autosome is almost always lethal to the embryo; an extra autosome is often catastrophic to surviving embryos. Aneuploidy of sex chromosomes (eg, X, XXX, XXY, and XYY) is less disastrous. Monosomies and trisomies are generally caused by mechanical accidents that increase or decrease the number of chromosomes in the gametes. The most common type of accident, meiotic *nondisjunction,* results from a disruption of chromosome movement during meiosis (see Fig 6-5).

Trisomy 21 syndrome, or Down syndrome, is the most common chromosomal syndrome in humans; it has an overall incidence of 1:800 live births. Clinical features of this syndrome have been well known since John Langdon Down originally described them in 1866.

The most important risk factor for having a child with Down syndrome is maternal age. The frequency of Down syndrome increases from approximately 1:1400 live births for mothers aged 20–24 years to approximately 1:40 live births for mothers aged 44 years. However, the frequency of Down syndrome is greater (1:1250) for mothers between 15 and 19 years of age than it is in the next-higher age range. Above age 50 years, the frequency is 1:11 live births. The eponym *Down syndrome* summarizes a clinical description of certain distinctive, if variable, phenotypic features whereas the karyotype describes the chromosomal constitution of the cells and tissues studied.

In more than 80% of Down syndrome cases, the genetic error occurs in meiosis I (see Chapter 5); and in more than 95% of cases, the error occurs in maternal rather than paternal meiosis. Approximately 5% of patients with Down syndrome have a *translocation* resulting from attachment of the long arm of chromosome 21 to the long arm of another acrocentric chromosome, usually 14 or 22. These translocations cause pairing problems during meiosis, and the translocated fragment of chromosome 21 appears in one of the daughter cells along with a normal chromosome 21. As in nondisjunction, the fragment becomes trisomic on fertilization. Trisomy of only the distal one-third of chromosome arm 21q is sufficient to cause the disorder. Genes that lie within the q22 band of chromosome 21 appear to be specifically responsible for the pathogenesis of Down syndrome.

Patients with Down syndrome may exhibit the following features:

- cognitive disabilities
- characteristic facies: oblique palpebral fissure, epicanthus, flat nasal bridge, and protruding tongue
- short, broad hands and wide space between first and second toes; characteristic dermatoglyphics
- hypotonia
- congenital heart disease
- immunologic, hematologic anomalies
- gastrointestinal anomalies
- atlantoaxial instability
- epilepsy
- Alzheimer disease
- short stature
- infertility
- dental hypoplasia

Table 6-6 Ocular Findings in Down Syndrome (Trisomy 21)

More common
Almond-shaped palpebral fissures
Upward-slanting palpebral fissures
Prominent epicanthal folds
Blepharitis, usually chronic, with cicatricial ectropion
Nasolacrimal duct obstruction
Strabismus, usually esotropic
Nystagmus (typically horizontal)
Aberrant retinal vessels (at optic disc margin)
Iris stromal hypoplasia
Brushfield spots
Cataract (congenital or acquired)
Myopia
Less common
Infantile glaucoma
Keratoconus
Optic nerve head abnormalities

Ophthalmic features of Down syndrome are presented in Table 6-6.

Leonard S, Bower C, Petterson B, Leonard H. Medical aspects of school-aged children with Down syndrome. *Dev Med Child Neurol.* 1999;41(10):683–688.

Mosaicism

Occasionally, an individual or a tissue contains two or more cell lines with distinctly different chromosomal constitutions. Such individuals or tissues are termed *mosaics.* Sometimes the peripheral blood, which is the usual source for chromosomal analysis, contains populations of cells with completely different chromosomal constitutions. One population of cells may be so infrequent that a second tissue, such as skin fibroblasts, must be analyzed to demonstrate the mosaicism.

The clinical effects of mosaicism are difficult to predict because the distribution of abnormal cells in the embryo is determined by the timing of the error and other variables. If mitotic nondisjunction immediately follows conception, the zygote divides into 2 abnormal cells: 1 trisomic and 1 monosomic. The monosomic cells rarely survive and may decrease in number or even disappear entirely over time. Mitotic nondisjunction may occur when the embryo is composed of a small population of cells. Thus, 3 populations of cells are established—1 normal and 2 abnormal—although some abnormal cell lines may be "discarded" or lost during development. If mitotic nondisjunction occurs at a more advanced stage of development, resulting abnormal populations constitute a minority of the embryo's cells, and mosaicism may have little or no measurable effect on development.

A small population of aneuploid mosaic cells may not have a direct effect on development. However, when cells of this type occur in the reproductive tissues of otherwise unaffected people, some of the gametes may carry extra chromosomes or may be missing some entirely. Consequently, mosaic parents tend to be at high risk for having chromosomally abnormal children.

The most common example of autosomal mosaicism is *trisomy 21 mosaicism*. Some patients with trisomy 21 mosaicism have the typical features of Down syndrome; others show no abnormalities in appearance or intelligence. The crucial variables seem to be the frequency and the embryologic distribution of the trisomic cells during early development, which do not necessarily correlate with the percentage of trisomic cells in any one tissue, such as peripheral blood.

Several types of sex chromosome mosaicism may occur. Again, the physical effects tend to vary, probably reflecting the quantity and distribution of the abnormal cells during development. For example, the cell population that lacks 1 of the X chromosomes can arise in a female embryo, leading to 45,X/46,XX mosaicism. In some cases, these patients develop normally; in other cases, some or all of the features of Turner syndrome appear. Similarly, the Y chromosome may be lost in some cells of a developing male embryo. This produces 45,X/46,XY mosaicism. Persons with X/XY mosaicism may develop as phenotypically unaffected males, as females with the features of Turner syndrome, or as individuals with physical characteristics intermediate between the sexes (*intersexes* or *pseudohermaphrodites*).

Important Chromosomal Aberrations in Ophthalmology

Short arm 11 deletion (11p13) syndrome: aniridia

Classic aniridia results from a defect in a gene that encodes a transcription factor needed for development of the eye. This developmental gene, *PAX6*, is located at 11p13. The *PAX6* gene product is a transcription factor required for normal development of the eye. Classic aniridia is a panophthalmic disorder characterized by the following features:

- iris absence or severe hypoplasia
- cataracts (usually anterior polar)
- keratitis due to limbal stem cell failure
- subnormal visual acuity
- congenital nystagmus
- foveal or macular hypoplasia
- optic nerve hypoplasia
- glaucoma
- strabismus
- ectopia lentis

When working with a new patient with aniridia, the ophthalmologist should, if possible, conduct a careful examination of the patient's parents for the variable expression of autosomal dominant aniridia. Although almost all cases of aniridia result from *PAX6* mutations, a rare autosomal recessive disorder called *Gillespie syndrome* (phenotype OMIM number 206700) also produces partial aniridia, as well as cerebellar ataxia, mental deficiency, and congenital cataracts.

Aniridia (often with cataract and glaucoma) can also occur sporadically in association with Wilms tumor, other genitourinary anomalies, and cognitive disability, the so-called *WAGR syndrome*. This complex of findings is called a *contiguous gene-deletion syndrome* because it results from a deletion involving nearby genes. Most affected patients have a karyotypically visible interstitial deletion of a segment of 11p13. Patients with aniridia that is *not* clearly part of an autosomal dominant trait, and those with coincident systemic malformations, should undergo chromosome analysis (karyotyping) and observation for possible Wilms tumor.

Mutations of *PAX6* have also been reported in Peters anomaly, autosomal dominant keratitis, and dominant foveal hypoplasia. The mechanism for disruption of normal embryology and the degenerative disease in aniridia and other *PAX6* disorders appears to be *haploinsufficiency,* which, in this case, is the inability of a single active allele to activate transduction of the developmental genes regulated by the *PAX6* gene product. In this way, aniridia is different from retinoblastoma and Wilms tumor, which result from an absence of both functional alleles at each of the homologous gene loci.

Landsend ES, Utheim ØA, Pedersen HR, Lagali N, Baraas RC, Utheim TP. The genetics of congenital aniridia—a guide for the ophthalmologist. *Surv Ophthalmol.* 2018;63(1): 105–113.

Long arm 13 deletion (13q14) syndrome: retinoblastoma

Retinoblastoma is one of several heritable childhood malignancies. Ocular tumors, which are usually noted before the age of 4 years, affect between 1 in 15,000 and 1 in 34,000 live births in the United States. The disease exhibits both hereditary occurrence (approximately 30%–40%), in which tumors tend to be bilateral and multicentric, and sporadic occurrence, in which unilateral and solitary tumors are the rule. Only about 10% of patients with hereditary retinoblastoma have a family history of the disease; the remaining 90% have a new mutation in their germ cells.

Retinoblastoma does not develop in approximately 10% of all obligate carriers of a germline mutation (ie, incomplete penetrance). In addition, a karyotypically visible deletion of part of the long arm of chromosome 13 occurs in 3%–7% of all cases of retinoblastoma. The larger this deletion is, the more severe is the phenotypic syndrome, which includes cognitive disabilities and developmental delays, microcephaly, hand and foot anomalies, and ambiguous genitalia.

Although the hereditary pattern in familial retinoblastoma is that of an autosomal dominant mutation, the defect is recessive at the cellular level. The predisposition to retinoblastoma is caused by hemizygosity of the retinoblastoma gene *(RB1)* within band 13q14. *RB1* is a member of a class of genes called *recessive tumor suppressor genes.* The RB protein regulates the cell cycle at the G_1 checkpoint. The alleles normally present at these loci help prevent tumor formation. At least 1 active normal allele is needed to prevent the cell from losing control of proliferation. Patients who inherit a defective allele from 1 parent are at greater risk for losing the other allele through a number of mechanisms. Thus, tumor formation in retinoblastoma is due to the loss of function of both normal alleles. Homozygous deletions within the 13q14 band have been noted in retinoblastomas derived from enucleated eyes.

The first step in tumorigenesis in retinoblastoma is a recessive mutation of 1 of the homologous alleles at the retinoblastoma locus by inheritance, germinal mutation, or somatic mutation. Hereditary retinoblastomas arise from a single additional somatic event in a cell that carries an inherited mutation, whereas sporadic cases require 2 somatic events. In approximately 50% of tumors, homozygosity for such a recessive mutation results from the mitotic loss of a portion of chromosome 13, including the 13q14 band. The 2 resulting mutant alleles at this locus allow the genesis of the tumor. Retinoblastoma, therefore, seemingly represents a malignancy caused by defective gene regulation rather than by the presence of a dominant mutant oncogene. Those who inherit a mutant allele at this locus have a high incidence of nonocular second tumors thought to be caused by the same mutation. Almost half of these tumors are osteosarcomas.

Knudson's 2-Hit Hypothesis and the Genetics of Retinoblastoma and the Phakomatoses

Knudson's hypothesis and the genetics of retinoblastoma

Study of the occurrence of unilateral and bilateral retinoblastoma led to the *2-hit hypothesis,* according to which some tumors arise from a single cell with de novo mutations in both copies of a key gene (*RB1* in retinoblastoma or other oncogenes in other diseases). Conversely, in an individual who has a germline mutation (first "hit") in every cell of their body, a second mutation ("hit") occurring spontaneously in a somatic cell(s) can result in single or multiple tumors (Fig 6-7). Knudson's hypothesis, now proven, is applicable to many cancers.

RB1 mutations occurring in a cone precursor cell result in retinoblastoma. In other cell lines, additional mutations in other genes (sometimes precipitated by radiation from radiotherapy or computed tomography [CT] scans) can lead to the development of other tumors, such as osteosarcoma, soft tissue sarcoma, and malignant melanoma. A cascade of mutations in other genes can also lead to increasing malignancy of a tumor.

With an autosomal dominant inheritance pattern, a germline mutation may be inherited from either parent. Alternatively, a child may inherit a germline mutation from an unaffected parent who has mutations in the cells producing eggs or, more often, in sperm. The risk of mutations in sperm increases with increasing age of the father. Guidelines for clinical screening and DNA testing of children at risk for retinoblastoma have recently been revised.

Skalet AH, Gombos DS, Gallie BL, et al. Screening children at risk for retinoblastoma: consensus report from the American Association of Ophthalmic Oncologists and Pathologists. *Ophthalmology.* 2018;125(3):453–458.

Genetics of the phakomatoses

As mentioned, Knudson's 2-hit hypothesis is applicable to many tumors, including the phakomatoses. The phakomatoses are a group of hereditary disorders characterized by hamartomas of the skin, eye, CNS, and viscera. Three disorders have traditionally been designated as phakomatoses: NF1 and NF2, von Hippel–Lindau syndrome, and tuberous sclerosis.

NF1 (von Recklinghausen disease) occurs with a germline mutation in the *NF1* gene, which produces neurofibromin. A second "hit," or mutation, can result in the development of neurofibromas in nerves, gliomas in the optic nerve, Lisch nodules (iris hamartomas),

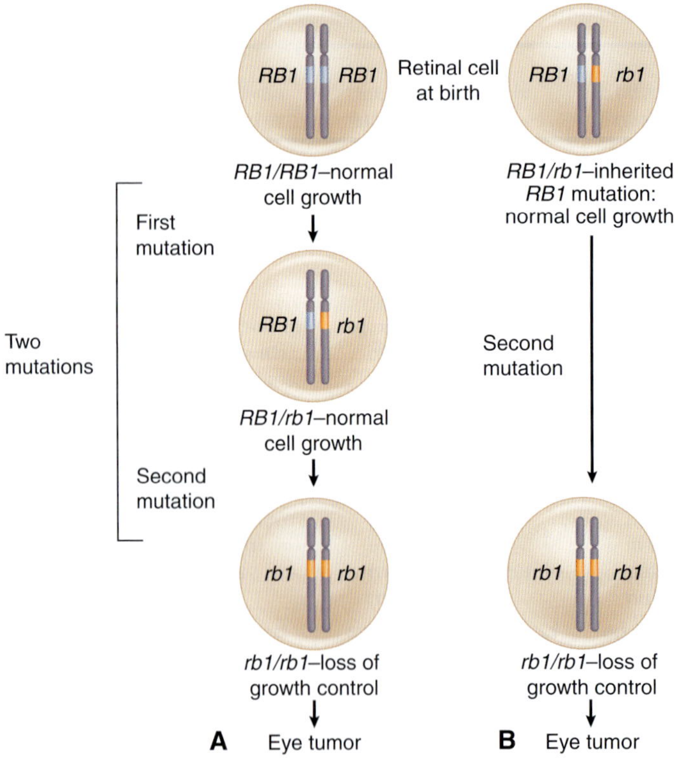

Figure 6-7 Comparison of sporadic retinoblastoma **(A),** where 2 independent mutations ("hits") in the *RB1* gene occur in a somatic cell, with hereditary retinoblastoma **(B),** where a germline mutation is present in every cell and second mutations can arise in multiple cells, leading to multiple tumors. *(Illustration by Cyndie C.H. Wooley.)*

café-au-lait spots in the skin, and other tumors. Genetic studies of isolated gliomas have found that these can arise from 2 hits in the *NF1* gene.

NF2 occurs with mutations in the *NF2* gene, which produces merlin (also called *schwannomin*). A second hit can result in acoustic neuromas, meningiomas, gliomas, ependymomas, and schwannomas.

Von Hippel–Lindau syndrome (also called *familial cerebello retinal angiomatosis)* occurs with germline mutations in the *VHL* tumor suppressor gene. Hypoxia inducible factor, a regulator of cell division and angiogenesis, is a target of the VHL protein. The syndrome is characterized by benign and malignant multisystem tumors, including retinal and CNS hemangioblastomas, clear cell renal carcinoma, pheochromocytoma, epidydimal cystadenoma, and pancreatic carcinoma.

Tuberous sclerosis is caused by mutation in either of 2 genes: *TSC1,* which produces the protein hamartin, and *TSC2,* which produces the protein tuberin. Each of these account for 50% of cases. The 2 proteins interact, forming a heterodimer in the cytoplasm. Tuberous sclerosis has many clinical features, including optic nerve or retinal tumors (astrocytic hamartoma), which may be flat or mulberry-like in appearance; cerebral tubers; ash-leaf skin lesions; subungual fibromas; and facial angiofibromas. In children, facial angiofibromas are thought to arise from second hits caused by exposure to UV radiation.

All of these genetic disorders can be inherited (with affected persons usually having multiple tumors) or sporadic (with affected persons having isolated tumors). The latter may occur from 2 hits in a somatic cell. One phakomatosis that is not inherited (possibly because germline mutations are not compatible with life) is Sturge-Weber syndrome (SWS; also called *encephalofacial angiomatosis*). SWS is caused by a somatic mutation in the *GNAQ* gene, which functions to control the development of blood vessels. SWS is characterized by vascular lesions that affect the skin; when the skin lesion is around the eyelids, there can also be vascular lesions of the choroid (hemangioma) and, in many cases, glaucoma. Glaucoma occurs either from trabeculodysgenesis or elevated episcleral venous pressure.

See BCSC Section 5, *Neuro-Ophthalmology*; Section 6, *Pediatric Ophthalmology and Strabismus*; and Section 12, *Retina and Vitreous,* for additional discussion of these disorders.

Racial and Ethnic Concentration of Genetic Disorders

Most genetic diseases occur without regard for the affected individual's racial or ethnic background. Some, however, are concentrated in certain population groups and may reflect a previous advantage of the mutation (particularly in the carrier state). For example, sickle cell carriers are more resistant to malaria and the disease is common in African-derived populations.

Tay-Sachs disease (GM_2 gangliosidosis type I), with its characteristic macular cherry-red spot, occurs predominantly in persons of Eastern European Jewish (Ashkenazic) ancestry. An estimated rate of 1 in 30 for carriers of this disorder in the Jewish population of New York City compares with an estimated carrier rate of 1 in 300 in non-Jewish Americans. Familial dysautonomia *(Riley-Day syndrome)*—characterized by alacrima, corneal hypoesthesia, exodeviation, and methacholine-induced miosis—also occurs more frequently in persons of Ashkenazic ancestry, as do *MAK (male germ cell–associated kinase)-associated RP, Gaucher disease,* and *Niemann-Pick disease.*

Several types of *achromatopsia* (complete color blindness) with *myopia* are common on the South Pacific island of Pingelap, affecting 5% of the Pingelapese population in the Caroline Islands of Micronesia. *Oguchi disease* is observed primarily, though not exclusively, in Japanese people. Similarly, *sickle cell hemoglobinopathies* are inherited largely among African Americans.

The prevalence of *oculocutaneous albinism* is high among the Kuna Indians in Panama. *Hermansky-Pudlak syndrome (HPS)* occurs with a higher frequency in persons of Puerto Rican ancestry. HPS is an autosomal recessive disorder characterized by oculocutaneous albinism, pulmonary interstitial fibrosis, easy bruising, and bleeding tendency, associated with a prolonged bleeding time and abnormal platelet aggregation.

Lyonization

In classical human genetics, females with a gene for a recessive disease or trait on only 1 X chromosome should have no manifestations of the defect. However, ophthalmic examples of structural and functional abnormalities in females heterozygous for supposedly recessive X-linked traits abound. Such *carrier states,* usually mild but occasionally severe, have been described in carriers of such diseases as

- choroideremia
- X-linked ocular albinism, or ocular albinism type 1 (also called *Nettleship-Falls ocular albinism*)
- X-linked RP
- X-linked sutural cataracts
- Lowe syndrome
- Fabry disease
- color vision defects of the protan and deutan types

See Figure 6-8 and Table 6-7.

Detection of these carrier states of the X-linked traits is clinically relevant, especially for sisters and maternal aunts of affected males. In 1961, geneticist Mary Lyon advanced an explanation for the unanticipated or partial expression of a trait by a heterozygous female. Briefly, in *lyonization* (X-chromosome inactivation), every somatic cell of a female has only 1 X chromosome that is actively functioning. The second X chromosome is inactive and forms a densely staining marginal nuclear structure demonstrated as a Barr body in a buccal smear or in "drumsticks," pedunculated lobules of the nucleus identified in about 5% of the leukocytes of the unaffected female. Inactivation of 1 X chromosome occurs randomly in early embryogenesis. The same X chromosome will be irreversibly inactive in every daughter cell of each of these "committed" primordial cells. The active gene is dominant at a cellular level. Thus, a heterozygous female for an X-linked disease will have 2 clonal cell populations (mosaic phenotype), 1 with normal activity for the gene in question and the other with mutant activity.

The proportion of mutant to normal X chromosomes inactivated usually follows a normal distribution, because presumably the inactivation in various cells is a random event. Thus, an average of 50% of paternal X chromosomes and 50% of maternal X chromosomes are inactivated. It is conceivable, however, that in some cases the mutant X is active in almost all cells; in other cases, the mutant X is inactivated in nearly all cells. By this mechanism, a female may express an X-linked disorder; and rare cases are known of women who have a classic color deficiency or X-linked ocular albinism, X-linked RP, or choroideremia.

Carriers of X-linked ocular albinism may have a mottled mosaic fundus: in the pigmented retinal epithelial cells, the normal X chromosome is active; in the nonpigmented cells, the mutant X is active. However, these distinguishing features of the carrier state are not always present. The possibility that the patient is a carrier cannot be entirely eliminated if a given sign is not present because in a female, chance inactivation of the

A B C D E

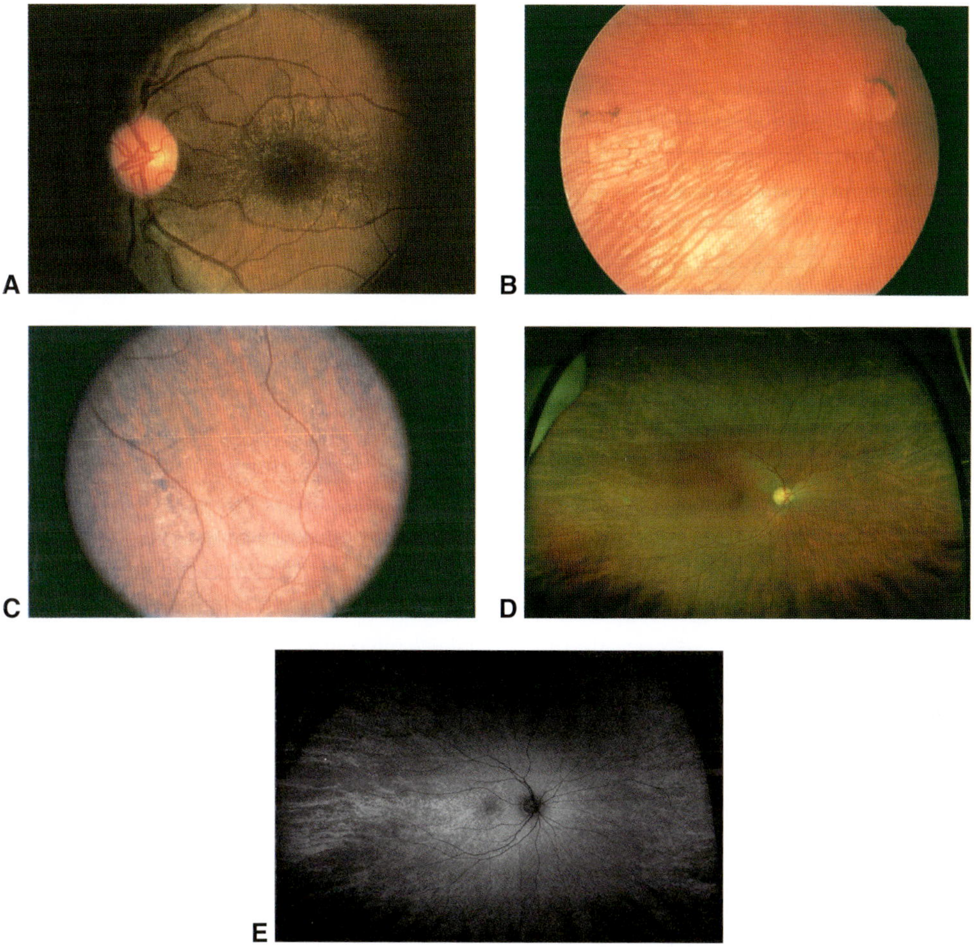

Figure 6-8 **A,** Yellow, "gold-dust" tapetal-like reflex in the left retina of a carrier for X-linked retinitis pigmentosa (RP). **B,** Nasal midperipheral retina in the left eye of a carrier for X-linked RP, showing patchy bone spicule–like pigment clumping. **C,** Peripheral retina from the left eye of a carrier of choroideremia, showing a "moth-eaten" fundus appearance from areas of hypopigmentation and hyperpigmentation. **D,** Wide-field fundus photograph, right eye, from a carrier for ocular albinism, showing a chocolate-brown pigmentation from areas of apparently enhanced pigmentation and clusters of hypopigmentation. **E,** Fundus autofluorescence image, right eye, from the same patient as in part D, showing mottled autofluorescence consistent with lyonization. *(Parts D and E courtesy of Elias Traboulsi, MD.)*

mutant X chromosome may have occurred in most of her primordial cells, which evolved into the specific tissue observed and may appear phenotypically normal. This subtlety is even more important in the evaluation of family members with X-linked disease if the phenotypic carrier state is age dependent; thus, even in obligate carrier females for Lowe syndrome, lenticular cortical opacities are not necessarily present before the third decade of life.

Table 6-7 Ocular Findings in Carriers of X-Linked Disorders

Disorder	Ocular Findings
S-cone (blue-cone) monochromatism	Abnormalities in cone function on ERG, psychophysical thresholds, and color vision testing
Choroideremia	"Moth-eaten" fundus pigmentary changes, with areas of hypopigmentation, mottling, and pigment clumping in a striated pattern near the equator
Congenital stationary night blindness with myopia	Reductions in ERG oscillatory potentials
Fabry disease	Whorl-like (verticillata) changes within the corneal epithelium
Lowe syndrome	Scattered punctate lens opacities on slit-lamp examination
Ocular albinism	Chocolate-brown clusters of pigment prominent in the midperipheral retina; mottling of macular pigment; iris transillumination
Red-green color vision deficiencies (protan and deutan)	Abnormally wide or displaced color match on a Nagel anomaloscope; decrease in sensitivity to red light in protan carriers (Schmidt sign)
X-linked retinitis pigmentosa	Regional fundus pigmentary changes, "gold-dust" tapetal-like reflex; ERG amplitude and implicit time abnormalities

ERG = electroretinogram.

Complex Genetic Disease: Polygenic and Multifactorial Inheritance

In chromosomal and mendelian (single-gene) disorders, genetic analysis of phenotypic, biochemical, or molecular parameters is imperative. However, a simple mode of inheritance cannot be assigned and a recurrence risk cannot be predicted for many common, normal characteristics or disorders for which genetic variability clearly exists. Such traits as stature, refractive error, intraocular pressure (IOP), central corneal thickness, and iris color are usually distributed as a continuous variation over a wide range without sharp distinction between normal and abnormal phenotypes. This normal distribution contrasts with the bimodal curve (or trimodal curve in codominant models) noted for conditions transmitted by a single gene. Such conditions are often termed *polygenic,* implying that they result from the operation of multiple collaborating genes, each with rather minor additive effects. Many of these common genes with small effect have been identified through GWAS. With the exception of AMD, the discovered genes account for only a small percentage of the genetic effect for the traits and diseases investigated.

The term *multifactorial inheritance* denotes a combination of genetic and environmental factors in the etiology of disease without specifying the nature of the genetic influence. Examples of disorders involving these factors in humans include refractive error, glaucoma, and AMD.

Counseling for recurrence may be difficult in this type of inheritance. Ideally, empirical data are summarized from exhaustive analyses of similarly affected families in the population. In general, the risk is intermediate between population risk and mendelian risk. For example, the population risk for primary open-angle glaucoma (POAG) is 2%–3%, whereas the risk for glaucoma in families with severe myocilin mutations is near 50%. The risk for first-degree relatives of POAG patients is approximately 20%. The more severe the abnormality in the index case, the higher the risk of recurrence of the trait in relatives, presumably because either a greater number of deleterious genes are at work or a fixed population of more harmful genes exists. The risk of recurrence in future children is increased when more than one member of a family is affected, which is not true for mendelian disorders. Such observations have been offered for various forms of strabismus, glaucoma, and significant refractive errors.

Finally, if the malformation or disorder has occurred in both paternal and maternal relatives, the recurrence risk is distinctly higher because of the sharing of multiple unspecifiable but potentially harmful genes in their offspring.

Pharmacogenetics

The study of heritable factors that determine how drugs are chemically metabolized in the body is called *pharmacogenetics.* This field addresses genetic differences among population segments that are responsible for variations in both the therapeutic and adverse effects of drugs. Investigations in pharmacogenetics are important not only because they may lead to more rational approaches to therapy, but also because they facilitate a deeper understanding of drug pharmacology. For further discussion, see Part V, Ocular Pharmacology.

The drug isoniazid provides an example of how pharmacogenetics works. This antituberculosis drug is normally inactivated by the liver enzyme acetyltransferase. A large segment of the population, which varies by geographic distribution, has a reduced amount of this enzyme; these individuals are termed *slow inactivators.* When they take isoniazid, the drug reaches higher-than-normal concentrations, causing a greater incidence of adverse effects. Family studies have shown that a reduced level of acetyltransferase is inherited as an autosomal recessive trait.

Several other well-documented examples demonstrate how pharmacogenetics works. An X-linked recessive trait, present in 10% of the African American male population, a high percentage of male Sephardic Jews (originally from around the Mediterranean Sea), and males from a number of other ethnic groups, causes a deficiency in the enzyme glucose-6-phosphate dehydrogenase in the erythrocytes of affected males. As a consequence, a number of drugs (including sulfacetamide, vitamin K, acetylsalicylic acid, quinine, chloroquine, dapsone, and probenecid) may produce acute hemolytic anemia in these individuals. Pharmacogenetic causes have also been ascribed to variations in response to ophthalmic drugs, such as the increased IOP noted in a segment of the population after prolonged use of topical corticosteroids.

Several drugs have been shown to cause greater reaction in children with Down syndrome than in children without the syndrome. As a result of hypersensitivity, some children with Down syndrome have died after systemic administration of atropine. This hypersensitivity is also found with topical use of atropine in some of these children. In these patients, atropine exerts a greater-than-normal effect on pupillary dilation. In several children with Down syndrome being treated for strabismus, hyperactivity occurred several hours after local instillation of echothiophate iodide, 0.125%.

One of the earliest examples of an inherited deficit in drug metabolism involved succinylcholine, a strong muscle relaxant that interferes with acetylcholinesterase, the enzyme that catabolizes acetylcholine at neuromuscular junctions. Normally, succinylcholine is rapidly destroyed by plasma cholinesterase (sometimes called *pseudocholinesterase*), so that its effect is short-lived—usually no more than a few minutes. Some individuals are homozygous for a recessive gene that codes for a form of cholinesterase with a considerably lower substrate affinity. Consequently, at therapeutic doses of succinylcholine, almost no destruction occurs, and the drug continues to exert its inhibitory effect on acetylcholinesterase, resulting in prolonged periods of apnea.

Clinical Management of Genetic Disease

Genetic disease may not be curable, but in most cases the patient benefits considerably from appropriate medical management by the physician. Such care should include all of the following steps.

Accurate Diagnosis

Unfortunately, because health care practitioners may not be as knowledgeable about genetic diagnoses as they are about other areas of medicine, many cases are not precisely diagnosed or, worse, are diagnosed incorrectly. A patient with deafness and pigmentary retinopathy may receive a diagnosis of rubella syndrome when the correct diagnosis is Usher syndrome. This latter syndrome, associated with RP, may not be recognized in patients with RP. In patients with RP and congenital polydactyly (surgically corrected in infancy), Bardet-Biedl syndrome may not be recognized. The correct diagnosis in such cases is important to ensure that the patient's educational and lifetime support needs are truly met.

Complete Explanation of the Disease

Patients are often very anxious when they do not understand the nature of their disease. Carefully explaining the disorder, as currently understood, will often dispel myths patients may have about their disease and their symptoms.

Virtually all genetic disorders confer burdens that may interfere with certain activities later in life. The appropriate time to discuss these burdens with patients and family members is often when they first ask about the consequences of a disease. Such explanations need to be tempered with empathy and an understanding of the possible emotional and psychological effects of this information.

Treatment of the Disease Process

Definitive cures—that is, reversing or correcting underlying genetic defects—are yet to emerge for most heritable disorders. However, some conditions in which metabolic defects have been identified can often be managed through 5 fundamental approaches:

1. dietary control
2. chelation of excessive metabolites
3. enzyme or gene-product replacements
4. vitamin and cofactor therapy
5. drug therapy to reduce accumulation of harmful products

Dietary control

Some genetic disorders affecting the eye that arise from an inborn error of metabolism can be managed effectively through dietary therapy. These conditions include homocystinuria, Refsum disease, gyrate atrophy, galactokinase deficiency, and galactosemia. Implementing a galactose-free diet can reverse some of the main clinical signs of galactosemia (eg, hepatosplenomegaly, jaundice, and weight loss). Progression of cortical cataracts can be avoided, and less extensive lens opacities may even regress with a galactose-free diet. Nevertheless, a lifelong galactose-restricted diet is recommended to limit complications.

Chelation of excessive metabolites

Disorders that result from enzyme or transport protein deficiencies may lead to the accumulation of a metabolite or metal that harms various tissues. For example, in Wilson disease (hepatolenticular degeneration), decreased levels of serum ceruloplasmin result in poor transport of free copper (Cu^{2+}) ions and in storage of copper in such tissues as the brain, liver, and cornea. Resultant clinical signs can be reversed, at least partially, after the administration of D-penicillamine, a chelator of Cu^{2+}. Other copper chelators, such as British anti-Lewisite (BAL), can be used, along with a copper-deficient diet, to reverse the clinical signs of Wilson disease.

Enzyme replacement therapy

Enzyme replacement therapy via plasma infusions in patients with Fabry disease has succeeded in temporarily decreasing plasma levels of the accumulated substrate ceramide trihexoside. The drugs are expensive (current costs at approximately $250,000 per year), presenting a barrier to successful treatment for many patients around the world. Enzyme replacement therapy for Fabry disease is not a cure, but it improves metabolism, curbs disease progression, and potentially reverses some symptoms.

Organ transplantation can be considered a form of regionalized enzyme replacement. In patients with cystinosis, cystine crystals accumulate in the kidneys. When a normal kidney, with its rich source of enzymes, is transplanted into a patient with cystinosis, cystine does not accumulate in the cells of the renal tubules and renal function tends to remain normal. In a complementary approach, stem cell transplantation is being investigated to treat various diseases, including those of the eye.

Vitamin therapy

Vitamin therapy appears to be of benefit in 2 autosomal recessive disorders. In at least some patients with homocystinuria, vitamin B_6 (pyridoxine) administration has decreased homocystine accumulation in plasma and reduced the severity of the disorder. Vitamin A and vitamin E therapy have been noted to benefit some patients with neurologic impairment due to abetalipoproteinemia; such therapy is also likely to slow or lessen the development and progression of retinal degeneration. More long-term therapeutic trials are necessary to better define the efficacy of vitamin therapy for these and perhaps other metabolic disorders.

Drug therapy

Various genetically determined disorders can be managed by use of an appropriate drug. For example, excess accumulation of uric acid in primary gout can be prevented or reduced either by blocking the activity of the enzyme xanthine oxidase with the drug allopurinol or by increasing excretion of uric acid by the kidneys with the use of probenecid. In familial hypercholesterolemia, the elevated serum cholesterol levels can often be reduced through the use of various cholesterol-lowering drugs or substances that bind bile acids in the gastrointestinal tract.

Appropriate management of sequelae and complications

Some of the sequelae of genetic diseases, such as glaucoma in Axenfeld-Rieger syndrome or cataracts in RP, can be managed successfully to preserve or partially restore vision. However, patients need to understand how treatment of the sequelae or complications may differ according to their individual situations.

Gene therapy

Clinical trials for a limited number of genes are under way; select viral mediated gene replacement for inherited retinal disease is available (see voretigene neparvovec-rzyl in Chapter 5). The ophthalmologist is obliged either to carefully search the online clinical trials databases and the published literature for treatment trials that the patient may qualify for; or to refer the patient to another professional who will conduct such a search for treatment trials for which the patient may qualify. (For a database of clinical studies, see www.clinicaltrials.gov.)

Genetic Counseling

> The ophthalmologist who understands the principles of human genetics has a foundation for counseling patients about their diseases.

Genetic counseling imparts knowledge of human disease, including a genetic diagnosis and its ocular and systemic implications. The genetic counseling process helps individuals, couples, and families understand the risk of occurrence or recurrence of the disorder within the family. It provides information about appropriate use and implications of available genetic testing, along with interpretation of results and reproductive options, as well as facts about therapies, research, and resources. Psychosocial issues are also an integral part of the discussion. Genetic counseling is nondirective and addresses ethical issues as well as ethnic and cultural diversity with sensitivity. All genetic counseling is predicated on the following essential requirements:

- *Accurate diagnosis:* To derive an accurate and specific diagnosis, the physician must be sufficiently aware of the range of human ocular pathology.
  - It is impossible to counsel or refer patients on the basis of "congenital nystagmus" or "color blindness" or "macular degeneration"; these are signs, not diagnoses.
- *Complete family history:* A family history will narrow the choices of possible inheritance patterns, but it may not necessarily exclude new mutational events, isolated occurrences of recessive diseases, and chromosomal rearrangements in individual circumstances.
  - The ophthalmologist should examine (or arrange to have examined) the parents, siblings, and other family members for mild manifestations of dominant diseases or characteristic carrier states in X-linked disorders.
  - Only an ophthalmologist will be cognizant of, and attentive to, the atypical findings that are observed in hereditary ocular disorders. For example, identification of 1 young adult with the findings of Usher syndrome—prelingual deafness; night blindness; visual field constriction; and, ultimately, deterioration of central vision—obligates the ophthalmologist to evaluate a younger sibling who is congenitally deaf but who "historically" has no eye problems. The probability is very high that the sibling has the same disease.
- *Understanding of the genetic and clinical aspects of the disorder:* The ophthalmologist should appreciate, perhaps more intimately than any other physician, how some clinically similar diseases inherited in the same pattern may be the result of different and even nonallelic defects. For example, the visual implications of, and prognoses for, tyrosinase-positive and tyrosinase-negative oculocutaneous albinism are considerably different.
  - Ocular albinism is an X-linked trait and very rare in females.
  - Some entities that are clinically similar may be inherited differently and thus have a different impact on various family members.
  - In another example, pseudoxanthoma elasticum is often a late-onset disease that has serious implications for cardiovascular disease, stroke, and gastrointestinal bleeding. Informed counseling falls short if the ophthalmologist advises an affected patient only about visual disability associated with angioid streaks without attention to the complete disease and the risks to other family members.

Issues in Genetic Counseling

It is important to remember that an individual affected by a heritable condition may have a homozygous recessive trait. Thus, the ophthalmologist should search for parental consanguinity or ambiguous parentage (nonpaternity, incest, occult adoption) or for a new mutation and should inquire about advanced paternal (or maternal grandparental) age. Heterogeneity may complicate the diagnosis. Somatic mutations also occur, as with segmental neurofibromatosis or unilateral unifocal retinoblastoma. Nonpenetrance or mild expressivity in other family members should be excluded through diligent examination. Chromosomal abnormalities and phenocopies caused by infections or drugs may account for the isolated affected person. Nonetheless, the ophthalmologist's obligation to explain the disorder begins with an accurate diagnosis and establishment of the mode of heritability.

The genetic counseling process is nondirective; the genetic counselor informs rather than advises. It is inappropriate, perhaps even unethical, for a counselor to tell the patient what to do (eg, not to have any children). Counselors recognize the ability of individuals and families to make appropriate decisions for themselves concerning their own health and reproductive choices in accordance with their personal beliefs and opinions, and they support them in the decision-making process.

In some instances, genetic testing for ocular disorders may provide individuals with information about their specific genetic mutation. While such testing can assist in the diagnosis and potentially give patients options to participate in clinical trials of new treatments, it may also identify carrier status and mutations in asymptomatic individuals who have known familial mutations, facilitating early diagnosis and subsequent intervention when available. The implications of these results require careful consideration and counseling, because the information can affect not just the individuals who underwent testing but other family members as well. Genetic testing requests need to be carefully evaluated for compliance with existing guidelines and position statements covering the related ethical issues. For example, genetic testing for an adult-onset condition in a child, on the parents' request when there is no immediate medical benefit for the child, is not indicated.

Reproductive Issues

With a genetic diagnosis, the counseling ophthalmologist should outline the options available for family planning. Some people may accept a high statistical risk and choose to have children. This decision is based on how they perceive the social and psychological challenges of the disorder. Attitude toward reproduction may be considerably different, for instance, for a female carrier of protanopia than for a female carrier of X-linked RP or choroideremia, even though the statistical risk for an affected son is the same for each carrier. Some may elect to delay childbearing in the hope of future medical advances. For a variety of personal and ethical considerations, others may opt for contraception, termination of pregnancy, sterilization, and/or adoption.

Artificial insemination by a donor is a useful option in family planning if the father has a dominant disease or if both parents are carriers of a biochemically detectable recessive disorder. However, it is clearly not applicable if the mother is the carrier of an X-linked or mitochondrial disorder or if the mother is the individual affected by an autosomal dominant mutation. Finally, donor eggs, donor embryos, and surrogate motherhood—where these options are available—may be alternatives for some families.

In some circumstances, an individual or a couple may use the results of genetic testing and consider prenatal testing or in vitro fertilization (IVF) technology with preimplantation genetic diagnosis (PGD) to avoid recurrence in their children. Knowledge of these options and of the potential ethical, social, and cultural issues they raise is important for clinicians.

Prenatal diagnosis

Prenatal diagnosis (PND) with amniocentesis or chorionic villus sampling (CVS) for biochemically identifiable disorders (eg, Tay-Sachs disease, many mucopolysaccharidoses, and more than 100 other diseases) is useful in the proper genetic scenarios.

Other possible indications for PND include

- advanced maternal age or positive results from prenatal screening, which both carry an increased risk of chromosomal abnormalities
- elevated maternal serum α-fetoprotein, suggesting a neural tube defect
- presence of soft markers or fetal abnormalities that could suggest a chromosomal abnormality or a genetic disease
- presence of a familial disease detectable by DNA analysis

Amniocentesis is usually performed at 15–16 weeks of gestation, when enough fluid and cells can be obtained for culture and the maternal risk of abortion is relatively low. The risk of spontaneous abortion or fetal morbidity from the procedure is approximately 0.5%. Earlier PND of chromosomal abnormalities, at about 10 weeks of gestation, is available through the use of CVS. In this procedure, tissue from the placenta is obtained under ultrasound visualization. It is then cultured and karyotyped in a manner similar to that used for amniocentesis. As a first-trimester procedure, CVS allows earlier diagnosis and can lead to earlier and thus safer pregnancy termination. The rate of spontaneous abortion associated with this procedure is estimated at 1%–2%.

Cell-free fetal DNA (cffDNA), sometimes called *noninvasive prenatal screening,* is a new technique to examine fetal DNA in the maternal bloodstream. CffDNA is being developed to allow PND without the risks associated with CVS or amniocentesis.

Couples who elect PND in the form of either CVS or amniocentesis may face considerable anxiety about complications, such as pregnancy loss, waiting time to obtain the genetic results, and, potentially, the difficult decision of whether to terminate an affected pregnancy—a dilemma that couples are aware they may face repeatedly with each consecutive pregnancy.

Preimplantation genetic diagnosis

Preimplantation genetic diagnosis (PGD) has the advantage of enabling selection of unaffected embryos through testing prior to implantation. Embryos are created using *intracytoplasmic sperm injection (ICSI),* in which a single sperm is injected into each egg in an attempt to achieve fertilization. On day 3, when each embryo consists of 6–8 cells, 1 cell (blastomere) is removed per embryo. DNA is extracted from these cells and amplified using fluorescent polymerase chain reaction (F-PCR) to make millions of copies of the relevant region of DNA. This region is then sequenced to provide a reliable diagnosis of the status of the genetic mutation in each embryo. Unaffected embryos are transferred to the uterus on day 4 or 5. Usually, no more than 1 or 2 embryos can be transferred, to avoid the possibility of multiple births.

PGD is acceptable to many couples and, for some, it represents a valuable alternative to PND. For some couples with a moral or religious objection to pregnancy termination and who are at risk of having a child with a genetic condition, this technique may provide the opportunity to have an unaffected child. However, PGD may be associated with stress and anxiety for couples similar to that discussed earlier. Other concerns include the high cost of IVF and genetic testing (often not covered by insurance) and the low IVF pregnancy rates. PGD has raised ethical issues about embryo destruction and sex selection. Furthermore, the issue of eugenics (selection for perceived favorable nonmedical traits) has also been debated. Just as diseases differ among individuals, so do the concerns and beliefs of different parents; thus, the acceptability of different reproductive technologies should be discussed with each couple.

Referral to Providers of Support for Persons With Disabilities

Individuals and families often receive considerable benefit from referral to local, regional, or national agencies, support groups, or foundations that provide services for those with a particular disease. These organizations include local and state agencies for the blind or visually impaired, special school education programs, and appropriate consumer groups. Particularly when a disability is chronic and progressive, these agencies or support groups can greatly aid the individual or family in adjusting to changing visual disabilities. They also allow individuals or families with a particular genetic disorder to meet others with the same condition, providing them with support and possible advice.

National Human Genome Research Institute website. Genetic counseling, support and advocacy groups online. www.genome.gov/11510370. Accessed November 14, 2021.

Online Mendelian Inheritance in Man website. www.ncbi.nlm.nih.gov/omim. Accessed November 14, 2021.

Recommendations for Genetic Testing of Inherited Eye Disease

The AAO Task Force on Genetic Testing has stated that when properly performed, interpreted, and acted upon, genetic tests can improve the accuracy of diagnosis, prognosis, and genetic counseling; can lead to reduced risk of disease recurrence in families at risk; and can facilitate the delivery of personalized care. Like other forms of medical intervention, genetic testing carries specific risks that vary from patient to patient and from family to family. The results of a genetic test may affect plans to have children, create guilt or anxiety, and complicate family relationships. For these reasons, skilled counseling should be provided to all individuals who undergo genetic testing in order to maximize benefits and minimize risks.

The task force's 7 recommendations are as follows:

1. Offer genetic testing to patients with clinical findings suggestive of a mendelian disorder whose causative gene(s) have been identified. If unfamiliar with such testing, refer the patient to a physician or counselor who is familiar with it. In all cases, ensure that the patient receives counseling from a physician with expertise in inherited disease or a certified genetic counselor.

2. Use Clinical Laboratories Improvement Amendments (CLIA)–approved laboratories for all clinical testing. When possible, use laboratories that include in their reports estimates of the pathogenicity of observed genetic variants that are based on a review of the medical literature and databases of disease-causing and non-disease-causing variants.
3. Provide a copy of each genetic test report to the patient so that she or he can independently seek mechanism-specific information, such as the availability of gene-specific clinical trials, should the patient wish to do so.
4. Avoid direct-to-consumer genetic testing and discourage patients from obtaining such tests themselves. Encourage the involvement of a trained physician, genetic counselor, or both for all genetic tests so that appropriate interpretation and counseling can be provided.
5. Avoid unnecessary parallel testing; order the most specific test(s) available, given the patient's clinical findings. Restrict massively parallel strategies like whole-exome sequencing and whole-genome sequencing to research studies conducted at tertiary care facilities.
6. Avoid routine genetic testing for genetically complex disorders like age-related macular degeneration and late-onset primary open-angle glaucoma until specific treatment or surveillance strategies have been shown in one or more published prospective clinical trials to be of benefit to individuals with specific disease-associated genotypes. In the meantime, confine the genotyping of such patients to research studies.
7. Avoid testing asymptomatic minors with untreatable disorders except in extraordinary circumstances. For the few cases in which such testing is believed to be warranted, the following steps should be taken before the test is performed: (a) the parents and child should undergo formal genetic counseling; (b) the certified counselor or physician performing the counseling should state his or her opinion in writing that the test is in the family's best interest; and (c) all parents with custodial responsibility for the child should agree in writing with the decision to perform the test.

AAO Task Force on Genetic Testing; Stone EM, Aldave AJ, Drack AV, et al. *Recommendations for Genetic Testing of Inherited Eye Diseases 2014.* Clinical Statement. San Francisco: American Academy of Ophthalmology; 2014. https://www.aao.org/clinical-statement/recommendations-genetic-testing-of-inherited-eye-d. Accessed November 14, 2021.

GTR: Genetic Testing Registry website. https://www.ncbi.nlm.nih.gov/gtr/. Accessed November 14, 2021.

Traboulsi EI, ed. *Genetic Diseases of the Eye.* 2nd ed. Oxford: Oxford University Press; 2012.

PART IV

Biochemistry and Metabolism

Introduction

Considerable progress has been made in understanding the biochemistry of vision over the past 15 to 20 years, as witnessed by the numerous reviews, research articles, and books published during this time. Part IV, Biochemistry and Metabolism, was written for practitioners and residents in ophthalmology, as well as for students and researchers seeking a concise picture of the current state of knowledge of the biochemistry of the eye. Recent growth in new information about vision biochemistry has been accompanied by increased specialization among ophthalmic researchers. These chapters cover most areas of research in ocular biochemistry, including tear film; cornea; aqueous humor, iris, and ciliary body; lens; vitreous; retina; retinal pigment epithelium; and free radicals and antioxidants. The text relates basic science to clinical problems that may be encountered during residency training and in subsequent practice.

CHAPTER 7

Tear Film

Highlights

- The precorneal tear film (ie, tear film) is the first ocular structure that light encounters. Because of the lower refractive index of air relative to that of the tear film, the air–tear film interface at the surface of the cornea constitutes a major refractive element of the eye, directing light toward the cornea.
- Evidence supports a 2-phase model of the tear film, in which a lipid layer overlies a mucoaqueous layer.
- Elevated tear film osmolarity is diagnostic of dry eye syndrome.
- There is mounting evidence that ocular surface inflammation is integral to the pathology of dry eye syndrome.

Overview

Human tears are distributed among the marginal tear strip (or *tear meniscus*) (Fig 7-1), the preocular film covering the exposed bulbar conjunctiva and cornea (*precorneal tear film,* also called *tear film*), and the conjunctival sac (between the eyelids and bulbar conjunctiva).

The primary functions of the precorneal tear film are to

- provide a smooth optical surface at the air–cornea interface
- allow diffusion of oxygen and other nutrients
- serve as a medium for removal of debris and protect the ocular surface

The tear film protects the cornea and ultimately the entire eye by carrying tear constituents and debris to the lacrimal puncta, providing a medium for antimicrobial agents (lysozyme and lactoferrin, among others) and immunoglobulins, and preventing desiccation of the ocular surface barrier.

Historically, the precorneal tear film was viewed as a 3-layer "sandwich" composed of distinct lipid, aqueous, and mucin layers. Evidence continues to support a 2-phase model of the tear film, in which a lipid layer overlies a mucoaqueous phase (Fig 7-2). Components of the tear film (lipids, mucins, proteins, and salts) may interact to prevent tear film evaporation and collapse; however, additional studies are needed to confirm this concept.

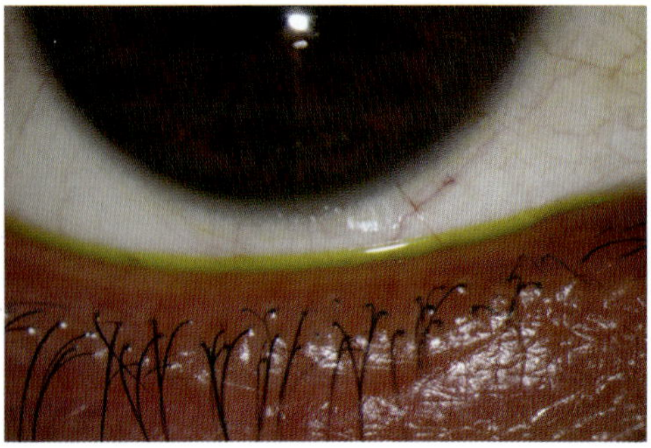

Figure 7-1 Clinical photograph of the tear lake at the lower eyelid margin, stained with fluorescein. A normal tear lake is approximately 1 mm above the eyelid margin. *(Courtesy of Vikram S. Brar, MD.)*

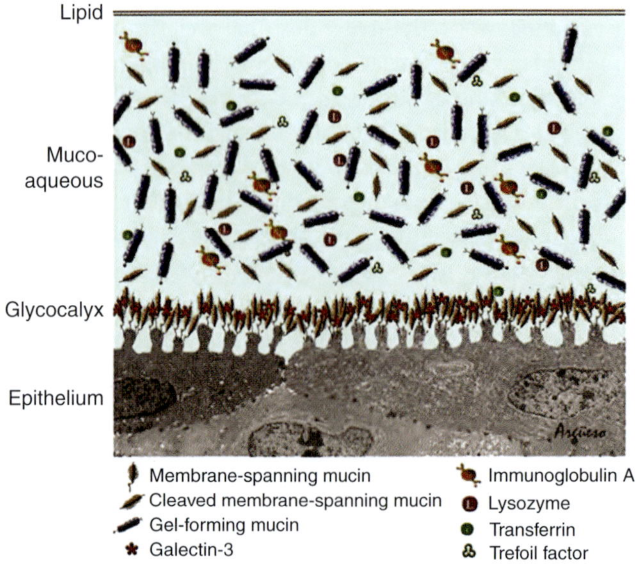

Figure 7-2 Two-phase model of the tear film. Schematic drawing of the structure of the tear film showing the outer lipid layer, the mucoaqueous layer, and the glycocalyx resting on the apical microvilli of the ocular surface epithelium. *(Reproduced with permission from Willcox MDP, Argüeso P, Georgiev GA, et al. TFOS DEWS II tear film report.* Ocul Surf. *2017;15(3):366–403.)*

Measurements of tear film thickness have differed widely, but more recent studies using optical coherence tomography (OCT) and reflectometry have found the tear film to be approximately 3.4 μm thick. The steady-state volume of tears is 7.4 μL for the unanesthetized eye and 2.6 μL for the anesthetized eye; this volume decreases with age. Some properties of the normal human tear film are given in Table 7-1.

Craig JP, Nelson JD, Azar DT, et al. TFOS DEWS II report executive summary. *Ocul Surf.* 2017;15(4):802–812.

Table 7-1 Approximate Properties of Normal Human Tear Film

Composition	Water	98.2%
	Solid	1.8%
Thickness	Total	3.4 μm
	Lipid layer	0.015–0.16 μm
Volume	Unanesthetized	7.4 μL
	Anesthetized	2.6 μL
Secretory rate	Unanesthetized	
	Schirmer	3.8 μL/min
	Fluorophotometry	0.9 μL/min
	Anesthetized	
	Schirmer	1.8 μL/min
	Fluorophotometry	0.3 μL/min
Turnover rate	Normal	12%–16%/min
	Stimulated	300%/min
Evaporation rate		0.06 μL/cm²/min
Osmolarity		296–308 mOsm/L
pH		6.5–7.6
Electrolytes (mmol/L)	Na^+	134–170
	K^+	26–42
	Ca^{2+}	0.5
	Mg^{2+}	0.3–0.6
	Cl^-	120–135
	HCO_3^-	26

Lipid Layer

The outermost layer of the tear film, or *lipid* layer, has the following functions:

- retards evaporation of the tear film
- contributes to the optical properties of the tear film because of its position at the air–tear film interface
- maintains a hydrophobic barrier *(lipid strip)* that prevents tear overflow by decreasing surface tension
- prevents damage to eyelid margin skin by tears

The lipid layer is approximately 43 nm thick and contains polar and nonpolar lipids in multilayers with a complex lipid composition. Polar amphiphilic phospholipids interact with the mucoaqueous layer, and a thick layer of nonpolar hydrophobic lipids occupies the outermost layer at the air–eye interface (Fig 7-3). These phospholipids are secreted primarily by the *meibomian (tarsal) glands,* which are located in the tarsal plate of the upper and lower eyelids and are supplied by parasympathetic nerves that are cholinesterase-positive and contain vasoactive intestinal polypeptide (VIP). Sympathetic and sensory nerves are present but sparsely distributed. Neuropeptide Y (NPY)–positive nerves are abundant. There are approximately 30–40 meibomian glands in the upper eyelid and 20–30 in the lower eyelid. Each gland orifice opens onto the skin of the eyelid margin,

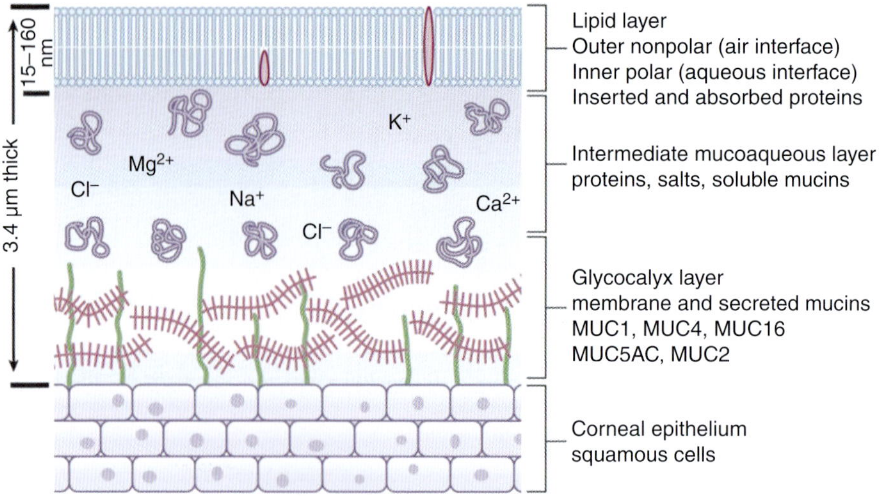

Figure 7-3 Schematic of the tear film demonstrating the lipid layer and distribution of nonpolar and polar lipids. Also shown is a proposed incorporation of proteins *(pink)* into the lipid layer. *(Modified with permission from Levin LA, Nilsson SFE, Ver Hoeve J, Wu SM.* Adler's Physiology of the Eye. *11th ed. Philadelphia: Elsevier/Saunders; 2011:361.)*

between the tarsal *gray line* and the mucocutaneous junction (see Chapter 1, Fig 1-27). The sebaceous glands of Zeis, located at the eyelid margin close to the eyelash roots, also secrete lipid, which is incorporated into the tear film. Clinically, tear film evaporation can be evaluated by assessing the tear breakup time (see BCSC Section 8, *External Disease and Cornea*).

The melting point of meibomian gland secretion ranges from 32°C to 40°C. With meibomian gland inspissation in chronic marginal blepharitis, the melting point is elevated, and the secretions become stagnant. In a study to determine whether tear film lipid layer thickness was altered after therapy with warm, moist compresses, samples of meibomian secretions from subjects without meibomian gland dysfunction (MGD) started to melt at 32°C, whereas secretion samples from subjects with MGD were found to begin melting at 35°C. Five minutes after initiation of compress therapy, the tear film lipid layer was shown to increase in thickness more than 80%.

Oral supplementation with omega-3 essential fatty acids (eg, fish oil) has been demonstrated to decrease symptoms associated with *dry eye syndrome (DES)* in women, presumably because of its direct effects on tear film fatty acids. However, research suggests that carotenoids and tocopherols in the oil or eicosanoids produced from the fatty acids of the oil may have a positive effect on inflammation (see the section Tear Dysfunction) and on differentiation of the meibomian gland cells.

Olson MC, Korb DR, Greiner JV. Increase in tear film lipid layer thickness following treatment with warm compresses in patients with meibomian gland dysfunction. *Eye Contact Lens.* 2003;29(2):96–99.

Mucoaqueous Layer

The functions of the mucoaqueous layer are as follows:

- transmits oxygen to the avascular corneal epithelium
- maintains a constant electrolyte composition over the ocular surface epithelium
- provides an antibacterial and antiviral defense
- smooths minute irregularities of the anterior corneal surface
- modulates corneal and conjunctival epithelial cell function
- converts the corneal epithelium from a hydrophobic to a hydrophilic layer, which is essential for the even and spontaneous distribution of the tear film
- interacts with the tear lipid layer to reduce surface tension, thereby stabilizing the tear film
- lubricates the eyelids as they pass over the globe

Aqueous Component

The core aqueous stratum is secreted by the main and accessory lacrimal glands (see Chapter 1, Fig 1-38). The main lacrimal gland is divided into 2 anatomical parts, the *orbital* and the *palpebral* lobes, by the lateral horn of the levator aponeurosis. The *glands of Krause,* which constitute two-thirds of the accessory lacrimal glands, are located in the lateral part of the upper fornix. A number of Krause glands are also present in the lower fornix. The *glands of Wolfring* are variably located along the proximal margin of each tarsus. The accessory lacrimal glands are structurally like the main lacrimal gland.

The main lacrimal gland is richly innervated by parasympathetic nerves containing the neurotransmitters acetylcholine and VIP. The sympathetic innervation is less dense than the parasympathetic and contains norepinephrine and NPY as neurotransmitters. The sensory nerves are sparsely supplied with the neurotransmitters substance P and calcitonin gene–related peptide (CGRP). The accessory lacrimal glands are densely innervated, but the majority of nerves are unidentified. Some of this innervation consists of nerves containing VIP, substance P, and CGRP.

The aqueous stratum consists of electrolytes, water, and proteins. *Electrolytes* and small molecules regulate the osmotic flow of fluids between the corneal epithelial cells and the tear film, buffer tear pH, and serve as enzyme cofactors in controlling membrane permeability. The sodium (Na^+) concentration of tears parallels that of serum; however, the concentration of potassium (K^+) is 5–7 times that of serum. Na^+, K^+, and chloride (Cl^-) regulate the osmotic flow of fluids from the cornea to the tear film and thereby contribute to corneal clarity. Bicarbonate (HCO_3^-) regulates tear pH. Other tear electrolytes (Fe^{2+}, Cu^{2+}, Mg^{2+}, Ca^{2+}, PO_4^{3-}) are enzyme cofactors.

> **CLINICAL PEARL**
>
> In some cases of corneal edema (eg, Fuchs dystrophy), hypertonic saline is used to help dehydrate the cornea.

Tear film solutes include urea, glucose, lactate, citrate, ascorbate, and amino acids. All enter the mucoaqueous layer of the tear film via the systemic circulation, and their concentrations parallel those of serum levels. Fasting tear glucose levels are 3.6–4.1 mg/mL in those with and those without diabetes mellitus. However, after a 100-mg oral glucose load, tear glucose levels exceed 11 mg/mL in 96% of diabetic persons tested.

Proteins in the mucoaqueous layer of the tear film include immunoglobulin (Ig) A and secretory IgA (sIgA). IgA is formed by plasma cells in interstitial tissues of the main and accessory lacrimal glands (see Chapter 1, Fig 1-39) and by the substantia propria of the conjunctiva. The secretory component is produced within lacrimal gland acini, and sIgA is secreted into the lumen of the main and accessory lacrimal glands. IgA plays a role in local host-defense mechanisms of the external eye, as shown by increased levels of IgA and IgG in human tears associated with ocular inflammation. Other immunoglobulins in tears are IgM, IgD, and IgE.

Vernal conjunctivitis causes elevated tear and serum levels of IgE, increased IgE-producing plasma cells in the giant papillae of the superior tarsal conjunctiva, and elevated histamine levels. Increased levels of tear histamine support the concept of conjunctival TC (tryptase and chymotryptic proteinase containing) mast-cell degranulation triggered by IgE–antigen interaction. TC mast cells are unique to the conjunctiva and are specifically sensitive to commercially available topical mast-cell stabilizers.

Levels of matrix metalloproteinase 9 (MMP-9) in the tear film have been shown to be elevated in patients with severe disorders affecting the ocular surface, including Sjögren syndrome and graft-vs-host disease, as well as in patients after laser in situ keratomileusis (LASIK). MMP-9 cleaves epithelial basement membrane components and tight-junction proteins. MMP-9 levels have been shown to parallel corneal staining severity and may represent a sign of late-stage DES. In addition, expression of intercellular adhesion molecule 1 (ICAM-1) has been shown to be upregulated on lymphocytes and/or vascular endothelial cells, resulting in lymphocytic migration to the lacrimal and conjunctival tissues in DES.

CLINICAL PEARL

Lymphocyte adhesion to ICAM is blocked by lifitegrast, a new therapeutic agent for dry eye syndrome (see the section Tear Dysfunction later in the chapter).

Lysozyme, lactoferrin, group II phospholipase A_2, lipocalins, and defensins are important antimicrobial constituents of the mucoaqueous layer. Interferon is also present; it inhibits viral replication and may be efficacious in limiting the severity of herpetic keratitis.

In addition, the mucoaqueous layer of the tear film contains a wide array of cytokines and growth factors, including transforming growth factor βs, epidermal growth factor, fibroblast growth factor β, interleukin 1α and 1β, and tumor necrosis factor α. These constituents may play a role in the proliferation, migration, and differentiation of corneal and conjunctival epithelial cells. They may also regulate wound healing of the ocular surface.

Mucin Component

The mucin component of the mucoaqueous layer coats the microplicae of the superficial corneal epithelial cells and forms a fine network over the conjunctival surface. In addition to mucin, it contains proteins, electrolytes, water, and carbohydrates in a polar *glycocalyx.* Mucins are glycoproteins; they have a protein backbone modified by the covalent addition of multiple long carbohydrate chains composed of repeating sugar molecules strung end to end (see Figs 7-2, 7-3).

Two main types of mucins are produced within the body: secreted and membrane-spanning. Secreted mucins are

- divided into gel-forming mucins and soluble mucins
- released into the extracellular environment
- secreted principally by the goblet cells of the conjunctiva

Membrane-spanning mucins (also called *membrane-anchored, membrane-bound, membrane-tethered mucins*) are

- embedded in the lipid bilayer of the cells
- expressed by the stratified squamous cells of the conjunctival and corneal epithelia

Some think that the membrane-spanning mucins help spread the secreted mucins across the ocular surface. Both are minimally secreted by the main lacrimal gland. Goblet cells produce mucin at a rate of 2–3 μL/day, which contrasts with the 2–3 mL/day of aqueous tear production.

Tear dysfunction may result when tear mucins are deficient in number (eg, in vitamin A deficiency and conjunctival destruction), excessive in number (eg, in hyperthyroidism; foreign-body stimulation; and allergic, vernal, and giant papillary conjunctivitis), or biochemically altered (eg, in keratoconjunctivitis).

CLINICAL PEARL

Mucous discharge differs in various conditions. For example, stringy, thin, and translucent mucus is characteristic of DES; globular and crusting mucus occurs in infection; and thick, tenacious, and stretchy strands of mucus are present in vernal conjunctivitis. See BCSC Section 8, *External Disease and Cornea,* for further discussion of these conditions.

Tear Secretion

Contrary to earlier belief—which ascribed basic secretion to the accessory lacrimal glands of Krause and Wolfring and reflex secretion to the main lacrimal gland—it is now thought that all lacrimal glands function as a unit in conjunction with the ocular surface and the brain. In addition, the cornea and conjunctiva can respond by secreting electrolytes, water, and mucins.

Although the meibomian glands are innervated, it is not known whether nerves mediate lipid secretion from these glands. Reflex tear secretion is neurally mediated and induced in response to physical irritation (ie, superficial corneal and conjunctival sensory stimulation by mechanical, thermal, or chemical means), psychogenic factors, and bright light. Induction of sensory nerves by a local neural reflex activates the parasympathetic and sympathetic nerves that innervate the tear glands and epithelia, causing secretion (Fig 7-4). Tear turnover rate has been demonstrated to be significantly lower in a symptomatic patient with dry eye (5%) than in an asymptomatic dry eye patient (12%).

A neural feedback mechanism for tear secretion has been widely accepted. The cornea and lacrimal gland are not directly connected; however, corneal damage profoundly affects the lacrimal gland, which, in turn, downregulates tear production. In the *vicious circle theory of DES,* this downregulation is due to the secretion of inflammatory cytokines that block neural signals for tear secretion (Fig 7-5). The feedback loop, initiated by inflammation on the surface of the eye, further suppresses or downgrades lacrimal gland function, creating a vicious circle that worsens DES (Fig 7-6).

Peptide and steroid hormones constitute another mechanism for stimulating tear secretion (in addition to nerves), as follows:

- Peptide hormones, including α-melanocyte-stimulating hormone (α-MSH) and adrenocorticotropic hormone (ACTH), stimulate protein secretion from the main lacrimal gland.

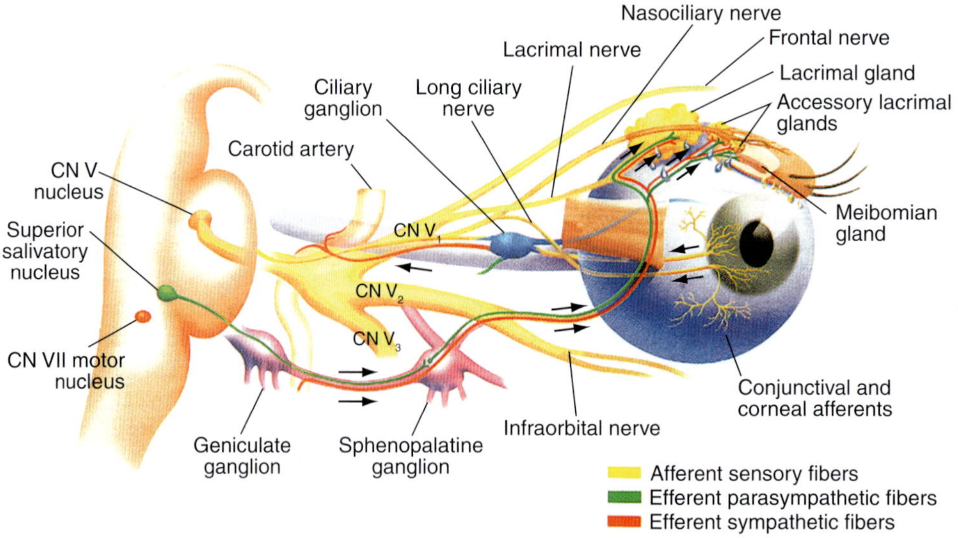

Figure 7-4 Sensory and motor nerves connecting the components of the lacrimal functional unit. Sensation (afferent) from the ocular surface is provided by branches of the long ciliary nerve of the ophthalmic division of cranial nerve V (CN V_1). Efferent fibers from both members of the autonomic nervous system stimulate lacrimal secretion at the main and accessory lacrimal glands. *(Modified with permission from Pflugfelder SC, Beuerman RW, Stern ME, eds.* Dry Eye and Ocular Surface Disorders. *New York: Marcel Dekker; 2004.)*

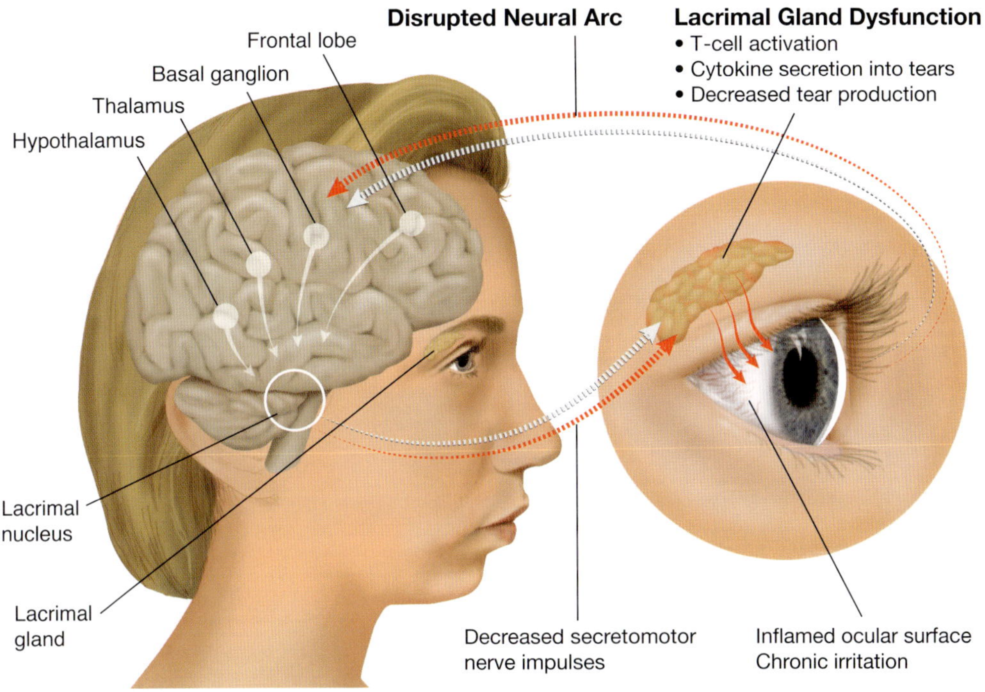

Figure 7-5 Disruption of the neural feedback loop in dry eye syndrome (DES). The *white lines* represent the normal pathway of the lacrimal functional unit. The *red lines* demonstrate disruption of the pathway. *(Illustration by Cyndie C.H. Wooley.)*

- Steroid hormones, specifically the androgens, stimulate secretion of sIgA from the main lacrimal gland and lipid from the meibomian glands.

Eyelid movement is important in tear film renewal, distribution, turnover, and drainage. As the eyelids close in a complete blink, the superior and inferior fornices are compressed by the force of the preseptal muscles, and the eyelids move toward each other, with the upper eyelid moving over the longer distance and exerting force on the globe. This force clears the anterior surface of debris and any insoluble mucin and expresses secretions from meibomian glands. The lower eyelid moves horizontally in a nasal direction and pushes tear fluid and debris toward the superior and inferior puncta. When the eyelids are opened, the tear film is redistributed. The upper eyelid pulls the mucoaqueous phase of the tear film by capillary action. The lipid layer spreads as fast as the eyelids move, so that no area of the tear film is left uncovered by lipid.

See BCSC Section 7, *Oculofacial Plastic and Orbital Surgery,* which discusses the lacrimal system in depth, with numerous illustrations.

Stern ME, Gao J, Siemasko KF, Beuerman RW, Pflugfelder SC. The role of the lacrimal functional unit in the pathophysiology of dry eye. *Exp Eye Res.* 2004;78(3):409–416.

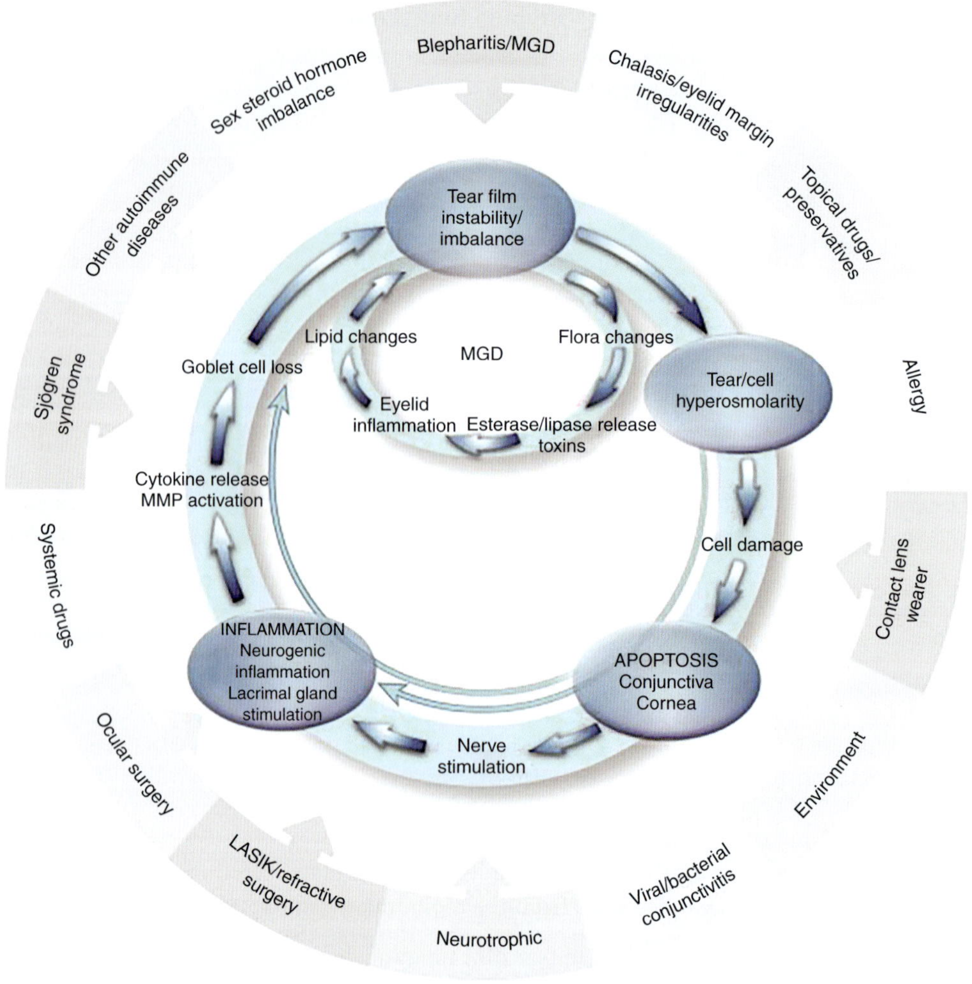

Figure 7-6 The vicious circle theory of DES. LASIK = laser in situ keratomileusis; MGD = meibomian gland dysfunction; MMP = matrix metalloproteinase. *(Modified with permission from Baudouin C, Aragona P, Messmer EM, et al. Role of hyperosmolarity in the pathogenesis and management of dry eye disease: proceedings of the OCEAN group meeting.* Ocul Surf. *2013;11(4):Fig 1.)*

Tear Dysfunction

A qualitative or quantitative abnormality of the tear film may occur as a result of

- change in the amount of tear film constituents
- change in the composition of the tear film
- uneven dispersion of the tear film because of corneal surface irregularities
- ineffective distribution of the tear film caused by eyelid–globe incongruity

The amount or composition of the tear film can change because of aqueous deficiency, mucin deficiency or excess (with or without associated aqueous deficiency), lipid abnormality (meibomian gland dysfunction), and/or ocular surface exposure. The inciting factors for a dysfunctional tear film are multifactorial (see Fig 7-6).

Increases in tear film osmolarity are diagnostic of DES and can be found in blepharitis and with contact lens use. The preocular tear film is dispersed unevenly with an irregular corneal or limbal surface (inflammation, scarring, dystrophic changes) or poor contact lens fit. Eyelid–globe incongruity results from congenital, traumatic, or neurogenic eyelid dysfunction or absent or dysfunctional blink mechanism and results in ineffective tear film distribution. Also, although overall hormone balance is unique to each person, estrogen and androgen deficiencies—combined with stress, pollution, and poor diet—produce a number of signs and symptoms, including dry eye, especially in postmenopausal women. In addition, the quality and quantity of the tear film diminish with age.

Diagnostic tests for tear dysfunction include tear breakup time, fluorescein staining, lissamine green staining, rose bengal staining, osmolarity testing, Schirmer test, tear meniscus evaluation, and MMP-9 testing.

There is increasing evidence that DES is associated with ocular surface inflammation (Fig 7-7). In various studies, adhesion molecule expression by conjunctival epithelial cells,

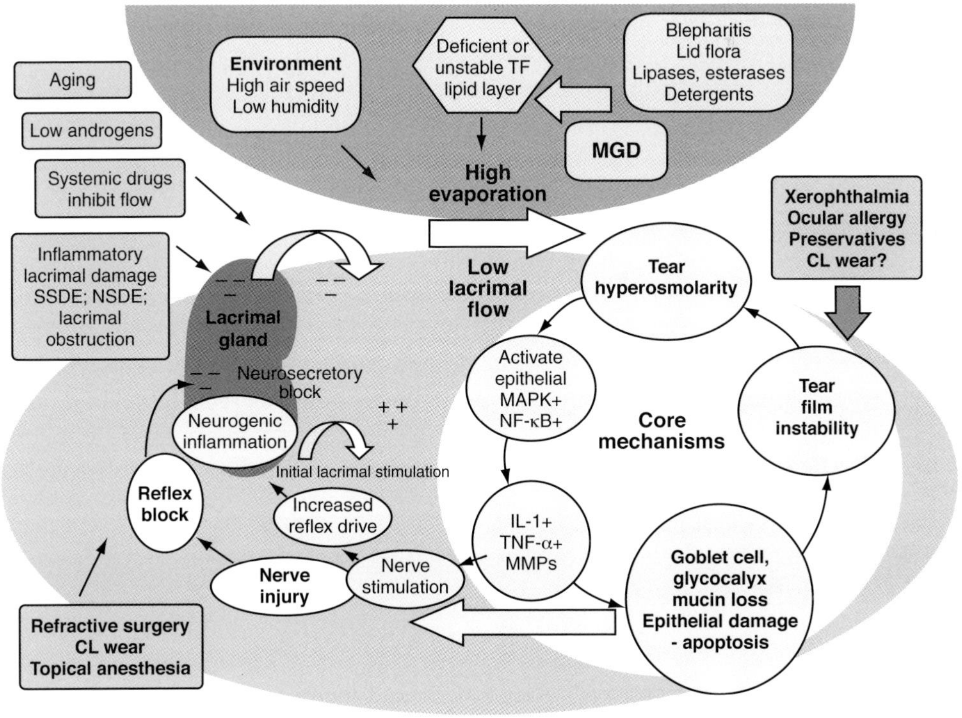

Figure 7-7 Ocular surface inflammation in DES. CL = contact lens; IL-1 = interleukin-1; MAPK = mitogen-activated protein kinase; MGD = meibomian gland dysfunction; MMPs = matrix metalloproteinases; NF-κB = nuclear factor kappa-light-chain-enhancer of activated B cells; NSDE = non–Sjögren dry eye; SSDE = Sjögren syndrome dry eye; TF = tear film; TNF-α = tumor necrosis factor alpha. *(Modified with permission from The definition and classification of dry eye disease: report of the Definition and Classification Subcommittee of the International Dry Eye WorkShop (2007).* Ocul Surf. *2007;5(2):75–92.)*

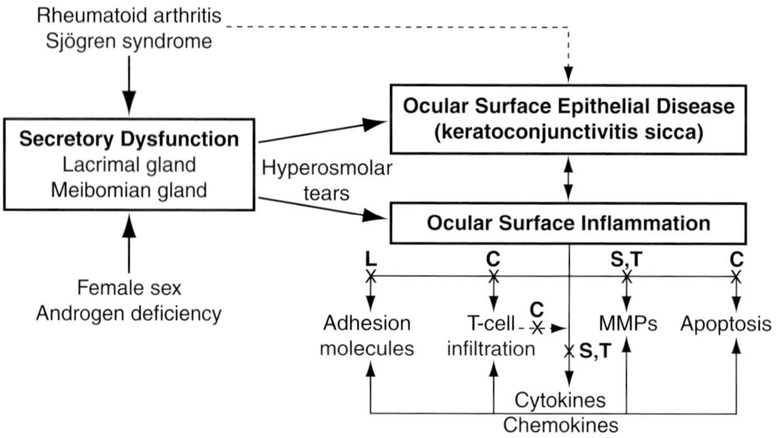

Figure 7-8 Targets of anti-inflammatory therapies for DES. C = cyclosporine A; L = lifitegrast; MMPs = matrix metalloproteinases; S = (cortico)steroids; T = tetracycline. *(Modified with permission from Pflugfelder SC. Antiinflammatory therapy for dry eye.* Am J Ophthalmol. *2004;137(2):340.)*

T-cell infiltration of the conjunctiva, and increases in soluble mediators (cytokines and proteases) in the tear film have been found in patients with DES. Preliminary clinical studies have shown that using tear substitutes to treat patients with DES may reduce tear osmolarity and improve ocular symptoms. Moreover, a variety of anti-inflammatory drugs (including corticosteroids, cyclosporine, lifitegrast, and doxycycline) have been used as therapy for DES and observed to improve the clinical symptoms of these patients (Fig 7-8).

Topical cyclosporine A emulsion and lifitegrast are approved by the US Food and Drug Administration for treating the inflammatory component of DES. Cyclosporine, a fungus-derived peptide emulsion, has been shown to be effective in stimulating aqueous tear production in patients with DES. Lifitegrast, a lymphocyte function–associated antigen-1 (LFA-1) antagonist that inhibits binding of ICAM-1 to LFA-1, has been shown to reduce inferior corneal staining and provided greater symptom relief in treated patients with DES than in control groups. No significant systemic or ocular adverse events (except for burning symptoms) were observed.

See also BCSC Section 8, *External Disease and Cornea,* which discusses DES in greater detail.

Willcox MDP, Argüeso P, Georgiev GA, et al. TFOS DEWS II tear film report. *Ocul Surf.* 2017;15(3):366–403.

CHAPTER 8

Cornea

Highlights

- Corneal avascularity is maintained by soluble vascular endothelial growth factor receptor 1.
- Corneal stem cells repopulate the desquamating epithelium. Recent research suggests that corneal stem cells exist in the central cornea as well as at the limbus.
- The corneal epithelium provides a barrier to diffusion of hydrophilic molecules; however, corneal proteoglycans confer hydrophilic properties to the stroma. Thus, when hydrophilic drugs are applied topically, the drug molecules must change their biochemical properties to reach the anterior chamber.
- Collagen fibrils and fibers (fibril bundles) within the corneal stroma maintain a regular arrangement with minimal variation in diameter. This uniformity is critical for corneal clarity.

Biochemistry and Physiology of the Cornea

Corneal avascularity is required in order to maintain optical clarity; further, avascularity contributes to the immune privilege of the cornea. Vascular endothelial growth factor A (VEGF-A), which is present in the cornea, is a potent angiogenic agent. Its actions are blocked by a soluble form of VEGF receptor 1 (also known as sflt-1). Suppression of this molecule has been shown to result in increased levels of unbound VEGF-A and in blood vessel growth in the cornea.

Because of the lack of blood vessels in the cornea, oxygen is provided to the cornea via the precorneal tear film, or *tear film* (which obtains oxygen from the air and eyelid vasculature), and aqueous humor. Glucose is the primary metabolic substrate for the epithelial cells, stromal keratocytes (corneal fibroblasts residing in the stroma), and endothelial cells. The stroma receives glucose primarily from the aqueous humor by carrier-mediated transport through the endothelium; the epithelium receives glucose by passive diffusion through the stroma and from the tear film. The precorneal tear film and limbal vessels supply approximately 10% of the glucose used by the cornea. Glucose is metabolized in the cornea by all 3 metabolic pathways:

- hexose monophosphate (HMP) shunt
- tricarboxylic acid (TCA) cycle
- glycolysis

In the epithelium and endothelium, the HMP pathway breaks down 35%–65% of the glucose, but the keratocytes of the stroma metabolize very little glucose via this pathway. The keratocytes lack 6-phosphogluconate dehydrogenase, an important enzyme in the HMP pathway. Pyruvic acid, the end product of glycolysis, is converted either to carbon dioxide and water (via the TCA cycle under aerobic conditions) or to lactic acid (under anaerobic conditions).

Production of lactic acid increases in conditions of oxygen deprivation, as in the case of tight-fitting contact lenses with low oxygen permeability. Accumulation of lactic acid in the cornea has detrimental consequences for vision, such as edema (due to an increase in an osmotic solute load) or stromal acidosis, which can change endothelial morphology and function.

Human corneas possess a remarkably high level of aldehyde dehydrogenase and transketolase. Together, these 2 proteins constitute 40%–50% of the soluble proteins in corneal stroma. Similar to enzyme crystallins of the lens, both aldehyde dehydrogenase and transketolase are thought to contribute to the optical properties of the cornea. Both proteins are also thought to protect corneal cells against free radicals and oxidative damage by absorbing ultraviolet B radiation.

The biomechanical properties of the cornea affect its functional responses. An understanding of these properties can help clinicians to better anticipate or understand the cornea's responses to stress and strain and also aid in diagnosing and treating corneal disease. The following clinically relevant principles have been confirmed:

- The paracentral and peripheral cornea are stiffer than the central cornea because of differing orientation and number of collagen fibrils.
- The elastic strength of the corneal stroma is greatest anteriorly and decreases posteriorly; thus, laser in situ keratomileusis (LASIK) flap creation and interruption of the anterior stromal lamellae are thought to disproportionately weaken the cornea and contribute to ectasia.
- The stiffness of the cornea increases with age, apparently as a result of natural collagen crosslinking.

Ambati BK, Nozaki M, Singh N, et al. Corneal avascularity is due to soluble VEGF receptor-1. *Nature.* 2006;443(7114):993–997.

Hjortdal JO. Regional elastic performance of the human cornea. *J Biomech.* 1996;29(7): 931–942.

Epithelium

The epithelium constitutes 5%–10% of the total corneal thickness. Surface projections (microvilli and microplicae) are present on the apical surface of the most superficial cell layer of epithelium. These projections are coated with filamentous material known as *glycocalyx.* Mucin glycoproteins, the major constituents of glycocalyx, are thought to promote both stability of the tear film and wettability of the corneal surface (Fig 8-1).

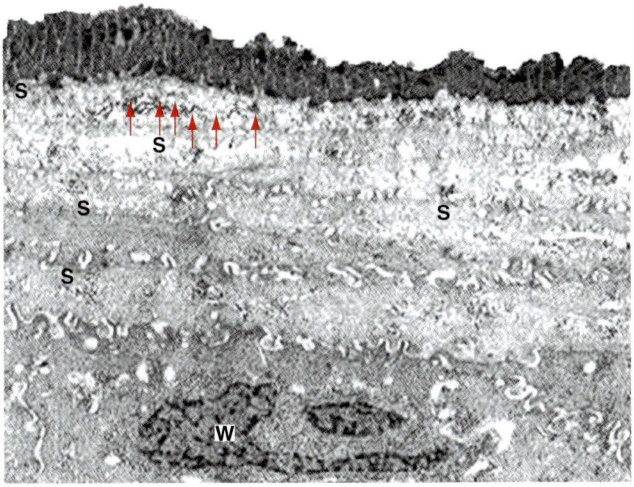

Figure 8-1 Electron micrograph of corneal epithelium stained for mucins. The glycocalyx *(dark area, at top)* interacts with the apices of the surface epithelial cells. Tight junctions *(arrows)* of adjacent epithelial cells are shown. S = surface cells; W = wing cells. *(Reproduced with permission from Levin LA, Nilsson SFE, Ver Hoeve J, Wu SM.* Adler's Physiology of the Eye. *11th ed. Philadelphia: Elsevier/Saunders; 2011:95.)*

Plasma membrane proteins and the lipids of corneal epithelial cells, similar to those of other cell types, are heavily glycosylated and play an important role in cell–cell adhesion as well as in adhesion of the basal cells of the corneal epithelium to the underlying basement membrane. The sugar residues of the plasma membrane glycoproteins and the glycolipids of corneal epithelium also play a role in wound-healing mechanisms; they do so by mediating corneal epithelial sheet migration over the wound surface following ocular injury. These residues also contribute to the pathogenesis of corneal infection by serving as attachment sites for microbes. The normal rate of epithelial cell migration is 2 mm per day and is adversely affected by preservatives in topical eyedrops.

Beginning with the discovery of the centripetal cell migration that occurs in the cornea, early studies on epithelial cell renewal led to the conclusion that the proliferative source of the corneal epithelium resides at the limbus. Interestingly, results of a more recent study suggest that corneal stem cells may also exist in the central cornea. The limbus is characterized by stromal invaginations known in humans as the *palisades of Vogt* (see Chapter 2, Fig 2-8A). These papillae-like projections show a distinctive vasculature with radially oriented arterial and venous components. The palisades of Vogt have been suggested as the reservoir that

- protects stem cells from traumatic and environmental insults
- allows epithelial–mesenchymal interactions
- provides access to chemical signals that diffuse from the rich underlying vascular network

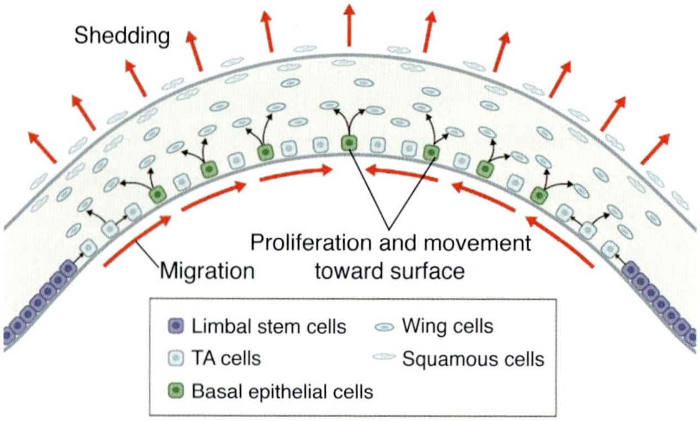

Figure 8-2 Desquamation of corneal epithelial cells. Stem cells migrate centrally from the limbus and give rise to transient amplifying (TA) cells and basal epithelial cells. *Arrows* indicate migration, differentiation, and desquamation pathways. *(Reproduced with permission from Levin LA, Nilsson SFE, Ver Hoeve J, Wu SM.* Adler's Physiology of the Eye. *11th ed. Philadelphia: Elsevier/Saunders; 2011:95.)*

Normal corneal epithelium remains in a steady state in which cell proliferation is necessary to replace cells lost by terminal differentiation and desquamation (Fig 8-2). While basal cells of the central cornea proliferate actively, basal cells at the limbus consist of a mixture of slow-cycling stem cells and their progeny, transient amplifying (TA) cells, which are affected by growth factors, cytokines, and extracellular matrix. During treatment of corneal wounds with cryopreserved amniotic membrane, TA cells are likely upregulated to enhance wound healing.

Penetration of the Corneal Epithelium

Hydrophilic molecules penetrate the epithelium poorly, but they may pass through tight junctions if the polar molecule has a mass lower than 500 Da. Hydrophilic drugs can also reach very high corneal penetration levels when the corneal epithelium is damaged or inflamed. The dissociation constant (also called *ionization constant*) is likewise important in determining a molecule's permeability across the cornea. To diffuse across the epithelium, organic molecules should be in an uncharged state. However, a charged molecule can more readily penetrate the stroma. To penetrate the cornea and enter the anterior chamber, therefore, an organic molecule should be able to dissociate at physiologic pH and temperature (ie, within the stroma).

Majo F, Rochat A, Nicolas M, Jaoudé GA, Barrandon Y. Oligopotent stem cells are distributed throughout the mammalian ocular surface. *Nature.* 2008;456(7219):250–254.

Bowman Layer

The Bowman layer is immediately beneath the epithelial basal lamina and is composed of randomly packed type I and type V collagen fibers that are 30 nm in diameter. The fibers are enmeshed in a matrix consisting of proteoglycans and glycoproteins. The Bowman layer is secreted during embryogenesis by the anterior stromal keratocytes and epithelium. It is acellular and does not regenerate when damaged.

It is thought that this layer, by virtue of its acellularity and packing distribution, serves to prevent exposure of stromal keratocytes to growth factors secreted by epithelial cells, such as transforming growth factor β. This effect is notable because, in excimer laser surgery (photorefractive keratectomy [PRK] or laser subepithelial keratomileusis [LASEK]), the Bowman layer is removed, along with anterior corneal stromal tissue. Corneal haze, a potentially significant postoperative complication of these procedures, is presumably due to absence of the Bowman layer and consequent keratocyte exposure to growth factors. In LASIK, by contrast, the Bowman layer is transected but retained; central corneal haze is thus extremely rare after this procedure.

Stroma

The stroma makes up approximately 90% of the total corneal thickness. Stromal cells, known as *keratocytes,* constitute 10%–40% of corneal volume, depending on age; loss of keratocyte density occurs with age. Usually, these cells reside between the collagen lamellae. The stroma is made up of roughly 200 lamellae, which are 1.5–2.5 µm thick and composed of collagen fibrils enmeshed in a matrix consisting of proteoglycans, proteins, and glycoproteins. The stromal fibrils within each lamella are narrow and uniform in diameter; in humans, the average fibril diameter is 30 nm. The stroma is less compact posteriorly, facilitating a deeper placement of intrastromal ring segments for keratoconus.

Collagen fibrils within each lamella run parallel to one another from limbus to limbus. The orientation of the lamellae with each other depends on the location within the stroma. The lamellae are obliquely oriented in the anterior third and perpendicular in the posterior two-thirds of the stroma (Fig 8-3). Also, collagen fibrils in each lamella are regularly spaced, with a center-to-center distance of 55–60 nm. The narrow and uniform diameter of collagen fibrils and their regular arrangement are characteristic of collagen of the corneal stroma and are necessary for the transparency of this tissue (Fig 8-4).

Type I is the major collagen component of the corneal stroma; it constitutes approximately 70% of the total stromal dry weight. Immunohistochemical and biochemical studies have demonstrated that normal adult corneal stroma also contains collagen types V, VI, VII, XII, and XIV. Type III collagen production is associated uniquely with stromal wound healing.

After collagen, proteoglycans are the second most abundant biological constituents of the cornea; they constitute approximately 10% of the dry weight of the cornea. Proteoglycans are the constituents that confer hydrophilic properties to the stroma. They are glycosylated proteins with at least 1 glycosaminoglycan (GAG) chain covalently bound to the protein core. GAGs are composed of repeating disaccharides. The GAGs found in corneal stroma include

- keratan sulfate
- chondroitin sulfate
- dermatan sulfate

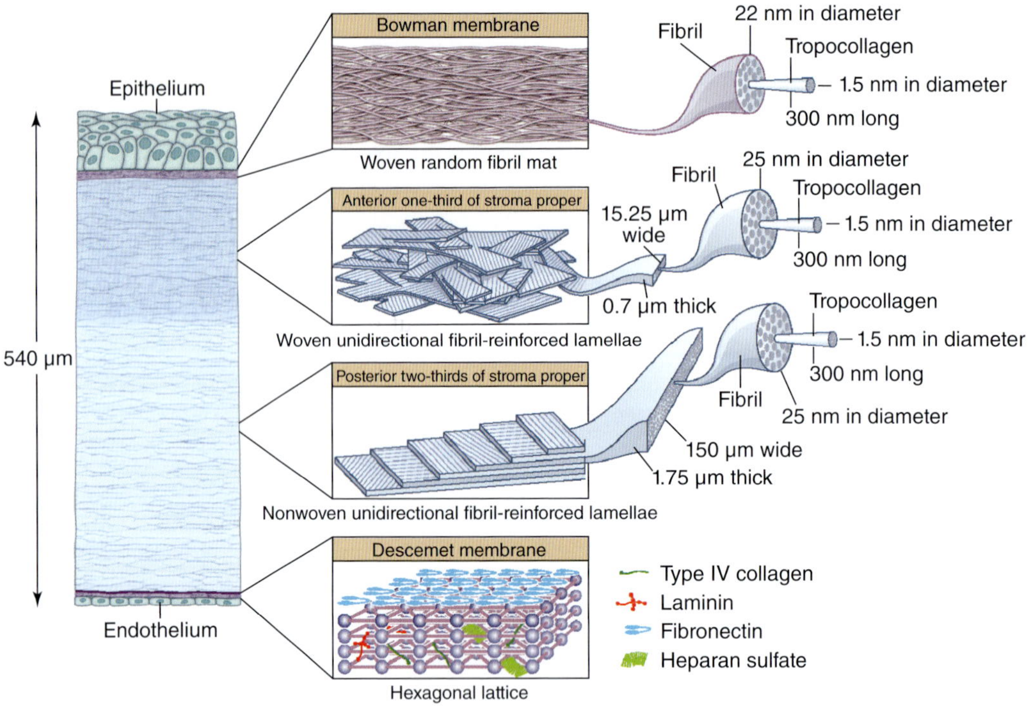

Figure 8-3 Orientation of stromal collagen fiber lamellae. The anterior stroma is more compact than the posterior stroma, particularly at the Bowman layer. *(Modified with permission from Levin LA, Nilsson SFE, Ver Hoeve J, Wu SM.* Adler's Physiology of the Eye. *11th ed. Philadelphia: Elsevier/Saunders; 2011:107.)*

Regulation of spacing between the stromal collagen fibrils is thought to result from highly specific interactions between the proteoglycans and the collagen fibrils. When these interactions are disturbed, the ability of the cornea to remain transparent is profoundly affected.

Matrix metalloproteinases (MMPs) are a family of Zn^{2+}-dependent enzymes responsible for degradation of the components of the extracellular matrix (including proteoglycans and various types of collagens) during normal development as well as in disease processes. Of the more than a dozen known metalloproteinases, only MMP-2 proenzyme has been found in the normal healthy cornea. However, after corneal injury, additional MMPs (including MMP-1, MMP-3, and MMP-9) are synthesized. The proteinase inhibitors of the cornea play a key role in corneal protection by restricting damage during corneal inflammation, ulceration, and wound healing. Many of these inhibitors are synthesized by resident cells of the cornea; some are derived from tears, aqueous humor, and limbal blood vessels.

Randleman JB, Dawson DG, Grossniklaus HE, McCarey BE, Edelhauser HF. Depth-dependent cohesive tensile strength in human donor corneas: implications for refractive surgery. *J Refract Surg.* 2008;24(1):S85–S89.

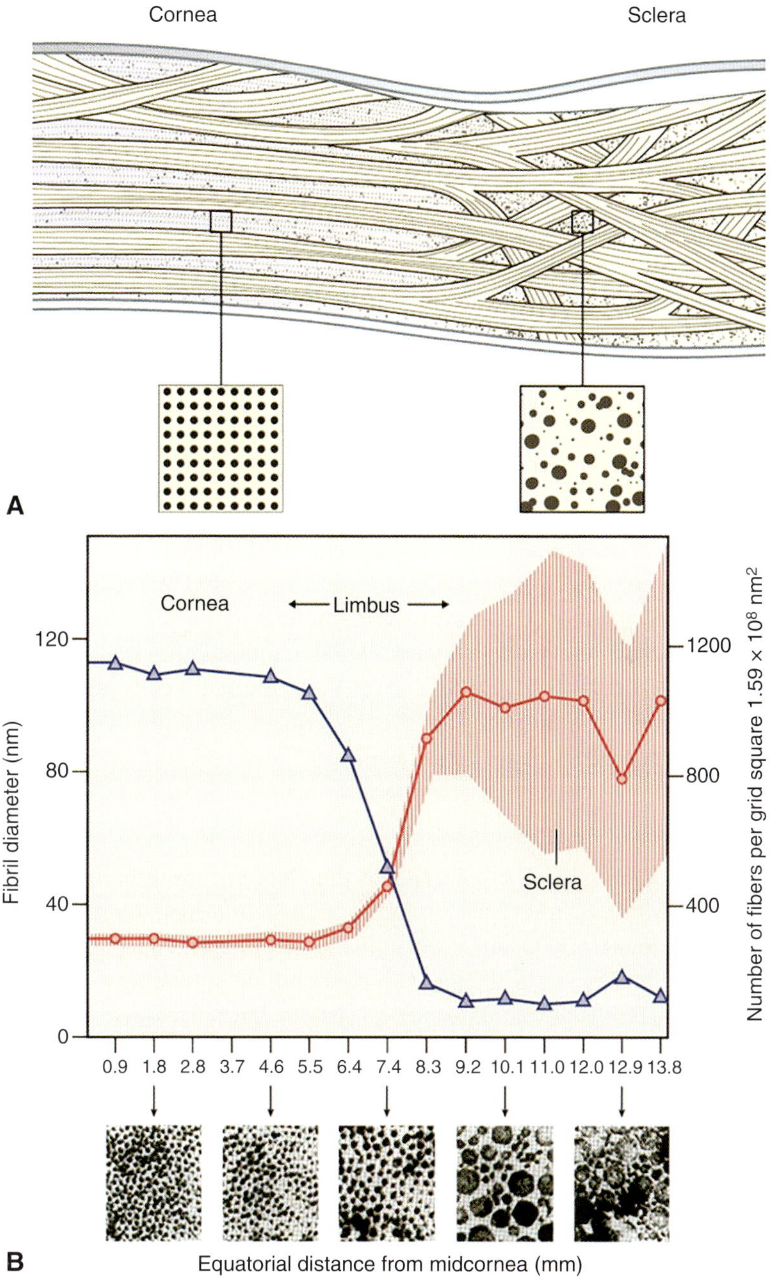

Figure 8-4 Cornea and sclera. **A,** Both are composed of similar collagen fibrils. However, fibril diameter and fiber density are consistent throughout the cornea, whereas in the sclera, they are not. **B,** The density of the fibers decreases in the sclera *(blue),* and the variation in fibril diameter increases *(red).* This heterogeneity contributes to the opacity of the sclera, as compared with the cornea, despite their similar collagen fiber composition. *(Modified with permission from Levin LA, Nilsson SFE, Ver Hoeve J, Wu SM.* Adler's Physiology of the Eye. *11th ed. Philadelphia: Elsevier/Saunders; 2011:117.)*

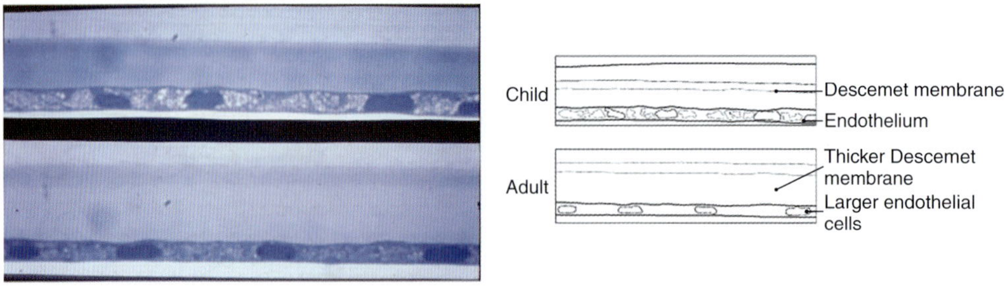

Figure 8-5 Thickening of the Descemet membrane with age as the posterior nonbanded layer is continuously produced. *(Courtesy of John Marshall.)*

Descemet Membrane and Endothelium

Descemet Membrane

The Descemet membrane is a specialized basement membrane, 10–12 µm thick, between the corneal endothelium and the posterior stroma. It is secreted by endothelium and comprises an anterior banded layer and a posterior nonbanded layer. The latter is secreted throughout life, which is the reason why the Descemet membrane is 3–4 times thicker in adulthood than at birth (Fig 8-5). Type IV is the most abundant collagen in the Descemet membrane. It has been hypothesized that the posterior-most 15 µm of stroma may represent a distinct, tough acellular layer (Dua layer).

Endothelium

The corneal endothelium, located posterior to the Descemet membrane, is a monolayer of hexagonal cells with a diameter of 20 µm. In young adult eyes, the normal endothelial cell count is approximately 3000/mm^2 centrally. The number of endothelial cells is higher in the periphery and decreases with age, with concomitant spreading and thinning of the remaining cells. The rate of physiologic corneal endothelial cell loss with normal aging has been reported to be 0.6% per year (Fig 8-6, Table 8-1).

Adjacent endothelial cells interdigitate in a complex way and form a variety of tight junctions, serving as a barrier to aqueous humor penetration, but desmosomes are never observed between normal cells. Approximately 20–30 short microvilli per cell extend from the apical plasma membrane into the aqueous humor. The endothelium functions both as a permeability barrier between the aqueous humor and the corneal stroma and as a pump to maintain the cornea in a dehydrated state by generating negative hydrostatic pressure, which also serves to hold free corneal flaps (eg, LASIK flaps) in place. The endothelium utilizes temperature-dependent Na^+,K^+-ATPase to maintain the hydration of the stroma at 78% and sustain corneal clarity. In vivo, the endothelium derives sufficient oxygen from the aqueous humor to maintain normal pump function.

If the endothelium is injured, healing occurs mainly via migration, rearrangement, and enlargement of the residual cells. Substantial cell loss or damage results in irreversible edema because human corneal endothelial cells have limited ability to divide after birth.

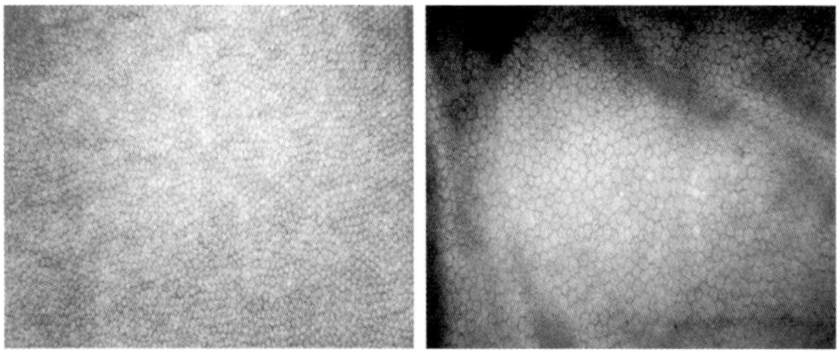

Figure 8-6 Corneal endothelium. Endothelial cells do not replicate. Over time, adjacent cells increase in size to accommodate for age-related endothelial cell loss. *Left:* Specular micrograph of the cornea of an 18-month-old infant. *Right:* Specular micrograph of the cornea of a healthy 74-year-old man. *(Modified with permission from Spalton DJ, Hitchings RA, Hunter PA, Tan JCH, Harry J.* Atlas of Clinical Ophthalmology. *3rd ed. St Louis: Mosby; 2005:151.)*

Table 8-1 Corneal Endothelial Cell Density

Parameter	Value
Density during first decade of life	4000 cells/mm^3
Average density at age 40 years	2600 cells/mm^3
Rate of cell loss	0.6% per year
Minimum density required for adequate function	400–700 cells/mm^3

Infiltration of polymorphonuclear leukocytes in response to severe corneal injury can induce endothelial cells to become fibroblastic and to synthesize a *retrocorneal fibrous membrane (RCFM).* RCFM forms between the Descemet membrane and the corneal endothelium and causes a significant decrease in visual acuity. Unlike normal corneal endothelial cells, which accumulate a limited amount of type I collagen protein, the fibroblastic cells isolated from the RCFM predominantly express type I collagen.

Panjwani N. Cornea and sclera. In: Harding JJ, ed. *Biochemistry of the Eye.* London: Chapman & Hall Medical; 1997:16–51.

CHAPTER 9

Aqueous Humor, Iris, and Ciliary Body

Highlights

- Aqueous humor is secreted by the nonpigmented ciliary epithelium (NPE) from a substrate of blood plasma.
- Aqueous humor is distinct from plasma, as it has low protein content and a high concentration of ascorbate.
- Ascorbate has antioxidant properties, and its high concentration in the aqueous protects intraocular structures by blocking ultraviolet (UV) light.
- The blood–aqueous barrier is composed of the tight junctions of the NPE, the iris vasculature, and the inner wall endothelium of the Schlemm canal.
- Disruption of the blood–aqueous barrier allows mixing of blood contents with ocular fluids, producing a plasmoid aqueous, as occurs in anterior uveitis.

Physiology of the Iris and Ciliary Body

The iris and ciliary body are the anterior parts of the uvea (also called *uveal tract*), which is continuous with the choroid posteriorly. The iris is a highly pigmented tissue that functions as a movable diaphragm between the anterior and posterior chambers of the eye to regulate the amount of light that reaches the retina. It is a delicate, dynamic structure that can make precise and rapid changes in pupillary diameter in response to light and specific pharmacologic stimuli. The ciliary body produces the aqueous humor, regulates its composition, and contributes to uveoscleral outflow, thereby directly influencing the ionic environment and metabolism of the cornea, lens, and trabecular meshwork.

The ciliary body is the main pharmacologic target in the treatment of glaucoma. Many of the agents used to lower intraocular pressure (IOP) in glaucoma, such as adrenergic and cholinergic drugs and prostaglandin analogues, work through receptors and their respective signal transduction pathways. The iris–ciliary body is rich in many types of receptors that bind to various ligands. Chapter 16 discusses these receptors and pharmacologic agents relevant to the treatment of glaucoma.

The ciliary body is a major contributor to the defense against oxidative stress, via molecules secreted into the aqueous humor, as discussed later in this chapter. It has the highest concentration of redox (oxidation-reduction) enzymes in the anterior segment. The ciliary body also contains proteins of the cytochrome P450 family, though only a small number compared with the liver. These enzymes are involved in detoxification, whereby they convert hydrophobic compounds to hydrophilic ones via hydroxylation. CYP2D6 is one such enzyme that metabolizes timolol. It is expressed in low levels in ocular tissues but is abundant in the liver.

See Chapter 2 of this volume for further discussion of the structures mentioned in this section.

Dynamics of the Aqueous Humor

Blood–Aqueous Barrier

The aqueous humor *(aqueous)* is a transparent fluid that fills the anterior and posterior chambers of the eye. It is the major nutrient source for the avascular lens and cornea and also serves as a medium for removal of waste products.

Ocular fluids are separated from blood by barriers formed by the tight junctions of epithelial cells and those of endothelial cells. These barriers are called either *blood–aqueous* or *blood–retina barriers,* depending on their location in the eye. Because of these barriers, the composition and amounts of all materials entering and leaving the eye can be carefully controlled. Perturbations of these *blood–ocular barriers* cause blood constituents to mix with ocular fluids; this mixing leads to plasmoid aqueous, retinal exudates, or retinal edema.

The blood–aqueous barrier is composed of the tight junctions of the following:

- nonpigmented ciliary epithelium
- iris vasculature
- inner wall endothelium of the Schlemm canal

This barrier restricts plasma proteins from entering the aqueous. Consequently, aqueous is essentially protein-free, which gives it a refractive index of 1.336 and allows optical clarity for transmission of light along the visual pathway. The blood–aqueous barrier, along with active transport systems, also allows increased levels of ascorbate and some amino acids in aqueous compared to levels in blood plasma. Breakdown of this barrier is discussed later in the chapter.

Aqueous Humor Formation and Secretion

The ciliary epithelium is a bilayer of polarized epithelial cells that line the surface of the ciliary body. The 2 cell layers are the nonpigmented epithelium (NPE), which faces the aqueous humor, and the pigmented epithelium (PE), which faces the ciliary stroma. These 2 layers are connected to each other at their apical membranes; their basal membranes face the aqueous and ciliary stroma. The NPE has tight junctions proximal to the apical plasma membrane that form part of the blood–aqueous barrier, thereby preventing paracellular transport from the ciliary stroma into the posterior chamber. In contrast, the PE cell layer is considered a leaky epithelium because it allows solutes to move through the space between the PE cells.

Aqueous humor is secreted by the NPE from a substrate of blood plasma. It is secreted at a flow rate of 2–3 μL/min, but this rate varies according to our circadian rhythm, dropping to 1.0 μL/min at night.

Aqueous enters the posterior chamber from the ciliary processes by means of active and passive physiologic mechanisms:

- *active:* energy-dependent secretion of certain ions and substrates
- *passive:* diffusion and ultrafiltration

The active process of aqueous secretion involves enzymes present in the NPE, such as sodium-potassium adenosine triphosphatase (Na^+,K^+-ATPase) and carbonic anhydrase (CA). Active secretion of sodium by Na^+,K^+-ATPase and accompanying anions creates high osmolarity on the basolateral (aqueous) side of the NPE, and this in turn promotes diffusion of water. In humans, CA is present in both PE and NPE. Its inhibitors reduce the rate of entry of sodium and bicarbonate into the aqueous, causing a reduction in aqueous flow. See Chapter 16 for further discussion.

Cotransport is the coupled transport of 2 chemical substances across a membrane, with one substance transported down its concentration gradient, which drives movement of the other substance against its concentration gradient. Symport and antiport are cotransport mechanisms. *Symporters* are membrane proteins that mediate the cotransport of molecules in the same direction, whereas *antiporters* mediate the cotransport of molecules in opposite directions. The systems' activities and cellular distributions along the membranes of PE and NPE cells determine unidirectional net secretion from the ciliary stroma to the posterior chamber, a process that involves 3 steps (Fig 9-1):

1. uptake of solute and water at the stromal surface by PE cells
2. transfer of solute and water from PE to NPE cells through gap junctions
3. transfer of solute and water by NPE cells into the posterior chamber

Likewise, it is thought that there is a mechanism for transporting solute and water from the posterior chamber back into the stroma. In this unidirectional reabsorption, another set of transporters may be involved in extruding sodium, potassium, and chloride back into the stroma.

Diffusion is the movement of solutes or ions across a membrane down the concentration or ionic gradient. In aqueous formation, ultrafiltration is the nonenzymatic component that depends on intraocular pressure (IOP), blood pressure, and the blood osmotic pressure in the ciliary body. Ultrafiltration decreases with increasing IOP.

IOP is maintained by continuous aqueous formation and drainage, which allow removal of metabolic waste products from the surrounding tissues. The factors determining IOP are summarized in the Goldmann equation and include

- rate of aqueous production
- resistance to outflow
- the pressure within the episcleral veins receiving drainage from the Schlemm canal

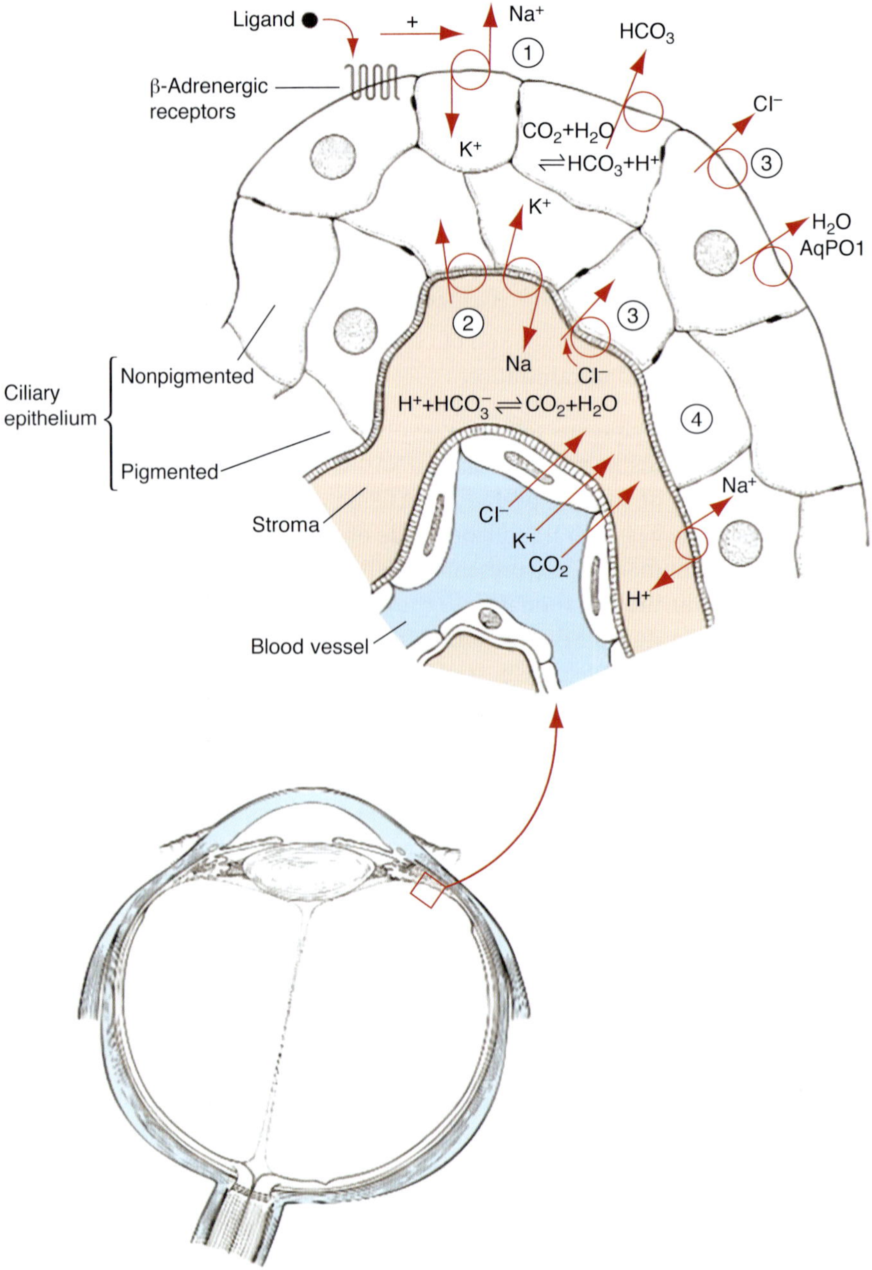

Figure 9-1 Production and secretion of aqueous humor. The oncotic pressure of the ciliary body stroma draws water toward the stroma from the neighboring blood vessel but also away from the posterior chamber. Thus, energy-dependent mechanisms (active transport) are needed to secrete water across the ciliary epithelium. This is accomplished by sodium-potassium adenosine triphosphatase (Na^+,K^+-ATPase), which pumps Na^+ into the posterior chamber. The resultant increase in osmolarity draws water into the posterior chamber via aquaporin channels. Within the epithelial layers, carbonic anhydrase provides hydrogen ions (H^+), which are exchanged with Na^+ to help provide a supply of sodium within the epithelium and drive the flow of water. Adrenergic stimulation has been reported to drive Na^+,K^+-ATPase. 1, Na^+,K^+ antiport; 2, K^+ channel; 3, Cl^- channel; 4, Na^+,H^+ antiport; AqPO1 = aquaporin channel 1. *(Adapted with permission from Forrester JV, Dick AD, McMenamin PG, Roberts F, Pearlman E.* The Eye: Basic Sciences in Practice. *4th ed. Edinburgh: Elsevier; 2016:224, Box 4-14.)*

Inhibitors of enzymatic processes decrease aqueous inflow by varying amounts, providing additional evidence of active secretory processes. For more information, see Chapter 16 of this volume and BCSC Section 10, *Glaucoma*.

CLINICAL PEARL

Carbonic anhydrase inhibitors and β-blockers are used systemically and topically in the treatment of glaucoma to reduce the rate of aqueous humor formation.

Composition of the Aqueous Humor

Table 9-1 summarizes the composition of the aqueous humor compared with that of plasma and vitreous. Aqueous secretion is not an ultrafiltrate of plasma (as was once speculated), because it is produced by energy-dependent processes in the epithelial layer of the ciliary body. This mode of production allows precise control to be maintained over composition of the fluid that bathes the structures essential for normal vision.

The ionic composition of the aqueous humor is determined by selective active transport systems (eg, Na^+,K^+-$2Cl^-$ symport, Cl^--HCO_3^- and Na^+,H^+ antiports, cation channels, water channels [aquaporin], Na^+,K^+-ATPase, K^+ channels, Cl^- channels, H^+-ATPase) that participate in secretion of aqueous humor by the NPE. Active secretion of ions and molecules leads to higher levels of ascorbate and some amino acids in aqueous than in plasma.

Molecular studies have shown that the secretory properties of the ciliary epithelium are not limited to ions and electrolytes but extend to a wide range of molecules with different molecular masses. Common features of many of these molecules are their local synthesis in the ciliary epithelium and their secretion by the NPE cells through the regulatory pathway into the aqueous humor. Among the proteins whose messenger RNA expression has been demonstrated are

- plasma proteins (eg, complement component C4, α_2-macroglobulin, selenoprotein P, apolipoprotein D, plasma glutathione peroxidases, angiotensinogen)
- proteinases (eg, cathepsin D, cathepsin O)

Table 9-1 Comparison of Components of Plasma, Aqueous Humor, and Vitreous

Components (mmol/kg H_2O)	Plasma	Aqueous	Vitreous
Na^+	146	163	144
Cl^-	109	134	114
HCO_3^-	28	20	20–30
Ascorbate	0.04	1.06	2.21
Glucose	6	3	3.4

From Macknight AD, MacLaughlin CW, Peart D, Purves RD, Carré DA, Civan MM. Formation of the aqueous humor. *Clin Exp Pharmacol Physiol.* 2000;27(1–2):100–106.

- cellular retinaldehyde–binding protein (CRALBP) and other components of the visual cycle
- neurotrophic factor (eg, PE-derived factor)
- neuropeptide-processing enzymes (eg, carboxypeptidase E, peptidylglycine-α-amidating monoxygenase)
- neuroendocrine peptides (eg, secretogranin II, neurotensin, galanin)
- bioactive peptides and hormones (eg, atrial natriuretic peptide, brain natriuretic peptide)

These findings support the view that the ciliary epithelium exhibits neuroendocrine properties that are directly related to the makeup of the aqueous humor and its regulation. The aqueous humor composition is in dynamic equilibrium, determined both by its rate of production and outflow and by continuous exchanges with the tissues of the anterior segment. The aqueous contains the following:

- inorganic ions and organic anions
- carbohydrates
- glutathione and urea
- proteins
- growth-modulatory factors
- oxygen and carbon dioxide

Yang W, Bradley JC, Reid TW, McCartney DL. Growth factors in aqueous humor. *Ophthalmology*. 2011;118(5):1003.

Inorganic Ions

The concentrations of sodium, potassium, and magnesium in the aqueous are similar to those in plasma, but the level of calcium in aqueous is only half that in plasma. The 2 major anions are chloride and bicarbonate. Phosphate is also present in the aqueous (aqueous-to-plasma ratio, ≈0.5 or lower), but its concentration is too low to have significant buffering capacity. Iron, copper, and zinc are all found in the aqueous humor at essentially the same levels as in plasma: approximately 1 mg/mL.

Organic Anions

Lactate is the most abundant organic anion in the aqueous, and its concentration there is always higher than that in plasma. The high lactate level in aqueous is a result of glycolytic metabolism, upon which the avascular lens depends.

Ascorbate (vitamin C) levels in aqueous are much higher (some 10–50 times higher) than those in plasma. Ascorbate has antioxidant properties, and its high concentration in the aqueous protects intraocular structures by blocking UV light.

Carbohydrates

Glucose concentration in the aqueous is roughly 50%–70% of that in plasma. The rate of entry of glucose into the posterior chamber is much more rapid than would be expected from its molecular size and lipid solubility, suggesting that the transport of glucose across the ciliary epithelium occurs by facilitated diffusion.

> **CLINICAL PEARL**
>
> In individuals with diabetes mellitus, glucose levels in the aqueous humor are increased. This leads to higher glucose concentrations in the lens, which has short-term refractive and longer-term cataract implications.

Inositol, which is important for phospholipid synthesis in the anterior segment, is found in the aqueous at a concentration approximately 10 times higher than that in plasma.

Glutathione and Urea

Glutathione, an important tripeptide with a reactive sulfhydryl group, is also found in the aqueous humor. Its concentration in primates ranges from 1 to 10 μmol/L. Blood contains a high concentration of glutathione; however, virtually all glutathione resides within the erythrocytes, and plasma has a low concentration of only 5 μmol/L or less. Glutathione stabilizes the oxidation-reduction (redox) state of the aqueous by reconverting ascorbate to its functional form after oxidation, as well as by removing excess hydrogen peroxide. Glutathione also serves as a substrate in the enzymatic conjugation by cytosolic enzymes; this process is involved in the cellular detoxification of electrophilic compounds. These enzymes (glutathione S-transferases) are important in protecting tissues from oxidative damage and oxidative stress and are highly concentrated in the ocular ciliary epithelium.

The concentration of urea in the aqueous is between 80% and 90% of that in plasma. This compound is distributed passively across nearly all biological membrane systems, and its high aqueous-to-plasma ratio indicates that this small molecule (molecular weight, 60) readily crosses the epithelial barrier. Urea is effective in hyperosmotic infusion treatment for glaucoma. However, mannitol (molecular weight, 182) is preferred to urea because urea crosses the epithelial barrier more easily.

Proteins

As stated earlier, the tight junctions of the NPE, along with other structures, establish the blood–aqueous barrier, which prevents diffusion of plasma proteins from the ciliary stroma into the posterior chamber; nevertheless, plasma proteins do enter the aqueous humor, possibly through the root and anterior surface of the iris. Normal aqueous contains approximately 0.02 g of protein per 100 mL, as compared with the typical plasma level of 7 g per 100 mL. The most abundant plasma proteins identified in aqueous humor are albumin and transferrin, which together may account for 50% of the total protein content.

In addition to the plasma proteins that enter the aqueous, there is compelling evidence that some proteins may be synthesized within the ciliary body and secreted directly into the aqueous humor. Molecular techniques (such as the screening of complementary DNA [cDNA] libraries constructed from intact human and bovine ciliary bodies) have enabled the isolation and identification of numerous protein-encoding genes. These studies, therefore, challenge the long-held view that plasma proteins in the aqueous humor are transported into the aqueous from outside the eye. Among the cDNA molecules isolated from the ciliary body are

- C4, a component of the classical complement pathway that participates in immune-mediated inflammatory responses
- α_2-macroglobulin, a carrier protein that is involved in proteinase inhibition, clearance, and targeting, as well as the processing of foreign peptides
- apolipoprotein D, which binds and transports hydrophobic substances, including cholesterol, cholesteryl esters, and arachidonic acid (AA)
- selenoprotein P, which has antioxidant properties

Proteinases and inhibitors

Several proteinases and proteinase inhibitors have also been identified in the aqueous humor. The proteinases include cathepsin D and cathepsin O, which are synthesized and secreted by the ciliary epithelial cells. Cathepsin D is involved in the degradation of neuropeptides and peptide hormones and has been found in high levels in the cerebrospinal fluid of patients with Alzheimer disease. Less is known about cathepsin O, which may be involved in normal cellular protein degradation and turnover.

Of the proteinase inhibitors, α_2-macroglobulin and α_1-antitrypsin are perhaps the most extensively studied. An imbalance in equilibrium between proteinases and proteinase inhibitors could alter aqueous humor composition, which may cause disease (eg, glaucoma).

Enzymes

Activators, proenzymes, and fibrinolytic enzymes are present in the aqueous and could play a role in the regulation of outflow resistance. Both plasminogen and plasminogen activator are found in human and monkey aqueous, but only traces of plasmin have been reported.

Neurotrophic and neuroendocrine proteins

The ciliary epithelia, which are derived from neuroectoderm, are functionally similar to neuroendocrine glands elsewhere in the body. The ciliary body has neuroendocrine peptides and neuroendocrine processing enzymes. Bioactive neuroendocrine markers, identified through human ciliary body cDNA subtraction studies, include neurotensin, angiotensin, endothelins, and natriuretic peptides; these markers are known to have systemic vascular hemodynamic effects and, by implication, may have similar roles in IOP regulation or aqueous secretion. The neuroendocrine properties of the ciliary epithelium may determine the composition of the aqueous humor, the diurnal (circadian) rhythm of aqueous humor secretion and IOP, the ciliary blood flow, and the immune privilege status of intraocular structures.

Coca-Prados M, Escribano J. New perspectives in aqueous humor secretion and in glaucoma: the ciliary body as a multifunctional neuroendocrine gland. *Prog Retin Eye Res.* 2007;26(3):239–262.

Growth-Modulatory Factors

The physical and chemical properties of the aqueous humor play a substantial role in modulating the proliferation, differentiation, functional viability, and wound healing of ocular tissues. These properties are largely influenced by several growth-promoting and differentiation factors that have been identified or quantified in aqueous humor, including the following:

- transforming growth factor βs 1 and 2 (TGF-β_1 and -β_2)
- acidic and basic fibroblast growth factors (aFGF and bFGF)
- insulin-like growth factor I (IGF-I)
- insulin-like growth factor binding proteins (IGFBPs)
- vascular endothelial growth factors (VEGFs)
- transferrin

The growth factors in the aqueous humor perform diverse, synergistic, and sometimes opposite biological activities. Normally, the lack of significant mitosis of the corneal endothelium and trabecular meshwork in vivo is probably controlled by the complex coordination of effects and interactions among the different growth-modulatory substances present in the aqueous humor (see Part V, Ocular Pharmacology).

Disruption in the balance among various growth factors, which occurs with the production of plasmoid aqueous humor as a result of breakdown of the blood–aqueous barrier, may explain the abnormal hyperplastic response of the lens epithelium and corneal endothelium observed in chronic inflammatory conditions and traumatic insults to the eye. Ultimately, however, the effect of a given growth factor on the aqueous humor is determined primarily by the growth factor's bioavailability. Bioavailability, in turn, depends on many factors, including the expression of receptors on target tissues, interactive effects of the growth factor with components of the extracellular matrix, and the levels of circulating and matrix-bound proteases.

Growth factor levels in the aqueous humor are altered in several disease states. Levels of IGFBPs are elevated fivefold in patients with diabetes mellitus without retinopathy, and IGF-I levels are elevated in patients with diabetic retinopathy. VEGF levels in the aqueous humor are elevated in eyes with acute nonarteritic ischemic optic neuropathy, whereas interleukin-2 concentration is reduced.

Micieli JA, Lam C, Najem K, Margolin EA. Aqueous humor cytokines in patients with acute nonarteritic anterior ischemic optic neuropathy. *Am J Ophthalmol.* 2017;177:175–181.

Vascular endothelial growth factors

The VEGF family of glycoproteins includes VEGF-A, -B, -C, and -D, as well as placental growth factor (PlGF). VEGF-A, the most thoroughly studied at present, has 9 isoforms and is the only VEGF family member induced by hypoxia. VEGF-A is a crucial regulator of vasculogenesis (embryologic blood vessel development from mesodermal elements) and a potent inducer of vascular permeability and angiogenesis (neovascularization). VEGF-C and VEGF-D regulate lymphangiogenesis. VEGF receptors (VEGFR) are tyrosine kinases.

Three VEGFRs have been identified:

- VEGFR-1 has high affinity for VEGF-A, VEGF-B, and PlGF. Functionally, it acts as a negative regulator of VEGF-A signaling by limiting the amount of ligand available to VEGFR-2.
- VEGFR-2 is the primary mediator of the mitogenic, angiogenic, and vascular permeability effects of VEGF-A.
- VEGFR-3 mediates the angiogenic effects of VEGF-C and VEGF-D on lymphatic vessels.

Although VEGF-A and its receptors are most studied in relation to the vascular endothelium, they are also present in other tissues and organ systems, a finding that underscores other possible physiological roles, such as retinal leukostasis and neuroprotection. In addition, VEGF-A may play a role in regulating IOP by elevating levels of nitric oxide (NO), which increases aqueous outflow facility. VEGF-A upregulates expression of endothelial NO synthase (eNOS), which produces NO; VEGF-A blockage may cause IOP elevation by decreasing NO production.

VEGF-A levels in ocular fluids are elevated not only in patients with active ocular neovascularization from proliferative diabetic retinopathy but also after central retinal vein occlusion and in eyes with iris neovascularization. The expression of VEGF is increased by hypoxia in retinal endothelial cells, retinal pericytes, Müller cells, retinal pigment epithelium cells, and the NPE cells of the ciliary body. Also, levels of VEGF-A in the aqueous humor increase in response to anterior segment ischemia in animal models, as well as in response to retinal hypoxia. Aqueous VEGF-A levels fall after intravitreal injection of anti-VEGF agents.

Karaman S, Leppänen VM, Alitalo K. Vascular endothelial growth factor signaling in development and disease. *Development.* 2018;145(14):1–8.

Penn JS, Madan A, Caldwell RB, Bartoli M, Caldwell RW, Hartnett ME. Vascular endothelial growth factor in eye disease. *Prog Retin Eye Res.* 2008;27(4):331–371.

Oxygen and Carbon Dioxide

Oxygen in the aqueous humor is derived from the blood supply to the ciliary body and iris, as the atmospheric oxygen flux across the cornea is negligible. Indeed, the corneal endothelium depends critically on the aqueous oxygen supply for the active fluid-transport mechanism that maintains corneal transparency. The lens and the endothelial lining of the trabecular meshwork also derive their oxygen supply from the aqueous. Oxygen is present in the aqueous humor at a partial pressure lower than that in arterial blood.

CLINICAL PEARL

Oxygen concentration in the aqueous humor may increase with age-related vitreous degeneration or after surgical removal of vitreous. Elevated oxygen concentration induces oxidative damage in the lens and trabecular meshwork and leads to an increased risk of nuclear sclerosis, cataract, and open-angle glaucoma after vitrectomy.

The carbon dioxide content of the aqueous ranges from about 40 to 60 mm Hg, contributing approximately 3% of the total bicarbonate. The relative proportions of carbon dioxide and bicarbonate determine the pH of the aqueous, which in most species ranges between 7.5 and 7.6. Carbon dioxide is continuously lost from the aqueous by diffusion across the cornea into the tear film and atmosphere.

Gong H, Tripathi RC, Tripathi BJ. Morphology of the aqueous outflow pathway. *Microsc Res Tech.* 1996;33(4):336–367.

Clinical Implications of Breakdown of the Blood–Aqueous Barrier

The blood–aqueous barrier may be disrupted in a number of conditions, including ocular trauma (mechanical, chemical, or physical), infection or inflammation, and ischemia, as well as with use of pharmacologic agents (eg, prostaglandin analogues, cholinesterase inhibitors). With compromise of the blood–aqueous barrier, the levels of inflammatory mediators, immunoglobulins, fibrin, and proteases rise, and the balance among the various growth factors is disrupted. The protein content of the aqueous humor increases, possibly as much as 10–100 times normal, especially in high-molecular-weight polypeptides.

The clinical sequelae include fibrinous exudate (with or without a macrophage reaction and formation of cyclitic membranes) and synechiae formation (peripheral and posterior), as well as an abnormal neovascular response, which further exacerbates breakdown of the blood–aqueous barrier. Chronic disruption of this barrier is implicated in the abnormal hyperplastic response of the lens epithelium, corneal endothelium, trabecular meshwork, and iris, and in the formation of complicated cataracts. Degenerative and proliferative changes may occur in various ocular structures as well. The use of anti-inflammatory steroidal and nonsteroidal drugs, cycloplegics, protease activators or inhibitors, growth factor and anti–growth factor agents, and even surgical intervention may be necessary to combat these events.

CHAPTER 10

Lens

Highlights

- The lens has an index of refraction of 1.390, which is higher than that of the surrounding media and a result of its high protein content.
- Proteins constitute 33% of the weight of the lens, which is 2–3 times higher than their concentration in other tissues in the body.
- The lens relies primarily on glycolysis to generate adenosine triphosphate (ATP). Alterations in this metabolic pathway have been implicated in the development of congenital cataract as well as diabetic cataract.

Overview

The lens is a transparent, avascular structure that, in concert with the cornea, focuses incident light onto the sensory elements of the retina. To do so, the lens must be transparent and must have an index of refraction higher than that of the surrounding fluids. The high refractive index is due to the high concentration of proteins—especially of soluble proteins called *crystallins*—in the lens cells. Furthermore, because there is little if any turnover of protein in the central region of the lens (where the oldest, denucleated cells are found), the proteins of the human lens must be extremely stable to remain functionally viable for a lifetime. Considering the lens's mode of growth and the stresses to which the lens is chronically exposed, it is remarkable that in most people, lenses retain good transparency until later in life; visually significant opacities typically develop by the sixth or seventh decade of life.

This chapter discusses the structure and chemical composition of the lens, as well as aspects of membrane function, metabolism, and regulatory processes within the lens. BCSC Section 11, *Lens and Cataract,* provides additional information about the lens, cataractogenesis, and cataract surgery.

Structure of the Lens

Capsule

The lens is enclosed in an elastic basement membrane called the *lens capsule* (Fig 10-1; see also Chapter 2, Fig 2-28). The capsule is acellular and is composed primarily of type IV collagen; it contains smaller amounts of other collagens and extracellular matrix

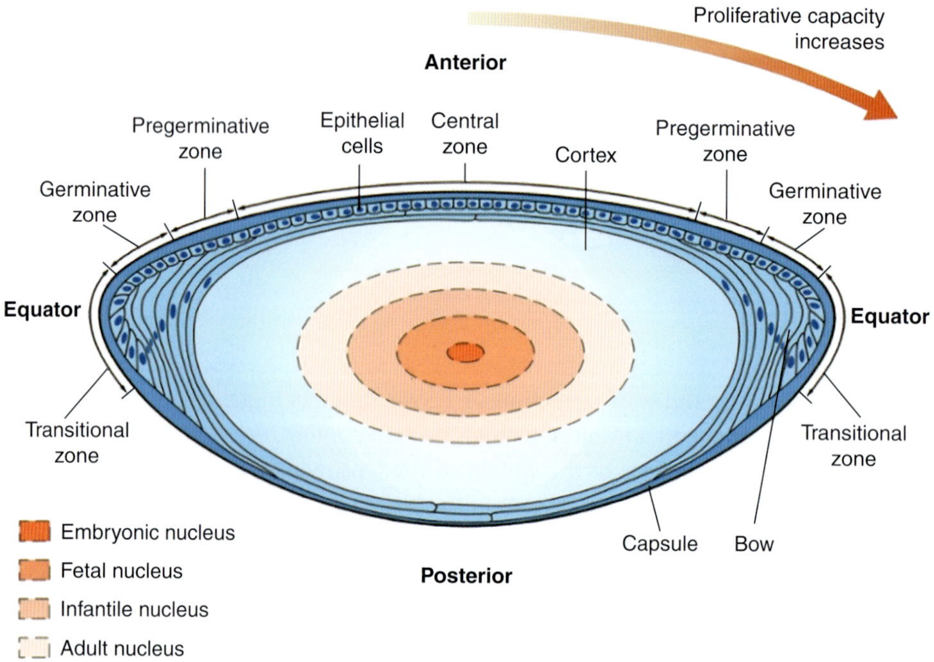

Figure 10-1 Cross section of the mammalian lens, demonstrating the central nucleus and its growth over time. Near the equator is the bow region, where the lens-fiber cells elongate until their 2 ends meet. At this point, they are fully mature and as they are pushed inward by newer fibers, they lose their nuclei and organelles, making up the lens cortex. There is no shedding of these fibers over time. Thus, the lens continues to increase in size throughout life. *(Reproduced with permission from Friedman NJ, Kaiser PK, Trattler WB.* Review of Ophthalmology. *3rd ed. Edinburgh: Elsevier; 2018:288.)*

components (including glycosaminoglycans, laminin, fibronectin, and heparan sulfate proteoglycan). The capsule is thicker on the anterior surface of the lens, where the epithelial cells continue to secrete capsular material throughout life. On the posterior surface of the lens, where there is no epithelium, the posterior fiber cells have limited capacity to secrete such material and the capsule is relatively thinner. The zonular fibers, from which the lens is suspended, insert into the capsule near the equator on both the anterior and posterior aspects. The capsule is not a barrier to diffusion of water, ions, small molecules, or proteins up to the size of serum albumin (which has a molecular weight of 68,000).

Epithelium

A single layer of epithelial cells covers the anterior surface of the lens. These cells have full metabolic capacity and play the primary role in regulating the water and ion balance of the entire lens. Although the cells of the central epithelium are not mitotically active, a germinative zone exists as a ring anterior to the equator, where the epithelial cells divide. The new cells migrate toward the equator and begin to differentiate into lens fibers (see Fig 10-1). In the adult lens, epithelial cells are not normally found posterior to the equator.

CLINICAL PEARL

In the adult lens, lens epithelial cell migration posterior to the equator results in the development of posterior subcapsular cataract. In pseudophakic patients, migration similar to this can result in the formation of posterior capsule opacity. Changes in intraocular lens design have limited such migration.

Cortex and Nucleus

Aside from the single layer of epithelial cells on its anterior surface, the lens is composed of lens fibers, which are long ribbonlike cells. These fibers are formed from epithelial cells at the lens equator; therefore, younger fibers are always exterior to older ones (see Fig 10-1 and Chapter 2, Fig 2-29). The lens structure can be equated with the growth rings of a tree: the oldest cells are in the center, and the progressively younger layers, or shells, of fiber cells are toward the periphery. Unlike the case with many tissues, no cells are sloughed from the lens, and cells produced before birth remain at the center of the lens throughout life. The fiber mass of the adult lens can be divided into the *cortex* (the outer fibers, laid down after approximately age 20 years) and the *nucleus* (the cells produced from embryogenesis through adolescence).

As new fiber cells elongate and differentiate into mature fibers, their cell nuclei form the *bow zone,* or *bow region,* at the lens equator (see Fig 10-1). Elongating fibers substantially increase their volume and surface area and express large amounts of both lens crystallins (discussed later) and a lens-fiber–specific membrane protein called the *major intrinsic protein (MIP).* As the fibers become fully elongated and make sutures at each end with fibers that have elongated from the opposite side of the lens, they become mature, terminally differentiated fiber cells. The cell nuclei disintegrate, as do mitochondria and other organelles. This process has been proposed to occur via *autophagy,* the degradation of the cell's own unneeded and/or damaged components via a defined intracellular process. There are several types of autophagy, and in each, the degradation is directed toward certain intracellular components:

- microautophagy: cytoplasmic material
- chaperone-mediated autophagy: proteins that can be recognized by a heat shock protein complex
- macroautophagy: cell organelles
- mitophagy (a type of macroautophagy): mitochondria

Elimination of cellular organelles is necessary in the central portion of the lens because such bodies are sufficiently large to scatter light and thereby degrade visual acuity. Also, with the loss of cell nuclei, the mature fibers lose the machinery required for synthesis of proteins.

Chai P, Ni H, Zhang H, Fan X. The evolving functions of autophagy in ocular health: a double-edged sword. *Int J Biol Sci.* 2016;12(11):1332–1340.

Costello MJ, Brennan LA, Basu S, et al. Autophagy and mitophagy participate in ocular lens organelle degradation. *Exp Eye Res.* 2013;116:141–150.

Chemical Composition of the Lens

Plasma Membranes

The chemical composition of lens-fiber plasma membranes suggests that they are both very stable and very rigid. A high saturated fatty acid content, a high cholesterol-to-phospholipid ratio, and a high concentration of sphingomyelin all contribute to the tight packing and low fluidity of the membrane. Although lipids make up only about 1% of the total lens mass, they constitute approximately 55% of the plasma membrane's dry weight; cholesterol is the major neutral lipid. As the lens ages, the protein-to-lipid and cholesterol-to-phospholipid ratios increase as a result of phospholipid loss, especially in the nucleus.

Lens Proteins

The lens has the highest protein content of any tissue in the body. In some species, more than 50% of lens weight is protein. Lens crystallins are a diverse group of proteins that are abundantly expressed in the cytoplasm of lens-fiber cells. They are thought to play crucial roles in providing the transparency and refractile properties essential to lens function. Crystallins constitute 90%–95% of total lens protein. In addition to crystallins, the lens has a full complement of enzymes and regulatory proteins that are present primarily in the epithelium and in immature fiber cells, where most metabolic activity occurs.

Crystallins

Crystallins are water-soluble proteins so named for their high abundance in the crystalline lens. Crystallins can be divided into 2 groups. One group includes α-crystallin and the β,γ-crystallin family, both of which seem to be present in all vertebrate lenses but have also been demonstrated in other ocular tissues. The second group consists of the taxon-specific crystallins, which are present only in certain species.

Andley UP. Crystallins in the eye: function and pathology. *Prog Retin Eye Res.* 2007; 26(1):78–98.

Slingsby C, Wistow GJ. Functions of crystallins in and out of lens: roles in elongated and post-mitotic cells. *Prog Biophys Mol Biol.* 2014;115(1):52–67.

α-Crystallin α-Crystallin is a member of the small heat shock protein family. Heat shock proteins are molecular chaperones; they stabilize partially folded proteins and prevent them from aggregating. Zinc ions enhance the chaperone function and stability of α-crystallin. Because protein aggregates in the lens scatter light and cause loss of transparency, the antiaggregative function of α-crystallin is crucial to the long-term maintenance of transparency in the fibers of the lens nucleus, where synthesis of new protein is impossible and protein molecules must exist for decades. Mutations in the α-crystallin gene result in premature cataract development; this has been confirmed in knockout models.

Berry V, Francis P, Ashwin Reddy M, et al. Alpha-B crystallin gene *(CRYAB)* mutation causes dominant congenital posterior polar cataract in humans. *Am J Hum Genet.* 2001;69(5):1141–1145.

Brady JP, Garland D, Duglas-Tabor Y, Robinson WG Jr, Groome A, Wawrousek EF. Targeted disruption of the mouse αA-crystallin gene induces cataract and cytoplasmic inclusion bodies containing the small heat shock protein αB-crystallin. *Proc Natl Acad Sci USA.* 1997;94(3):884–889.

β,γ-Crystallins β,γ-Crystallins are divided into 2 groups, β-crystallins and γ-crystallins, on the basis of molecular mass and isoelectric points. β-Crystallins exist as polymers, and γ-crystallins are monomeric. The specific functions of the β,γ-crystallins are unknown. Acquired posttranslational modifications of β-crystallins have been associated with cataract formation. Most expression of γ-crystallins occurs early in development; thus, they tend to be most concentrated in the nuclear region of the lens. Given their compact and symmetric structures (which can pack very densely), γ-crystallins tend to be highly concentrated in aged, hard lenses, which have little to no accommodative ability.

Taxon-specific crystallins In addition to the α-crystallin and β,γ-crystallins found in all vertebrate lenses, other proteins are abundantly expressed in various phylogenetic groups. Taxon-specific crystallins have not been demonstrated in humans. However, they are present in the developing eye of other species. Most taxon-specific crystallins are oxidoreductases, which bind pyridine nucleotides, and their presence in the lens significantly increases the concentration of the bound nucleotides. Reduced nucleotides absorb ultraviolet (UV) light and may protect the retina from UV-induced oxidation.

Cytoskeletal and membrane proteins

Although most proteins in the normal lens are water soluble, several important structural proteins can be solubilized only in the presence of chaotropic agents or detergents. These water-insoluble proteins include the cytoskeletal elements *actin* (actin filaments), *vimentin* (intermediate filaments), and *tubulin* (microtubules), as well as 2 additional proteins called *filensin* and *phakinin.* The last 2 proteins have been found only in lens-fiber cells and compose a cytoskeletal structure, the *beaded filament,* which is unique to the lens. The filamentous structures of the cytoskeleton provide structural support to the cells and play crucial roles in processes such as differentiation, motility and shape change, and organization of the cytoplasm. Mutations of the beaded filament have been shown to result in congenital cataract formation.

Lens-fiber membranes have 1 quantitatively dominant protein, MIP. MIP is expressed only in lens-fiber cells and was earlier thought to be a gap-junction protein. In fact, it is not a connexin but rather an aquaporin—a member of a large, diverse family of proteins involved in regulating water transport. MIP has been reported to function as a water channel and to play a role in cell adhesion. Mutations in the *MIP* gene lead to cataract formation.

Chepelinsky AB. Structural function of MIP/aquaporin 0 in the eye lens; genetic defects lead to congenital inherited cataracts. *Handb Exp Pharmacol.* 2009;(190):265–297.

Jakobs PM, Hess JF, FitzGerald PG, Kramer P, Weleber RG, Litt M. Autosomal-dominant congenital cataract associated with a deletion mutation in the human beaded filament protein gene BFSP2. *Am J Hum Genet.* 2000;66(4):1432–1436.

Posttranslational modifications to lens proteins

The proteins of the lens are some of the longest-lived in the body; the oldest ones (in the center of the lens nucleus) are synthesized before birth. As would be expected, these proteins become structurally modified in various ways: oxidation of sulfur and aromatic residue side chains, inter- and intrapolypeptide crosslinking, glycation, racemization, phosphorylation, deamidation, and carbamylation. Many of these modifications occur early in life and are probably part of a programmed modification of the crystallins that is required for their long-term stability and functionality. There is evidence that certain of these processes (phosphorylation, thiol oxidation) are reversible and may serve a regulatory function, although this hypothesis remains to be proved.

It is known that as the proteins age (particularly in some cataracts), certain oxidative modifications accumulate, which contributes to the crosslinking of crystallin polypeptides, alterations in fluorescent properties, and an increase in protein-associated pigmentation. In particular, the formation of disulfide crosslinks in the proteins of the lens nuclear region is associated with the formation of protein aggregates, light scattering, and cataract.

Transparency and Physiologic Aspects of the Lens

Lens Transparency

Transparency of the lens depends on the precise organization and maintenance of its elements. This is accomplished structurally by the orderly spatial distribution of the lens fibers and by the tight connections formed between them via specialized interdigitations (Fig 10-2). Light scatter is reduced by the minimized space between cells. Scatter is also diminished by the loss of nuclei and organelles as the lens fibers elongate and approach the visual axis. Light scatter alters lens transparency, thereby affecting vision. Loss of transparency can have beneficial effects. In the aging lens, accumulation of yellow chromophores protects the retina from shorter wavelengths of light.

The cornea and aqueous humor protect the retina from wavelengths below the visible spectrum. The visible spectrum refers to the part of the electromagnetic spectrum that is perceived as light, with wavelengths normally considered to range from 400 nm to 700 nm. Wavelengths shorter than 400 nm are referred to as *UV light.* Wavelengths of 300 nm or below are blocked by the cornea and by ascorbate (vitamin C), which is present at high levels in the aqueous humor. Wavelengths of 360 nm or below are blocked by the lens (Fig 10-3).

Lens Physiology

Because of its avascularity and its mode of growth, the lens faces some unusual physiologic challenges. All nutrients must be obtained from the surrounding fluids. Likewise, all waste products must be released into those fluids. Most of the cells of the adult lens have reduced metabolic activity and lack the membrane machinery to regulate ionic homeostasis independently. Understanding how the lens maintains ionic balance and how solutes move from cell to cell throughout the lens is crucial to comprehending the normal biology of the organ and the maintenance of lens transparency.

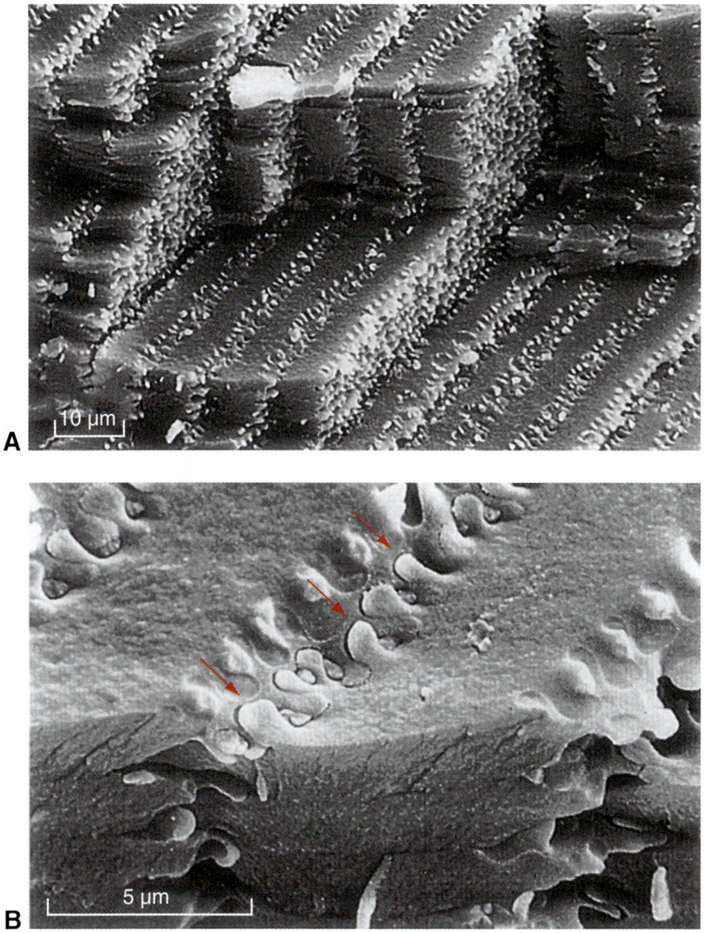

Figure 10-2 Scanning electron micrographs depicting the relationship between hexagonal packing of lens fibers **(A)** and interdigitation (*arrows* in **B**). *(Reproduced with permission from Kessel RG, Kardon RH.* Tissues and Organs: A Text-Atlas of Scanning Electron Microscopy. *San Francisco: WH Freeman; 1979.)*

In the normal lens, sodium (Na^+) levels are low (≈10 mmol/L), and potassium (K^+) levels are high (≈120 mmol/L). In the aqueous humor, Na^+ levels are approximately 150 mmol/L, and K^+ levels are about 5 mmol/L. When normal regulatory mechanisms are abrogated, K^+ leaks out of the lens and Na^+ floods in, followed by chloride (Cl^-). Water then enters in response to the osmotic gradient, causing loss of transparency by disrupting the normally smooth gradient of refractive index, as can occur following traumatic violation of the lens capsule.

The ionic balance in the lens is maintained primarily by Na^+,K^+-ATPase (also called *sodium-potassium pump*), an intrinsic membrane protein complex that hydrolyzes adenosine triphosphate (ATP) to transport Na^+ out of and K^+ into the lens (Fig 10-4). Functional Na^+,K^+-ATPase pumps are found primarily at the anterior surface of the lens, in the epithelium and the outer, immature fibers. Studies using ouabain, a specific inhibitor of

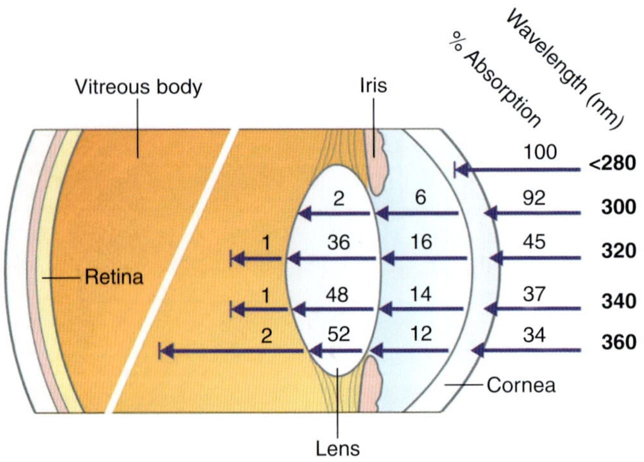

Figure 10-3 Blockage of ultraviolet light by the cornea, aqueous humor, and lens. *(Reproduced with permission from Levin LA, Nilsson SFE, Ver Hoeve J, Wu SM.* Adler's Physiology of the Eye. *11th ed. Philadelphia: Elsevier/Saunders; 2011:114.)*

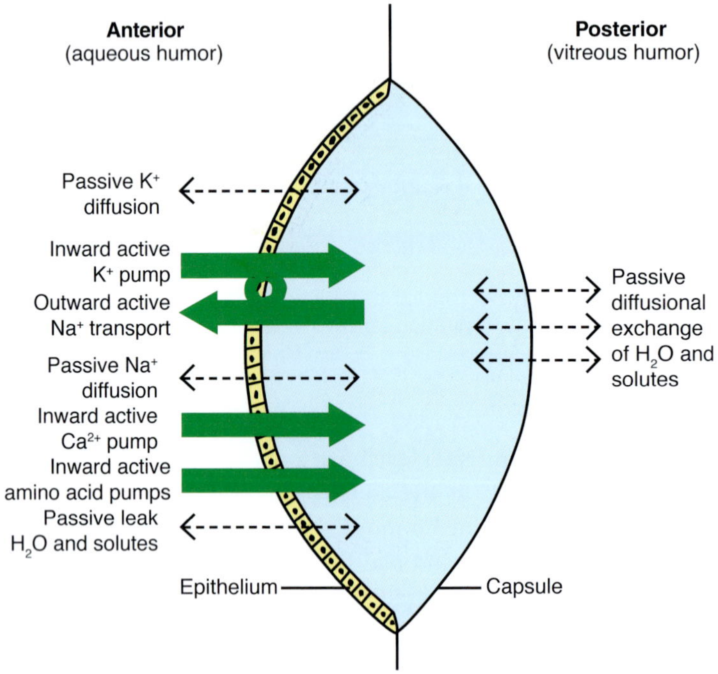

Figure 10-4 The pump–leak hypothesis of pathways of solute movement in the lens. The major site of active-transport mechanisms is the anterior epithelium. Passive diffusion occurs over both surfaces of the lens. *(Modified with permission from Paterson CA, Delamere NA. The lens. In: Hart WM Jr, ed.* Adler's Physiology of the Eye. *9th ed. St Louis: Mosby; 1992:365.)*

Na^+,K^+-ATPase, have established the pump's role as the primary determinant of the normal ionic state of the lens. Lens cells also contain membrane channels that pass ions; in particular, K^+-selective channels have been studied by patch-clamp techniques and found to be present primarily in the epithelial cells.

Communication between lens cells is provided by gap junctions, which are thought to account for most ion and small-molecule movement between cells. In fact, the density of gap junctions in the lens-fiber cells is greater than that in all other cells in the body. True gap junctions occur in the lens and are composed of members of the connexin family.

Lens Metabolism and Formation of Sugar Cataracts

Energy Production

Energy, in the form of ATP, is produced in the lens primarily through *glycolysis* in metabolically active cells in the anterior lens. This process is required because the oxygen tension in the lens is much lower than that in other tissues, given that oxygen reaches the avascular lens only via diffusion from the aqueous humor.

Most of the glucose entering the lens is phosphorylated to glucose-6-phosphate by hexokinase, the rate-limiting enzyme of the glycolytic pathway. Under normal conditions, most glucose-6-phosphate passes through glycolysis, wherein 2 molecules of ATP are formed per original molecule of glucose. A small proportion of glucose-6-phosphate is metabolized through the *pentose phosphate pathway* (also called *hexose monophosphate shunt*). This pathway is activated under conditions of oxidative stress because it is responsible for replenishing the supply of nicotinamide adenine dinucleotide phosphate (NADPH) that becomes oxidized through the increased activity of glutathione reductase under such conditions (Fig 10-5).

Carbohydrate Cataracts

Much research on lens carbohydrate metabolism has been stimulated by interest in *sugar cataracts,* which are associated with diabetes mellitus and galactosemia. True diabetic cataract is a rapidly developing bilateral snowflake cataract (see Fig 5-19 in BCSC Section 11, *Lens and Cataract*) that appears in the lens cortex of persons with poorly controlled type 1 diabetes mellitus. Individuals with type 2 diabetes mellitus do not typically develop this type of cataract but do have a higher prevalence of age-related cataract with a slightly earlier onset. It is likely that for these patients, the diabetes is simply an additional factor contributing to the development of age-related cataracts.

Defects in galactose metabolism also cause cataracts. Classic galactosemia is caused by a deficiency of galactose-1-phosphate uridyltransferase. Infants with this inborn error of metabolism develop bilateral cataracts within a few weeks of birth unless milk (lactose) is removed from the diet. Cataracts are also associated with a deficiency of galactokinase. Under certain conditions in which sugar levels are elevated significantly, some glucose (or galactose) is metabolized through the *polyol pathway,* also known as the *sorbitol pathway* (see Fig 10-5). Aldose reductase is the key enzyme for the pathway, and it converts

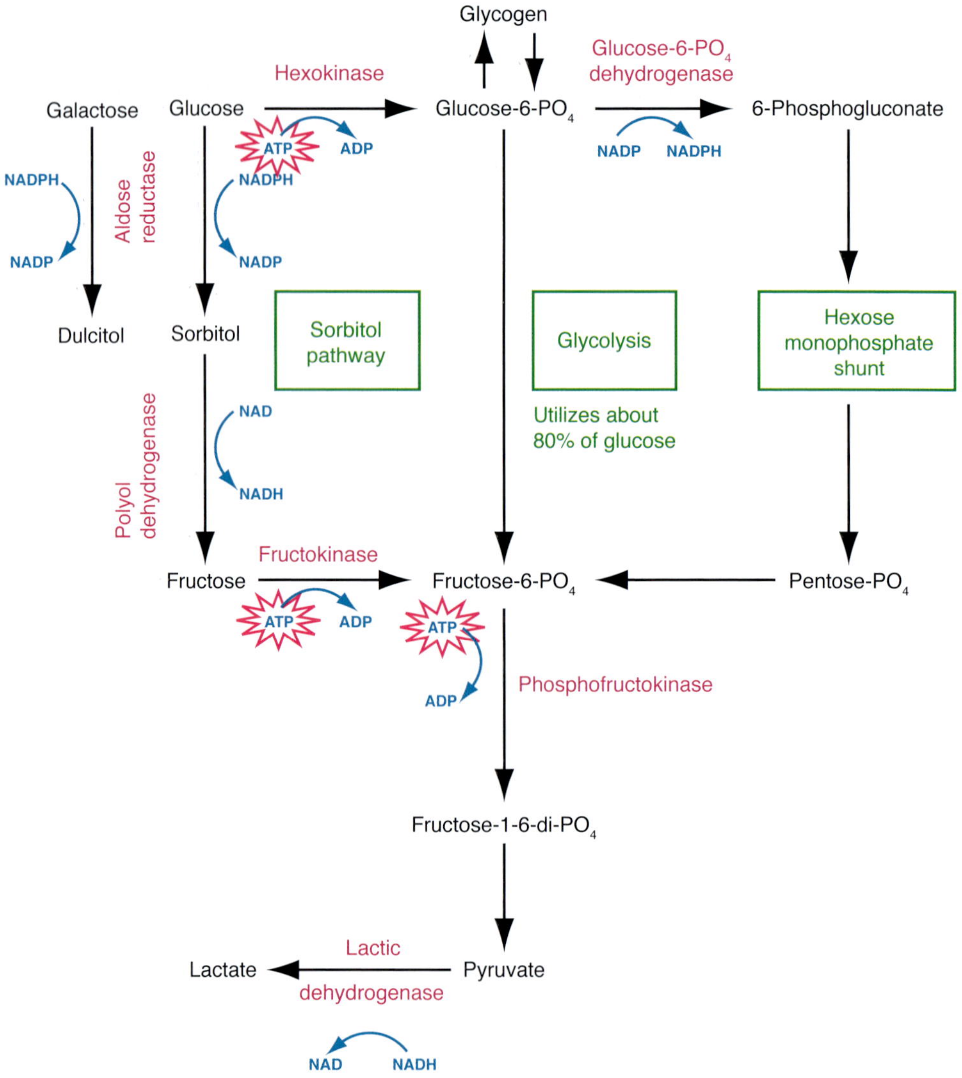

Figure 10-5 Glucose metabolism in the lens. Energy (ATP) from glucose is derived primarily through glycolysis. Alternatively, glucose can participate in the hexose monophosphate shunt (also called *pentose phosphate pathway*), generating nicotinamide adenine dinucleotide phosphate (NADPH) for oxidation-reduction (redox) reactions. In cases of hyperglycemia or galactosemia, the polyol pathway (also called *sorbitol pathway*) has been implicated in the formation of cataract. *(Adapted with permission from Hart WM Jr, ed.* Adler's Physiology of the Eye: Clinical Application. *9th ed. St Louis: Mosby; 1992:362.)*

the sugars into the corresponding sugar alcohols. Because aldose reductase has a very high K_m (apparent affinity constant) value—that is, low affinity—for glucose (or galactose), under normal conditions little or no activity occurs through this pathway. Under hyperglycemic conditions, however, aldose reductase competes with hexokinase for glucose (or galactose).

Studies using animal models have established the importance of the polyol pathway in experimental sugar cataracts. Animals with diabetes mellitus (either natural or induced) develop cataracts that are associated with the presence of sorbitol in the lens and with the influx of water. The osmotic hypothesis may account for these findings. According to this hypothesis, the activity of aldose reductase is central to the pathology by serving to increase the sorbitol content of the lens. Sorbitol is largely unable to penetrate cell membranes and thus is trapped inside the cells. Because its further conversion to fructose by polyol dehydrogenase is slow, sorbitol builds up in lens cells under conditions of hyperglycemia such that it creates an osmotic pressure that draws water into the lens, swelling the cells, damaging membranes, and causing cataract.

Hejtmancik JF, Riazuddin SA, McGreal R, Liu W, Cvekl A, Shiels A. Lens biology and biochemistry. *Prog Mol Biol Transl Sci.* 2015;134:169–201.

CHAPTER 11

Vitreous

Highlights

- The vitreous represents up to 80% of the volume of the eye.
- Vitreous liquefaction has been associated with loss of vitreous ascorbate and the development of posterior vitreous detachment.
- Pars plana vitrectomy increases the diffusion of oxygen in the posterior segment of the eye. The resultant increase in oxidative stress has been implicated in the acceleration of cataract formation after vitrectomy.

Overview

During formation of the eye, the *primary vitreous* contributes the hyaloid artery, which nourishes the developing anterior segment and lens. Failure of the vitreous to regress following this stage leads to pathology of the anterior and/or posterior segment. See BCSC Section 12, *Retina and Vitreous,* for further discussion of persistent fetal vasculature (also called *persistent hyperplastic primary vitreous*). The *secondary vitreous* consists of a gel matrix representing the largest structure of the eye and is routinely seen on clinical examination. The *tertiary vitreous* gives rise to the zonular fibers. See Chapter 4 for additional discussion of development of the vitreous.

In adulthood, the vitreous is less dynamic than during ocular development and acts as a conduit for nutrients and other solutes between the lens and the vitreous and for fluid to and across the retina (Fig 11-1). It occupies a volume of 4 mL and has an osmotic pressure and index of refraction (1.334) similar to those of the aqueous humor. Its viscosity, however, is almost twice that of water. The basic physical structure of the vitreous is that of a gel composed of a collagen framework interspersed with molecules of hydrated hyaluronan, also known as *hyaluronic acid.* The hyaluronan contributes to the viscosity of the vitreous humor and is thought to help stabilize the collagen network.

The relative amounts of collagen determine whether the vitreous is a liquid or a gel. The rigidity of the gel is greatest in regions of highest collagen concentration: the peripheral (cortical) vitreous and the vitreous base. The collagen fibrils confer resistance to tensile forces and give plasticity to the vitreous; the hyaluronan resists compression and confers viscoelastic properties. Degeneration of these fibrils occurs in most of the population and may lead to retinal pathology.

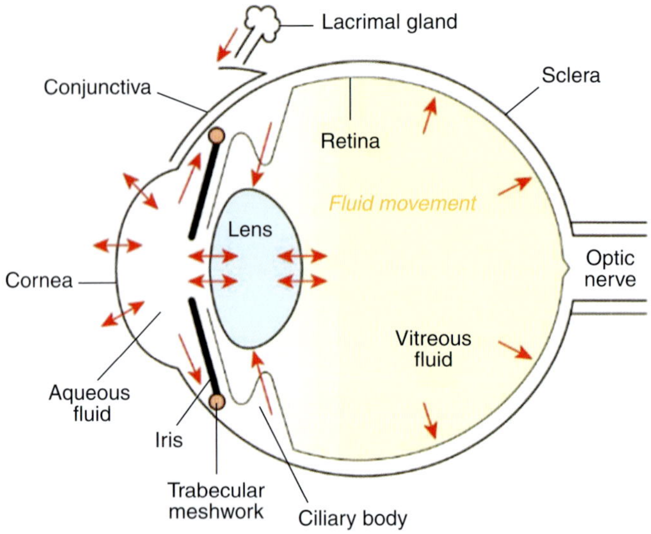

Figure 11-1 Fluid transport in the eye facilitated by aquaporin channels. The *red arrows* indicate exchange between the lens and the vitreous, as well as flow of fluid to and eventually across the retina, where this movement contributes to retinal adhesion. *(Reproduced with permission from Forrester JV, Dick AD, McMenamin PG, Roberts F, Pearlman E.* The Eye: Basic Sciences in Practice. *4th ed. St Louis: Saunders; 2016:233.)*

Composition

The vitreous is composed primarily of water (≈98%) and macromolecules (0.15%), including collagen, hyaluronan, and soluble proteins. There are very few resident cells in the vitreous; these are called *hyalocytes* (see Fig 11-4). In addition to the 2 major structural components, collagen and hyaluronan, several noncollagenous structural proteins and glycoproteins have been identified in the vitreous; these include chondroitin sulfate (versican), opticin, VIT1, and fibrillin. The human vitreous also contains hyaluronidase and at least 1 matrix metalloproteinase (MMP-2, or *gelatinase*), suggesting that turnover of vitreous structural macromolecules can occur.

Collagen

At present, 19 types of collagen are known, and the genes for several more have been identified. Tropocollagen, the smallest molecular unit of the various collagen types, is arranged in a specific pattern to create collagen fibrils. Aggregation of fibrils, sometimes of different types, gives rise to collagen fibers. Vitreous collagen fibers are composed of 3 different collagen types (Fig 11-2):

- Type II fibrils are the major structural component of the fiber and are also found in cartilage.
- Type IX fibrils, found on the surface of the fiber, act to shield type II collagen fibrils and prevent them from fusing together, which can lead to condensation of vitreous collagen.
- Type V/XI fibrils, located in the core of collagen fibers, likely participate in the initial stages of fiber formation.

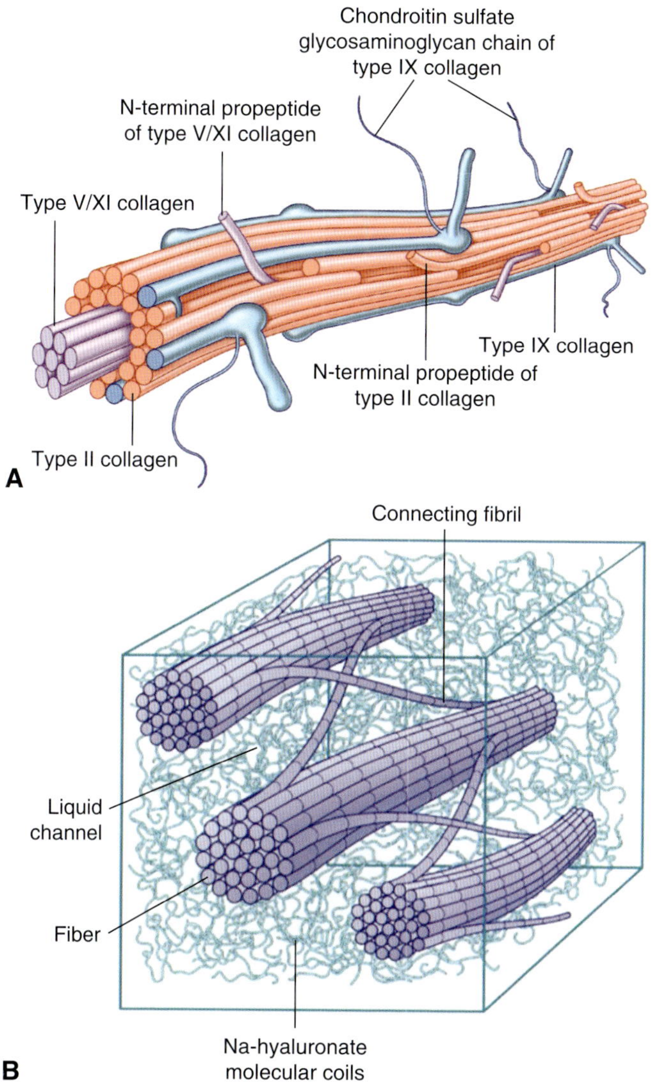

Figure 11-2 **A,** Model for the structure of a collagen fiber from the vitreous. Type II collagen *(red)* forms the major structure of the vitreous, accounting for three-quarters of the total vitreous collagen. Type IX collagen *(blue),* the second most common collagen found in the vitreous, lies on the surface of the fiber. Type IX collagen is proposed to protect type II collagen from degeneration. Type V/XI collagen *(purple)* is present in the core of the fibril and functions in fibrillogenesis. **B,** Vitreous collagen fibrils are organized into bundles surrounded by sodium hyaluronate. *(Part A modified with permission from Schachat AP, Wilkinson CP, Hinton DR, Sadda SR, Widemann P.* Ryan's Retina. *6th ed. Amsterdam: Elsevier; 2018:545. Part B reproduced with permission from Lund-Andersen H, Sander B. The vitreous. In: Levin LA, Nilsson SFE, Ver Hoeve J, Wu SM, eds.* Adler's Physiology of the Eye. *11th ed. St Louis: Saunders; 2011:167.)*

The vitreous collagens are closely related to the collagens of hyaline cartilage. They differ from the collagens (types I, III, XII, and XIV) commonly found in scar tissue and in tissues such as dermis, cornea, and sclera.

Collagen fibers are condensed in the peripheral vitreous, which comprises the cortical vitreous and has a thickness of approximately 100–300 µm. The vitreoretinal interface exists between the cortical vitreous and the internal limiting membrane (ILM). Interaction between the collagen fibers of the cortical vitreous (known as the *posterior hyaloid* over the posterior pole) and the ILM is mediated by laminin, fibronectin, and the proteoglycan chondroitin sulfate, among others (Fig 11-3). The adhesion of cortical vitreous to the ILM is relatively weak in the posterior pole compared with adhesion in the region near the vitreous base, where the fibers are firmly anchored to the peripheral retina and pars plana.

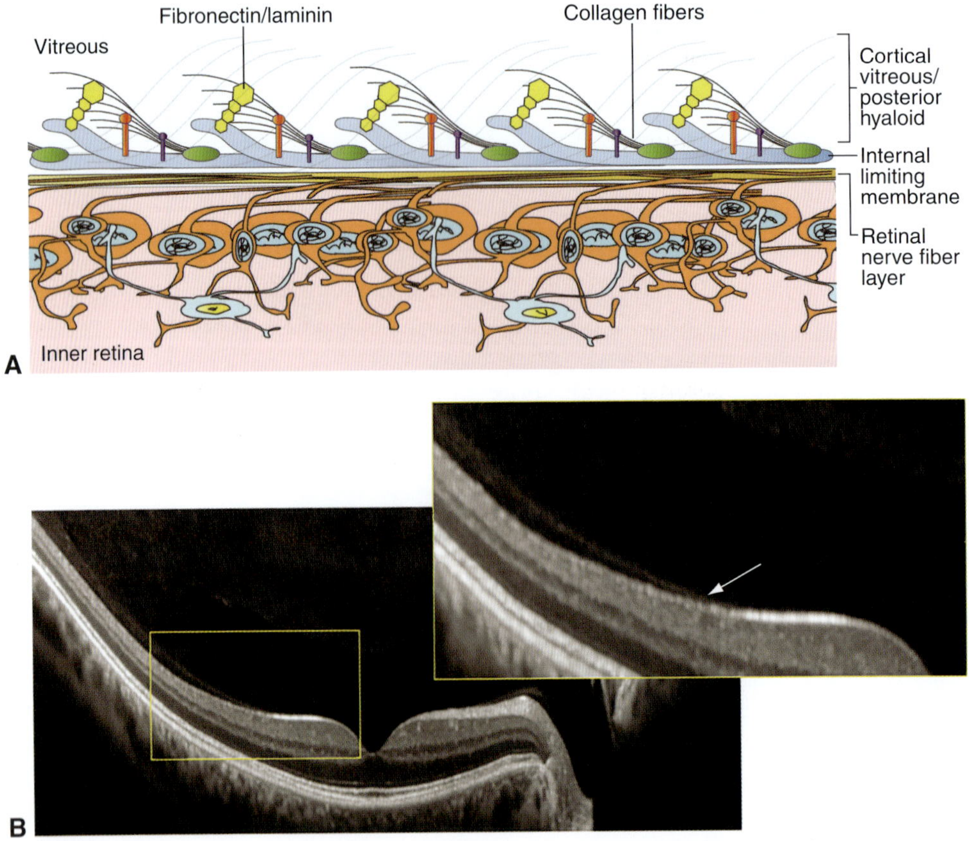

Figure 11-3 Vitreoretinal interface. **A,** Condensed collagen fibers in the peripheral vitreous form the cortical vitreous, which, over the posterior pole, is also known as the *posterior hyaloid.* The vitreoretinal interface lies between the collagen fibers of the posterior hyaloid and the internal limiting membrane (ILM). Interaction between the cortical collagen fibers and the ILM occurs via several macromolecules, including laminin and fibronectin. Pharmacologic cleavage of these connections facilitates posterior vitreous detachment. **B,** Optical coherence tomography scan of the vitreoretinal interface *(arrow).* *(Part A reproduced with permission from Barak Y, Ihnen MA, Schaal S. Spectral domain optical coherence tomography in the diagnosis and management of vitreoretinal interface pathologies.* J Ophthalmol. *2012;2012:876472. Part B courtesy of Vikram S. Brar, MD.)*

CLINICAL PEARL

While the posterior pole bolsters relatively weak vitreoretinal adhesion, the cortical vitreous maintains firmer attachment around the optic nerve. The collagen fiber anchors in this area are the last to separate as posterior vitreous detachment (PVD) occurs. A complete or partial ring within the posterior hyaloid is often visualized over the optic nerve as an indicator of PVD and creates a shadow on the retina, manifesting clinically as floaters.

Fichard A, Kleman JP, Ruggiero F. Another look at collagen V and XI molecules. *Matrix Biol.* 1995;14(7):515–531.

Le Goff MM, Bishop PN. Adult vitreous structure and postnatal changes. *Eye (Lond).* 2008; 22(10):1214–1222.

Russell SR, Shepherd JD, Hageman GS. Distribution of glycoconjugates in the human retinal internal limiting membrane. *Invest Ophthalmol Vis Sci.* 1991;32(7):1986–1995.

Hyaluronan and Chondroitin Sulfate

Hyaluronan is present in nearly all vertebrate connective tissues and is nontoxic and nonimmunogenic. It is a polysaccharide (glycosaminoglycan, or GAG) that has a repeating unit of glucuronic acid and *N*-acetylglucosamine. At physiologic pH, hyaluronan is a weak polyanion because of the ionization of the carboxyl groups present in each glucuronic acid residue. This ionization, together with the GAG residues, confers a negative charge on hyaluronan. The negative charge attracts sodium and thereby water, resulting in hydration of the vitreous. Production of hyaluronan begins around the time of birth, when the corresponding hydration has been proposed to contribute to vitreous transparency and growth of the eye.

In free solution, hyaluronan occupies an extremely high volume relative to its weight and may fill all the space in the vitreous except for that occupied by the collagen fibers (see Fig 11-2B). Hyaluronan molecules of the vitreous may undergo lateral interactions with one another, and such interactions may be stabilized by noncollagenous proteins. Both the concentration and the molecular weight of hyaluronan in the vitreous vary, depending on the species and on the location in the vitreous body, with higher concentrations typically found in the posterior pole.

Chondroitin sulfate is also a GAG, but unlike hyaluronan, it is sulfated. Chondroitin sulfate plays an independent role in maintaining the ultrastructure of the vitreous. Versican is the predominant form of chondroitin sulfate in the vitreous, where it interacts with hyaluronan. Versican has been reported to participate in the formation of the vitreous gel.

CLINICAL PEARL

Mutations in the *VCAN* gene, which encodes versican, have been implicated in Wagner syndrome. Affected patients have an optically empty vitreous with peripheral condensation and retinal degeneration (see also BCSC Section 12, *Retina and Vitreous*).

Kloeckener-Gruissem B, Bartholdi D, Abdou M-T, Zimmermann DR, Berger W. Identification of the genetic defect in the original Wagner syndrome family. *Mol Vis.* 2006;12:350–355.

Theocharis DA, Skandalis DA, Noulas AV, Papageorgakopoulou N, Theokaris AD, Karamanos NK. Hyaluronan and chondroitin sulfate proteoglycans in the supramolecular organization of the mammalian vitreous body. *Connect Tissue Res.* 2008;49(3):124–128.

Soluble and Collagen Fiber–Associated Proteins

Many proteins remain in solution after the collagen fibers and other insoluble elements present in the vitreous gel are removed by filtration or centrifugation. Serum albumin is the major soluble vitreous protein, followed by transferrin. Other proteins include neutrophil elastase inhibitor (which may play a role in resisting neovascularization) and tissue plasminogen activator (which may have a fibrinolytic role in the event of vitreous hemorrhage). The concentration of serum proteins in the vitreous gel depends on the integrity of the retinal vasculature and the degree of intraocular inflammation. Consequently, if the blood–ocular barrier is compromised, the concentration of soluble proteins within the vitreous cavity can rise dramatically.

Some structural proteins are specifically associated with the collagen fibers. These include a leucine-rich repeat glycoprotein called *opticin,* which is produced in the posterior nonpigmented ciliary epithelium (NPE), and another glycoprotein called *VIT1.* Both opticin and VIT1 are thought to play key roles in the structure of collagen fibers and to interact with proteoglycans within the vitreous.

Zonular Fibers

Some zonular fibers are present in the anterior vitreous and can be observed by electron microscopy. However, most of these fibers form the zonular apparatus, which is the structural connection between the lens and the ciliary body. The major structural protein of these fibers is a large linear protein named *fibrillin,* which has an unusually high cysteine content.

CLINICAL PEARL

Defects in fibrillin are present in patients with Marfan syndrome, some of whom experience spontaneous lens subluxation and premature vitreous liquefaction, which can lead to retinal detachment.

Low-Molecular-Weight Solutes

Ions and organic solutes in the vitreous originate from adjacent ocular tissues and blood plasma. The barriers that control their entry into the vitreous include the following:

- vascular endothelium of iris vessels
- nonpigmented epithelium of the ciliary body

- inner wall endothelium of the Schlemm canal
- vascular endothelium of retinal vessels
- retinal pigment epithelium (RPE)

Together, these structures constitute the blood–ocular barrier. The concentrations of sodium (Na^+) and chloride (Cl^-) in the vitreous are similar to those in plasma, but the concentration of potassium (K^+) is higher than that in plasma, as is that of ascorbate.

Bishop PN. Structural macromolecules and supramolecular organisation of the vitreous gel. *Prog Retin Eye Res.* 2000;19(3):323–344.

Mayne R, Brewton RG, Ren Z-X. Vitreous body and zonular apparatus. In: Harding JJ, ed. *Biochemistry of the Eye.* London: Chapman & Hall Medical; 1997:135–143.

Hyalocytes

Under normal physiologic conditions, the vitreous cavity has very few cells. The predominant cell type identified is the hyalocyte (Fig 11-4). The highest concentration of these cells occurs at the vitreous base and in the posterior cortical vitreous. Hyalocytes possess phagocytic properties, process antigens, and thereby regulate the immunologic response within the vitreous cavity. A process similar to anterior chamber–associated immune deviation (ACAID) occurs in the vitreous cavity (VCAID) and is likely mediated by hyalocytes.

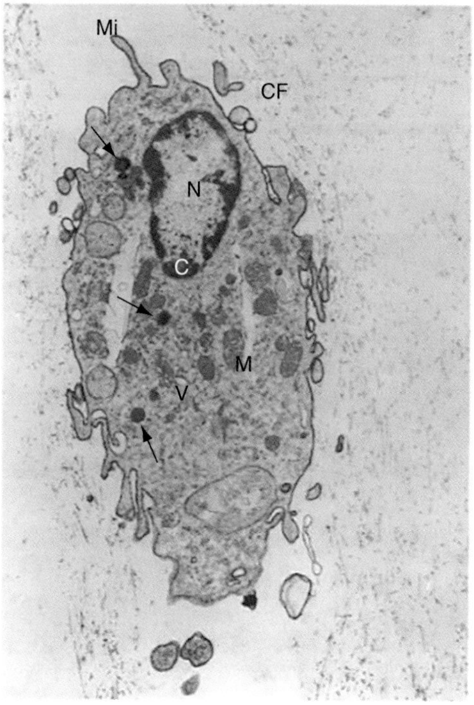

Figure 11-4 Hyalocyte within the cortical vitreous. *Arrows* indicate granules. C = chromatin; CF = collagen fibril; M = mitochondria; Mi = microvilli; N = nucleus; V = vacuoles. *(Modified with permission from Schachat AP, Wilkinson CP, Hinton DR, Sadda SR, Widemann P.* Ryan's Retina. *6th ed. Amsterdam: Elsevier; 2018:551.)*

CLINICAL PEARL

In specimens obtained after PVD, hyalocytes have been found on the surface of the retina, where they contribute to formation of idiopathic epiretinal membranes (also known as *macular pucker* or *cellophane maculopathy.*)

Sakamoto T, Ishibashi T. Hyalocytes: essential cells of the vitreous cavity in vitreoretinal pathophysiology? *Retina.* 2011;31(2):222–228.

Biochemical Changes With Aging and Disease

Vitreous Liquefaction and Posterior Vitreous Detachment

The human vitreous gel undergoes progressive liquefaction beginning around 40 years of age, so that typically by age 80–90 years, more than half of the vitreous is liquid. A crucial step in the process of vitreous liquefaction is the breakdown of the thin (12–15-nm) collagen fibrils into smaller fragments. Implicated in this process is reduced shielding of type II collagen fibrils due to the age-related exponential loss of type IX collagen. Some proteolytic enzymes, such as plasminogen, may have elevated vitreous concentrations with increasing age, but others, such as MMP-2 (matrix metalloproteinase-2), do not.

The fragments aggregate into thicker fibers, or *fibrillar opacities,* which are visible with low-power slit-lamp microscopy. As liquefaction proceeds, the collagen fibers become condensed into the residual gel phase and are absent from (or in low concentration in) the liquid phase. In terms of hyaluronan concentration or molecular weight, there are no differences between the gel and liquid phases. With increasing age, a weakening of adhesion occurs at the vitreoretinal interface, which lies between the cortical vitreous gel and the ILM. These combined processes eventually result in posterior vitreous detachment (PVD) in approximately 50% of individuals after 50 years of age.

PVD is a separation of the cortical vitreous gel from the ILM as far anteriorly as the posterior border of the vitreous base; the separation does not extend into the vitreous base owing to the unbreakable adhesion between the vitreous and retina in that zone (Fig 11-5). PVD is often a sudden event, during which liquefied vitreous from the center of the vitreous body passes through a hole in the posterior vitreous cortex, at its attachment to the optic nerve, and then dissects the residual cortical vitreous away from the ILM. As the residual vitreous gel collapses anteriorly within the vitreous cavity, retinal tears sometimes occur in areas where the retina is more strongly attached to the vitreous than the surrounding retina can withstand, which subsequently can result in rhegmatogenous retinal detachment. Anomalous PVD can lead to the formation of epiretinal membranes and macular holes (see BCSC Section 12, *Retina and Vitreous*).

Bishop PN, Holmes DF, Kadler KE, McLeod D, Bos KJ. Age-related changes on the surface of vitreous collagen fibrils. *Invest Ophthalmol Vis Sci.* 2004;45(4):1041–1046.

Fincham GS, James S, Spickett C, et al. Posterior vitreous detachment and the posterior hyaloid membrane. *Ophthalmology.* 2018;125(2):227–236.

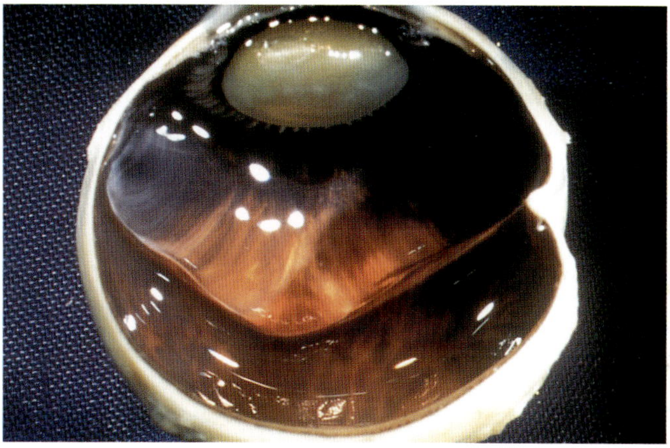

Figure 11-5 Posterior vitreous detachment (PVD). Gross photograph of an eye with PVD. The vitreous gel remains anchored anteriorly at the vitreous base, having separated from the posterior pole. *(Courtesy of Hans E. Grossniklaus, MD.)*

Myopia

Myopia is associated with faster liquefaction and earlier development of PVD. Vitreous samples taken from myopic eyes exhibit a higher concentration of MMP-2. MMPs are proteases involved in remodeling extracellular matrices, such as the vitreous. Physiologically, MMPs can facilitate cell differentiation, proliferation, and migration. Pathologically, they participate in inflammatory responses and promote angiogenesis. Premature vitreous liquefaction may be a result of increased MMP activity, leading to vitreoretinal pathologies in myopic individuals.

Zhuang H, Zhang R, Shu Q, et al. Changes of TGF-β2, MMP-2, and TIMP-2 levels in the vitreous of patients with high myopia. *Graefes Arch Clin Exp Ophthalmol.* 2014; 252(11):1763–1767.

Vitreous as an Inhibitor of Angiogenesis

Numerous studies have shown that the normal vitreous is an inhibitor of angiogenesis. This inhibitory activity is decreased in proliferative diabetic retinopathy. However, the molecular basis of the phenomenon remains poorly understood. Known inhibitors of angiogenesis, such as thrombospondin 1 and pigment epithelium–derived factor, are present within the mammalian vitreous and may inhibit angiogenesis in healthy eyes. The vitreous protein opticin also suppresses angiogenesis in mouse models of retinal neovascularization. In contrast, the level of vascular endothelial growth factor (VEGF), a promoter of angiogenesis, is markedly elevated in the vitreous of patients with proliferative diabetic retinopathy, a condition in which the vitreous also acts as a scaffold for retinal neovascularization.

Le Goff MM, Lu H, Ugarte M, et al. The vitreous glycoprotein opticin inhibits preretinal neovascularization. *Invest Ophthalmol Vis Sci.* 2012;53(1):228–234.

Physiologic Changes After Vitrectomy

Most of the changes in ocular physiology that occur after vitrectomy result from altered viscosity in the vitreous cavity; when the vitreous is removed, the viscosity decreases between 300- and 2000-fold. Consequently, growth factors and other compounds, such as antibiotics, transfer between the posterior and anterior segments more easily and are also cleared more quickly from the eye. This effect is proportional to the change in diffusion coefficient, which is of the same magnitude as the change in viscosity.

Fluid currents that move solutes even more rapidly may be present (see Fig 11-1). In particular, oxygen movement is accelerated. The oxygen gradient that exists between the well-oxygenated anterior segment and the posterior segment under normal physiologic conditions is abolished. This leads to increased oxygen tension in the vitreous cavity. Under physiologic conditions, vitreous ascorbate combines with oxygen, forming dehydroascorbate and water. However, after vitrectomy, oxygen levels exceed the capacity of ascorbate, leading to increased oxidative stress at the posterior pole of the lens and the development of cataract (Fig 11-6).

Holekamp NM, Shui YB, Beebe DC. Vitrectomy surgery increases oxygen exposure to the lens: a possible mechanism for nuclear cataract formation. *Am J Ophthalmol.* 2005;139(2):302–310.

Shui YB, Holekamp NM, Kramer BC, et al. The gel state of the vitreous and ascorbate-dependent oxygen consumption: relationship to the etiology of nuclear cataracts. *Arch Ophthalmol.* 2009;127(4):475–482.

Injury With Hemorrhage and Inflammation

Injury to the eye can result in inflammation and, in many cases, intraocular hemorrhage. If blood penetrates the vitreous cortex, platelets come into contact with vitreous collagen, aggregate, and initiate clot formation. The clot in turn stimulates a phagocytic inflammatory reaction, and the vitreous becomes liquefied in the area of a hemorrhage. The subsequent inflammatory reaction varies in degree for unknown reasons and may result in proliferative vitreoretinopathy (see also BCSC Section 12, *Retina and Vitreous*).

Streeten BAW, Wilson DJ. Disorders of the vitreous. In: Garner A, Klintworth GK, eds. *Pathobiology of Ocular Disease: A Dynamic Approach.* 2nd ed. 2 vols. New York: M. Dekker; 1994:701–742.

Genetic Disease Involving the Vitreous

Stickler syndrome is most commonly due to a mutation in the gene *COL2A1,* which codes for type II collagen, a major component of vitreous collagen fibers. Affected patients have an optically empty vitreous due to premature liquefaction with peripheral condensation, which may induce retinal detachment (see also BCSC Section 12, *Retina and Vitreous*). Mutations in both the α_1(II) and α_1(XI) collagen chains have been shown to be responsible for this syndrome.

Wagner syndrome is another condition in which patients present with an optically empty vitreous and have an increased risk of retinal detachment. As mentioned earlier in

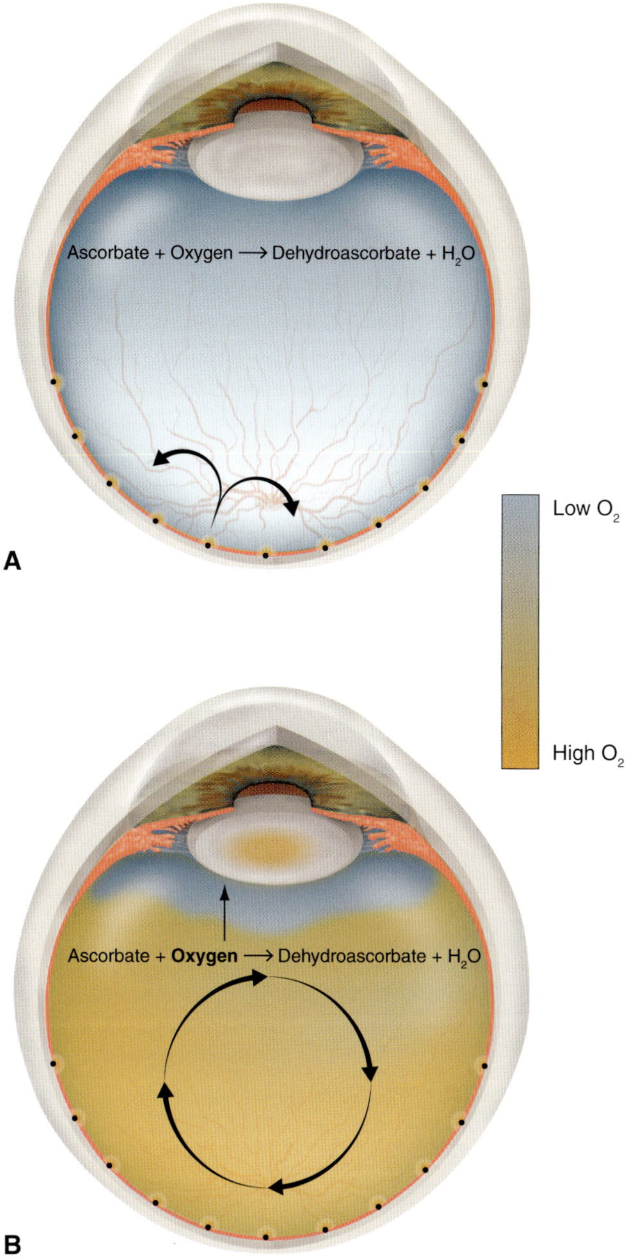

Figure 11-6 The role of ascorbate in the vitreous cavity. **A,** The vitreous acts as a barrier to the diffusion of oxygen within the posterior segment. The available ascorbate binds with oxygen, forming dehydroascorbate, which is taken up by surrounding cells. **B,** In postvitrectomized eyes, the amount of oxygen exceeds the capacity for clearance, leading to the production of reactive compounds that create oxidative stress in the lens, which in turn accelerates cataract formation. *(Illustration by Cyndie C.H. Wooley.)*

this chapter, these patients have mutations in the *VCAN* gene, encoding versican, which participates in formation of the vitreous gel.

Robin NH, Moran RT, Ala-Kokko L. *Stickler Syndrome.* GeneReviews [Internet]. Seattle, WA: University of Washington, Seattle; 1993–2019.

Enzymatic Vitreolysis

Considerable interest exists in enzyme preparations that can be injected into the vitreous cavity to aid in clearing blood from the vitreous and inducing PVD. Enzymes that have been proposed for injection include hyaluronidase, plasmin, dispase, and chondroitinase. Clinical trials with hyaluronidase and collagenase failed to induce PVD. However, ocriplasmin, which cleaves fibronectin and laminin (see Fig 11-3), was better able to induce PVD than placebo and demonstrated efficacy in nonsurgical management of vitreomacular traction and macular holes. Subsequently, there have been reports describing retinal changes on optical coherence tomography and altered electroretinogram following administration of ocriplasmin.

Fahim AT, Khan NW, Johnson MW. Acute panretinal structural and functional abnormalities after intravitreous ocriplasmin injection. *JAMA Ophthalmol.* 2014;132(4):484–486.

Gandorfer A. Enzymatic vitreous disruption. *Eye (Lond).* 2008;22(10):1273–1277.

Stalmans P, Benz MS, Gandorfer A, et al. Enzymatic vitreolysis with ocriplasmin for vitreomacular traction and macular holes. *N Engl J Med.* 2012;367(7):606–615.

Tibbetts MD, Reichel E, Witkin AJ. Vision loss after intravitreal ocriplasmin: correlation of spectral-domain optical coherence tomography and electroretinography. *JAMA Ophthalmol.* 2014;132(4):487–490.

CHAPTER 12

Retina

Highlights

- The retina has the highest rate of oxygen consumption of any tissue in the human body because of its high metabolic activity.
- Retinal neurons (photoreceptor, bipolar, horizontal, amacrine, and ganglion cells), glial cells (Müller cells, astrocytes, and microglia), and vascular cells (endothelial cells and pericytes) together form a functional neurovascular unit that converts light into a neural signal.
- Light induces hyperpolarization, leading to a cascade of reactions in the photoreceptor outer segments called *phototransduction,* which converts light energy into an electrical impulse.
- Rods are highly sensitive and can be stimulated by a single photon, whereas cone photoreceptors can adapt to a wider range of light intensities.
- Gene mutations affecting components of the phototransduction pathway lead to inherited retinal dystrophies with varying clinical phenotypes.

Overview

Two laminar structures line the back of the eye: the retinal pigment epithelium (RPE) and the neural retina. This chapter discusses the neurosensory retina; the RPE is discussed in Chapter 13. These laminar structures arise from an invagination of the embryonic optic cup that folds the neuroectodermal layer into apex-to-apex contact with itself, creating the subretinal space (Fig 12-1). The 2 layers form a hemispheric shell on which the visual image is focused by the anterior segment of the eye. The retina is composed of neural, glial, and vascular components.

The neural retina contains multiple types of cells (see also Chapter 2):

- photoreceptors (rods and 3 types of cones)
- bipolar cells (rod on-bipolar cells and cone on- and off-bipolar cells)
- interneurons (horizontal and amacrine cells)
- ganglion cells and their axons, which form the retinal nerve fiber layer and the optic nerve
- glial cells, including astrocytes, Müller cells, and microglia

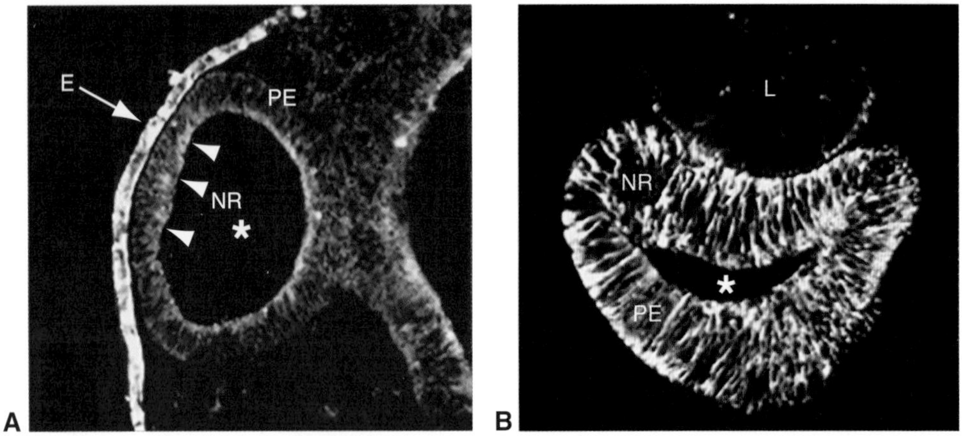

Figure 12-1 Development of the retina and the retinal pigment epithelium. **A,** Apposition of the surface ectoderm (E) with the inner wall of the optic cup *(arrowheads);* the neural retina (NR) is separated from the outer wall and the pigment epithelium (PE) by the subretinal space *(*)*. **B,** Further invagination of the optic cup with induction of the overlying lens (L) by the NR. The intervening subretinal space separates the NR from the PE. *(Modified with permission from Ryan SJ, Ogden TE, Hinton DR, Schachat AP, Wilkinson CP.* Retina. *3rd ed. St Louis: Mosby; 2001:5.)*

Photoreceptors and Phototransduction

Phototransduction is the process by which photosensitive cells in the retina convert light energy into an electrical impulse that is transmitted to the brain. Rods and cones are highly polarized photoreceptor cells that capture energy from photons and generate a neural response. Rods are highly sensitive and can be stimulated by a single photon. Cones are less sensitive than rods, but they can adapt to a wider range of light intensities and respond more rapidly to repetitive stimulation.

Rod Phototransduction

Most of our knowledge of phototransduction comes from information known about rods, which are sensitive nocturnal light detectors. Considerably more biochemical material can be obtained from rods than from cones because rods are much more numerous in most retinas. In addition, rods contain far more membrane (ie, surface area) than do cones, which contributes to the rods' greater sensitivity.

The outer segment of photoreceptors contains all the components required for phototransduction. It is composed primarily of plasma-membrane material organized into discs flattened perpendicular to the long axis of the outer segment (see Chapter 2, Fig 2-33). There are approximately 1000 discs within a rod outer segment and 1 million membrane-bound rhodopsin molecules in each disc. The discs float within the cytoplasm of the outer segment like a stack of coins disconnected from the plasma membrane. The discs contain the protein machinery to capture and amplify light energy. This abundance of outer-segment membrane increases the number of rhodopsin molecules, which can absorb light. Some deep-sea fish, which need considerable sensitivity to detect small amounts of light, rely on longer rod segments than those found in humans.

Rhodopsin is a freely diffusible membrane protein with 7 helical loops that is embedded in the lipid membrane (Fig 12-2). Rhodopsin absorbs green light best at wavelengths of approximately 510 nm. It absorbs blue and yellow light less well and is insensitive to longer wavelengths (red light). Rhodopsin is tuned to this part of the electromagnetic spectrum by its amino-acid sequence and by the binding of its chromophore 11-*cis*-retinal (also called 11-*cis*-retinaldehyde), which creates a molecular antenna.

The plasma membrane of the outer segment contains the cationic cyclic nucleotide–gated (CNG) channels, which are gated by cyclic guanosine monophosphate (cGMP). This channel controls the flow of sodium (Na^+) and calcium (Ca^{2+}) ions into the outer segment. In the dark, Na^+ and Ca^{2+} flow in through the channel, which is kept open by cGMP. Ionic balance is maintained by Na^+,K^+-ATPase (also called *sodium-potassium pump*) in the inner segment and a Na^+,K^+-Ca^{2+} exchanger in the outer-segment membrane, both of which

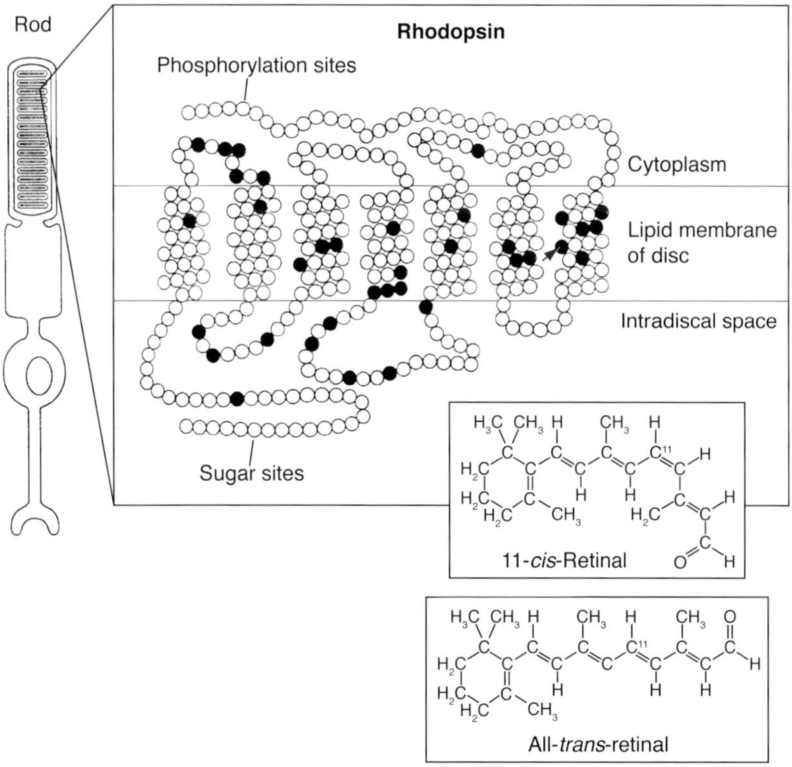

Figure 12-2 The rhodopsin molecule is embedded in the lipid membrane of the outer segment with 7 helical loops. Each circle represents an amino acid, and the highly conserved ones are shown in *black*. The *red arrow* represents the lysine to which the vitamin A chromophore is linked. Phosphorylation sites occur on the cytoplasmic and sugar attachment sites on the intradiscal (extracellular) ends of the rhodopsin molecule. Insets show the structures of 11-*cis*-retinal and all-*trans*-retinal. *(Courtesy of Peter Gouras, MD.)*

require metabolic energy. This flow of ions sets up the circulating dark current that keeps the photoreceptor's membrane potential in a relatively depolarized state. The depolarized state of the photoreceptors causes a steady release of the transmitter glutamate from its synaptic terminal in the dark (Fig 12-3).

Light activation of rhodopsin starts a series of reactions that lead to hyperpolarization of the photoreceptor's membrane potential (Fig 12-4). Once rhodopsin absorbs a quantum of light, the 11-*cis* double bond of retinal is reconfigured (creating all-*trans*-retinal, also called all-*trans*-retinaldehyde), and the opsin molecule undergoes a series of rapid configurational changes to an activated state known as *metarhodopsin II.* Light-activated rhodopsin triggers a second molecule, transducin, by causing an exchange of guanosine diphosphate (GDP) for guanosine triphosphate (GTP) (see Fig 12-4A). One rhodopsin molecule can activate 100 transducin molecules, amplifying the reaction. Activated transducin excites a third protein, cGMP phosphodiesterase (PDE), which hydrolyzes cGMP to 5′-noncyclic GMP. The decrease in cGMP closes the CNG channels, which stops entry of Na^+ and Ca^{2+} and hyperpolarizes the rod. Hyperpolarization stops the release of glutamate from the synaptic terminal.

When the light is extinguished, the rod returns to its dark state as the reaction cascade turns off. Recovery of the dark current requires that the catalytically active components of the phototransduction cascade be fully quenched and cGMP resynthesized to allow opening of the CNG channels. Rhodopsin is inactivated by phosphorylation at its C-terminal end by rhodopsin kinase and subsequent binding to arrestin (see Fig 12-4B). Inactivation of rhodopsin is aided by recoverin, a highly conserved Ca^{2+}-binding protein found in both rods and cones. Transducin is inactivated by the hydrolysis of GTP to GDP via transducin's intrinsic GTPase activity, which reduces PDE activity. Closure of the CNG channels with light activation also causes a drop in intracellular Ca^{2+} levels, which in turn stimulates retinal guanylate cyclase (also called *guanylyl cyclase*), the enzyme that synthesizes cGMP from GTP; the enzyme's action is assisted by guanylate cyclase–assisting proteins (see Fig 12-4C). As cGMP levels increase, the CNG channels open and the rod is depolarized again. The corresponding rise in intracellular Ca^{2+} levels inhibits retinal guanylate cyclase activity to its dark level.

"Rim" proteins

The discs of rod outer segments differ from those of cones in that they are disconnected from the outer plasma membrane. The rim of each rod disc has a collection of proteins. Two such proteins are peripherin and rod outer segment protein 1 (ROM1), which play a role in the development and maintenance of the disc's curvature. Peripherin and ROM1 are also found in cone outer segments. Another protein in rod discs is ABCA4, an ATP-binding cassette (ABC) transporter. It is a transmembrane protein involved in the energy-dependent transport of substrates from the disc lumen to the rod cytosol. ABCA4 is unique to rod discs and is not found in cones. It functions as a transporter of all-*trans*-retinal.

Tsybovsky Y, Molday RS, Palczewski K. The ATP-binding cassette transporter ABCA4: structural and functional properties and role in retinal disease. *Adv Exp Med Biol.* 2010; 703:105–125.

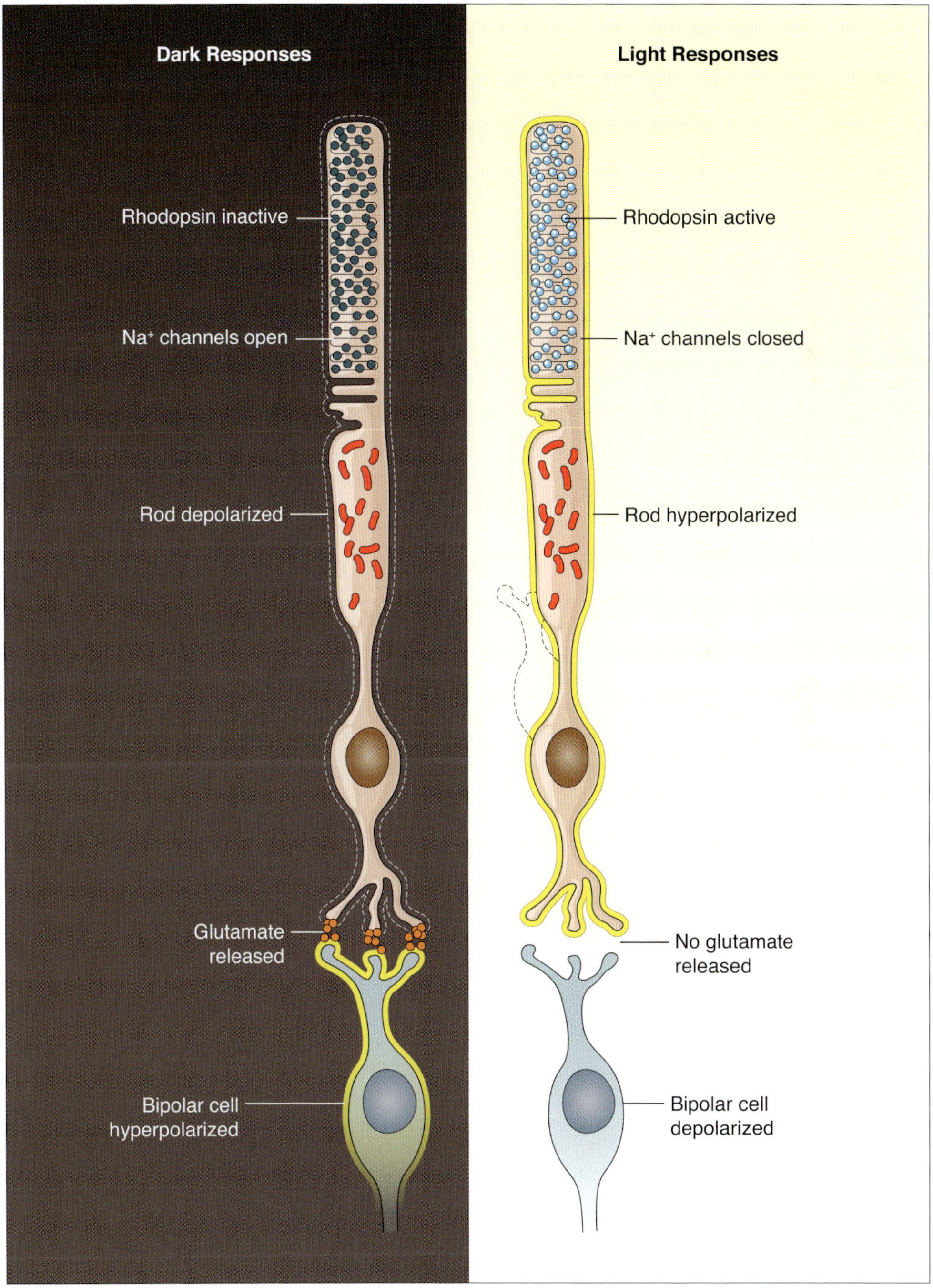

Figure 12-3 Dark current and light response. *(Left)* In the dark, rhodopsin is inactive; the cyclic nucleotide–gated (CNG) channels in the outer segment are open; and the rod is depolarized with a steady release of glutamate from its axonal terminal. *(Right)* Rhodopsin is activated by light, which leads to closing of the CNG channels, rod membrane hyperpolarization, and inhibition of glutamate release from the axon terminal. *(Illustration by Mark Miller.)*

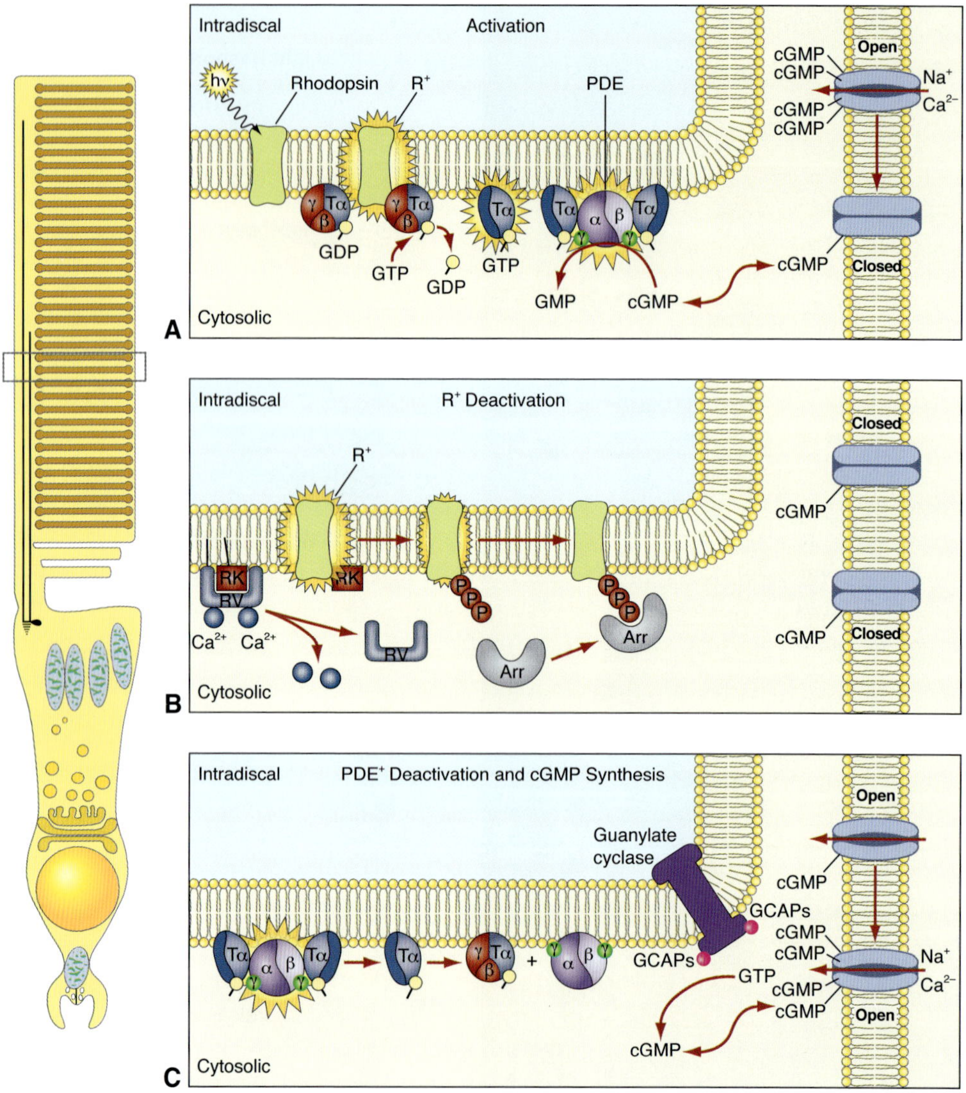

Figure 12-4 Schematic representation of the phototransduction cascade in photoreceptor outer segments. **A,** Light-activated rhodopsin (R^+) causes levels of cGMP to be reduced via transducin-disinhibited phosphodiesterase (PDE), leading to closure of cGMP voltage–gated channels (CNG) and subsequent hyperpolarization of the photoreceptor cell. **B,** R^+ is deactivated through phosphorylation (indicated by Ps) and the binding of the protein arrestin (Arr). Phosphorylation is mediated by rhodopsin kinase (RK), which is regulated by recoverin (RV). RV dissociates from RK as calcium levels decrease following closure of cGMP voltage–gated channels. Arrestin binds to phosphorylated R^+, completing the process. **C,** cGMP levels are restored through deactivation of transducin (T) via its intrinsic GTPase activity. PDE activity then decreases and guanylate cyclase activity increases, allowing cGMP levels to rise and opening the voltage-gated channels. cGMP = cyclic guanine monophosphate; GCAP = guanylate cyclase–activating protein; GDP = guanosine diphosphate; GTP = guanosine triphosphate; $T\alpha$, $T\beta$, $T\gamma$ = subunits of transducin. *(Redrawn from Ryan SJ, Schachat AP, Wilkinson CP, Hinton DR, Sadda SR, Wiedemann P.* Retina. *5th ed. London: Saunders/Elsevier; 2013:Fig 14-4.)*

Energy Metabolism of Photoreceptor Outer Segments

Adenosine triphosphate (ATP) is necessary to drive the reactions that control the ionic current generators as well as the transporters in the outer segment. Because only the inner, and not the outer, segment contains mitochondria, oxidative metabolism is confined to the former. The outer segment is responsible for glycolysis, including the hexose monophosphate pathway and the phosphocreatine shuttle, which produces ATP and GTP and modulates nicotinamide adenine dinucleotide phosphate (NADPH). NADPH reduces retinal to retinol before it is returned to the RPE for isomerization, and it reduces glutathione, which protects against oxidative stress.

Cone Phototransduction

Qualitatively, the phototransduction of cones resembles that of rods. Light-activated cone opsins initiate an enzymatic cascade that hydrolyzes cGMP and closes cone-specific cGMP–gated cationic channels on the outer-segment membrane. Cone phototransduction is comparatively insensitive but fast and capable of adapting significantly to ambient levels of illumination. The greater the ambient light level is, the faster and more temporally accurate is the response of a cone. Speed and temporal fidelity are important for all aspects of cone vision. This is one reason visual acuity improves progressively with increased illumination. Because of their ability to adapt, cones are indispensable to good vision. A person without cones loses the ability to read and see colors and can be legally blind. In comparison, lost rod function is a less severe visual problem, except under scotopic conditions.

Several factors contribute to light adaptation. For example, higher levels of illumination bleach away photopigments, making the outer segment less sensitive to light. As light levels increase, so does the noise level, which reduces sensitivity. Biochemical and neural feedback speed up the cone response. This feedback must be increased as light intensity increases and the cone absorbs more and more light. All the processes that turn off the rod response are probably stronger in cones.

Cones also show neurally mediated negative feedback. Horizontal cells of the inner nuclear layer synapse antagonistically back onto cones, releasing γ-aminobutyric acid (GABA), an inhibitory neurotransmitter. When light hyperpolarizes a cone, the cone hyperpolarizes neighboring horizontal cells. This effect inhibits the horizontal cells, stopping the release of GABA, which depolarizes (disinhibits) the cone by a recurrent synapse. This depolarization antagonizes the hyperpolarization produced by light and restores the cone to its resting state. Depolarization occurs with a synaptic delay so that its main effect is on the later response of the cone. Horizontal-cell feedback occurs with strong stimuli, preventing the cone from being overloaded. The feedback also turns off the cone response more quickly, enabling the cone to respond rapidly to a new stimulus. *Flicker fusion threshold* is the frequency of a repetitive stimulus at which it appears to be a completely steady light stimulus. This threshold is much higher in cones (approximately 100 Hz) than in rods (approximately 30 Hz).

Trivariant color vision

To see colors, mammals must have at least 2 different spectral classes of cones. Most humans with normal vision have 3 types of cones and consequently a 3-variable color vision (3 cone opsins) system:

- short-wavelength-sensitive cones (termed *S cones*), which detect only color by comparing their signals with those of the M cones; this mechanism creates blue-yellow color vision
- middle-wavelength-sensitive cones (termed *M cones*), which detect high-resolution achromatic (black and white) contrast
- long-wavelength-sensitive cones (termed *L cones*), which evolved in primates to enhance color vision; this mechanism creates red-green color vision

Both L and M cones contribute to achromatic and chromatic contrast. Therefore, both are more numerous than S cones in the human retina.

Most color vision defects involve red-green discrimination and the genes coding for the L- and M-cone opsins. These genes are in tandem on the X chromosome. There is 1 copy of the L-cone opsin gene at the centromeric end of the X chromosome, and there are 1–6 copies of the M-cone gene arranged in a head-to-tail tandem array. Normally, only the most proximal of these 2 genes is expressed. Most color vision abnormalities are caused by unequal crossing over between the L- and M-cone opsin genes. This inequality creates hybrid opsins that have different spectral absorption functions, which are usually less ideal than those of normal opsins. Some males have a serine-to-alanine substitution at amino acid 108 on the cone opsin gene, which allows more sensitivity to red light. Potentially, females with both the serine-containing and the alanine-containing opsins could have tetravariant color vision.

Photoreceptor Gene Defects Causing Retinal Degeneration

Gene mutations involving the phototransduction pathway lead to inherited retinal dystrophies with varying degrees of visual impairment. These mutations can disrupt physiology in different ways; they can alter the transduction cascade, protein folding, or localization of the affected protein. Retinitis pigmentosa (RP), Leber congenital amaurosis (LCA), and Stargardt disease are among the most prevalent inherited retinal dystrophies. Autosomal dominant RP (ADRP) can be caused by more than 100 different mutations in the rhodopsin gene *(RHO)*. The most common *RHO* mutation is P23H (responsible for 10% of RP cases in the United States), which causes the rhodopsin protein not to fold properly and instead to accumulate in the rough endoplasmic reticulum. Generally, *RHO* mutations affecting the intradiscal area and amino-terminal end of rhodopsin result in less severe defects than do mutations affecting the cytoplasmic region and the carboxyl tail. Alterations in the middle of the gene, coding for the transmembrane regions of rhodopsin, result in moderately severe defects. Relatively uncommon mutations have been reported in the rhodopsin gene that cause autosomal recessive RP (ARRP) and a stationary form of nyctalopia. See Tables 12-1 through 12-4 for other gene mutations that cause inherited retinal dystrophies.

Molday RS. Photoreceptor membrane proteins, phototransduction, and retinal degenerative diseases. Friedenwald Lecture. *Invest Ophthalmol Vis Sci.* 1998;39(13):2491–2513.

Table 12-1 Rod-Specific Gene Defects

Protein(s) Affected	Corresponding Retinal Disease
Rod transducin	A dominant mutation in the *GNAT1* gene causes congenital stationary night blindness, Nougaret type, the oldest-known form of AD stationary nyctalopia. Transducin becomes continuously activated, an example of constitutively active rods that do not degenerate.
Rod cGMP phosphodiesterase	Defects in either the α-subunit (PDEA) or β-subunit (PDEB) of cGMP phosphodiesterase (rod PDE) cause ARRP. These are nonsense mutations that truncate the catalytic domain of the protein. An H258D mutation in PDEB also causes dominant stationary nyctalopia.
Rod cGMP–gated channel	Null mutations of the rod cGMP–gated channel β-subunit cause ARRP.
Arrestin, rhodopsin kinase	A mutation either in the gene *SAG* (2q37), which encodes arrestin, or in *GRK1* (13q34), which encodes rhodopsin kinase, causes Oguchi disease, a form of stationary nyctalopia.
Guanylate cyclase	Null mutations of the guanylate cyclase gene cause LCA, a childhood AR form of RP. LCA shows genetic heterogeneity.
Rod ABC transporter	Mutations in the *ABCA4* gene cause recessive defects of ABC transporter proteins, which cause Stargardt disease.

ABC = adenosine triphosphate–binding cassette; AD = autosomal dominant; AR = autosomal recessive; ARRP = autosomal recessive retinitis pigmentosa; cGMP = cyclic guanosine monophosphate; LCA = Leber congenital amaurosis; RP = retinitis pigmentosa.

Table 12-2 Cone- and Rod-Specific Gene Defects

Protein Affected	Corresponding Retinal Disease or Condition
Peripherin/RDS	There is substantial allelic heterogeneity in the peripherin/RDS gene *(PRPH2)*. Defects cause several dominantly inherited retinal degenerations that range from ADRP to macular degeneration, pattern macular dystrophy, vitelliform macular dystrophy, butterfly macular dystrophy, and fundus flavimaculatus.
Rod outer segment protein 1	Double-heterozygotic mutations in both the *ROM1* and the peripherin genes cause digenic RP. A *ROM1* gene defect alone has been reported in a patient with vitelliform macular dystrophy.
Myosin VIIA	Myosin VIIA is a protein found in cochlear hair cells and in the cilium connecting the rod inner and outer segments. A heterozygous null mutation in a form of myosin VIIA causes Usher syndrome type 1. Affected patients have early and profound deafness, vestibular areflexia at birth, and ARRP.

ADRP = autosomal dominant retinitis pigmentosa; *PRPH2* = peripherin 2.

Table 12-3 Cone-Specific Gene Defects

Protein Affected	Corresponding Retinal Disease
Cone cGMP–gated channel	A homozygous defect in the cone cGMP–gated channel α-subunit causes achromatopsia, loss of all cone function.
L- and M-cone opsins	Mutations in the genes coding for L- and M-cone opsins cause defects that lead to S-cone (or blue-cone) monochromatism. These defects occur only in males because of the gene's location on the X chromosome. Defects in all 3 cone opsins lead to achromatopsia, also known as *rod monochromatism.*
L- or M-cone opsins	Defects in one or the other of the X-linked L- or M-cone opsin genes cause red-green color deficiencies, almost exclusively in males.

cGMP = cyclic guanosine monophosphate; L cone = long-wavelength-sensitive cone; M = middle-wavelength-sensitive cone.

Table 12-4 Ubiquitously Expressed Genes Causing Retinal Degeneration

Protein Affected	Corresponding Retinal Disease
Rab escort protein 1	Mutations in *CHM,* the gene encoding Rab escort protein 1 (REP-1), cause choroideremia, an X-linked disease. The protein is involved in prenylating Rab proteins, a process that facilitates their binding to cytoplasmic membranes and promoting vesicle fusion. Photoreceptors, the RPE, and/or the choroid must be uniquely vulnerable for this process to occur.
Ornithine aminotransferase	Homozygous mutations in the ornithine aminotransferase gene *(OAT)* cause gyrate atrophy. Ornithine aminotransferase enzyme breaks down ornithine, which, in high concentrations, seems to be toxic to the RPE.
Microsomal triglyceride transfer protein	Homozygous defects in microsomal triglyceride transfer protein *(MTTP)* cause abetalipoproteinemia, or Bassen–Kornzweig syndrome, characterized by ARRP and an inability to absorb fat. The condition is treatable with fat-soluble vitamins.
Peroxin	Homozygous defects in *PEX1* cause infantile Refsum disease, with RP, cerebellar ataxia, polyneuropathy, anosmia, hearing loss, and cardiomyopathy. Infantile Refsum disease represents the least-severe disease in a spectrum of familial disorders involving mutations in the *PEX* genes, which code for peroxins, proteins necessary for peroxisome biogenesis.
Phytanoyl-CoA hydroxylase	Homozygous defects in *PHYH,* the gene encoding phytanoyl-CoA hydroxylase, cause Refsum disease, characterized by RP, cerebellar ataxia, and peripheral polyneuropathy. The enzyme, located in peroxisomes, degrades phytanic acid. Elevated levels of phytanic acid are toxic to the RPE. Patients with Refsum disease may be treated with a phytanic acid–restricted diet.

Classes of Retinal Cells

The retina contains 3 broad classes of cells (Fig 12-5):

- neurons (photoreceptor, bipolar, horizontal, amacrine, and ganglion cells)
- glial cells (Müller cells, astrocytes, microglia)
- vascular cells (endothelial cells and pericytes)

The major route of information flow from photoreceptors to the optic nerve consists of a 3-neuron chain—photoreceptor cell to bipolar cell to ganglion cell. Horizontal cells and amacrine cells are interneurons that regulate the flow of information. Glial cells and vascular elements support the neuronal components.

Neurons

Bipolar cells

Retinal bipolar cells receive neural signals from photoreceptors (discussed earlier in the chapter) and convey them to the inner retina. Separate bipolar cells exist for cones and rods. Morphologically, there are 9–12 different kinds of cone bipolar cells but only 1 type of rod bipolar cell. Functionally, in the cone pathway there are *on-bipolar* and *off-bipolar* cells (Fig 12-6). On-bipolar cells are optimized to detect increases in light intensity, and off-bipolar cells detect decreases in light intensity. When light hyperpolarizes a cone, the on-bipolar cell is excited (turned on), and the off-bipolar cell is inhibited (turned off). When a shadow depolarizes the cones, the opposite occurs (see Fig 12-3).

Some cone bipolar cells synapse only with L cones and others only with M cones (see the section "Trivariant color vision"), a differentiation that is necessary for color vision. In

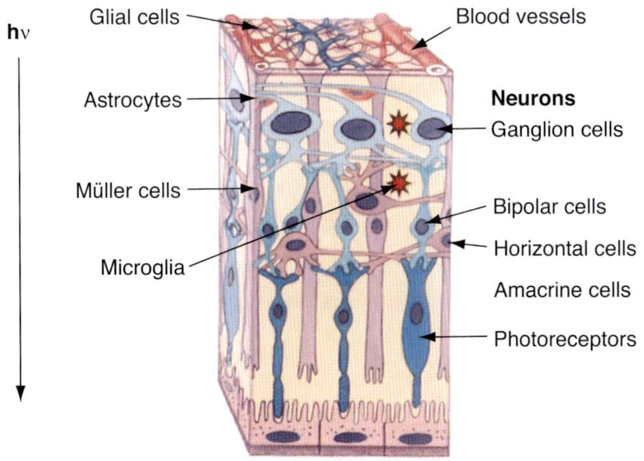

Figure 12-5 Schematic of the 3 major classes of retinal cells: glial cells (Müller cells, astrocytes, and microglia); neurons (photoreceptor, bipolar, horizontal, amacrine, and ganglion cells); and vascular cells (pericytes and endothelial cells). *(Reproduced with permission from Gardner TW, Antonetti DA, Barber AJ, LaNoue KF, Levison SW. Diabetic retinopathy: more than meets the eye.* Surv Ophthalmol. *2002;47(Suppl 2):S253–S262. Fig 1.)*

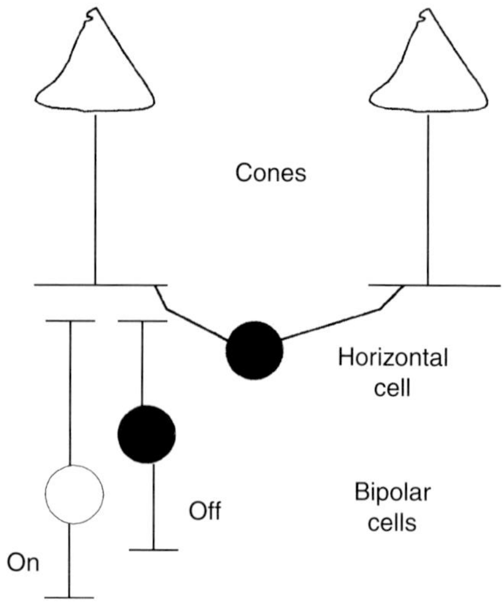

Figure 12-6 Basic circuitry of the cones. Separate on- and off-bipolar cells contact each cone. In the fovea, a cone has midget bipolar cells contacting only a single cone, and usually a single ganglion cell, for high spatial acuity. Horizontal cells are antagonistic neurons between cones. Absorbing light hyperpolarizes the cone; this, in turn, hyperpolarizes the horizontal cell, which resembles an off-bipolar cell. *(Courtesy of Peter Gouras, MD.)*

the fovea, some cone bipolar cells (midget bipolar cells) synapse with a single L or M cone, which allows the highest spatial acuity. This cone selectivity is preserved throughout the ganglion cell layer. Selectivity for L- or M-cone inputs is transmitted by a tonic responding system of small ganglion cells. Separate L- and M-cone on-bipolar cells and off-bipolar cells transmit a faster, phasic signal to a parallel system of larger ganglion cells. Rods and probably S cones have only on-bipolar cells. Thus, neither rods nor S cones are involved in high spatial resolution. S cones are involved in color vision; rods, in dim light (night vision).

Horizontal cells

Horizontal cells are antagonistic interneurons that provide negative feedback to photoreceptors (see Figs 12-5, 12-6). The dendrites of horizontal cells synapse with cones. One type of horizontal cell modulates L and M cones; another type modulates mainly S cones. The dendrites of horizontal cells receive glutamate from cones and rods and release GABA back onto them. This process provides negative feedback. When light causes the cone to hyperpolarize and stop its transmitter release, the neighboring horizontal cells are also hyperpolarized (turned off). This effect stops the release of GABA from the horizontal cell onto the cone, consequently depolarizing the cone. This feedback inhibition allows visualization of low-contrast details against background luminance.

Amacrine cells

Like horizontal cells, amacrine cells are inhibitory interneurons. Cone amacrine cells mediate antagonistic interactions among on-bipolar, off-bipolar, and ganglion cells. Rod bipolar cells do not usually synapse directly with ganglion cells but rather send their signal to amacrine cells, which then deliver the signal to on- and off-bipolar ganglion cells. Thus, rod signals undergo additional synaptic delays before they reach the ganglion cell output.

Ganglion cells

The functional division of the cone pathway into on and off channels begins at the first synapse (between the cones and the on-bipolar or off-bipolar cells). This division is preserved across the pathway to the higher visual centers. On-bipolar cells synapse with on-ganglion cells and off-bipolar cells with off-ganglion cells. Midget ganglion cells, a special type of ganglion cell with small dendritic trees, are dominant in the central macula. They have a 1:1:1 ratio with cones and midget bipolar cells, allowing high spatial resolution.

Ganglion cells can be divided into 3 subgroups: (1) tonic cells driven by L or M cones; (2) tonic cells driven by S cones; and (3) phasic cells. The tonic system transmits signals from the cones that are relatively well maintained for the duration of the light or dark stimulus. The phasic system transmits signals at the beginning or end of a light stimulus, producing a brief or transient response.

Tonic cells driven by either L or M cones include small cells concentrated in the fovea (responsible for high acuity) and other cells located extrafoveally. They mediate both high spatial resolution and color vision. Tonic cells driven by S cones are designed to detect successive color contrast, for example, blue-yellow or gray-brown borders. These ganglion cells are excited by short waves entering and long waves leaving their receptive fields. Phasic cells are larger, less concentrated in the fovea, and faster conducting than the other ganglion cells. Phasic cells may be important in movement detection.

Glial Cells

Müller cells are glial in origin and form a supporting element in the neural retina extending from the inner segments of the photoreceptors to the internal limiting membrane (ILM), which is formed by their end feet. They buffer the ionic concentrations in the extracellular space, enclose the subretinal space by helping form the external limiting membrane (ELM), and may play a role in vitamin A metabolism of cones.

The other nonneural, or neuroglial, cells of the retina are *macroglia* (mainly astrocytes) and *microglia.* Macroglia

- provide physical support to neuronal and vascular cells
- regulate the ionic and chemical composition of the extracellular milieu
- participate in the blood–retina barrier
- form the myelin sheath of the optic nerve (This function is performed by oligodendrocytes, which are macroglia that are similar to Schwann cells in the peripheral nervous system. Because the myelination does not usually extend into the retina, these glial cells are not found in the retina.)
- guide neuronal migration during development
- exchange metabolites with neurons

Microglia are related to tissue macrophages and are activated when retinal homeostasis is disturbed. These cells mediate immune responses in the central nervous system.

Vascular Cells

In addition to neural and glial cells, the retina contains blood vessels with endothelial cells and pericytes. Pericytes surround the endothelial cells and are modified smooth muscle cells that play a role in autoregulation of retinal blood vessels. Endothelial cells form the blood–retina barrier; pericytes structurally support the endothelium and suppress proliferation, loss of which leads to increased permeability and development of microaneurysms.

The neuronal, glial, and vascular components of the retina together form a functional neurovascular unit. Ophthalmoscopically, the vascular components are the only visible part of the retina. The neural retina lacks pigment (except for foveal xanthophyll) and is transparent, thus allowing the passage of light through the inner retinal layers. Conditions such as diabetic retinopathy are categorized on the basis of clinically evident vascular changes. Despite the clinical emphasis on vascular changes, there is strong evidence of neuronal dysfunction early in the disease process, even prior to the detection of clinically evident disease.

Gardner TW, Antonetti DA, Barber AJ, LaNoue KF, Levison SW. Diabetic retinopathy: more than meets the eye. *Surv Ophthalmol.* 2002;47(Suppl 2):S253–S262.

Retinal Electrophysiology

Changes in the light flux on the retina produce electrical changes in all retinal cells, including the RPE and Müller cells, as well as neurons. These electrical changes result from ionic currents that flow when ion-specific channels are opened or closed. These currents reach the vitreous and the cornea, where they can be detected noninvasively and form the basis of the electroretinogram (ERG) (Figs 12-7, 12-8). The currents are initiated by the ionic response started in the rods and cones. This response influences the ionic current *directly* by changes in Na^+, K^+, and Ca^{2+} fluxes and *indirectly* by synaptic modification of second-order retinal neurons. The ionic changes are due to shifts in the photoreceptors' conductivity of Na^+, K^+, and Ca^{2+}; this conductivity is facilitated by the CNG channels (see Fig 12-4).

As discussed previously, light hyperpolarizes cones and rods. The cone response is rapid; it turns off while the light is still on and overshoots the dark potential (see Fig 12-7). The rod response is more prolonged and turns off very slowly. Darkness depolarizes the

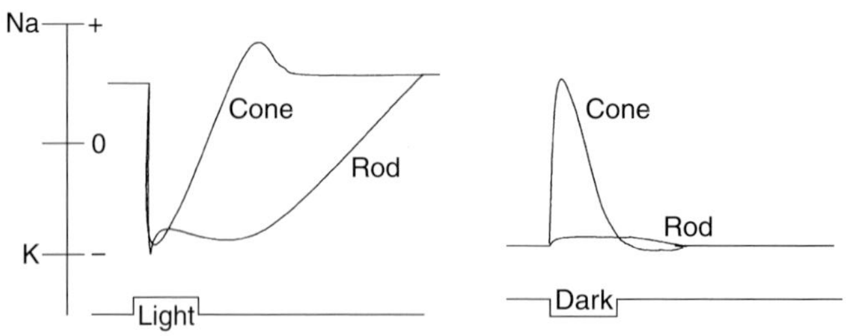

Figure 12-7 Electroretinogram (ERG) showing the responses of a rod and a cone to a pulse of light and a pulse of darkness. The light pulse hyperpolarizes both photoreceptors. The rod responses are prolonged. The cone responses turn off quickly, even while the pulse of light is on. Darkness rapidly depolarizes the cone but has only a small effect on the slower rod response.

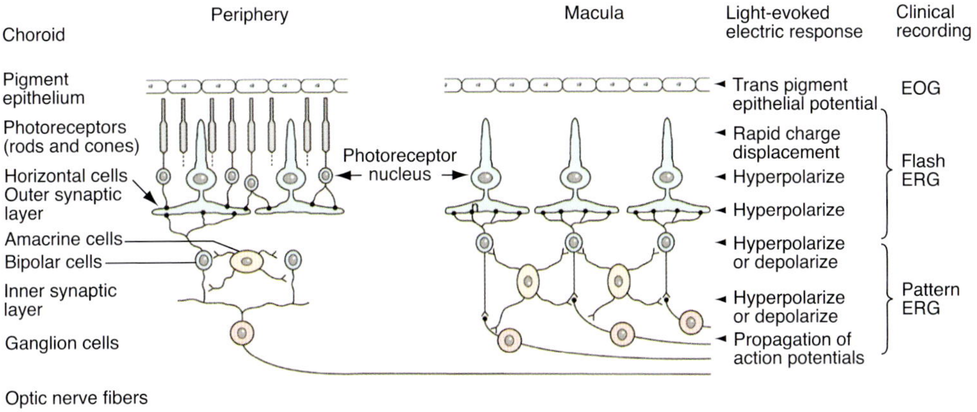

Figure 12-8 Origins of measurable electrical signals from the retina. EOG = electro-oculogram; ERG = electroretinogram. *(Modified with permission from Forrester JV, Dick AD, McMenamin PG, Roberts F, Pearlman E.* The Eye: Basic Sciences in Practice. *4th ed. St Louis: Saunders; 2016:297.)*

cone and has little influence on the rod, which is saturated at high light levels and too slow to respond to the shadow.

See BCSC Section 12, *Retina and Vitreous,* for detailed discussion of ERGs and retinal responses.

CHAPTER 13

Retinal Pigment Epithelium

Highlights

- The retinal pigment epithelium (RPE) is derived embryologically from the same neural anlage as the neurosensory retina.
- Although it has no photoreceptive or neural function, the RPE is essential for the viability of photoreceptor cells and the choriocapillaris and thus for vision.
- Mutation of the gene *RPE65,* which encodes the enzyme (RPE65 isomerohydrolase) that converts all-*trans*-retinyl ester to 11-*cis*-retinol, causes Leber congenital amaurosis (LCA). *RPE65* is the target of a treatment approved by the US Food and Drug Administration (FDA) that uses an adeno-associated virus to deliver the gene to the RPE of LCA patients.
- Autophagy is a homeostatic process whereby the cell degrades its own damaged components and recycles the products. In the RPE, this is essential for management of phagocytosed outer segments as well as for turnover of its components.

Overview of RPE Structure

The RPE is a monolayer of neuroectoderm-derived epithelial cells, located between the highly vascular choriocapillaris and the photoreceptor outer segments (Figs 13-1, 13-2). Embryologically, it is derived from the same neural anlage as the neurosensory retina. The retina and RPE develop as an invagination of the embryonic optic cup that folds the neuroectodermal layer into apex-to-apex contact with itself. The outer layer forms the RPE and the inner layer forms the neurosensory retina. The intervening area remains throughout life as a potential space and is the plane of separation for retinal detachment.

In humans, there are approximately 4–6 million RPE cells per eye. On the apical surface of RPE cells are long microvilli that interdigitate with the outer segments of photoreceptor cells (see Figs 13-1, Fig 13-2). These cells are joined near their apical side by tight junctions that establish polarity, block the passage of water and ions, and constitute the outer blood–retina barrier. The RPE basal surface, which is adjacent to the Bruch membrane (an extracellular matrix between the RPE and the choriocapillaris), has many infoldings that increase the surface area available for the exchange of solutes (see Fig 13-1).

In addition to the organelles found in most cells (eg, the nucleus, Golgi apparatus, smooth and rough endoplasmic reticulum, and mitochondria), RPE cells contain melanin

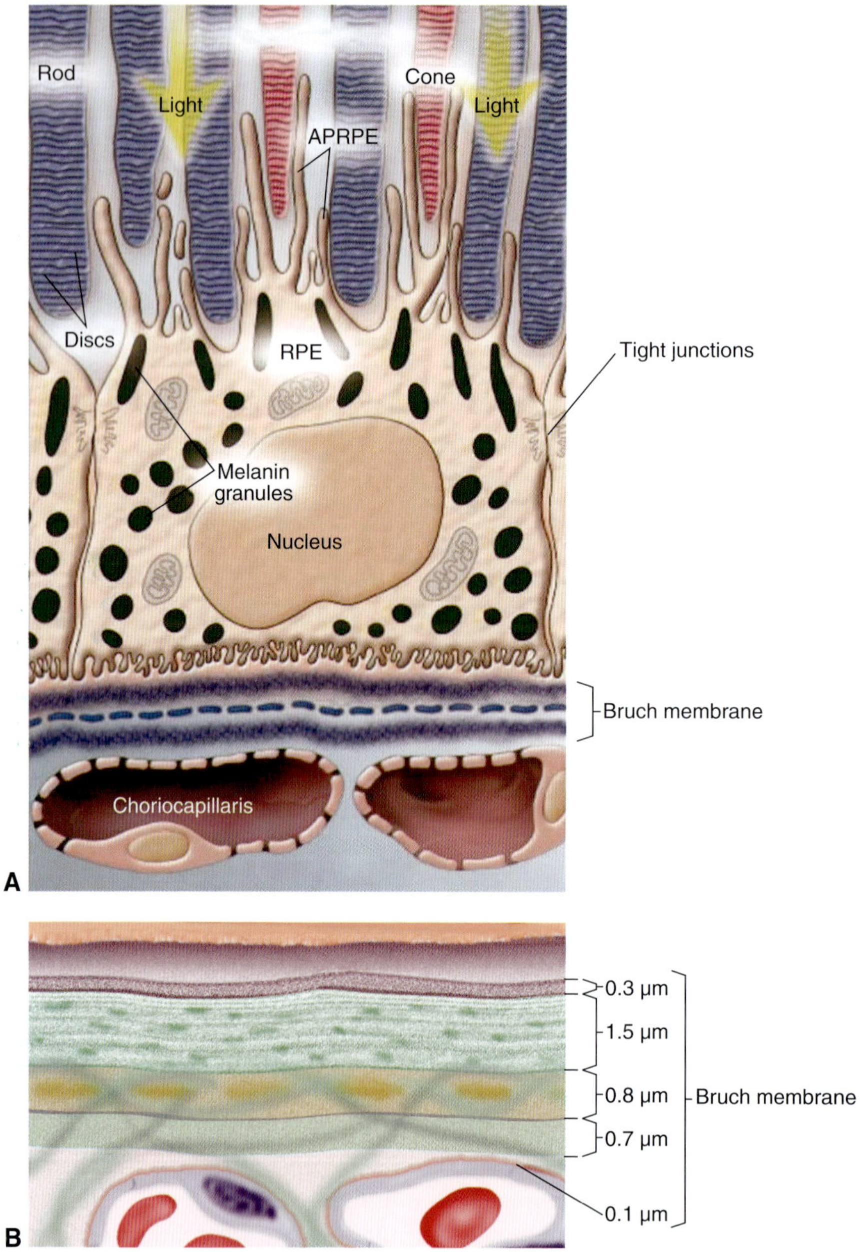

Figure 13-1 The retinal pigment epithelium (RPE) and Bruch membrane. **A,** The Bruch membrane separates the RPE from the choriocapillaris. Note the interdigitation of the apical processes of the RPE with the photoreceptor outer segments as well as the infoldings of the basal surface. **B,** The thickness of the different layers of Bruch membrane is demonstrated (starting from the top): basement membrane of the RPE, inner collagenous layer, elastic layer, outer collagenous layer, and basement membrane of the choriocapillaris. APRPE = apical processes of the RPE. *(Part A modified courtesy of University of Rochester; part B illustration by Daniel Casper, MD, PhD.)*

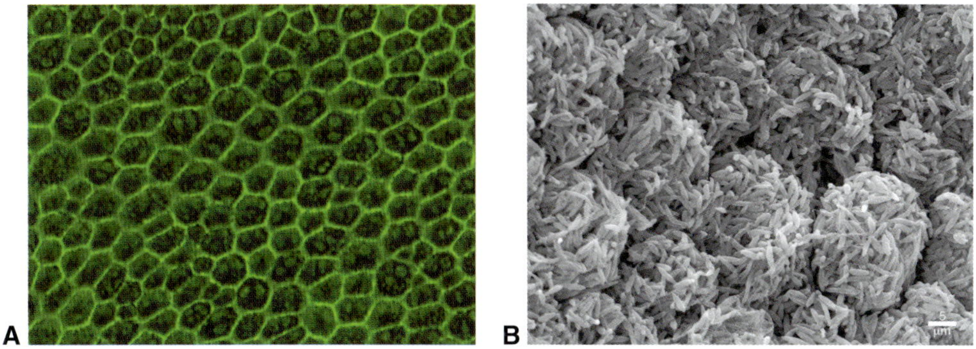

Figure 13-2 RPE. **A,** Monolayer of cultured RPE cells grown to confluence shows the polygonal appearance of the RPE cells (phase microscopy, ×25). **B,** Scanning electron micrograph of RPE cells demonstrates the apical microvilli. *(Parts A and B reproduced with permission from Handa JT. Cell biology of the retinal pigment epithelium. In: Schachat AP, ed.* Ryan's Retina. *6th ed. Edinburgh: Elsevier; 2017: Figs 18.1 and 18.4.)*

granules and phagosomes, reflecting their role in light absorption and phagocytosis (discussed later in the chapter). The RPE is particularly rich in microperoxisomes, suggesting that it is active in detoxifying the large number of free radicals and oxidized lipids generated in this highly oxidative and light-rich environment.

Biochemical Composition

Biochemically, the RPE is a dynamic and complex cell. It must meet demands for its own active metabolism, its extraordinary phagocytic function, and its role as a biological filter for the neurosensory retina. These processes impose a very high energy requirement on the RPE; not surprisingly, RPE cells contain all the enzymes of the 3 major biochemical pathways: glycolysis, the Krebs cycle, and the pentose phosphate pathway. Glucose is the primary carbon source used for energy metabolism and for conversion to protein. Although the RPE does make a minor contribution to the glycosaminoglycan- and proteoglycan-containing interphotoreceptor matrix, glucose is not converted to glycogen in the RPE. Glucosamine, fucose, galactose, and mannose are all metabolized to some extent in the RPE, although mannose seems to be passed on almost directly to the photoreceptors.

More than 80% of the wet weight of the RPE is contributed by water. Proteins, lipids, and nucleic acids contribute most of the remaining weight.

Proteins

Nearly 850 proteins have been identified in the RPE. Many proteins found in other cells are also present in the RPE. These include hydrolytic enzymes such as glutathione, peroxidase, catalase, and superoxide dismutase, which are important for detoxification. The cytoskeletal proteins actin, myosin, α-actinin, fodrin, and vinculin are also present in both the RPE and other cells.

Some proteins found in the RPE and other cells are localized differently in the RPE. A well-known example of such a protein is Na^+,K^+-ATPase (also called *sodium-potassium pump*), which has a unique location in RPE cells. In most polarized epithelial cells, Na^+,K^+-ATPase is localized to the basolateral membrane, but in the RPE this enzyme is found on the apical membrane. The sodium-potassium pump uses energy derived from adenosine triphosphate (ATP) hydrolysis to transport sodium (Na^+) and potassium (K^+) against their electrochemical gradients. It is thought that the apical location of Na^+,K^+-ATPase in the RPE maintains the balance of Na^+ and K^+ in the subretinal space. RPE cells also contain proteins whose polarity has been shown to be reversed compared with the polarity of other epithelial cells; examples include an isoform of neural cell adhesion molecule (NCAM-140) and folate receptor α.

Some proteins are expressed only in the RPE. One such protein, RPE-specific protein 65 kDa (RPE65), is an obligate component of the isomerization and hydrolysis of vitamin A, which is required for regeneration of visual pigment (described later in Vitamin A Regeneration).

Lipids

Lipids account for approximately 3% of the wet weight of the RPE; about half are phospholipids. Phosphatidylcholine and phosphatidylethanolamine make up more than 80% of the total phospholipid content. In general, levels of saturated fatty acids are higher in the RPE than in the adjacent outer segments. The saturated fatty acids palmitic acid and stearic acid are used for retinol esterification and for energy metabolism by the RPE mitochondria. The level of polyunsaturated fatty acids, such as docosahexaenoic acid (22:6, n–3), is much lower in the RPE than in the outer segments, although the level of arachidonic acid is relatively high. A number of studies have suggested that the retina may be spared the effects of essential fatty acid deficiency because the RPE efficiently sequesters fatty acids from the blood. The RPE actively conserves and efficiently reuses fatty acids, thus preventing their loss as waste products.

Nucleic Acids

RNA is synthesized continually by the RPE. This is required to produce the numerous enzymes that are necessary for cell metabolism, phagocytosis of shed discs, and maintenance of the retinoid pathway and transport functions.

Major Physiologic Roles of the RPE

The RPE has a number of physiologic roles (Fig 13-3). Crucial among these functions are

- vitamin A regeneration, which is integral to sustaining vision
- phagocytosis of shed photoreceptor outer-segment discs
- biological filter for the neurosensory retina through transport of necessary nutrients and ions to photoreceptor cells and removal of waste products from photoreceptors

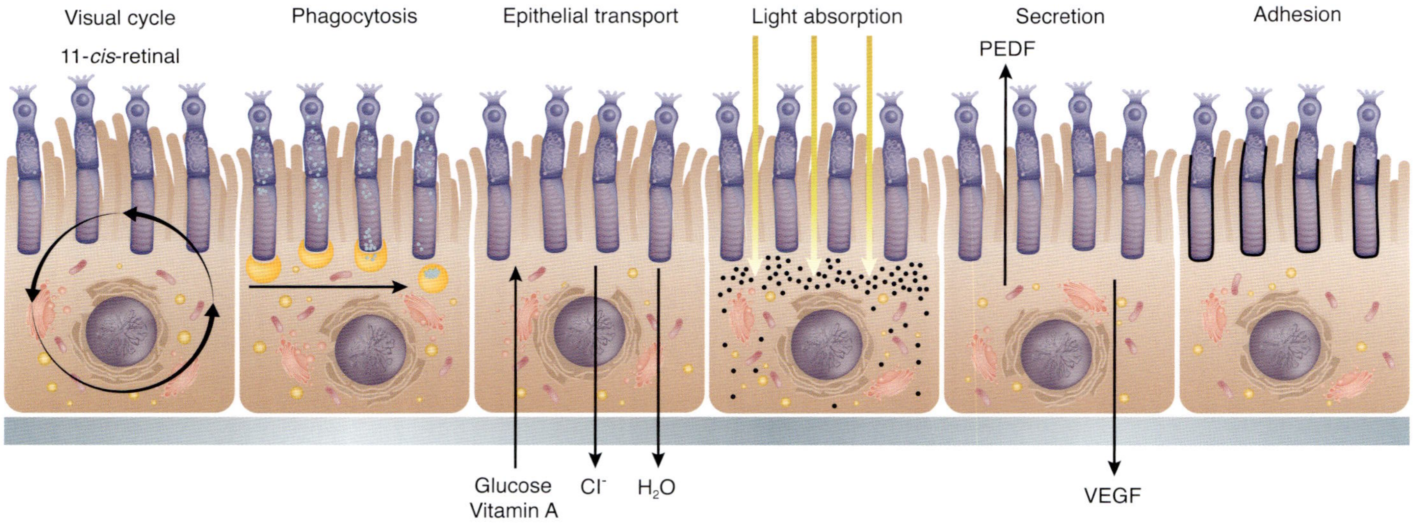

Figure 13-3 Physiologic functions of the RPE. Additional functions (not shown) include its role in synthesis and remodeling of the interphotoreceptor matrix, formation of the outer blood–retina barrier, and formation of the basal lamina of Bruch membrane. PEDF = pigment epithelium–derived factor; VEGF = vascular endothelial growth factor. *(Illustration by Cyndie C.H. Wooley.)*

- absorption of scattered and out-of-focus light via pigmentation
- adhesion of the retina
- secretion of humoral and growth factors

These functions are discussed briefly in the following sections. Other important functions subserved by the RPE include its role in synthesis and remodeling of the interphotoreceptor matrix, formation of the outer blood–retina barrier, and formation of the basal lamina of Bruch membrane.

Vitamin A Regeneration

The RPE, second only to the liver in its concentration of vitamin A, plays a major role in the uptake, storage, and mobilization of vitamin A. The RPE supplies the photoreceptor outer segments with vitamin A, which is tethered to rhodopsin in rods and to the 3 different cone opsins (red, green, and blue). Although the different opsins have specific absorption spectra, vitamin A changes its configuration identically in response to the particular wavelength of light (see Chapter 12).

The basic function of the RPE cell is to generate 11-*cis*-retinal (also called 11-*cis*-retinaldehyde) (Fig 13-4). Light-induced activation of rhodopsin leads to isomerization of 11-*cis*-retinal to all-*trans*-retinal and initiates the phototransduction cascade. Light-activated rhodopsin releases all-*trans*-retinal and must bind with another 11-*cis*-retinal to be ready for activation by the next photon of light. The free all-*trans*-retinal isomer undergoes a series of enzymatic reactions, called the *visual cycle* or *retinoid cycle,* to regenerate 11-*cis*-retinal. The visual cycle ensures a steady supply of 11-*cis*-retinal for the opsins for maintaining vision and requires close interaction between the RPE and photoreceptor outer segments. Similar processes occur in all photoreceptors; the process specific to rods is discussed below.

Free all-*trans*-retinal is cleared from the rod discs by ABCA4, an ATP-binding cassette (ABC) transporter protein. After transport from the rod discs to the cytosol of the outer segments, all-*trans*-retinal is enzymatically reduced to all-*trans*-retinol by retinol dehydrogenase. All-*trans*-retinol is rapidly released by photoreceptor cells to the interphotoreceptor matrix, where it binds to interphotoreceptor retinoid-binding protein (IRBP). RPE cells contain cellular retinol-binding protein 1 (CRBP1), which promotes the uptake of all-*trans*-retinol into the RPE. The RPE also obtains vitamin A from the blood, where it is complexed with retinol-binding protein (RBP) and transthyretin. Phagocytosis of shed photoreceptor outer-segment discs (see the following section) by the RPE also allows recycling of vitamin A.

Within the RPE cells, CRBP1-bound all-*trans*-retinol is enzymatically esterified by lecithin retinol acyltransferase (LRAT). The resultant retinyl ester is hydrolyzed and isomerized to the 11-*cis* configuration by the retinoid isomerohydrolase RPE65. 11-*cis*-Retinol is then oxidized to 11-*cis*-retinal by 11-*cis*-retinol dehydrogenase. The newly formed 11-*cis*-retinal is released from RPE cells to the interphotoreceptor matrix. From there it is transported by IRBP (IRBP binds both retinol and retinal forms) to the photoreceptor outer-segment discs to generate another visual transduction cycle.

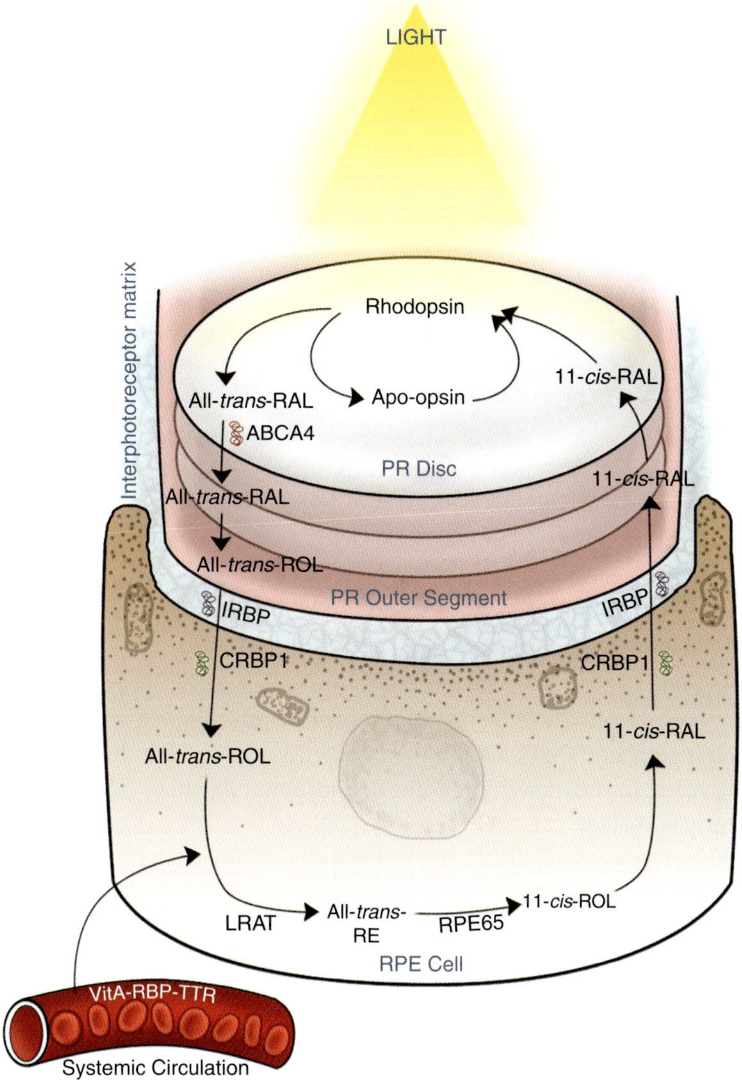

Figure 13-4 The visual cycle (also known as *retinoid cycle*) involves a series of reactions in the photoreceptor outer segments and RPE to regenerate 11-*cis*-retinal (also known as 11-*cis*-retinaldehyde). 11-*cis* Retinal attaches to a lysine residue on rhodopsin. When the complex absorbs light, 11-*cis*-retinal transforms into all-*trans*-retinal via a process known as *photoisomerization.* This induces a conformational change in the attached rhodopsin molecule, activating the second-messenger system and initiating the phototransduction cascade within the photoreceptor. The all-*trans*-retinal is shed from rhodopsin and transported by ABCA4 from the rod disc to the cytosol, where it is converted to all-*trans*-retinol. Then, all-*trans*-retinol is delivered to the RPE via interphotoreceptor retinoid-binding protein (IRBP), which acts as a shuttle and also shields the cell membranes from the membranolytic retinoid molecules. Once in the RPE, this molecule is esterified by lecithin retinol acyltransferase (LRAT). The resultant retinyl ester is converted to 11-*cis*-retinol by the isomerohydrolase RPE65. 11-*cis*-Retinol is then oxidized to 11-*cis*-retinal by retinol dehydrogenase (RDH) and shuttled back to the photoreceptor outer-segment discs by IRBP to participate in another visual cycle. ABCA4 = ATP-binding cassette transporter protein; Apo-opsin = apo-rhodopsin; CRBP1 = cellular retinol-binding protein 1; PR = photoreceptor; RAL = retinal; RBP = retinol-binding protein; RE = retinyl ester; ROL = retinol; TTR = transthyretin; VitA = vitamin A. *(Modified with permission from Singh RSJ, Kim JE. Visual cycle modulation. In: Lim J, ed.* Age-related Macular Degeneration. *3rd ed. Boca Raton, FL: CRC Press; 2012:330.)*

CLINICAL PEARL

Because vitamin A intermediaries are membranolytic, they require shuttles or are esterified to protect the plasma membrane of the photoreceptors and RPE. Mutations in the genes that encode the corresponding shuttles and enzymes have been identified in many inherited retinal diseases. Mutations of the *ABCR* gene, which encodes the ABC transporter protein ABCA4, lead to Stargardt disease. Mutation of the retinoid isomerohydrolase RPE65 gene *(RPE65),* which encodes the RPE65 protein, causes Leber congenital amaurosis (LCA) (see Table 13-1). RPE65 isomerohydrolase is the target of an FDA-approved treatment that uses an adeno-associated virus to deliver the *RPE65* gene to the RPE of patients with LCA.

Testa F, Maguire AM, Rossi S, et al. Three-year follow-up after unilateral subretinal delivery of adeno-associated virus in patients with Leber congenital amaurosis type 2. *Ophthalmology.* 2013;120(6):1283–1291.

Phagocytosis of Shed Photoreceptor Outer-Segment Discs

The RPE plays a crucial role in turnover of the photosensitive membrane of rod and cone photoreceptors (Fig 13-5). Each photoreceptor cell sheds approximately 100 outer-segment discs per day. Because many photoreceptors interdigitate with a single RPE cell, each RPE cell ingests and digests more than 4000 discs daily. The shedding event follows a circadian rhythm: in rods, shedding is most vigorous at dawn; in cones, shedding occurs most vigorously at dusk.

The shed outer-segment discs are encapsulated in phagosomes (see Fig 13-5C; see also Chapter 2, Fig 2-45), which in turn fuse with lysosomes and are digested. During degradation of the discs, building blocks are recycled into photoreceptors for use in the synthesis and assembly of new discs. The lipofuscin characteristic of the RPE is derived from the photosensitive membranes and is responsible for generating the signal detected in fundus autofluorescence imaging (Fig 13-6).

As detailed earlier in the chapter, phototransduction causes release of free all-*trans*-retinal, which is transported from the outer-segment discs into the outer-segment cytosol by ABCA4. In certain disease states (eg, Stargardt disease), the free all-*trans*-retinal is not readily cleared from the outer-segment discs by ABCA4. The excess all-*trans*-retinal combines with phosphatidylethanolamine (PE) in the disc lipid bilayer, forming *N*-retinylidene-PE (*N*-ret-PE). Elevated *N*-ret-PE and all-*trans*-retinal undergo a secondary nonenzymatic condensation in the outer segments to yield A2PE-H2. The distal outer segments containing A2PE-H2 and elevated all-*trans*-retinal and *N*-ret-PE are phagocytosed by the RPE as part of the normal disc-renewal process, but the RPE is unable to fully degrade the nonphysiologic load. This leads to the accumulation of toxic retinal fluorophores like A2E (derived from A2PE-H2), which damage the RPE.

Transport

The health and integrity of retinal neurons depend on a well-regulated extracellular environment. A crucial function of the RPE that contributes to this regulation is control of the

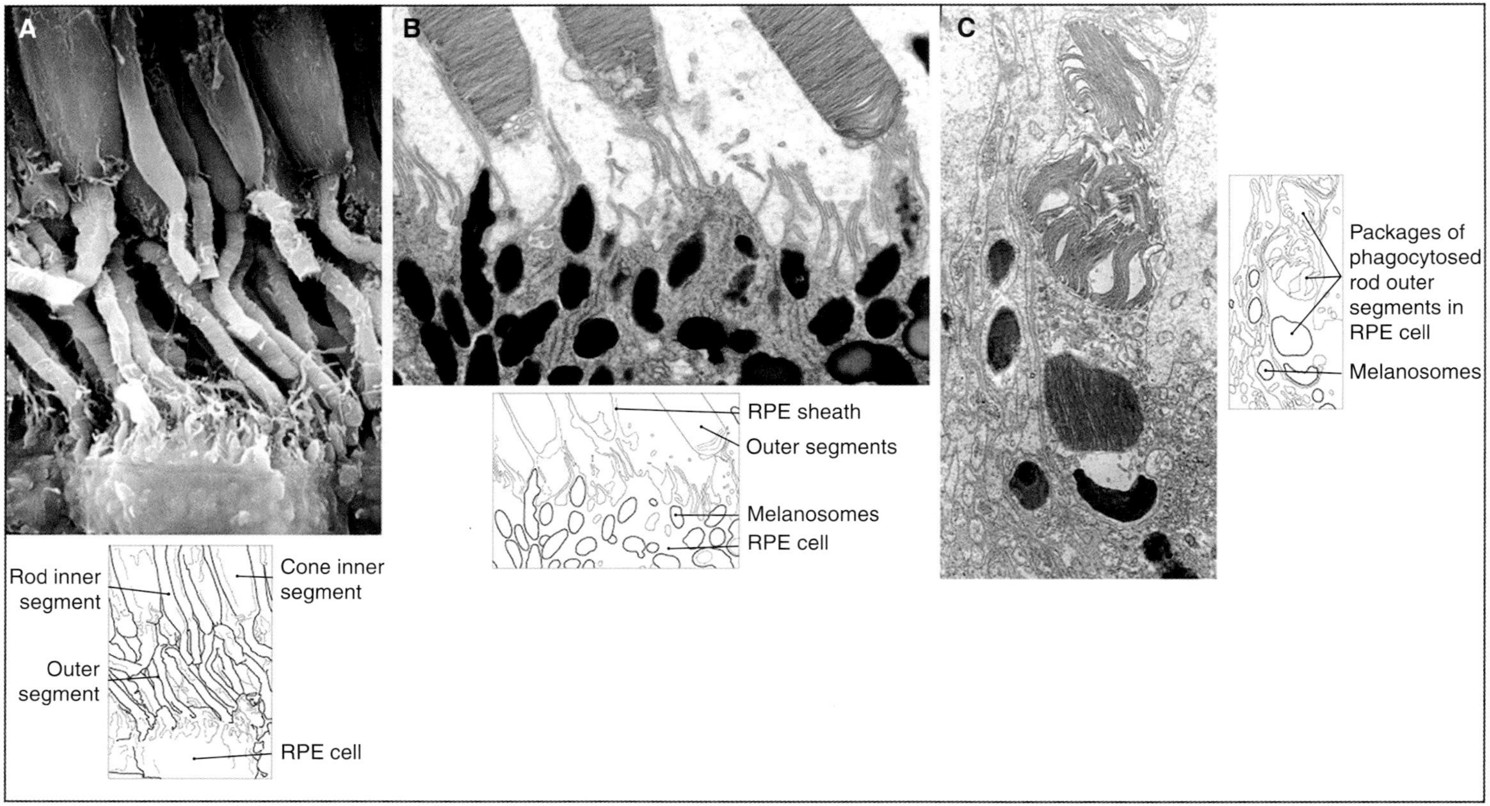

Figure 13-5 RPE. **A,** Interdigitization of the apical processes of the RPE with photoreceptors in the subretinal space. **B,** RPE apical microvilli surround photoreceptor outer segments. Cytosolic melanin granules are also shown. **C,** Phagocytosed photoreceptor outer segments within the RPE. *(Reproduced with permission from Spalton D, Hitchings R, Hunter P.* Atlas of Clinical Ophthalmology. *3rd ed. New York: Elsevier/Mosby; 2005:403.)*

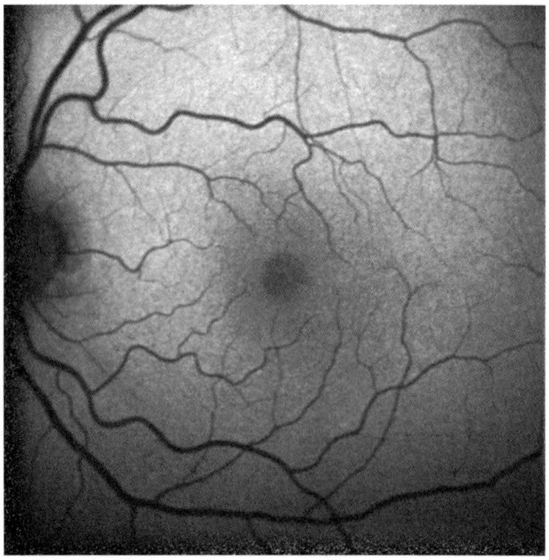

Figure 13-6 Example of fundus autofluorescence imaging, which is facilitated by lipofuscin molecules present within the RPE. Changes in fundus autofluorescence patterns reflect disorders of the RPE in the presence of hyperfluorescence and atrophic RPE in the presence of hypofluorescence (see BCSC Section 12, *Retina and Vitreous*). *(Courtesy of Vikram S. Brar, MD.)*

volume and composition of fluid in the subretinal space through transport of ions, fluid, and metabolites. The distribution of transport proteins residing in the apical and basolateral membrane domains of the cell is asymmetric, and this allows the epithelium to carry out vectorial transport. The membrane proteins remain in their proper location because of tight junction proteins. The polarity of the cell is maintained because of the intracellular molecular machinery that synthesizes new proteins and delivers them preferentially to the apical or basolateral cell membranes. Cytoskeletal proteins are fundamental in determining cell polarity and regulating transport.

The aqueous environment of the subretinal space is actively maintained by the ion-transport systems of the RPE, which regulate transport of a variety of ions (K^+, Ca^{2+}, Na^+, Cl^-, and HCO_3^-). This transport is vectorial in most cases; for example, Na^+ is actively transported from the choriocapillaris toward the subretinal space, whereas K^+ is transported in the opposite direction. The apical membrane of the RPE appears to be the major locus of this transport. As mentioned previously, ouabain-sensitive Na^+,K^+-ATPase is present at the apical, but not the basal, side. Similarly, an active bicarbonate-transport system appears to be located in the apical RPE membrane. High carbonic anhydrase activity seems to be associated with both the apical and basal sides of the cell.

Net ionic fluxes in the RPE are responsible for the transepithelial electrical potential that can be measured across the RPE apical membrane—a potential that is rapidly modified in the presence of a variety of metabolic inhibitors (eg, ouabain and dinitrophenol). Ion gradients across the RPE drive the transport of water from the subretinal space to the choriocapillaris. The RPE also transports lactic acid produced by metabolic activity in the retina away from the subretinal space. Active vectorial transport systems for other retinal metabolites (eg, taurine, methionine, and folate) have also been demonstrated. The RPE, therefore, appears to be important for maintaining the ionic environment of the subretinal space, which in turn is responsible for maintaining the integrity of the RPE–photoreceptor interface. The trans-RPE potential is the basis for the electro-oculogram (EOG), which is the most common electrophysiologic test for evaluating the RPE (see Chapter 12, Fig 12-8).

Pigmentation

A characteristic feature of the RPE is the presence of melanin pigment. Pigment granules are abundant in the cytoplasm of adult RPE cells, predominantly in the apical and midportions of the cell (see Fig 13-5B). During development, activation of the tyrosinase promoter triggers the onset of melanogenesis in this cell and marks the commitment of the neuroectoderm to become RPE. Although most melanogenesis occurs before birth, melanin production in the RPE occurs throughout life, albeit at a slow rate. As humans age, the melanin granules fuse with lysosomes; thus, the fundus of an older person is less pigmented than that of a young person. Clinically, this is most evident in the peripheral fundus.

The exact role of melanin within cells remains speculative. One universally recognized function of melanin is to act as a neutral-density filter in scattering light. In so doing, melanin may have a protective role. But even in the minimally pigmented fundus, visual acuity can be 20/20. Visual problems in persons with albinism are attributable to foveal hypoplasia, not optical scatter. When melanin levels are below a critical level, as in oculocutaneous albinism, there is aberrant neuronal migration in the visual pathway (more contralateral projections of ganglion cells), incomplete foveal development, low vision, nystagmus, and strabismus.

Melanin is also a free-radical stabilizer and can bind many toxins and drugs (such as chloroquine and hydroxychloroquine). Some regard this feature as protective; others think that it contributes to tissue toxicity.

CLINICAL PEARL

In addition to its functions as a neutral-density filter in scattering light and as a free-radical stabilizer, melanin within the RPE absorbs the light delivered to the eye during laser photocoagulation of the retina. The absorbed energy is transferred to the surrounding tissues as heat. The outer retina is damaged, and the ensuing inflammatory reaction creates an adhesion between the retina and the RPE. Because of the high blood flow of the choroid, the heat typically dissipates, with minimal to no damage to the choroid.

Retinal Adhesion

The subretinal space is never bridged by tissue, and yet the neural retina remains firmly attached to the RPE throughout life. The RPE is crucial to maintaining retinal adhesion. Detachment of the photoreceptors from the RPE can lead to permanent morphologic and functional changes in the retina.

Numerous factors keep the retina in place. These include passive hydrostatic forces, interdigitation of outer segments and RPE microvilli, active transport of subretinal fluid, and the complex structure of the interphotoreceptor matrix and its binding properties (van der Waals forces). In pathologic conditions, retinal adhesion can diminish, and detachment of the retina occurs. Detachment does not occur simply because there is a hole in the retina or a leak in the RPE; there must be either positive traction pulling the neural retina or positive forces pushing fluid into the subretinal space that overwhelms the removal capacity of the RPE.

> **CLINICAL PEARL**
>
> In certain cases of rhegmatogenous retinal detachment, pneumatic retinopexy can be used to repair the detached retina. This technique involves injection of a gas bubble into the vitreous cavity. The patient's head is positioned so that the gas bubble lies over the retinal break. The RPE pumps out the subretinal fluid while the gas bubble occludes the retinal break and prevents additional fluid from entering the subretinal space. This allows reattachment of the retina; laser retinopexy can then be done.

Secretion

A number of growth factors, cytokines, and immune modulators are secreted by the RPE and are essential for maintaining the physiologic function of the photoreceptors and the choriocapillaris. Examples include PEDF (pigment epithelium–derived factor) and CNTF (ciliary neurotrophic factor), which prevent photoreceptor cell death; VEGF (vascular endothelial growth factor), which maintains choroidal vascular endothelium; and TIMP (tissue inhibitor of metalloproteinases), which maintains the extracellular matrix.

The Role of Autophagy in the RPE

Autophagy is a normal homeostatic mechanism whereby the cell degrades its own damaged components and recycles the degradation products for continued cell survival. In RPE cells, autophagic machinery, which includes phagosomes and lysosomes, is abundant. Autophagy is essential to the RPE for management of phagocytosed outer segments and for turnover of its own components. Because RPE cells do not divide under normal conditions, autophagy is also important for quality control of intracellular components. Dysregulated autophagy is involved in the pathophysiology of diseases such as age-related macular degeneration, glaucoma, and photoreceptor loss in retinal detachment. Drugs that inhibit autophagy (eg, chloroquine) lead to RPE and photoreceptor damage.

The RPE in Disease

The RPE is vital for normal visual function. Genetic defects unique to the RPE may produce retinal degenerations and disorders. Table 13-1 presents some of these conditions.

RPE cells have been found to play a role in nongenetic ophthalmic conditions as well. Defects in the pump mechanism of the RPE have been proposed as the cause of central serous chorioretinopathy. In certain pathologic conditions, RPE cells, which normally do not divide, detach from the basement membrane and become migratory. On contact with the vitreous and/or transforming growth factor β (TGF-β), these cells undergo metaplasia, acquiring myofibroblast qualities. Proliferative vitreoretinopathy (PVR) is an example of

Table 13-1 RPE-Specific Gene Defects

Protein Affected	Corresponding Retinal Degenerations and Disorders
RPE65 isomerohydrolase	Homozygous defects in the *RPE65* gene, which encodes the RPE65 isomerohydrolase, cause LCA. LCA usually has an autosomal recessive pattern. Null mutations of the guanylate cyclase gene (see Chapter 12) also cause LCA. The protein is the target of an FDA-approved treatment using an adeno-associated virus to deliver the gene to the RPE of patients with LCA.
Bestrophin	Heterozygous missense mutations of the bestrophin gene *(BEST1)* produce Best disease. The encoded protein bestrophin functions as a chloride channel, found on the basolateral surface of the RPE.
TIMP3	Heterozygous point mutations of the *TIMP3* gene produce Sorsby macular dystrophy. The TIMP3 protein is an inhibitor of a metalloproteinase that regulates the extracellular matrix, where it acts as an antiangiogenesis factor.
CRALBP	Homozygous defects of the gene *RLBP1,* which encodes cellular retinaldehyde-binding protein, cause retinitis punctata albescens. This protein facilitates 11-*cis*-retinal formation and shields the plasma membrane from the potential lytic effects of its aldehyde moiety.
11-*cis*-Retinol dehydrogenase	A mutation in *RDH5,* the gene encoding 11-*cis*-retinol dehydrogenase, causes fundus albipunctatus, a form of stationary nyctalopia. This enzyme forms 11-*cis*-retinal from 11-*cis*-retinol.
EFEMP1	A single heterozygous, nonconservative mutation of the gene *EFEMP1* (EGF-containing fibrillin-like extracellular matrix protein) causes Malattia Leventinese (Doyne honeycomb dystrophy), a dominant form of macular degeneration. It is uncertain whether the protein is unique to the RPE.

LCA = Leber congenital amaurosis; RPE = retinal pigment epithelium.

such a condition. In PVR, the metaplastic RPE cells form contractile membranes on the surface of the retina, leading to retinal detachment. PVR is the most common cause of retinal redetachment after surgery. See BCSC Section 12, *Retina and Vitreous,* for further discussion.

Marmor MF, Wolfensberger TJ, eds. *The Retinal Pigment Epithelium: Function and Disease.* New York: Oxford University Press; 1998:103–134.

Parapuram SK, Chang B, Li L, et al. Differential effects of TGFβ and vitreous on the transformation of retinal pigment epithelial cells. *Invest Ophthalmol Vis Sci.* 2009;50(12):5965–5974.

CHAPTER 14

Reactive Oxygen Species and Antioxidants

Highlights

- Oxidative stress has a causal role in many vision-threatening diseases, including cataract, glaucoma, diabetic retinopathy, and age-related macular degeneration.
- Oxidative processes play a central role in the development of nuclear sclerosis. The lens utilizes glutathione, among other antioxidant mechanisms, to combat oxidative stress.
- The Age-Related Eye Disease Study (AREDS) confirmed the role of antioxidants in slowing the progression of macular degeneration.
- Antioxidants may prevent the development of primary open-angle glaucoma and visual field defects.
- Targeting oxidative pathways affords new therapeutic interventions for some of the most common ophthalmic diseases.

Overview

Under physiologic conditions, reactive oxygen species (ROS) participate in normal biochemical processes, where they either act as intermediaries or function as second messengers. Also, ROS can be generated by exogenous influences, such as exposure to ultraviolet (UV) light or cigarette smoking. Oxidative stress occurs when the production of ROS exceeds their degradation.

Unchecked, ROS injure cell membranes and DNA, leading to tissue damage and cell death. ROS, like free radicals, react with unsaturated fatty acids that are present within cells and cell membranes, forming lipid peroxides. The oxidation of membrane phospholipids has been hypothesized to increase the permeability of cell membranes and/or inhibit membrane ion pumps. This loss of barrier function is thought to lead to edema, disturbances in electrolyte balance, and elevation of intracellular calcium levels, all of which contribute to cell malfunction and, potentially, to cell death. Free radical–mediated DNA damage can also lead to cell death through induction of apoptosis.

The resultant loss of cells leads to dysfunction in the eye, whether at the level of the trabecular meshwork and retinal ganglion cells (RGCs) in glaucoma, the inner retina in diabetic retinopathy, or the outer retina in age-related macular degeneration (AMD).

Reactive Oxygen Species

Sources of Reactive Oxygen Species

Reactive oxygen species are generated from metabolic processes, inflammatory responses, and exposure to UV light. ROS include hydrogen peroxide (H_2O_2) and singlet oxygen ($^1O_2$), as well as lipid peroxides and reactive carbohydrates such as ketoamine and keto-aldehyde groups. Free radicals, another group of ROS, possess an unpaired electron that makes them highly reactive toward other molecular species.

Exogenous sources of ROS include UV light and tobacco smoke. Endogenous sources include the *electron transport chain* in mitochondria and, as part of our innate immune response by neutrophils and macrophages, *respiratory burst,* where superoxide anion ($O_2^{\bullet-}$) and the hydroxyl radical (OH•) form to attack pathogens (Fig 14-1). The nicotinamide adenine dinucleotide phosphate (NADPH) oxidases (Nox) constitute an enzyme family that functions primarily to produce ROS and is expressed in many cells. Table 14-1 presents some important ROS.

Toxicity from ROS leads to cell death. ROS may directly induce DNA damage, resulting in cell death via apoptosis. Cell death can also occur through loss of the barrier function of the plasma membrane via a process known as *lipid peroxidation.* Structures with a high concentration of polyunsaturated fatty acids (PUFAs) are particularly susceptible to lipid peroxidation.

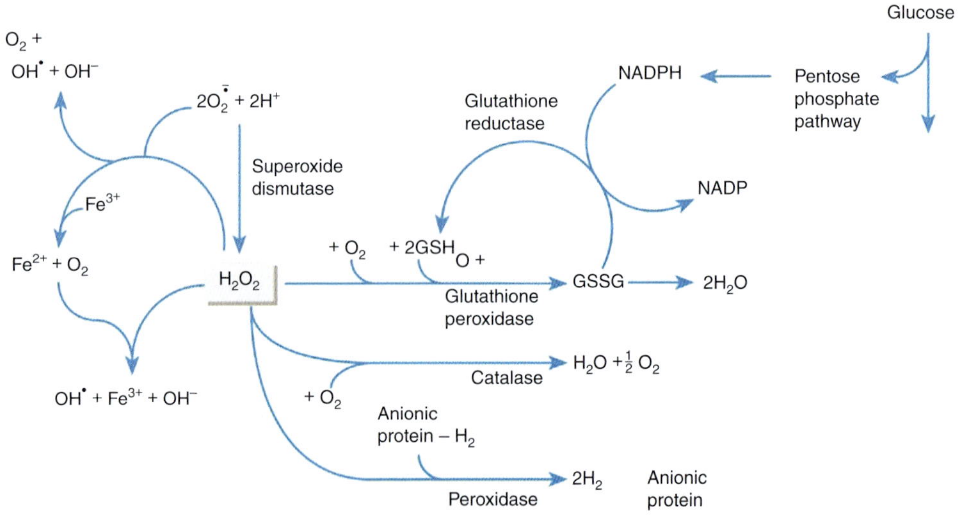

Figure 14-1 Generation and detoxification of reactive oxygen species. *Left,* Generation of hydroxyl radicals (OH•) through the reaction of iron with the superoxide anion ($O_2^{\bullet-}$) and hydrogen peroxide (H_2O_2). *Center,* Conversion of $O_2^{\bullet-}$ into H_2O_2 and the 3 subsequent pathways involved in eliminating it via (1) glutathione peroxidase; (2) catalase; and (3) peroxidase. *Right,* The role of the glucose-initiated pentose phosphate pathway in providing reduced glutathione (GSH) for redox reactions. GSSG = oxidized glutathione; $NADP^+$ = nicotinamide adenine dinucleotide phosphate; NADPH = reduced $NADP^+$. *(Modified with permission from Forrester JV, Dick AD, McMenamin PG, Roberts F, Pearlman E.* The Eye: Basic Sciences in Practice. *4th ed. St Louis: Saunders; 2016:194.)*

Table 14-1 ROS and Antioxidant Pathways

ROS	ROS Source	Antioxidants Involved in Detoxification
Superoxide anion ($O_2^{\cdot -}$)	Electron transport chain (mitochondria), respiratory burst (neutrophils), xanthine oxidase	Superoxide dismutase
Hydroxyl radical (OH•)	Electron transport chain (mitochondria), respiratory burst (neutrophils)	Catalase and peroxidase
Hydrogen peroxide (H_2O_2)	Electron transport chain (mitochondria), respiratory burst (neutrophils), superoxide dismutase	Catalase and peroxidase, glutathione peroxidase
Singlet oxygen ($^1O_2$)	Photo-oxidation	Carotenoids (quenching)

ROS = reactive oxygen species.

Lipid Peroxidation

Lipid peroxidation occurs via auto-oxidation and photo-oxidation. Random oxidation of lipids occurs by the process of *auto-oxidation,* a free radical chain reaction usually described as a series of 3 steps:

1. initiation
2. propagation
3. termination

During the initiation step, fatty acids are converted to an intermediate radical following removal of an allylic hydrogen. The propagation step follows immediately, and the fatty acid radical intermediate reacts with oxygen at both ends to produce fatty acid peroxy radicals (ROO•); this process is known as *lipid peroxidation.* Thus, a new fatty acid radical is formed, which again can react with oxygen. As long as oxygen is available, a single free radical can cause oxidation of thousands of fatty acids. A termination reaction, in which 2 radicals form a nonradical product, can interrupt the chain reaction. Auto-oxidation is also inhibited by free radical scavengers such as vitamin E, which cause termination reactions (Fig 14-2).

PUFAs are susceptible to auto-oxidation because their allylic hydrogen atoms are easily removed by several types of initiating radicals. The primary products of auto-oxidation formed during the propagation step are hydroperoxides (ROOH), which may decompose, especially in the presence of trace amounts of transition metal ions (eg, ferrous [reduced iron, Fe^{2+}] or cupric [reduced copper, Cu^{1+}]), to create ROO•, OH•, and oxy radicals (RO•).

In *photo-oxidation,* by contrast, oxygen is activated by light to form $^1O_2$, which in turn reacts with unsaturated fatty acids or other cellular constituents. The most widely accepted mechanism of $^1O_2$ generation involves exposure of a photosensitizer to light in the presence of normal triplet oxygen ($^3O_2$). Photo-oxidation can be inhibited by $^1O_2$ quenchers such as carotenoids (see the section Carotenoids) (see Fig 14-2).

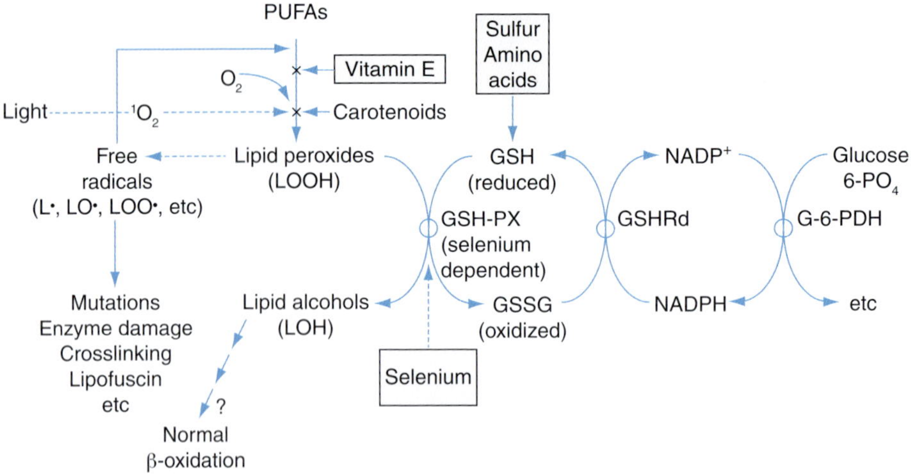

Figure 14-2 Mechanisms by which several antioxidants protect against oxidative damage. *Upper left,* Free radicals lead to the formation of lipid peroxides. Vitamin E inhibits this auto-oxidation process by scavenging free radical intermediates. Carotenoids inhibit photo-oxidation by quenching singlet oxygen ($^1O_2$). *Center,* If lipid hydroperoxides are formed, they can be reduced by glutathione peroxidase (GSH-Px), which requires selenium as a cofactor. If these protective enzymes are not fully active, more free radicals are formed by the breakdown of lipid peroxides, which in turn leads to additional oxidation of polyunsaturated fatty acids. G-6-PDH = glucose-6-phosphate dehydrogenase; GSH = glutathione; GSHRd = glutathione reductase; GSSG = oxidized glutathione; $NADP^+$ = nicotinamide adenine dinucleotide phosphate; NADPH = reduced $NADP^+$; PUFAs = polyunsaturated fatty acids. *(Courtesy of F. J. G. M. van Kuijk, MD, PhD.)*

Lipid peroxidation causes not only direct damage to the cell membrane but also secondary damage to cells through its breakdown products. Lipid peroxides are unstable, and they break down to form many aldehydes, such as malondialdehyde and 4-hydroxyalkenals. These aldehydes can quickly react with proteins, inhibiting the proteins' normal functions. Both the lens and the retina are susceptible to such oxidative damage.

Reactive Oxygen Species and Defense Mechanisms

Although the eye is constantly exposed to light, it is protected from the consequences of UV-light exposure via various mechanisms employed by different ocular structures. The cornea and the lens prevent different wavelengths of UV light from reaching the retina (see Chapter 10, Fig 10-3). The high concentration of ascorbate (vitamin C) in the aqueous and vitreous also acts to block UV light and participates in cellular antioxidant pathways.

Cellular components are protected from ROS by antioxidant mechanisms. Cells contain enzymes that neutralize ROS and the toxic metabolites formed by the interaction between ROS and cellular components (see Fig 14-1). These enzymes include superoxide dismutase (SOD), catalase, glutathione reductase, and glutathione peroxidase (GSH-Px); they are discussed later in the chapter. The transcription factor *nuclear factor erythroid 2-related factor 2* (Nrf2) regulates expression of numerous antioxidant genes and is upregulated under oxidative stress. Nrf2 is a potential therapeutic target, and induction of Nrf2 enhanced RGC survival in experimental models of oxidative stress generated by ischemia–reperfusion injury.

The cell is also protected from ROS by compartmentalizing these species, preventing their contact with intracellular components. An example of this is the electron transport chain, which is contained within the walls of the mitochondria. However, some reactive species may leak out of their enzyme-binding sites or escape antioxidant enzymes, causing damage to cellular components such as proteins, membrane lipids, and DNA. In addition, any free iron (Fe^{2+}) present may catalyze formation of OH• from superoxide and H_2O_2 (see Fig 14-1).

CLINICAL PEARL

Formation of H_2O_2 by free iron (Fe^{2+}) is the mechanism underlying damage to structures in the eye in siderosis bulbi and hemosiderosis bulbi. The former is due to iron released into the eye from a retained intraocular foreign body; the latter, from the breakdown of hemoglobin molecules in cases of intraocular hemorrhage. In both conditions, excess Fe^{2+} can accumulate in the trabecular meshwork, neurosensory retina, and retinal pigment epithelium (RPE), leading to secondary dysfunction. See BCSC Section 11, *Lens and Cataract,* and Section 12, *Retina and Vitreous,* for additional discussion of siderosis bulbi.

Oxidative Damage to the Lens and Protective Mechanisms

As stated earlier, ROS are generated by metabolic processes, inflammatory responses, and exposure to UV light. The lens relies almost entirely on anaerobic metabolism and is shielded from the immune system. Thus, the major source of ROS in the lens is exposure to UV light. Although most UVB radiation (<320-nm wavelength) striking the human eye is absorbed either by the cornea or by the ascorbate present at high levels in the aqueous humor, a certain amount reaches the lens epithelium, where it can cause damage. UVA light (320–400-nm wavelength) can penetrate more deeply into the lens, where it can react with various chromophores to generate H_2O_2, $O_2^{\bullet -}$, and $^1O_2$.

Although repair and regeneration mechanisms are active in the lens epithelium and superficial cortex, no such mechanisms exist in the deep cortex and the nucleus, where any damage to lens proteins and membrane lipids is irreversible. One result of this damage can be crosslinking and insolubilization of proteins, leading to loss of transparency (see Chapter 10 in this volume and BCSC Section 11, *Lens and Cataract*). The lens contains unusually high levels of protein sulfhydryl groups that must exist almost entirely in the reduced state for the tissue to remain transparent. The young, healthy lens possesses a variety of effective antioxidant systems to protect against oxidative stress. These defenses include the enzymes glutathione reductase, GSH-Px, catalase, and SOD (see Fig 14-1).

Glutathione (GSH), concentrated at the lens epithelium, acts as a major scavenger of ROS in the lens. With age, levels of GSH decline significantly in the human lens, particularly in the nucleus. Studies have indicated that a cortical–nuclear barrier may exist in the mature human lens, which inhibits the free flow of GSH to the nucleus. As a result, the human lens nucleus becomes more susceptible to oxidative damage and cataract formation with age.

The free radical scavengers ascorbate and vitamin E, also present in the lens, work in conjunction with GSH and the GSH oxidation-reduction (redox) cycle to protect against oxidative damage (see Fig 14-2). Carotenoids that can quench $^1O_2$ also exist in the lens. Epidemiologic (observational) studies have shown that individuals with higher levels of plasma antioxidants, particularly vitamin E, have a reduced risk of cataract, especially nuclear cataract. However, 3 prospective randomized placebo-controlled clinical trials—Age-Related Eye Disease Study (AREDS); Age-Related Eye Disease Study 2 (AREDS2); and the Vitamin E, Cataract, and Age-Related Maculopathy Trial (VECAT)—found that high-dose formulations of antioxidants neither prevented the development nor slowed the progression of age-related cataracts.

Age-Related Eye Disease Study Research Group. A randomized, placebo-controlled clinical trial of high-dose supplementation with vitamins C and E and beta carotene for age-related cataract and vision loss: AREDS report no. 9. *Arch Ophthalmol.* 2001;119(10):1439–1452. [Erratum appears in *Arch Ophthalmol.* 2008;126(9):1251.]

Age-Related Eye Disease Study 2 (AREDS2) Research Group; Chew EY, SanGiovanni JP, Ferris FL, et al. Lutein/zeaxanthin for the treatment of age-related cataract: AREDS2 randomized trial report no. 4. *JAMA Ophthalmol.* 2013;131(7):843–850.

Cetinel S, Semenchenko V, Cho JY, et al. UV-B induced fibrillization of crystallin protein mixtures. *PLoS One.* 2017;12(5):e0177991.

McNeil JJ, Robman L, Tikellis G, Sinclair MI, McCarty CA, Taylor HR. Vitamin E supplementation and cataract: randomized controlled trial. *Ophthalmology.* 2004;111(1):75–84.

Vulnerability of the Retina to Reactive Oxygen Species

Experimental data have shown that retinal photoreceptors degenerate when exposed to oxidative challenges such as hyperbaric oxygen, iron overload, or injection of lipid peroxide into the vitreous humor. In addition, the retina degenerates when antioxidant defenses are reduced, which presumably increases lipid peroxidation even in the absence of unusual oxidative stress. The retina has several distinctive characteristics that make it vulnerable to damage from lipid peroxidation; 4 of them are considered here:

- Vertebrate rod outer segments are susceptible to damage by oxygen because of their high levels of PUFAs. Their phospholipids contain docosahexaenoic acid, the most highly polyunsaturated fatty acid occurring in nature. It is well established that PUFAs are sensitive to peroxidation in proportion to their number of double bonds.
- Rod inner segments are very rich in mitochondria. The majority of endogenous ROS are produced by the mitochondrial electron transport chain, which may leak activated oxygen species.
- The abundant oxygen supply through the choroid and the retinal vessels elevates the risk of oxidative damage. Vertebrate retinas maintained in vitro showed at least

a sevenfold-higher rate of oxygen consumption per milligram of protein than all other tissues tested (except the adrenal gland). The oxygen tension is highest at the choroid and decreases toward the inner segments of the retina.
- There are many chromophores in the outer retina. Light exposure may trigger photo-oxidative processes mediated by $^1O_2$.

Intense light at levels that may be encountered in daily life is phototoxic to the retina. Even though the cornea absorbs UV radiation, the retinas of young people are exposed to UV light in the range of 350–400 nm (young lenses transmit these wavelengths). As the lens yellows with age, it can block wavelengths of up to approximately 430 nm. Because the adult lens absorbs nearly 100% of light below 400 nm, little or no UV light reaches the retina in older people.

Antioxidants in the Retina and Retinal Pigment Epithelium

As mentioned earlier, several antioxidant mechanisms have been established in biological systems, including free radical scavenging, quenching of $^1O_2$, and enzymatic reduction of ROOH. Antioxidants found in vertebrate retinas and RPE include the following:

- selenium
- GSH
- selenium-dependent GSH-Px
- non–selenium-dependent GSH-Px (glutathione-S-transferase)
- vitamin E
- SOD
- catalase
- carotenoids

See Figure 14-2, which depicts the relation between some of these antioxidants and the protective mechanisms.

Yu BP. Cellular defenses against damage from reactive oxygen species. *Physiol Rev.* 1994;74(1): 139–162.

Selenium, Glutathione, and Glutathione Peroxidase

The role of GSH (discussed earlier in the chapter) is depicted in Figures 14-1 and 14-2. The primary enzyme involved in GSH-mediated detoxification of peroxides is GSH-Px, which is selenium dependent. The highest concentration of selenium in the human eye is present in the RPE: 100–400 ng in the RPE cells of a single human eye, up to 10 times as many as in the retina (40 ng). The selenium level in the human retina remains constant with age; in the human RPE, however, the level increases with age.

González de Vega R, García M, Fernández-Sánchez ML, González-Iglesias H, Sanz-Medel A. Protective effect of selenium supplementation following oxidative stress mediated by glucose on retinal pigment epithelium. *Metallomics.* 2018;10(1):83–92.

Vitamin E

Vitamin E scavenges free radicals, thus terminating the propagation step (described earlier in the chapter) and leading to interruption of the auto-oxidation reaction. A detailed study of the vitamin E content of microdissected parts of vertebrate eyes showed that the RPE is rich in vitamin E relative to photoreceptors and that photoreceptors are rich in vitamin E relative to most other cells in the eye. Furthermore, vitamin E levels in human retinal tissues increase with age until the sixth decade of life, after which they decrease. This decrease coincides with the age at which the incidence of AMD increases in the population.

Friedrichson T, Kalbach HL, Buck P, van Kuijk FJ. Vitamin E in macular and peripheral tissues of the human eye. *Curr Eye Res.* 1995;14(8):693–701.

Superoxide Dismutase and Catalase

Superoxide dismutase catalyzes the dismutation of superoxide to H_2O_2, which is further reduced to water by catalase or peroxidase. Two types of SOD are isolated from mammalian tissues: (1) copper-zinc SOD (CuZnSOD), the cytoplasmic enzyme, which is inhibited by cyanide; and (2) manganese SOD (MnSOD), the mitochondrial enzyme, which is not inhibited by cyanide. SOD activity and polymorphisms have been implicated in AMD in certain populations.

Catalase catalyzes the reduction of H_2O_2 to water. At present, information on catalase activity in the retina is limited. Total retinal catalase activity has been found to be very low but detectable in rabbits. A protective role for catalase has been reported in rats with retinal ischemia–reperfusion injury, where it prevented RGC loss and preserved function as shown by electroretinography. In addition, treatment with catalase was shown to be protective against hyperglycemia-induced oxidative stress in cell culture and animal models.

Anand A, Sharma NK, Gupta A, Prabhakar S, Sharma SK, Singh R. Superoxide dismutase1 levels in North Indian population with age-related macular degeneration. *Oxid Med Cell Longev.* 2013;2013:365046.

Chen B, Tang L. Protective effects of catalase on retinal ischemia/reperfusion injury in rats. *Exp Eye Res.* 2011;93(5):599–606.

Kowalski M, Bielecka-Kowalska A, Oszajca K, et al. Manganese superoxide dismutase (MnSOD) gene (Ala-9Val, Ile58Thr) polymorphism in patients with age-related macular degeneration (AMD). *Med Sci Monit.* 2010;16(4):CR190–196.

Ohta Y, Yamasaki T, Niwa T, Niimi K, Majima I, Ishiguro I. Role of catalase in retinal antioxidant defence system: its comparative study among rabbits, guinea pigs, and rats. *Ophthalmic Res.* 1996;28(6):336–642.

Ascorbate

In many species, ascorbate (vitamin C) is found throughout the eye in concentrations that are high relative to those in other tissues. In addition to blocking UV light in the aqueous humor, ascorbate is thought to function synergistically with vitamin E to terminate free radical reactions. Vitamin C functions as an electron donor, reducing oxidized elements and molecules. It has been proposed that vitamin C can react with the vitamin E radicals formed when vitamin E scavenges free radicals. Vitamin E radicals are then regenerated to form native vitamin E. The vitamin C radicals resulting from this regeneration can be reduced by nicotinamide adenine dinucleotide (NADH) reductase, with NADH as the electron acceptor. Ascorbate is found at high levels in the aqueous humor as well as in the vitreous, where it also functions to reduce oxygen levels (see Chapter 11, Fig 11-6).

Buettner GR. The pecking order of free radicals and antioxidants: lipid peroxidation, alpha-tocopherol, and ascorbate. *Arch Biochem Biophys.* 1993;300(2):535–543.

Reddy VN, Giblin FJ, Lin LR, Chakrapani B. The effect of aqueous humor ascorbate on ultraviolet-B-induced DNA damage in lens epithelium. *Invest Ophthalmol Vis Sci.* 1998; 39(2):344–350.

Rose RC, Bode AM. Ocular ascorbate transport and metabolism. *Comp Biochem Physiol A Comp Physiol.* 1991;100(2):273–285.

Carotenoids

Carotenoids (xanthophylls) have been proposed to play various roles in biological systems, including limiting chromatic aberration at the fovea of the retina and quenching of $^1O_2$. Beta carotene, the precursor of vitamin A, can act as a free radical trap at low oxygen tension. Studies of postmortem human retinas have shown that carotenoids make up the yellow pigment in the macula. Two carotenoids, *lutein* and *zeaxanthin,* are present in the macula and located in the Henle fiber layer. In humans, zeaxanthin is concentrated primarily in the fovea, whereas lutein is dispersed throughout the retina. Interestingly, little beta carotene is present in the human eye. Furthermore, carotenoids are present only in the retina and are absent from the RPE. In the peripheral retina, lutein and zeaxanthin are concentrated in rod outer segments and may act as antioxidants to protect against short-wavelength visible light. Figure 14-3A shows the localization of antioxidants in the human macula and peripheral retina, and Figure 14-3B shows their localization in a cross section of the peripheral retina.

Chew EY, Clemons TE, Agrón E, et al. Long-term effects of vitamins C and E, beta-carotene, and zinc on age-related macular degeneration. AREDS report no. 35. *Ophthalmology.* 2013;120(8):1604–1611.

Khachik F, Bernstein PS, Garland DL. Identification of lutein and zeaxanthin oxidation products in human and monkey retinas. *Invest Ophthalmol Vis Sci.* 1997;38(9):1802–1811.

The Role of Oxidative Stress in Vision-Threatening Ophthalmic Diseases

Reactive oxygen species and oxidative stress have been directly implicated in the pathogenesis of several diseases that are the leading causes of blindness, including glaucoma, diabetic retinopathy, and AMD. In many cases, the onset of oxidative damage may precede the clinical manifestation of these conditions.

In addition to their role in the diseases discussed in the following sections, oxidative mechanisms are involved in numerous diseases of the anterior and posterior segments and are central in many inherited diseases of the eye. Future research and treatment will

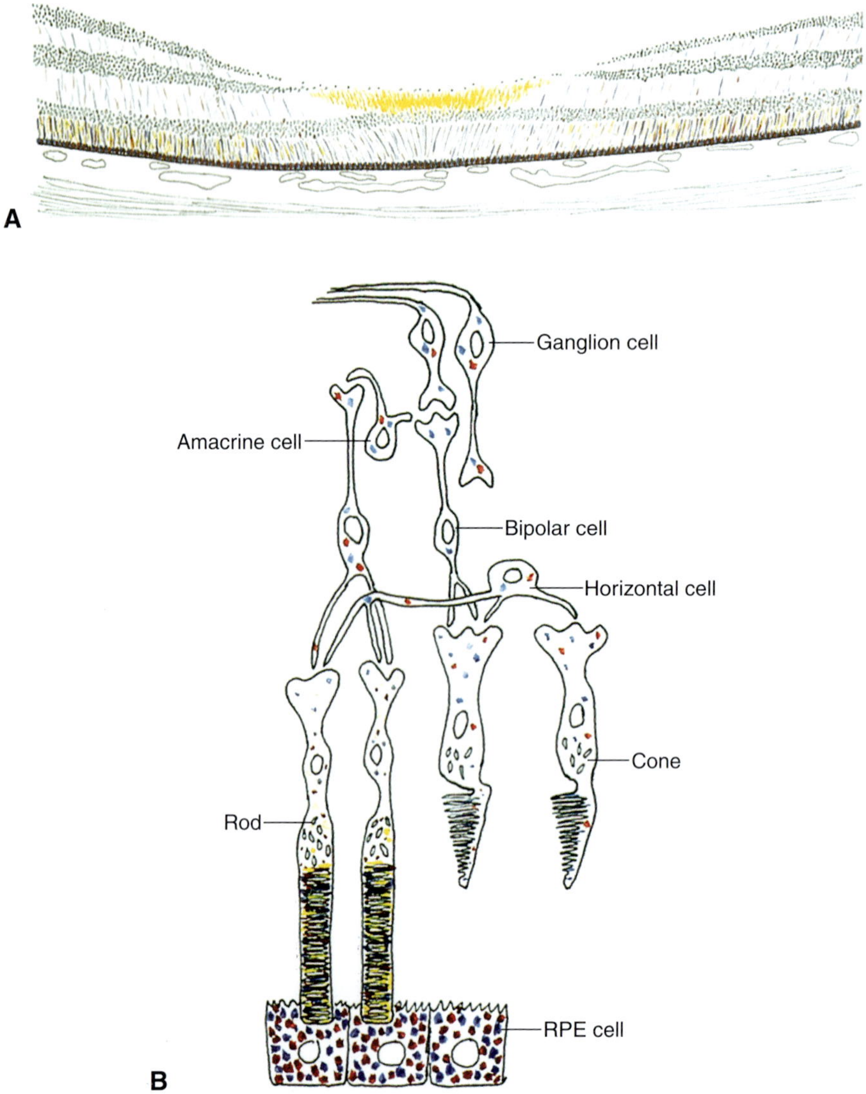

Figure 14-3 **A,** Localization of antioxidants in the human macula and peripheral retina. Vitamin E *(blue)* and selenium *(red)* are concentrated primarily in the retinal pigment epithelium (RPE). In the macula, carotenoids *(yellow)* are present in the Henle fiber layer; in the peripheral retina, they are also present in the rods. **B,** Localization of antioxidants in a cross section of the peripheral retina. Vitamin E and selenium remain concentrated mainly in the RPE but are also enriched in the rod outer segments. Carotenoids have been found in rod outer segments in the peripheral retina. *(Illustrations by J. Woodward, MD; courtesy of F. J. G. M. van Kuijk, MD, PhD.)*

target these mechanisms, directly and indirectly, to aid in the management of their related conditions.

Ung L, Pattamatta U, Carnt N, Wildinson-Berka JL, Liew G, White AJR. Oxidative stress and reactive oxygen species: a review of their role in ocular disease. *Clin Sci (London).* 2017;131(24):2865–2883.

Glaucoma

Reactive oxygen species' involvement in glaucoma may pertain to their effect on the trabecular meshwork and RGCs. An increasing body of evidence suggests that trabecular dysfunction occurs following exposure of the trabecular meshwork to ROS. In addition, several reports have demonstrated the development of oxidative stress and cell loss when RGCs in culture are exposed to increased pressure.

Population-based studies on the effect of dietary antioxidants have shown conflicting results in glaucoma, and earlier studies failed to show a benefit of these antioxidants. However, a more recent study, with longer follow-up, demonstrated that the risk of developing primary open-angle glaucoma (POAG) was 20% lower in participants who consume more foods high in antioxidants. Furthermore, in patients with POAG, a similar diet reduced the risk of development of paracentral visual field defects by 44%. The mechanism of such an effect has been suggested to involve aberrant nitric oxide pathways.

Benoist d'Azy C, Pereira B, Chiambaretta F, Dutheiul F. Oxidative and anti-oxidative stress markers in chronic glaucoma: a systematic review and meta-analysis. *PLoS One*. 2016;11(12):e0166915.

Kang JH, Willett WC, Rosner BA, Buys E, Wiggs JL, Pasquale LR. Association of dietary nitrate intake with primary open-angle glaucoma: a prospective analysis from the Nurses' Health Study and Health Professionals Follow-up Study. *JAMA Ophthalmol.* 2016;134(3):294–303.

Diabetic Retinopathy

Diabetic retinopathy is the leading cause of blindness worldwide in adults aged 20 to 64 years. Several metabolic pathways, initiated by hyperglycemia and lack of insulin signaling, generate oxidative stress and are implicated in the development of diabetic retinopathy:

- polyol pathway
- protein kinase C (PKC) pathway
- hexosamine pathway

Advanced glycation end products (AGEs) result from nonenzymatic glycation of various molecules (proteins, lipids, nucleic acids) and exist in foods prepared at very high temperatures. AGEs interact with specific cell surface receptors, which then signal intracellular inflammatory pathways, leading to generation of ROS.

ROS can lead to long-term changes via epigenetic modification, especially in mitochondrial DNA. This may partly explain the phenomenon of metabolic memory, wherein beneficial effects of past tight metabolic control persist for a period, reducing the progression of retinopathy, as demonstrated by the Diabetes Control and Complications Trial (DCCT). Conversely, in patients with poor metabolic control, epigenetic modifications may allow diabetic retinopathy to progress even after intensive control has been achieved. Most data supporting a role for antioxidants in diabetic retinopathy have come from cell culture or animal models. One clinical trial evaluated the role of the PKC inhibitor ruboxistaurin, which reduced vision loss and the need for macular laser therapy in comparison to controls in patients with diabetic retinopathy.

CLINICAL PEARL

Radiation retinopathy is an example of retinal damage from ROS. Clinically, the retinal findings in this condition are comparable to those of diabetic retinopathy. Diabetic retinopathy and complications of radiation retinopathy, such as macular edema and retinal neovascularization, are therefore managed similarly.

Aiello LP, Vignati L, Sheetz MJ, et al; PKC-DRS and PKC-DRS2 Study Groups. Oral protein kinase c β inhibition using ruboxistaurin: efficacy, safety, and causes of vision loss among 813 patients (1,392 eyes) with diabetic retinopathy in the Protein Kinase C β Inhibitor-Diabetic Retinopathy Study and the Protein Kinase C β Inhibitor-Diabetic Retinopathy Study 2. *Retina*. 2011;31(10):2084–2094.

Li C, Miao X, Li F, et al. Oxidative stress-related mechanisms and antioxidant therapy in diabetic retinopathy. *Oxid Med Cell Longev*. 2017;2017:9702820.

Reichstein D. Current treatments and preventive strategies for radiation retinopathy. *Curr Opin Ophthalmol.* 2015;26(3):157–166.

Van Puyvelde K, Mets T, Njemini R, Beyer I, Bautmans I. Effect of advanced glycation end product intake on inflammation and aging: a systematic review. *Nutr Rev.* 2014; 72(10):638–650.

Age-Related Macular Degeneration

Age-related macular degeneration (AMD) represents the leading cause of blindness in the Western world. Risk factors related to oxidative mechanisms include sunlight exposure, smoking, and to some extent genetics. Several models demonstrate the protective effect of antioxidants in this condition. AREDS and AREDS2 represent 2 of the largest prospective randomized clinical trials studying the effects of antioxidants on the eye, especially the development of lenticular opacity and the development and progression of AMD. No data confirmed a role for oral supplements in the development of cataract; however, both trials supported the role of antioxidants in limiting the progression of AMD in high-risk patients. See BCSC Section 12, *Retina and Vitreous,* for further discussion of AREDS.

Age-Related Eye Disease Study 2 Research Group. Lutein + zeaxanthin and omega-3 fatty acids for age-related macular degeneration: the Age-Related Eye Disease Study 2 (AREDS2) randomized clinical trial. *JAMA*. 2013;309(19):2005–2015.

Shaw PX, Stiles T, Douglas C, et al. Oxidative stress, innate immunity, and age-related macular degeneration. *AIMS Mol Sci*. 2016;3(2):196–221.

PART V

Ocular Pharmacology

Introduction to Pharmacologic Principles

This chapter reviews the general principles of pharmacology and includes discussion of special features of the eye that facilitate or impede ocular therapy.

Pharmacokinetics

Pharmacokinetics concerns the movement of a drug through the body, including the absorption, distribution, metabolism, and excretion of that drug. To achieve a therapeutic effect, a drug must reach its site of action in sufficient concentration. The concentration at the site of action is a function of the following:

- route of administration
- amount administered
- extent and rate of absorption at the administration site
- distribution and binding of the drug in tissues
- movement by bulk flow in circulating fluids
- transport between body compartments
- biotransformation
- excretion

Pharmacokinetics and dose together determine *bioavailability,* or concentration of the active drug at the therapeutic site.

Pharmacodynamics

Pharmacodynamics concerns the biological activity and clinical effects of a drug—the drug action after distribution (pharmacokinetics) of the active agent to the therapeutic site. Included within the area of pharmacodynamics are the tissue receptor for the drug and the intracellular changes initiated by binding of the active drug with the receptor. The pharmacodynamic action of a drug is often described using the receptor for that drug; for example, a drug may be categorized as an α-adrenergic agonist or a β-adrenergic antagonist.

Pharmacotherapeutics

Pharmacotherapeutics is the study of the uses of drugs in reaching a given clinical endpoint, such as the prevention or treatment of disease. The therapeutic dose may vary for any patient and is related to the patient's age, sex, race, other currently prescribed medications, and preexisting medical conditions. Pharmacotherapeutics is covered in Chapter 16.

Toxicity

Toxicity refers to the adverse effects of either medications or environmental chemicals, including poisoning. Toxicity may be influenced by pharmacokinetics and/or pharmacodynamics (the biochemical and physiological effects of a drug/agent). For example, topically applied ophthalmic medications are readily absorbed through the mucous membranes of the eye and nasopharynx, as well as through the iris and ciliary body. Topical absorption avoids the first-pass metabolism of the liver and increases systemic bioavailability. Therefore, the systemic toxicity of these medications may be greater than expected relative to the total topical dose.

The importance of pharmacokinetics and its influence on potential toxicity can be illustrated by the pediatric population. Drug metabolism and excretion are less developed in neonates and infants than in adults. For example, in early neonatal life, the drug-metabolizing activities of the cytochrome P450–dependent, mixed-function oxidases and the conjugating enzymes are approximately 50%–70% of those in adults. A second example is the formation of glucuronide, which does not reach adult levels until the third or fourth year of life. Similarly, the glomerular filtration rate is low in young infants, reaching the adult value by 6–12 months of life. Therefore, drug doses and dosing schedules must be adjusted appropriately in pediatric populations to avoid toxicity.

Local toxicity of topical drugs is more common than systemic toxicity. Local toxicity may be a type I immunoglobulin E (IgE)–mediated hypersensitivity reaction, or it may represent a delayed hypersensitivity reaction to either the medication itself or its associated preservatives.

Preservatives and toxicity

Preservatives commonly used in ophthalmic preparations include quaternary cationic surfactants such as benzalkonium chloride and benzododecinium bromide; mercurial agents such as thimerosal, chlorobutanol, and parahydroxybenzoates; and aromatic alcohols. The preservatives used in ophthalmic solutions can be toxic to the ocular surface following topical administration; they can also enhance the corneal permeability of various drugs.

Preservatives have been developed that use different methods to reduce the toxic effect on the ocular surface. One method allows the preservative to dissipate upon exposure to light or to the ions in the tear film. Two examples of preservatives using this method are stabilized oxychloro complex, which breaks down to sodium chloride and water, and sodium perborate, which breaks down to hydrogen peroxide before becoming oxygen and hydrogen. Theoretically, these "disappearing preservatives" should have no toxic effect on the corneal surface.

Other preservative systems may be less toxic to the ocular surface than quaternary cationic surfactants such as benzalkonium chloride. One such system is an ionic buffer containing borate, sorbitol, propylene glycol, and zinc that breaks down into innate elements upon encountering the cations in the tear film. Polyquaternium-1, another preservative system, is a cationic polymer of quaternary ammonium structures that lacks a hydrophobic region. Although polyquaternium-1 is a detergent, human corneal epithelial cells tend to repel the compound.

To completely eliminate toxicity from preservatives, some topical ophthalmic products are available preservative-free, in single-use containers.

Pharmacologic Principles and Elderly Patients

Pharmacologic principles apply differently to elderly patients. Compared with younger patients, elderly patients have less lean body mass because of a decrease in muscle bulk, less body water and albumin, and an increased relative percentage of adipose tissue. These physiologic differences alter tissue binding and distribution of a drug. Human renal function declines with age; both hepatic perfusion and enzymatic activity are variably affected as well. Older patients tend to take more medications for chronic conditions than do younger patients, and many of the drugs they use are processed simultaneously by their already-compromised metabolic systems.

According to the National Kidney Foundation, the average estimated glomerular filtration rate (GFR) in different age groups is as follows:

- 20–29 years: 116 mL/min/1.73 m^2
- 30–39 years: 107 mL/min/1.73 m^2
- 40–49 years: 99 mL/min/1.73 m^2
- 50–59 years: 93 mL/min/1.73 m^2
- 60–69 years: 85 mL/min/1.73 m^2
- 70 years and older: 75 mL/min/1.73 m^2

The pharmacokinetic processing of drugs in elderly patients is thus significantly altered, extending the effective half-life of most medications. The pharmacodynamic action of a drug is often independently potentiated in these patients. The increase in both drug effect and adverse effects occurs even when the dose is decreased in consideration of these pharmacokinetic differences. Thus, the pharmacotherapeutic effects and toxicity of a medication may be altered simply by the aging process, independent of drug dosage. Accordingly, the selection of a specific therapeutic agent should be guided by the general health and age of the individual, as well as by concomitant medication used by the patient.

Awwad S, Mohamed Ahmed AHA, Sharma G, et al. Principles of pharmacology in the eye. *Br J Pharmacol.* 2017;174(23):4205–4223.

Pharmacokinetics: The Route of Drug Delivery

Topical Administration: Eyedrops

Most ocular medications are administered topically as eyedrops. This route of administration maximizes the anterior segment concentrations while minimizing systemic toxicity. The drug gradient, from the concentrated tear reservoir to the relatively barren corneal and conjunctival epithelia, forces a passive route of absorption (Fig 15-1).

Retention of topical agents

Some features of topical ocular therapy limit treatment effectiveness. Very little of an administered drop is retained by the eye. When a 50-μL drop is delivered from a conventional commercial dispenser, the volume of the tear lake rises from 7 μL to only 10 μL in the blinking eye of an upright patient. Thus, at most, 20% of the administered drug is retained (10 μL/50 μL). A rapid turnover of fluid also occurs in the tear lake—16% per minute in the undisturbed eye—with even faster turnover if the drop elicits reflex tearing. Consequently, for slowly absorbed drugs, at most only 50% of the drug that was initially

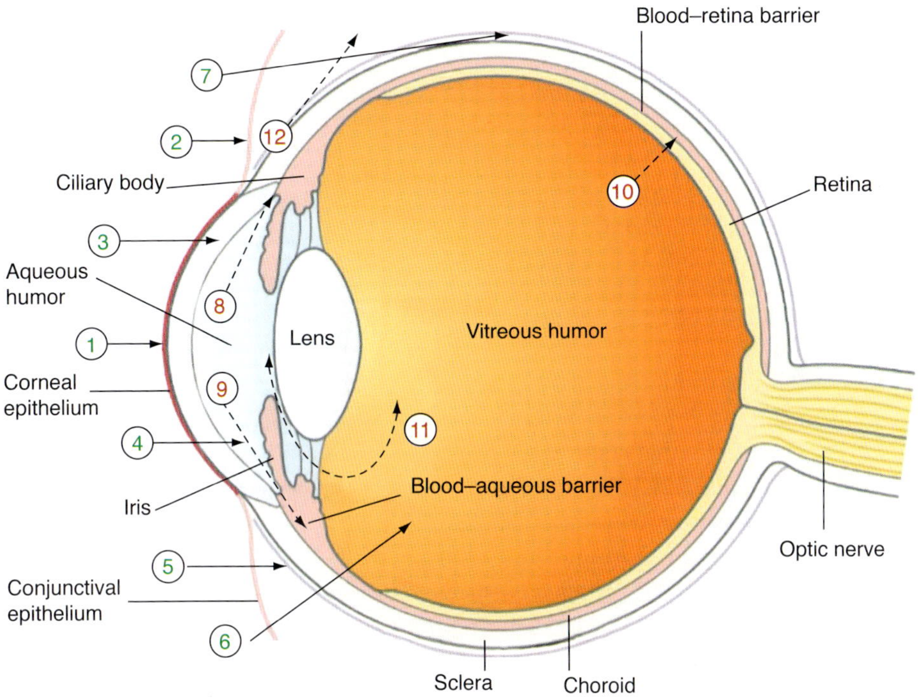

Delivery routes
1. Transcorneal
2. Transconjunctival
3. Intrastromal
4. Intracameral
5. Subconjunctival
6. Intravitreal
7. Sub-Tenon

Elimination pathways (from)
8. Trabecular meshwork and Schlemm canal
9. Uvea
10. Blood–retina barrier
11. Anterior hyaloid to posterior chamber or vice versa
12. Subconjunctival and/or episcleral space

Figure 15-1 Diagram of the eye with common drug delivery routes and elimination pathways. *Delivery routes:* (1) Transcorneal route from the tear film across the cornea into the anterior chamber; (2) transconjunctival route across the conjunctiva, sclera, and anterior uvea into the posterior chamber; (3) intrastromal route directly into corneal stroma; (4) intracameral route directly into anterior chamber; (5) subconjunctival route from the anterior subconjunctival space across the sclera and anterior uvea into the posterior chamber or across the sclera, choroid, retinal pigment epithelium (RPE), and retina into the anterior vitreous; (6) intravitreal drug injection directly into the vitreous; (7) sub-Tenon route from the posterior sub-Tenon space across the sclera, choroid, RPE, and retina into the posterior vitreous; *absorption pathways:* (8) elimination of drug in the aqueous humor across the trabecular meshwork and Schlemm canal into the systemic vascular circulation; (9) elimination of drug in the aqueous humor across the uvea into the systemic vascular circulation; (10) elimination of drug in the vitreous humor across the blood–retina barrier to the systemic vascular circulation; (11) drug elimination from the vitreous across the anterior hyaloid to the posterior chamber or vice versa; (12) drug elimination from subconjunctival and/or episcleral space to systemic lymphatic or vascular circulation. *(Modified with permission from Levin LA, Nilsson SFE, Ver Hoeve J, Wu SM.* Adler's Physiology of the Eye. *11th ed. Philadelphia: Elsevier/Saunders; 2011:113.)*

retained in the tear reservoir, or 10% of the original dose (50% of the 20% of the delivered medication), remains 4 minutes after instillation, and only 17%, or 3.4% of the original dose, remains after 10 minutes.

The amount of time that a drug remains in the tear reservoir and tear film is called the *residence time* of a medication. This time is affected not only by drug formulation but also by the timing of subsequent medication, tear production, and drainage.

Some simple measures have been shown to improve ocular absorption of materials that do not traverse the cornea rapidly:

- Patients using more than 1 topical ocular medication should be instructed to allow 5 minutes between instillation of drops; otherwise, the second drop may simply wash out the first.
- Blinking also diminishes a drug's effect by activating the nasolacrimal pump mechanism, forcing fluid from the lacrimal sac into the nasopharynx, and creating a negative sac pressure that empties the tear lake (see BCSC Section 7, *Oculofacial Plastic and Orbital Surgery*). Patients can circumvent this loss of drug reservoir either by compressing the nasolacrimal duct through application of digital pressure at the medial canthus or by closing their eyes for 5 minutes after instillation of each drop. These 2 measures will prevent emptying of the tear lake and will reduce systemic toxicity by decreasing absorption through the nasal mucosa. Nasolacrimal occlusion will increase the absorption of topically applied materials and decrease systemic absorption and potential toxicity (Fig 15-2).
- Tear reservoir retention and drug contact time can also be extended either by increasing the viscosity of the vehicle or by using drug delivery objects such as contact lenses, collagen shields, and inserts.

Topical medications that are absorbed by the nasal mucosa can attain significant levels in the blood. One or 2 drops of a topical medication may provide a significant systemic dose of that drug. For example, a 1% solution of atropine has 1 g/100 mL, or 10 mg/1 mL. A simpler way of remembering this conversion is to add a 0 to the drug percentage to change the value to milligrams per milliliter. As there are 20 drops per milliliter (up to 40 in some

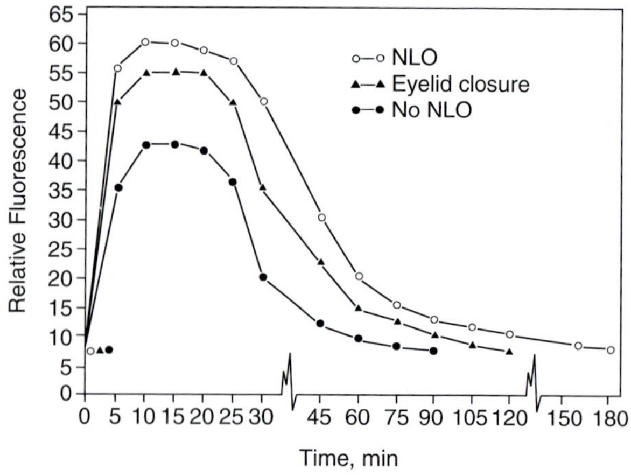

Figure 15-2 Relative fluorescence in the anterior chamber at various times after application: with nasolacrimal occlusion (NLO), with 5 minutes of eyelid closure, or with no intervention (no NLO).

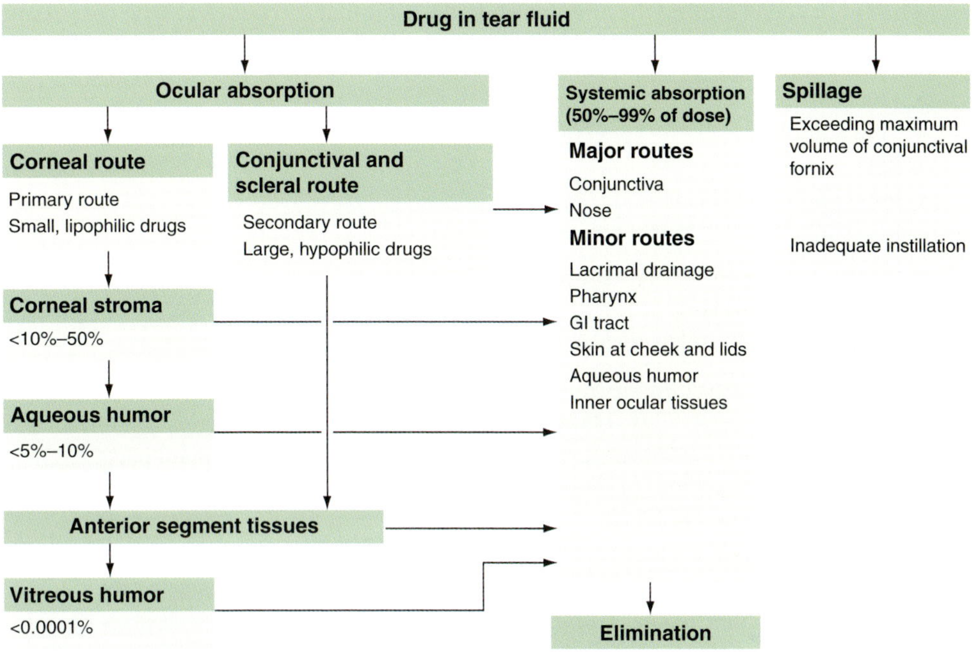

Figure 15-3 Pharmacokinetics of topical eyedrop drug delivery. GI tract = gastrointestinal tract. *(Modified with permission from Levin LA, Nilsson SFE, Ver Hoeve J, Wu SM.* Adler's Physiology of the Eye. *11th ed. Philadelphia: Elsevier/Saunders; 2011:113.)*

newer, small-tip dispensers), there is ¼–½ mg of 1% atropine per drop. If this drop is given bilaterally, up to 1 mg of active agent is available for systemic absorption, although the actual amount absorbed is limited by dilution and the washout effect of tears (Fig 15-3).

Absorption of topical agents

Because the contact time of topical medication is short, the rate of transfer from the tear fluid into the cornea is crucial. The corneal epithelium and endothelium have tight junctions that limit paracellular passage of molecules. To enter the anterior segment, topically applied medication must first pass through hydrophobic/lipophilic cell membranes in the corneal epithelium, then through the hydrophilic/lipophobic stroma, and finally through the hydrophobic/lipophilic cell membranes in the endothelium. Thus, topical ophthalmic drug formulations must be both lipophilic and hydrophilic. As nonionic particles are more lipophilic than ionic particles are, they pass through the cellular phospholipid membranes more readily. The pH of the medication can be manipulated to adjust the percentage of the drug that is in the ionized form and the nonionized form to optimize the rate of drug penetration. Mechanical disruption of the epithelial barrier in corneal abrasion or infection also increases the rate of intraocular drug penetration.

Similar considerations apply to the conjunctiva. However, the permeability of the conjunctiva to small water-soluble molecules is thought to be 20 times that of the cornea. Perilimbal conjunctiva thus offers an effective transscleral route for delivery of drugs to anterior segment structures.

The factors determining the amount of medication that can penetrate the cornea are

- concentration and solubility in the delivery vehicle
- viscosity
- lipid solubility
- pH
- ionic and steric forms
- molecular size
- chemical structure and configuration
- vehicle
- surfactants (also called *surface-active agents*)

In addition, reflex tearing and the binding of the active medication to proteins in tears and tissue affect drug bioavailability. Many preservatives used in topical drops are surfactants that can alter the barrier effect of the corneal epithelium and increase drug permeability.

Drug concentration and solubility

In order for a sufficient amount of a drug to pass through the corneal barriers, it may be necessary to load the tear reservoir with concentrated solutions (eg, by selecting pilocarpine, 4%, instead of pilocarpine, 1%). A practical limit to exploiting these high concentrations is reached when the high tonicity of the resulting solutions elicits reflex tearing or when drugs that are poorly water-soluble reach their solubility limits and precipitate. A drug with adequate solubility in an aqueous solution can be formulated as a solution, whereas a drug with poor solubility may need to be provided in a suspension.

A *suspension* is a mixture of a substance with poor solubility and a dispersion medium in which the substance is evenly distributed. A suspension requires agitation so that the active medication is redistributed before administration. Suspensions may be more irritating to the ocular surface than solutions are, a factor that may affect the choice of drug formulation. Prednisolone acetate and brinzolamide are 2 examples of a topical suspension.

An *emulsion* is similar to a suspension in that it is also a mixture of 2 components; however, the components are immiscible (not susceptible to being mixed) liquids. External force or an emulsifying agent is required to maintain the stability of the emulsion. Compared with solutions, emulsions have the advantages of increased contact time (because of the adsorption of nanodroplets on the corneal surface) and greater bioavailability. An emulsion typically has a cloudy appearance, but in contrast with a suspension, shaking the container before instillation is not necessary. Since emulsions are more viscous than solutions, patients may experience a foreign-body sensation after instillation. Difluprednate and cyclosporine are examples of a topical emulsion.

> Because the units of concentration or dilution of solution are not standardized, students of pharmacology need to familiarize themselves with conversions between different units. The solution's labeled percentage (%) represents the amount of active
>
> *(Continued)*

ingredient in the number of grams per 100 mL of solution (eg, 1% = 1 g/100 mL, or 1000 mg/100 mL, or 10 mg/1 mL). The solution concentration may also be presented in a dilution ratio. For example, a 1:1000 solution has 1 g of active ingredient per 1000 mL solution, or 1000 mg/1000 mL, or 1 mg/1 mL. Converting this ratio to a percentage, a 1:1000 solution equals a concentration of 0.1 g/100 mL, or 0.1%.

Viscosity

The addition of high-viscosity substances such as methylcellulose and polyvinyl alcohol (PVA) to a drug increases drug retention in the inferior cul-de-sac, aiding drug penetration. An example is timolol maleate formulated in gellan gum or xanthan gum, both of which are a high-molecular-weight, water-soluble, anionic polysaccharide that thickens on contact with the tear film, maintaining therapeutic levels and allowing the dosing to be decreased to once daily.

Improvement in ocular drug delivery is observed when drug viscosity is in the range of 1–15 cP (1 cP = 1 millipascal-second [mPas]); the optimal viscosity is 12–15 cP. Increases in viscosity above this level do not appear to proportionally increase the drug concentration in aqueous. In fact, formulations with higher levels of viscosity cause ocular surface irritation, resulting in reflex blinking, lacrimation, and increased drainage of the applied formulation. They may also inhibit product–tear mixing and distort the ocular surface. Products with viscosity levels that are too high may impart a sticky feeling, cause blurring of vision, and be uncomfortable for patients to use.

Lipid solubility

Lipid solubility is more important than water solubility in promoting penetration.

Studies of the permeability of isolated corneas to families of chemical compounds show that lipid solubility is more important than water solubility in promoting penetration. To determine the solubility of a drug or group of drugs, researchers ascertain the ratio of lipid solubility to water solubility for each compound in the series by (1) measuring the phase separation of a drug between 2 solvents—1 lipid-soluble and 1 water-soluble (eg, octanol and water); and (2) calculating the ratio of the drug concentration in the 2 compartments (partition coefficient). Drugs with greater relative lipid solubility have a higher partition coefficient. For example, the permeability coefficient is 70 times higher for substituted ethoxzolamides with high lipid solubility than for those of low lipid solubility. Drugs with higher levels of lipid solubility and higher partition coefficients have increased penetration of cell membranes. Compared with the parent molecules, prodrugs, such as various prostaglandin analogues, with ester or amide moieties achieve lipophilicity that is 2-fold to 3-fold higher and in vitro corneal permeability that is enhanced 25- to 40-fold. However, compounds with excessively high partition coefficients are often poorly soluble in tears. Experimental studies of substituted compounds must account for the effects of the substituents on potency, solubility, and the permeability coefficient.

pH and ionic charge

Many eye medications are alkaloids, or weak bases, and are most stable at an acidic pH. The buffer system used should have a capacity adequate to maintain pH within the stability range for the duration of the product shelf life. The pH range that a patient can tolerate is narrow. A large difference between the pH of a topical solution and that of tears may result in ocular irritation and stimulate reflex tearing that dilutes or washes away the topical drops. Thus, the buffer capacity should be adequate for stability but minimized to allow the overall pH of the tear fluid to be disrupted only momentarily upon instillation. Drugs such as tropicamide, cyclopentolate, atropine, and epinephrine exist in both charged and uncharged forms at the slightly alkaline pH of tears (pH 7.4). The partition coefficients, and therefore drug penetration, can be increased by raising the pH of the water phase, thereby increasing the proportion of drug molecules in the more lipid-soluble, uncharged form.

Surfactants

Many preservatives used in topical drops to prevent bacterial contamination are surfactants (also called *surface-active agents*) that alter cell membranes in the cornea as well as in bacteria, reducing the barrier effect of the corneal epithelium and increasing drug penetration. For example, a 0.1% carbachol solution containing 0.03% benzalkonium chloride can elicit the same miotic response as a 2% solution without this preservative.

Reflex tearing

Ocular irritation and secondary tearing wash out the drug reservoir in the tear lake and reduce the contact time of the drug with the cornea. Reflex tearing occurs when topical medications are not isotonic and when they have a nonphysiologic pH or contain irritants.

Binding of medication

Tear and ocular surface proteins, as well as ocular melanin, may bind topical or systemic medication, making the drug unavailable or creating a slow-release reservoir. This binding may alter the lag time, or onset, of a medication as well as the peak effect and duration of action, and it can cause local toxicity that occurs after discontinuation of the medication. One example of this effect is the retinal toxicity that progresses even after discontinuation of the aminoquinoline antimalarial drugs chloroquine and hydroxychloroquine. The latter is also often used in the management of autoimmune diseases such as lupus and rheumatoid arthritis.

Topical Administration: Ointments

Another strategy for increasing the contact time of ocular medications is through the use of ointments. Commercial oil-based ointments usually consist of petrolatum and mineral oil. The mineral oil allows the ointment to melt at body temperature. Both ingredients are also effective lipid solvents. However, most water-soluble medications are insoluble in the ointment and are present as microcrystals. Only those microcrystals on the surface of the ointment dissolve in the tears; the rest are trapped until the ointment melts. Such protracted, slow release may prevent the drug from reaching a therapeutic level in the tears. Only when the drug has high lipid solubility (which allows it to diffuse through the ointment) and some water solubility can it escape from the ointment into both the corneal epithelium and the tears. Fluorometholone, chloramphenicol, and tetracycline are examples of drugs that achieve higher aqueous levels when administered as ointment than as drops.

Local Administration

Periocular injections

Injection of medication beneath the conjunctiva or the Tenon capsule allows drugs to bypass the conjunctival and corneal epithelial barriers and absorb passively down a concentration gradient across the sclera and into intraocular tissues (see Fig 15-1). Subconjunctival, sub-Tenon, and retrobulbar injections all allow medications to reach therapeutic levels behind the lens–iris diaphragm. The Tenon capsule is a lipophilic barrier, and if a hydrophilic drug is injected into the sub-Tenon space, it can penetrate intraocular tissue more quickly than topical application can. This approach is especially useful for drugs with low lipid solubility (such as penicillin), which do not penetrate the eye adequately when given topically. Subconjunctival injections create a reservoir of drug that can be slowly released into the tear film.

Injections can also be helpful in delivering medication closer to the local site of action—for example, posterior sub-Tenon injections of steroids for cystoid macular edema (CME) or subconjunctival injection of fluorouracil (5-FU) after trabeculectomy. Retrobulbar and peribulbar injections also act directly at the site of delivery. These techniques are typically used for delivery of ophthalmic anesthesia and are covered in BCSC Section 11, *Lens and Cataract.* Other examples of local, injectable medications are botulinum toxin, used in the treatment of benign essential blepharospasm and hemifacial spasm, as well as for strabismus; and retrobulbar alcohol, used as therapy for chronic pain in blind eyes. See BCSC Section 10, *Glaucoma,* for further discussion of local application of antifibrotic agents in filtering surgery.

Intraocular medications

Intraocular injection of drugs instantly delivers effective concentrations at the target site. Although this route of administration may reduce systemic adverse effects, ocular adverse effects, which can include transient ocular hypertension and inflammation/infection, may be more pronounced. Clinicians must take great care to avoid the use of preserved medications and to control the concentration of intraocular drugs so that the delicate internal structures of the eye are protected from toxicity. Also, clinicians should strictly adhere to standard aseptic technique for the preparation and injection of intraocular medication so that infection is prevented. There are 2 types of intraocular injections: intracameral, or injection into the anterior chamber; and intravitreal, or injection into the vitreous cavity. Examples of substances and medications delivered via intraocular routes are presented in Table 15-1.

Intracameral injection of an antibiotic, administered at the end of cataract surgery to prevent endophthalmitis, has been reported. These injections have the advantage of reducing the need for postoperative dosing of medications. Cefuroxime, a broad-spectrum cephalosporin, is commonly used for this purpose. However, single-dose solution of cefuroxime is unavailable in the United States, and strict aseptic compounding protocol for reconstitution and dilution needs to be followed. Vancomycin is effective against methicillin-resistant *Staphylococcus aureus* (MRSA) but also needs to be diluted before injection. Further, the

Table 15-1 Examples of Medications Delivered by Intracameral and Intravitreal Routes

Route of Administration	Clinical Application
Intracameral	
Antibiotics (eg, cefuroxime, moxifloxacin, vancomycin)	Prevent endophthalmitis in cataract surgery
Acetylcholine	Constrict pupil in intraocular surgery
Carbachol	Same as above
Balanced salt solution	Intraocular surgery, re-form anterior chamber
Ophthalmic viscosurgical devices (OVDs)	Same as above
Epinephrine (preservative- and bisulfite-free[a])	Dilate pupil in intraocular surgery
Phenylephrine 1%/ketorolac 0.3%	Maintain pupil dilatation in intraocular surgery (added to irrigation solution)
Lidocaine (preservative-free)	Intraocular surgery, anesthesia
Trypan blue	Stain anterior capsule in cataract surgery
Tissue plasminogen activator (tPA) (off-label use)	Assist fibrinolysis of fibrin in anterior chamber and subretinal hemorrhage
Intravitreal	
Anti–vascular endothelial growth factor	Choroidal neovascularization, diabetic retinopathy, diabetic macular edema, retinal vein occlusion
Corticosteroids (eg, triamcinolone acetonide; sustained-release intraocular implants such as dexamethasone in poly(lactic-*co*-glycolic acid) (PLGA) matrix and fluocinolone acetonide in a polyvinyl acetate/silicone laminate)	Cystoid macular edema, diabetic macular edema, retinal vein occlusion, posterior uveitis, postoperative inflammation
Foscarnet injection	Cytomegalovirus retinitis
Ganciclovir injection	Same as above
Silicone oil	Vitreoretinal surgery
Intraocular gases	Same as above
Perfluorocarbon	Same as above
Various antibiotics	Intraocular infection

[a] Preservative-free epinephrine with 0.1% bisulfite ampules of 1:1000 epinephrine can be safely injected intracamerally if it is diluted 1:4 with either balanced salt solution (BSS) or fortified BSS (BSS Plus).

theoretical risk of inducing drug resistance with indiscriminate use of vancomycin is a concern. Another option is diluting preservative-free topical moxifloxacin—a broad-spectrum, fourth-generation fluoroquinolone—for intracameral use. It is important that antibiotic solutions prepared for intracameral injection be free of preservatives or other additives. Cases of toxic anterior segment syndrome (TASS) have been reported after the use of antibiotics with preservatives or with dosing errors.

A regulated, compounded preservative-free formulation of triamcinolone acetonide 15 mg/mL, moxifloxacin hydrochloride 1 mg/mL, and vancomycin 10 mg/mL is available for administration into the anterior vitreous after intraocular lens implantation through the zonule via the ciliary sulcus. Controlled studies on the safety and efficacy of this formulation are lacking. In 2017, the US Food and Drug Administration (FDA) received an adverse event report concerning a patient in whom bilateral hemorrhagic occlusive retinal vasculitis (HORV) developed after this formulation was administered in each eye at the conclusion of cataract surgery procedures performed 2 weeks apart. HORV is a rare but potentially blinding complication that has occurred in patients who received intraocular injections of vancomycin formulations at the end of otherwise uncomplicated cataract surgery.

Intravitreal injection is the most common form of intraocular drug delivery. These injections are most often used to manage patients with complications of diabetic retinopathy (diabetic macular edema) and age-related macular degeneration (choroidal neovascularization). They are also used in the treatment of uveitis, endophthalmitis, and other conditions. For example, for retinal vascular diseases, various agents are available that target vascular endothelial growth factor (VEGF). Intravitreal delivery can result in a relevant systemic concentration, as evidenced by the effects noted in fellow eyes in clinical trials. For discussion of individual agents used for intravitreal injection, see Chapter 16 in this volume and BCSC Section 12, *Retina and Vitreous.*

Ho AC, Scott IU, Kim SJ, et al. Anti-vascular endothelial growth factor pharmacotherapy for diabetic macular edema: a report by the American Academy of Ophthalmology. *Ophthalmology.* 2012;119(10):2179–2188.

Wen JC, McCannel CA, Mochon AB, Garner OB. Bacterial dispersal association with speech in the setting of intravitreous injections. *Arch Ophthalmol.* 2011;129(12):1551–1554.

Witkin AJ, Chang DF, Jumper JM, et al. Vancomycin-associated hemorrhagic occlusive retinal vasculitis: clinical characteristics of 36 eyes. *Ophthalmology.* 2017;124(5):583–595.

Yeh S, Albini TA, Moshfeghi AA, Nussenblatt RB. Uveitis, the Comparison of Age-related Macular Degeneration Treatments Trials (CATT), and intravitreal biologics for ocular inflammation. *Am J Ophthalmol.* 2012;154(3):429–435.

Systemic Administration

Just as the tight junctions of the corneal epithelium and endothelium limit anterior access to the interior of the eye, similar barriers limit access through vascular channels. The vascular endothelium of the retina, like that of the brain, is nonfenestrated and knitted together by tight junctions. Although both the choroid and the ciliary body have fenestrated vascular endothelia, the choroid is effectively sequestered by the retinal pigment epithelium (tight junctions); and the ciliary body, by its nonpigmented epithelium (tight junctions).

Compared with medications with lower lipid solubility, drugs with higher lipid solubility more readily penetrate the blood–ocular barrier. Thus, chloramphenicol, which is highly lipid-soluble, penetrates 20 times better than does penicillin, which has poor lipid solubility.

The ability of systemically administered drugs to gain access to the eye is also influenced by the degree to which they are bound to plasma proteins. Only the unbound form can cross the blood–ocular barrier. Sulfonamides are lipid-soluble but penetrate poorly because, at therapeutic levels, more than 90% of the medication is bound to plasma proteins. Similarly, compared with methicillin, oxacillin has reduced penetration because of its increased binding of plasma protein. Because bolus administration of a drug exceeds the binding capacity of plasma proteins and leads to higher intraocular drug levels than can be achieved by a slow intravenous drip, this approach is used for the administration of antibiotics in order to attain high peak intraocular levels.

Sustained-release oral preparations

The practical value of sustained-release preparations is substantial. For example, a single dose of acetazolamide will reduce intraocular pressure for up to 10 hours, whereas a single dose of sustained-release acetazolamide will produce a comparable effect that lasts 20 hours. A sustained-release medication offers a steadier blood level of the drug, avoiding marked peak concentrations and low concentrations, and reduces the frequency of administration.

Intravenous injections

Intravenously injected agents can be administered for diagnostic effect. Sodium fluorescein and indocyanine green are 2 agents used for retinal angiography to aid in the diagnosis of retinal and choroidal diseases.

Intravenous agents are also used therapeutically in ophthalmology. Although intravitreal injections have replaced intravenous therapy for postoperative endophthalmitis, continuous intravenous administration of an antibiotic is an effective way of maintaining therapeutic intraocular levels in endogenous infection (see BCSC Section 12, *Retina and Vitreous*).

The barriers and reservoir effects of the eye affect the pharmacodynamics of antibiotics such as ampicillin, chloramphenicol, and erythromycin. When given as a single intravenous bolus, each of these drugs penetrate the eye with a higher initial intraocular level than when given by continuous infusion and maintain comparable bioavailability for 4 hours. The intraocular penetration of a drug may be better in the inflamed eye than in the healthy eye because of the disruption of the blood–aqueous and blood–retina barriers that occurs with inflammation. This disruption is demonstrated by the leakage of fluorescein from inflamed retinal vessels into the vitreous during angiography.

Studies in rabbit eyes found that the bioavailability of intravenous ampicillin, tetracycline, and dexamethasone differed in various structures of the rabbit eye, with the highest levels of these medications found in the sclera and conjunctiva, followed by the iris and ciliary body, and finally the cornea, aqueous humor, choroid, and retina. Very low levels appeared in the lens and vitreous. No marked differences in vascular distribution of the drugs was shown, however. The tissue bioavailability is determined by the vascularity of the tissue and the barriers existing between the blood and that tissue.

Intramuscular injections

In ophthalmology, intramuscular injection of drugs is used less frequently than topical, oral, or intravenous administration of medications. Notable exceptions include intramuscular injection of prostigmine in the diagnosis of myasthenia gravis and botulinum toxin, given for local effect, in facial dystonias and in some cases of strabismus.

Cholkar K, Patel SP, Vadlapudi AW, Mitra AK. Novel strategies for anterior ocular drug delivery. *J Ocular Pharmacol Ther.* 2013;29(2):106–123.

Gaudana R, Ananthula HK, Parenky A, Mitra AK. Ocular drug delivery. *AAPS J.* 2010;12(3): 348–360.

Ocular Drug Design and Methods of Delivery

New ocular drugs are designed with a focus on specificity of action and safety, with delivery systems aimed at improving convenience and therefore patient compliance. Each of the following approaches responds to a specific problem in ocular pharmacokinetics.

Prodrugs

Ophthalmic prodrugs are therapeutically inactive derivatives of drug molecules that are designed to be activated by enzymatic systems within the eye in order to improve ocular penetration. These derivatives are usually synthesized by conjugation of a specific promoiety to the parent drug via ester or amide. The ester and amide ophthalmic prodrugs are hydrolyzed by esterase and amidases to the active molecules as they permeate through the cornea or conjunctiva. Permeability across the cornea is also improved by the increased lipid solubility of the prodrug. Prostaglandin analogues are successful examples of this drug delivery strategy. Latanoprost, travoprost, and tafluprost are prostaglandin analogues that interact with the prostaglandin FP receptor. They require hydrolyzation prior to becoming active compounds in the eye.

Valacyclovir hydrochloride is an antiviral prodrug that, when taken orally, is easily absorbed through the gastrointestinal tract and quickly converted to the active form of acyclovir. Likewise, famciclovir is a prodrug of the active antiviral penciclovir.

Sustained-Release Delivery

Ocular inserts

Eyedrop therapy involves periodic delivery of relatively large quantities of a drug to overcome low ocular bioavailability due to various factors, such as tearing and blinking, nasolacrimal drainage, conjunctival blood and lymph flow, metabolic degradation, and corneal and blood–aqueous barriers. The high peak drug levels attained with bolus dosing can cause local and systemic side effects, such as induced accommodation producing brow ache, which can occur after pilocarpine use. In addition, drug concentration in the eye can vary significantly because of variations in application technique and patient adherence to dosing amounts and schedules. Thus, there is a need for an efficient delivery system that can provide controlled release of a drug with a reduced dosing frequency.

Devices have been developed that deliver an adequate supply of medication at a steady-state level, achieving beneficial effects with fewer adverse effects. In the 1970s, the first steady-state drug delivery system, a nonbiodegradable insert designed to deliver pilocarpine at a steady rate of 40 µg/hr, became available. This device was discontinued as the use of pilocarpine decreased. Ocular inserts currently in development or under investigation are cylindrical in shape and are placed in the fornix for prolonged drug release. They can be categorized as soluble or insoluble:

- *Soluble* inserts release the drug via interaction between the polymeric matrix of the device and the tear film. Removal of these inserts is unnecessary.

- *Insoluble* inserts may achieve a more constant rate of drug release than soluble inserts, but removal of the device is required.

Ocular inserts have the advantages of prolonged and steady delivery of drugs, which can improve patient compliance. However, they have the potential for patient discomfort such as foreign-body sensation.

Implants

To circumvent the repeated injections that are required with intraocular injection of a drug, various implantable devices were developed for sustained drug delivery. The first-available sustained-release implant was the ganciclovir intravitreal implant for treatment of cytomegalovirus (CMV) retinitis. An ethylene vinyl acetate disc with a PVA coating served as the drug reservoir. The thickness of the PVA lid regulated the delivery of ganciclovir to the target tissue. After surgical implantation, the device delivered a steady source of ganciclovir for 5–8 months. The ganciclovir intravitreal implant was discontinued after the patent expired in 2015. Current intraocular sustained-release products approved by the FDA include 2 fluocinolone acetonide intravitreal implants (0.59 mg and 0.19 mg) and a dexamethasone intravitreal implant.

The 0.59-mg fluocinolone acetonide implant, a nonbiodegradable intraocular polymer implant requiring surgical placement in the pars plana region, is approved by the FDA for the treatment of chronic noninfectious posterior uveitis. It was designed to release fluocinolone acetonide at a nominal initial rate of 0.6 μg/d, decreasing over the first month to a steady state between 0.3 and 0.4 μg/d over approximately 30 months.

The 0.19-mg fluocinolone implant, delivered by intravitreal injection, has a nonbioerodable tube of polyimide and a permeable membrane of PVA at one end that releases the medication. It was approved by the FDA for the treatment of diabetic macular edema in patients who are not steroid responders. The implant releases fluocinolone acetonide at an average rate of 0.2 μg/d for 36 months.

The 0.7-mg dexamethasone implant is a biodegradable poly(lactic-*co*-glycolic acid) (PLGA) matrix loaded with dexamethasone for injection into the vitreous cavity. The polymer degrades to lactic acid and glycolic acid, and dexamethasone is slowly released within the vitreous cavity. The implant is indicated for the treatment of macular edema secondary to retinal vein occlusion, noninfectious posterior uveitis, and diabetic macular edema. Various biodegradable and nonbiodegradable implants designed for sustained release of single or multiple medications are under development.

Intraocular lenses and other sustained-release systems

Sustained-release systems that use biodegradable polymers entrapped with triamcinolone acetonide or antibiotics and are attached to the periphery or haptics of an artificial intraocular lens are under investigation to prevent intraocular infection and control postoperative intraocular inflammation. Other research efforts include development of an intraocular lens prepared with biomaterials that not only allow high transmittance at visible wavelengths but also can be loaded with dexamethasone to achieve sustained release of this drug after cataract surgery.

Intraocular sustained-release devices are being studied as alternatives to glaucoma medical therapy that has been shown to have poor patient compliance. Products under investigation include injectable sustained-release biodegradable implants through which various hypotensive medications can be delivered into the anterior chamber or supraciliary space or beneath the conjunctiva to achieve a sustained reduction of intraocular pressure for months.

Collagen Corneal Shields

Collagen corneal shields are useful as a delivery system to prolong the contact between a drug and the cornea. For the creation of these shields, porcine scleral tissue is extracted and molded into contact lens–like shields. Drugs can be incorporated into the collagen matrix during the manufacturing process, absorbed into the shield during rehydration, or applied topically while the shield is in the eye. Because the shield dissolves in 12, 24, or 72 hours, depending on the manufacturing process for collagen crosslinking, the drug is released gradually into the tear film, and high concentrations are maintained on the corneal surface and in the conjunctival cul-de-sac.

Recent attempts to create collagen shields have focused on using metal oxide nanoparticles as agents for collagen crosslinking. In one study, an initial rapid release, or *burst release,* due to adsorption of the drug on the shields, was followed by a constant release over the next 13 days, which was due to diffusion of the drug from the collagen matrix. Additional crosslinking with ultraviolet light achieved a slower rate of drug release.

Collagen shields have been used for the early management of bacterial keratitis, as well as for antibiotic prophylaxis. They have also been used to promote epithelial healing after ocular surgery, trauma, or spontaneous erosion. Despite these therapeutic benefits, collagen shields are poorly tolerated because they are very uncomfortable.

Agban Y, Lian J, Prabakar S, Seyfoddin A, Rupenthal ID. Nanoparticle cross-linked collagen shields for sustained delivery of pilocarpine hydrochloride. *Int J Pharm.* 2016;501(1–2): 96–101.

New Technologies in Drug Delivery

Contact lenses

Ongoing research approaches for contact lens (CL) drug delivery systems focus on improving the residence time of the drug at the surface of the eye to enhance bioavailability and to provide more convenient and efficacious therapy. Various techniques are used to incorporate the drug into the CL body, including

- soaking the CL in drug solution
- incorporating monomers able to interact with target drugs into the CL hydrogels
- incorporating drug-loaded colloidal nanoparticles into the matrix of the CL
- using a molecular imprinting technique in which the components of the hydrogel network are organized such that high-affinity binding sites for the drug are created

These CL delivery systems need to be designed so that they also preserve the transparency required for vision and the oxygen permeability necessary for corneal health. One way to maintain transparency is by lathing the encapsulated drug-polymer film in the periphery of the CL hydrogel.

Guzman-Aranguez A, Colligris B, Pintor J. Contact lenses: promising devices for ocular drug delivery. *J Ocular Pharmacol Ther.* 2013;29(2):189–199.

Punctal plug–mediated delivery

Various punctal plug–mediated drug delivery systems are currently under clinical investigation. The design of these delivery systems generally includes a cylindrical polymeric core loaded with the drug compound, an impermeable shell, and a cap (or head portion of the plug exposed to the tear film) with pores from which the drug is released by diffusion. Most examples of punctal plug systems show nearly constant drug-release rates for drug molecules. Delivery of drugs by punctal plug has several potential advantages over administration via eyedrops, including lack of exposure to preservatives, dose reduction, controlled release of the drug at an optimum rate, and improved patient compliance. Limitations include ocular irritation, itching, discomfort, increased lacrimation, and spontaneous extrusion of the plug.

Gel-forming drops

Gel-forming drops use pentablock copolymers as a vehicle for topical drug delivery. The drug is added to a nonviscous polymer drop. After the drop is in contact with the surface of the eye, the drop reacts upon exposure to body temperature and transforms into a gel.

Encapsulated cell technology

Encapsulated cell technology has been applied to the delivery of therapeutic agents for treatment of retinal diseases. This technology involves encapsulation of cells within a semipermeable polymer capsule that secretes therapeutic material into the vitreous. The device is implanted in the vitreous cavity and secured to the sclera.

Liposomes

Liposomes are synthetic lipid microspheres that serve as multipurpose vehicles for the topical delivery of drugs, genetic material, and cosmetics. They are produced when phospholipid molecules interact to form a bilayer lipid membrane in an aqueous environment. The interior of the bilayer consists of the hydrophobic fatty-acid tails of the phospholipid molecule, whereas the outer layer is composed of hydrophilic polar-head groups of the molecule. A water-soluble drug can be dissolved in the aqueous phase of the interior compartment; a hydrophobic drug can be intercalated into the lipid bilayer itself. However, the routine use of liposome formulation for topical ocular drug delivery is limited by the short shelf life of these products, their limited drug-loading capacity, and difficulty with stabilizing the preparation.

Nanotechnology

Nanotechnology has been increasingly applied in medication design to protect active molecules and provide sustained drug delivery. Methods for transporting hydrophilic and lipophilic drugs and genes include the use of biodegradable nanoparticles such as nanospheres, nanocapsules, and nanomicelles; the colloidal dispersion of nanoparticles as nanosuspension; and the use of nanoemulsion. These methods are modeled after the molecular structure of viruses.

The physical process of moving charged molecules by an electrical current is called *iontophoresis.* This procedure places a relatively high concentration of a drug locally, where it can achieve maximum benefit with little waste or systemic absorption. Animal studies have demonstrated that iontophoresis increases penetration of various antibiotics and antiviral drugs across ocular surfaces into the cornea and the interior of the eye. However, patient discomfort, ocular tissue damage, and necrosis restrict the widespread use of this mode of drug delivery.

Microelectromechanical systems

Drug delivery devices based on microelectromechanical systems (MEMS) are under investigation to provide antiangiogenic therapy for age-related macular degeneration and steroid therapy for chronic uveitis. These devices are implanted in a manner similar to that used for current glaucoma tube shunts and deliver multiple microdoses of a drug directly into the vitreous cavity through a pars plana cannula. The device contains a drug reservoir with a refill port, a battery, electronics, and an electrolysis chamber to deliver the desired dose.

Pharmacodynamics: The Mechanism of Drug Action

Most drugs act by binding to and altering the function of regulatory macromolecules, usually neurotransmitter receptors, hormone receptors, or enzymes. Binding may be a reversible association mediated by electrostatic and/or van der Waals forces, or it may involve formation of a covalent intermediate. If the drug–receptor interaction stimulates the receptor's natural function, the drug is termed an *agonist.* Stimulation of an opposing effect characterizes an *antagonist.* Corresponding effectors of enzymes are termed *activators* and *inhibitors.* This terminology is crucial to understanding Chapter 16.

The relationship between the initial drug–receptor interaction and the drug's clinical dose-response curve may be simple or complex. In some cases, the drug's clinical effect closely reflects the degree of receptor occupancy on a moment-to-moment basis. Such is usually the case for drugs that affect neural transmission or for drugs that are enzyme inhibitors. In contrast, some drug effects lag hours behind receptor occupancy or persist long after the drug is gone. Such is the case with many drugs acting on hormone receptors, because their effects are often mediated through a series of biochemical events.

In addition to differences in timing of receptor occupancy and drug effects, the degree of receptor occupancy can differ considerably from the corresponding drug effect. For example, because the amount of carbonic anhydrase present in the ciliary processes is 100 times that required to support aqueous secretion, more than 99% of the enzyme must be inhibited before secretion is reduced. On the other hand, some maximal hormone responses occur at concentrations well below those required for receptor saturation, indicating the presence of "unbound receptors."

Pharmacogenetics: The Influence of Genetic Variation on Drug Efficacy and Toxicity

Genetic polymorphisms in genes encoding drug-metabolizing enzymes, drug transporters, and receptors contribute, at least in part, to the wide interindividual variability in drug response and adverse drug reactions. *Pharmacogenetics* is the study of the influence of genetic variation on drug efficacy or toxicity, focusing on single genes. The term is often used interchangeably with *pharmacogenomics,* which is the study of how genetic makeup affects an individual's response to drugs; in other words, the focus is on many genes. Pharmacogenetics can be broadly divided into (1) the study of genetic variations that affect drug metabolism (pharmacokinetics); and (2) the study of genetic variations that affect drug targets (pharmacodynamics).

Thus far, some small-scale studies have demonstrated an association between various genotypes or haplotypes and response to drug therapies for 2 major eye disorders, age-related macular degeneration and glaucoma, but the results are conflicting. One example is the relationship between single nucleotide polymorphisms (SNPs) in genes and the response to latanoprost, specifically, SNPs in the genes coding for matrix metalloproteinases and SNPs in the prostaglandin F2α receptor gene *(PTGFR).* Another example is the pharmacogenetic relationship between polymorphisms in specific genes and the different levels of drug efficacy in the treatment of exudative age-related macular degeneration.

Although translation of pharmacogenetic and pharmacogenomic data into clinical practice would provide significant opportunities to increase the safety and efficacy of pharmacotherapy, consensus (social, ethical, and economical) on issues such as genetic discrimination needs to be reached and such issues addressed by regulatory agencies. Clinicians must be aware of the ethical, legal, and social issues associated with genetic testing.

Shastry BS. Genetic diversity and medicinal drug response in eye care. *Graefes Arch Clin Exp Ophthalmol.* 2010;248(8):1057–1061.

CHAPTER 16

Ocular Pharmacotherapeutics*

Highlights

- Off-label drug use is common in ophthalmology. Certain off-label uses are even the predominant treatment options or standard of care for some conditions.
- Compounded pharmaceuticals are used to treat numerous ophthalmic diseases. Practicing ophthalmologists should be up-to-date with current state and federal pharmacy regulations concerning compounded pharmaceuticals.
- The drugs carbachol, 0.01%, and acetylcholine, 1%, are administered intracamerally to induce miosis. Acetylcholine is faster acting; however, carbachol is 100 times more effective and longer lasting. In addition, carbachol can lower intraocular pressure.
- There is no evidence that the ophthalmic administration of fluoroquinolones affects weight-bearing joints in the pediatric population.
- Topical povidone-iodine solution (5%) is the only drug that has had a significant effect on postsurgical endophthalmitis. Povidone-iodine can be safely given to patients with an allergy to contrast agents or shellfish; these patients have likely developed hypersensitivity reactions to specific proteins of the food itself (eg, seafood) or to the contrast medium rather than to the iodine in the compound.
- Topical proparacaine reportedly does not inhibit the growth of *Staphylococcus, Candida,* or *Pseudomonas;* thus, it may be preferred to other drugs for corneal anesthesia before scraping a corneal ulcer for a culture.

*This chapter may include information on pharmaceutical applications that are not considered community standard, that are approved for use only in restricted research settings (ie, investigational drugs), or that reflect indications not approved in US Food and Drug Administration (FDA) labeling (ie, off-label use). For example, many ophthalmic uses of medications, including most antibiotics and antifungal drugs compounded for systemic treatment of ocular infections such as keratitis and endophthalmitis, are off-label. Many antifungal drugs are used off-label on the basis of in vitro and animal data because human data for unusual infectious agents are often limited. **The FDA has stated that it is the responsibility of the physician to determine the FDA status of each drug or device he or she wishes to use and to use it with appropriate, informed patient consent in compliance with applicable law. (The legal aspect of medical therapy varies by country and region. For example, the General Medical Council [GMC] in the United Kingdom recognizes that a physician has a moral duty toward all of his or her patients that may affect the choice of appropriate medical therapy under tight budgetary restrictions.)**

The reader is encouraged to consult the books and website given in the following reference list for more information on many of the topics covered in this chapter.

Bartlett JD, Jaanus SD, eds. *Clinical Ocular Pharmacology.* 5th ed. St Louis: Butterworth-Heinemann/Elsevier; 2008.

Brunton LL, Hilal-Dandan R, Knollmann BC, eds. *Goodman & Gilman's The Pharmacological Basis of Therapeutics: Digital Edition.* 13th ed. New York: McGraw-Hill; 2018.

Fraunfelder FT, Fraunfelder FW. *Drug-Induced Ocular Side Effects.* 7th ed. New York: Elsevier; 2014.

Murray L, ed. *Physicians' Desk Reference.* 72nd ed. Montvale, NJ: Thomson PDR; 2018.

Physicians' Desk Reference for Ophthalmic Medicines. 42nd ed. Montvale, NJ: Thomson PDR; 2012.

U.S. Food and Drug Administration. Drugs@FDA: FDA-approved drugs. www.accessdata.fda.gov/scripts/cder/daf/. Accessed November 14, 2021.

Legal Aspects of Medical Therapy

The US Food and Drug Administration (FDA) has statutory authority to approve the marketing of prescription drugs and to specify the uses of these drugs. The FDA's Office of Prescription Drug Promotion reviews and regulates prescription drug advertising and promotion through surveillance activities and issuance of enforcement letters to pharmaceutical manufacturers, whereas the Federal Trade Commission regulates advertising and promotion for over-the-counter drugs. The FDA has created a 3-step process for human testing of new drugs before they are approved for marketing:

- *Phase 1:* After animal and in vitro studies, human testing begins. This process involves trials with 10–80 people for collection of toxicology data and pharmacokinetic data on dosage range, absorption, and metabolism.
- *Phase 2:* Randomized controlled clinical trials involving a minimum of 50–100 affected people are conducted to determine safety and effectiveness of the drug.
- *Phase 3:* Controlled and uncontrolled trials evaluate the overall risk–benefit relationship and provide an adequate basis for physician labeling. The data gathered from these tests are then submitted as part of a new drug application for marketing.

The FDA's approval of each drug and its specific uses ("on-label" prescribing) are based on documentation submitted by manufacturers that supports the safety and efficacy of the drug. Although the FDA is committed to making drugs available as rapidly as possible, the process of bringing a new product to market requires extensive research and development and millions of dollars.

Once approved for a specific use(s), a drug may be prescribed by individual physicians for other indications and/or patient populations. For example, doxycycline, typically prescribed to treat infection, can also be used to treat ocular rosacea (based on its inhibition of matrix-metalloproteinases). Off-label drug use, defined as prescribing a drug for an indication or employing a dosage or dose form that has not been approved through the FDA process, is common. An off-label use may even be the predominant treatment option for a given clinical condition. Although off-label use of a drug may already be the standard of care for a certain medical condition, drug proprietors may never seek FDA approval for the new indication because of financial reasons.

In ophthalmology, many common drugs are used off-label. Some examples are listed in Table 16-1. One of the most commonly used medications, topical prednisolone, has not been approved by the FDA for postoperative care. Use after cataract surgery is thus an off-label application.

Although off-label drug use per se does not violate federal law, prescribing physicians remain liable to malpractice actions with their use. In particular, unapproved use of a drug that does not adhere to an applicable *standard of care* places a practitioner in a difficult legal position. However, if other physicians, similarly situated, would have prescribed in the same manner, a *standard of care* can be met in most jurisdictions. In equivocal cases where standard of care is uncertain, informed consent should be considered.

Expanded access refers to the clinical use of investigational new drugs (INDs) prior to FDA approval. Clinical use of INDs in this setting is typically requested for patients with terminal conditions who either do not qualify for the clinical trial or may succumb to their illness before the drug obtains approval. The treating physician must ensure that the company is willing to provide the drug/device and agrees with the treatment plan.

Table 16-1 Common Drugs Used Off-label in Ophthalmology

Drug	Indications
Bevacizumab, an antiangiogenic drug	Used as an intravitreal injection for numerous neovascular ocular diseases
Acetylcysteine (10% or 20%)	Used as a mucolytic drug in filamentary keratopathy and as an anticollagenase drug in severe alkali injuries
Tissue plasminogen activator (tPA)	Used as an intravitreal injection for thrombolysis and fibrinolysis
Fluorouracil (5-FU)	Improves the outcomes of glaucoma filtering surgery
Mitomycin C (MMC)	Improves the outcomes of glaucoma filtering surgery and treats ocular surface neoplasia
Cyclosporine A 2% compounded solution	Used in high-risk corneal transplants and in severe vernal, ligneous, and autoimmune keratopathies
Doxycycline	Used in ocular rosacea
Edetate disodium (salt of EDTA)	Used in band keratopathy
Hyaluronic acid	Used as a viscoelastic material for re-formation of the anterior chamber
Fibrin sealant	Used to adhere the conjunctival graft to the scleral bed in pterygium resection
Triamcinolone acetonide[a]	The preparation Kenalog is used in intravitreal and sub-Tenon injections of triamcinolone acetonide for a variety of conditions, including macular edema, anterior/intermediate uveitis, and retinal vein occlusions

[a]The preservative-free formulation of triamcinolone acetonide (Triesence) is FDA-approved for intraocular use.

Compounded Pharmaceuticals

Compounded pharmaceuticals are used to treat numerous ophthalmic diseases during both surgical and diagnostic office procedures. Compounding is defined by the US Pharmacopeia (USP) as "the preparation, mixing, assembling, altering, packaging, and labeling of a drug, drug-delivery device, or device in accordance with a licensed practitioner's prescription, medication order, or initiative based on the practitioner/patient/pharmacist/compounder relationship in the course of professional practice."

The Pharmacy Compounding Accreditation Board (PCAB) accredits pharmacies that provide evidence of adherence to quality standards for pharmacy compounding. The PCAB requires proper licensure with state and federal regulatory authorities, appropriate training of personnel, and facilities and methods that permit aseptic compounding of sterile preparations and meet the USP guidelines. Compounding pharmacies are also regulated by state boards of pharmacy and the FDA.

The 2013 Drug Quality and Security Act created a new 2-tiered regulatory structure for compounding pharmacies and the products they distribute. The law defines government oversight authority over large-volume compounding facilities, preserving a pathway for ophthalmologists to access certain compounding drugs for office use. Under the law:

- In accordance with section 503A of the Food, Drug, and Cosmetic Act (FDCA), traditional compounding pharmacies require a patient-specific prescription for all drugs compounded. Oversight of these pharmacies remains primarily a state function unless the FDA receives a complaint.
- According to section 503B of the FDCA, new outsourcing facilities do not require a prescription, but they must meet higher federal safety, sterility, and quality control standards than conventional drug manufacturing plants, while being subject to similar regular federal inspections.

Although ensuring the safety and sterility of compounded products is important, maintaining practitioner access to essential compounded products for office use is crucial. Unfortunately, the implementation of the new system and its regulation have been uncertain and costly. State rules for 503A compounding pharmacies still prevent some small, local compounders (including hospital pharmacies) from providing ophthalmologists with supplies of fortified antibiotics and other commonly compounded drugs for urgent cases. Shipment of compounded medications across state lines is more difficult because the compounder must have an in-state pharmacy license. In addition, costly, extensive baseline testing required for each of the compounded products shortens the compendium list. Finally, although the FDA has dropped its 5-day expiration rule and allows 503B pharmacies to determine the expiration dates on biologics, additional expensive testing regimens are required on the part of compounders to substantiate a longer shelf life on the label.

To help the clinician be proactive about compounding drugs, the American Academy of Ophthalmology (AAO) issued the following recommendations for the sourcing of drugs used in intravitreal injection:

1. Select a compounding pharmacy that is accredited by the PCAB and adheres to quality standards for aseptic compounding of sterile medications set forth by USP Chapter 797.

2. Record the lot numbers of the medication vial and the syringes in the patient record or a log, in case they need to be tracked.

These recommendations were made after the 2011 outbreaks of infectious endophthalmitis associated with compounded bevacizumab. Practicing ophthalmologists should stay up-to-date with current state and federal pharmacy regulations concerning compounding pharmaceuticals. The AAO and many subspecialty societies send e-mail alerts and provide updates on regulations and legislation to their members.

Compliance

Noncompliance with a physician's prescribed therapeutic regimen is a serious obstacle to patient care. Although much of the research on noncompliance in ophthalmology has been conducted in patients who required medical therapy for glaucoma, the findings can be applied to medical therapy for other ophthalmic conditions.

Medication compliance is different from adherence. Medication *compliance* is the act of taking medication as prescribed, whereas medication *adherence* is the act of filling new prescriptions or refilling prescriptions on time. Generally, the degree of compliance reported by patients is lower than their actual compliance. The degree of adherence to treatment is poor with chronic ophthalmic diseases, similar to adherence with other chronic diseases. Concurrent medical conditions or disabilities may also interfere with compliance or adherence. The list of factors that contribute to noncompliance or nonadherence is long. Selected examples are presented in Table 16-2.

Depending on the factors identified, reasonable options for improving compliance or adherence include patient education about the disease or medical therapy, simplification of the medical regimen, maximized cost reduction, and recruitment of support from family members. Although positive effects of these interventions have not been proven, noncompliance can lead to unnecessary disease progression, additional medical costs and physician visits, and unneeded change or escalation of therapy. Clinicians can play an active role in improving compliance and preventing these outcomes.

Tsai JC. A comprehensive perspective on patient adherence to topical glaucoma therapy. *Ophthalmology*. 2009;116(suppl 11):S30–S36.

Table 16-2 Factors Contributing to Noncompliance or Nonadherence to Therapy

Advanced age
Lower economic status
High medication cost
Limited health insurance
Patient's forgetfulness
Anxiety with disease and treatment
Poor comprehension of disease
Misunderstanding of instructions
Fear of becoming dependent on medication
Complexity and length of treatment
Concurrent medical conditions or disabilities
Adverse effects

Cholinergic Drugs

Several commonly used ophthalmic medications affect the activity of acetylcholine receptors in synapses of the somatic and autonomic nervous systems (Fig 16-1). These receptors are found in

- the motor end plates of the extraocular and levator palpebrae superioris muscles (supplied by somatic motor nerves)
- the cells of the superior cervical (sympathetic) ganglion and the ciliary and sphenopalatine (parasympathetic) ganglia (supplied by preganglionic autonomic nerves)
- parasympathetic effector sites in the iris sphincter and ciliary body and in the lacrimal, accessory lacrimal, and meibomian glands (supplied by postganglionic parasympathetic nerves)

Although all cholinergic receptors are by definition responsive to acetylcholine, they are not homogeneous and can be classified by their responses to 2 drugs: muscarine and nicotine (Table 16-3). *Muscarinic receptors* are found in the end organs of the parasympathetic autonomic system. *Nicotinic receptors* are found in the postganglionic neurons of both the sympathetic and parasympathetic systems, in striated muscle (the end organ of

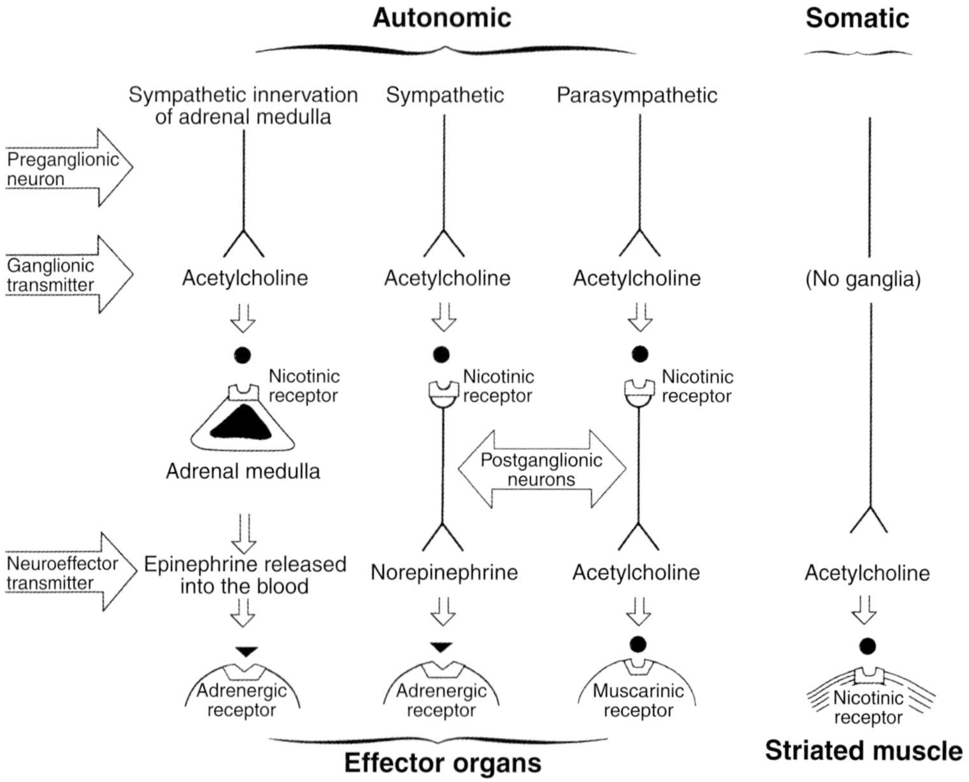

Figure 16-1 Summary of the neurotransmitters released and the types of receptors found within the autonomic and somatic nervous systems. *(Reproduced with permission from Mycek MJ, Harvey RA, Champe PC, eds.* Pharmacology. *2nd ed. Lippincott's Illustrated Reviews. Philadelphia: Lippincott-Raven; 1997:32.)*

Table 16-3 **Cholinergic and Adrenergic Receptors**[a]

Receptors	Agonists	Blocking Agents
Cholinergic (sphincter)	Acetylcholine	
Muscarinic	Muscarine	Atropine
Nicotinic	Nicotine	D-Tubocurarine
Adrenergic (dilator)	Norepinephrine	
Alpha[b]	Phenylephrine	Phentolamine and phenoxybenzamine
α_1	Phenylephrine	Prazosin, thymoxamine, dapiprazole
α_2	Apraclonidine	Yohimbine
Beta	Isoproterenol	Propranolol and timolol
β_1	Tazolol	Betaxolol
β_2	Albuterol	Butoxamine

[a] The cholinergic agonists and the adrenergic blockers listed cause miosis; the adrenergic agonists and the cholinergic blockers listed cause dilation.
[b] The prefixes α_1 and α_2 have been proposed for postsynaptic and presynaptic α-adrenoceptors, respectively. According to the present view, the classification into α_1 and α_2 subtypes is based exclusively on the relative potencies and affinities of agonists and antagonists, regardless of their function and localization.

the somatic system), and in the adrenal medulla. Cholinergic drugs may be further divided into the following groups (Fig 16-2):

- direct-acting agonists, which act on the receptor to elicit an excitatory postsynaptic potential
- indirect-acting agonists, which increase endogenous acetylcholine levels at the synaptic cleft by inhibiting acetylcholinesterase
- antagonists, which block the action of acetylcholine on the receptor

Muscarinic Drugs

Direct-acting agonists

Topically applied, direct-acting agonists have 3 actions:

- They cause contraction of the iris sphincter, which not only constricts the pupil *(miosis)* but also changes the anatomical relationship of the iris to both the lens and the chamber angle.
- They cause contraction of the circular fibers of the ciliary muscle, relaxing zonular tension on the lens equator and allowing the lens to shift forward and assume a more spherical shape *(accommodation).*
- They cause contraction of the longitudinal fibers of the ciliary muscle, producing tension on the scleral spur (opening the trabecular meshwork) and facilitating aqueous outflow. Contraction of the ciliary musculature also produces tension on the peripheral retina, occasionally resulting in a retinal tear or even rhegmatogenous detachment.

Acetylcholine does not penetrate the corneal epithelium well, and it is rapidly degraded by acetylcholinesterase (Fig 16-3). Thus, it is not used topically. Acetylcholine, 1%, and

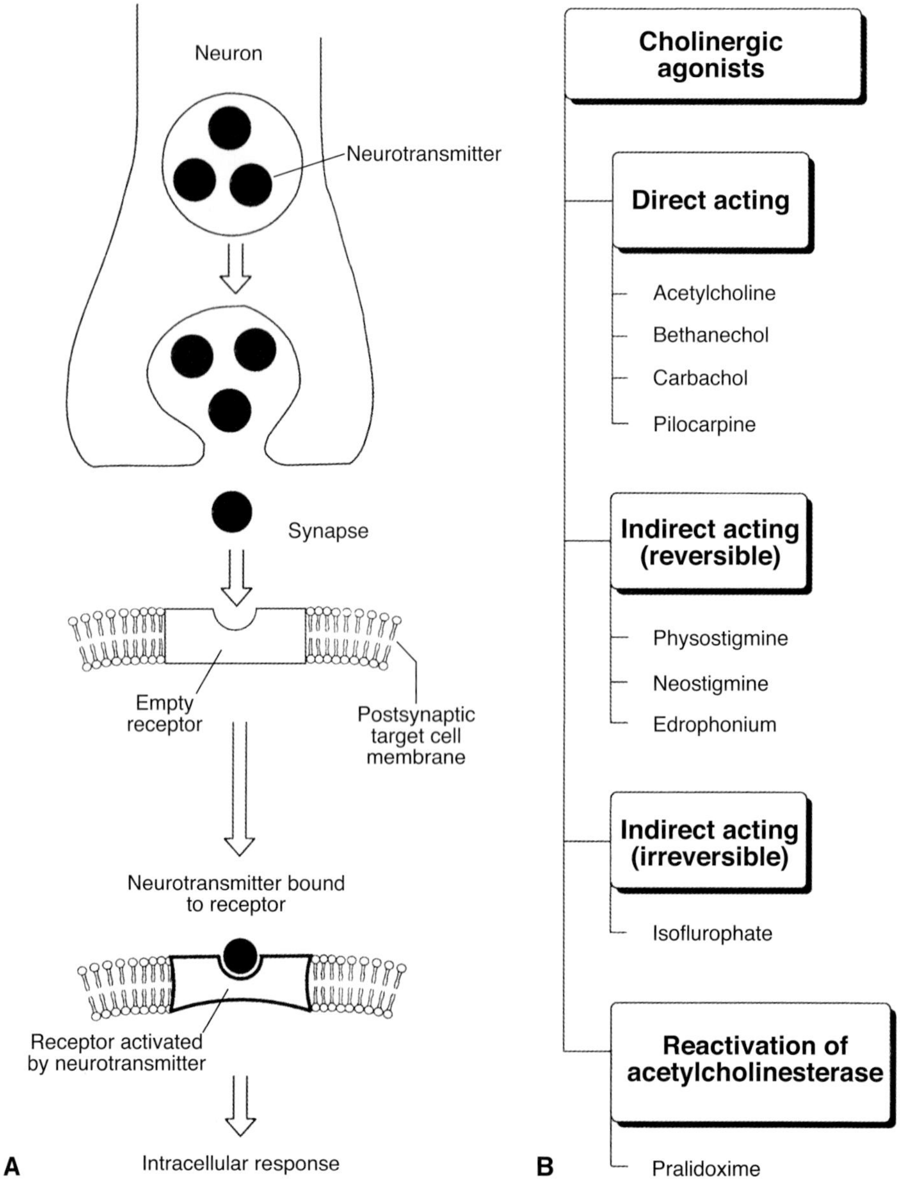

Figure 16-2 **A,** Neurotransmitter binding triggers an intracellular response. **B,** Summary of cholinergic agonists. *(Reproduced with permission from Harvey RA, Champe PC, eds.* Pharmacology. *Lippincott's Illustrated Reviews. Philadelphia: Lippincott; 1992:30, 35.)*

carbachol, 0.01%, are available for intracameral use in anterior segment surgery. These drugs produce prompt and marked miosis.

The onset of intracameral acetylcholine, 1%, is more rapid than that of intracameral carbachol; acetylcholine acts within seconds of instillation, but the effect is short-lived. The drug is not stable in aqueous form and, as mentioned previously, is rapidly broken down by acetylcholinesterase in the anterior chamber. When administered similarly,

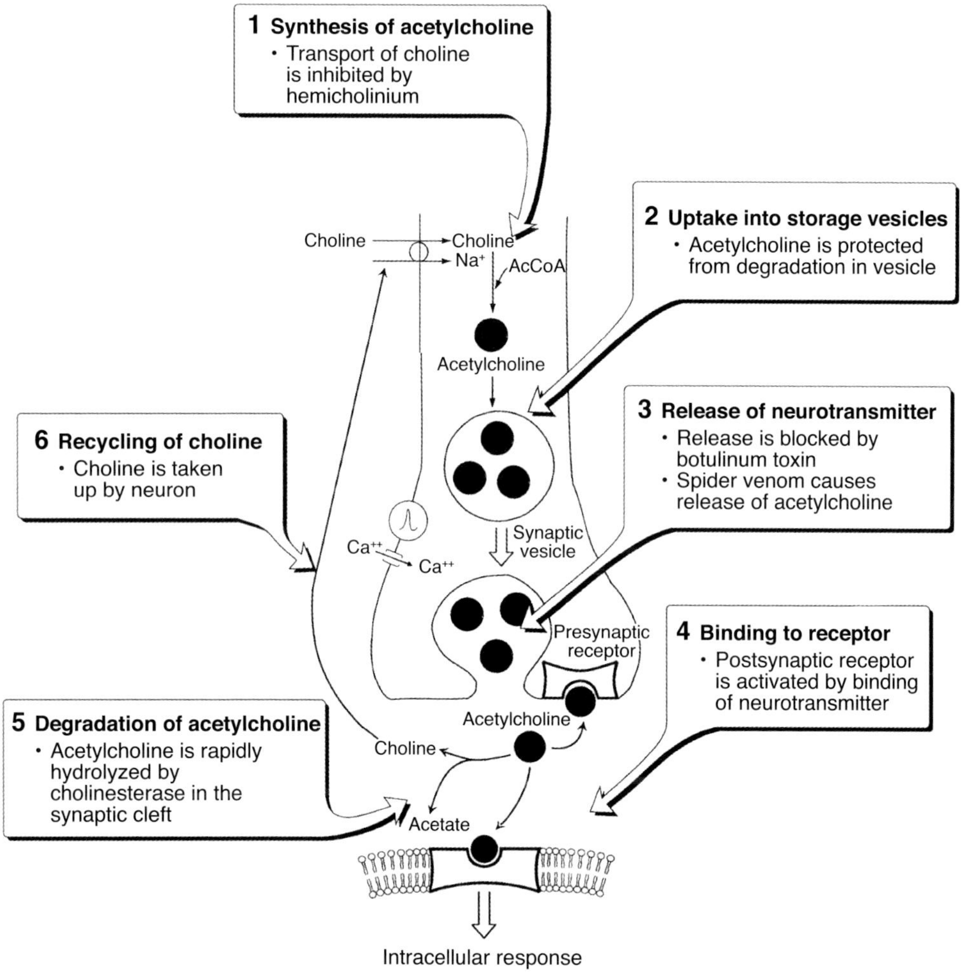

Figure 16-3 Synthesis and release of acetylcholine from the cholinergic neuron. AcCoA = acetyl coenzyme A. *(Reproduced with permission from Mycek MJ, Harvey RA, Champe PC, eds.* Pharmacology. *2nd ed. Lippincott's Illustrated Reviews. Philadelphia: Lippincott-Raven; 1997:37.)*

intracameral carbachol, 0.01%, is 100 times more effective and longer lasting than acetylcholine, 1%. Maximal miosis is achieved within 5 minutes and lasts for 24 hours. In addition, carbachol, 0.01%, is an effective hypotensive drug that lowers intraocular pressure (IOP) during the crucial 24-hour period after surgery.

Pilocarpine, 0.12%, is used diagnostically to confirm an Adie tonic pupil, a condition in which the parasympathetic innervation of the iris sphincter and ciliary muscle is defective because of the loss of postganglionic fibers. Denervated muscarinic smooth muscle fibers in the affected segments of the iris exhibit supersensitivity and respond well to this weak miotic, whereas the normal iris does not.

Pilocarpine, 0.25%, 0.5%, 1%, 2%, 3%, or 4% (4 times daily), and carbachol, 1.5% or 3% (2 times daily), are used in the treatment of primary open-angle glaucoma (POAG) because they lower IOP by facilitating outflow (Table 16-4). Use of pilocarpine beyond 2%

Table 16-4 Miotics

Generic Name	Trade Name	Strengths
Cholinergic drugs		
Carbachol	Isopto Carbachol	1.5%, 3%
Pilocarpine HCl	Isopto Carpine	0.25%, 1%, 2%, 4%
	Available generically	0.5%, 1%, 2%, 3%, 4%
Pilocarpine HCl ointment	Pilopine HS gel	4%
Cholinesterase inhibitors		
Physostigmine	Available generically	1 mg/mL ampule
Echothiophate iodide[a]	Phospholine Iodide	0.125%

[a] Not available for ophthalmic use in the United States.

is not more effective and may even cause a paradoxical increase in IOP in some cases of angle-closure glaucoma because this strong miotic may induce anterior movement of the lens–iris diaphragm. This is a concern particularly in cases of secondary angle closure attributed to anterior rotation of the ciliary body and choroidal edema (eg, malignant glaucoma [also referred to as *aqueous misdirection*] and topiramate-induced angle closure, respectively).

Miotic therapy can also be used (1) to treat elevated IOP in patients with primary angle-closure glaucoma in which the anterior chamber angle remains occludable despite laser iridotomy; and (2) as prophylaxis for angle closure before iridotomy, but not as a long-term substitute for laser iridotomy (see BCSC Section 10, *Glaucoma,* for additional information).

Miosis, cataractogenesis, and induced myopia are generally unwelcome adverse effects of muscarinic therapy. Although the broad range of retinal dark adaptation usually compensates sufficiently for the effect of miosis on vision during daylight hours, patients taking these drugs may be visually incapacitated in dim light. In addition, miosis often compounds the effect of axial lenticular opacities; thus, many patients with cataracts are unable to tolerate miotics. Furthermore, older patients with early cataracts have visual difficulty in scotopic conditions, and the miosis induced by cholinergic drugs may increase the risk of falls. Younger patients may have difficulty with miotics as well. For example, patients younger than 50 years may manifest disabling myopia and induced accommodation because of drug-induced contraction of the ciliary body, which increases the convexity of the lens and shifts the lens forward. Other complications observed with use of higher concentrations of miotics include iris cysts and retinal detachment due to ciliary body contraction and traction on the pars plana.

Systemic adverse effects of muscarinic agonists include salivation, diarrhea, urinary urgency, vomiting, bronchial spasm, bradycardia, and diaphoresis. However, systemic adverse effects are rare following topical use of direct-acting agonists. For example, a slowly dissolving pilocarpine gel used at bedtime minimizes the unwanted adverse effects of the agent and is useful for younger patients, patients with symptoms of variable myopia or intense miosis, older patients with lens opacities, and patients who have difficulty complying with more frequent dosing regimens.

Ciliary muscle stimulation can help manage accommodative esotropia. The near response is a synkinesis of accommodation, miosis, and convergence. As discussed previously, muscarinic agonists contract the ciliary body and induce accommodation as an adverse effect. Therefore, the patient does not need to accommodate at near, which decreases not only the synkinetic convergence response but also the degree of accommodative esotropia.

Indirect-acting agonists

Indirect-acting muscarinic agonists (cholinesterase inhibitors) have the same actions as direct-acting muscarinic agonists, although they have a longer duration of action and are frequently more potent. These medications react with the active serine hydroxyl site of cholinesterases, forming an enzyme–inhibitor complex that renders the enzyme unavailable for hydrolyzing acetylcholine.

There are 2 classes of cholinesterase inhibitors:

- *reversible inhibitors,* such as physostigmine (available as a powder for compounding and as a solution for injection), neostigmine, and edrophonium
- *irreversible inhibitors,* such as echothiophate (phospholine iodide, no longer available for ophthalmic use in the United States); diisopropyl phosphorofluoridate (no longer available for ophthalmic use in the United States), which phosphorylates both the acetylcholinesterase of the synaptic cleft and the butyrylcholinesterase (pseudocholinesterase) of plasma; and demecarium bromide (no longer available for ophthalmic use in the United States)

The duration of inhibitory action is determined by the strength of the bond between the inhibitor and the enzyme. Inhibitors that are organic derivatives of phosphoric acid (eg, organophosphates such as echothiophate) undergo initial binding and hydrolysis by the enzyme, forming a phosphorylated active site. Such a covalent phosphorus–enzyme bond is extremely stable and hydrolyzes very slowly. Because of the marked differences in their duration of action, organophosphate inhibitors are irreversible inhibitors.

The action of phosphorylating cholinesterase inhibitors can be reversed by treatment with oxime-containing compounds. Oxime pralidoxime—though useful in the treatment of acute organophosphate poisoning (eg, insecticide exposure)—is of little value in reversing the marked reduction of plasma butyrylcholinesterase activity that occurs with long-term irreversible cholinesterase-inhibitor therapy.

Patients receiving long-term irreversible cholinesterase-inhibitor therapy such as echothiophate may experience toxic reactions from systemic absorption of local anesthetics containing ester groups (eg, procaine), which are normally inactivated by plasma cholinesterase. Administration of the muscle relaxant succinylcholine during induction of general anesthesia is also hazardous in these patients because the drug will not be metabolized and will prolong respiratory paralysis.

Phosphorylating cholinesterase inhibitors may also cause local ocular toxicity. In children, cystlike proliferations of the iris pigment epithelium may develop at the pupil margin, which can block the pupil. For unknown reasons, cyst development can be minimized by concomitant use of phenylephrine (2.5%) drops. In adults, cataracts may develop, or preexisting opacities may progress. Interestingly, such cataracts are rare in children, and significant epithelial cysts are rare, if they occur at all, in adults.

Antagonists

Topically applied muscarinic antagonists, such as atropine, react with postsynaptic muscarinic receptors and block the action of acetylcholine. Paralysis of the iris sphincter, coupled with the unopposed action of the dilator muscle, causes pupillary dilation, or *mydriasis* (Table 16-5). Mydriasis facilitates examination of the peripheral lens, ciliary body, and retina. Muscarinic antagonists are approved for therapeutic use in the treatment of anterior uveitis in adults because they reduce contact between the posterior iris surface and the anterior lens capsule, thereby preventing the formation of iris–lens adhesions, or *posterior synechiae.* Topically applied muscarinic antagonists also reduce permeability of the blood–aqueous barrier and are useful for treating ocular inflammatory disease. Atropine and cyclopentolate have been approved by the FDA for use in pediatric patients but not for all indications.

Muscarinic antagonists also paralyze the ciliary muscles, which helps relieve pain associated with iridocyclitis; inhibit accommodation for accurate refraction in children

Table 16-5 Mydriatics and Cycloplegics

Generic Name	Trade Name	Strengths	Onset of Action	Duration of Action
Phenylephrine HCl	AK-Dilate	Solution, 2.5%, 10%	30–60 min	3–5 h
	Altafrin	Solution, 2.5%, 10%		
	Mydfrin	Solution, 2.5%		
	Neofrin	Solution, 2.5%		
	Neo-Synephrine	Solution, 2.5%		
	Available generically	Solution, 2.5%, 10%		
Hydroxyamphetamine hydrobromide, 1%		Available as powder for compounding	30–60 min	3–5 h
Atropine sulfate	Atropine-Care	Solution, 1%	45–120 min	7–14 d
	Isopto Atropine	Solution, 1%		
	Available generically	Solution, 1%		
		Ointment, 1%		
Cyclopentolate HCl	AK-Pentolate	Solution, 1%	30–60 min	1–2 d
	Cyclogyl	Solution, 0.5%–2%		
	Cylate	Solution, 1%		
	Available generically	Solution, 1%, 2%		
Homatropine hydrobromide	Isopto Homatropine	Solution, 2%, 5%	30–60 min	3 d
	Homatropaire	Solution, 5%		
Scopolamine hydrobromide	Isopto Hyoscine	Solution, 0.25%	30–60 min	4–7 d
Tropicamide	Mydral	Solution, 0.5%, 1%	20–40 min	4–6 h
	Mydriacyl	Solution, 1%		
	Tropicacyl	Solution, 0.5%, 1%		
	Available generically	Solution, 0.5%, 1%		
Cyclopentolate HCl/ phenylephrine HCl[a]	Cyclomydril	Solution, 0.2%/1%	30–60 min	1–2 d
Hydroxyamphetamine hydrobromide/ tropicamide[b]	Paremyd	Solution, 1%/0.25%	20–40 min	4–6 h

[a] A dilute combination agent for infant examinations.
[b] Used for dilating the pupil; cannot be used to test for Horner syndrome.

(cyclopentolate, atropine); and treat ciliary block (malignant) glaucoma. However, use of cycloplegic drugs to dilate the pupils of patients with POAG may elevate IOP, especially in patients who require miotics for pressure control. Therefore, use of short-acting medications and monitoring of IOP in patients with severe optic nerve damage are advised.

In situations requiring complete cycloplegia, such as the treatment of iridocyclitis (scopolamine, homatropine, or atropine for adults) or the full refractive correction of accommodative esotropia, more potent drugs are preferred. Although a single drop of atropine has some cycloplegic effect that lasts for days, 2 or 3 instillations a day may be required to maintain full cycloplegia for pain relief from iridocyclitis. It may become necessary to change medications if atropine elicits a characteristic local irritation with swelling and maceration of the eyelids and conjunctival injection (hyperemia). When mydriasis alone is necessary to facilitate examination or refraction, drugs with a shorter residual effect are preferred because they allow faster return of pupil response and reading ability.

Systemic absorption of topical muscarinic antagonists can cause dose-related toxicity, especially in children, for whom the dose is distributed within a smaller body mass. A combination of central and peripheral effects, including flushing, fever, tachycardia, constipation, urinary retention, and even delirium, can result. Mild cases may require only discontinuation of the drug, but severe cases can be treated with intravenous physostigmine (approved for adults and children), slowly titrated until the symptoms subside. Physostigmine is used because it is a tertiary amine (uncharged) and can cross the blood–brain barrier.

Administration of atropine for systemic effect blocks the oculocardiac reflex, a reflex bradycardia that is sometimes elicited during ocular surgery by manipulation of the conjunctiva, the globe, or the extraocular muscles. The reflex can also be prevented at the afferent end by retrobulbar anesthesia, although it can occur during administration of the retrobulbar block.

Nicotinic Drugs

Indirect-acting agonists

Edrophonium is the only cholinesterase inhibitor that ophthalmologists administer in a dose high enough to work as an indirect-acting nicotinic agonist. Edrophonium is a short-acting competitive inhibitor of acetylcholinesterase that binds to the enzyme's active site but does not form a covalent link with it. It is used in the diagnosis of myasthenia gravis, a neuromuscular disease caused by autoimmunity to acetylcholine receptors (nicotinic receptors) in the neuromuscular junction and characterized by muscle weakness and marked fatigability of skeletal muscles. This disease may manifest primarily as ptosis and diplopia. In patients with myasthenia gravis, the inhibition of acetylcholinesterase by edrophonium allows acetylcholine released into the synaptic cleft to accumulate to levels that can act through the reduced number of acetylcholine receptors. Because edrophonium also augments muscarinic transmission, muscarinic adverse effects (vomiting, diarrhea, urination, and bradycardia) may occur unless 0.4–0.6 mg of atropine is co-administered intravenously (see BCSC Section 5, *Neuro-Ophthalmology*).

Another drug used in the diagnosis of myasthenia gravis is neostigmine methylsulfate, a longer-acting intramuscular drug. The longer duration of activity allows the examiner to assess specific complex endpoints, such as orthoptic measurements.

Antagonists

Nicotinic antagonists are neuromuscular blocking agents that facilitate intubation for general anesthesia (Table 16-6). There are 2 types of nicotinic antagonists:

- *nondepolarizing agents,* including curare-like drugs such as rocuronium, vecuronium, gallamine, and pancuronium, which bind competitively to nicotinic receptors on striated muscle but do not cause contraction
- *depolarizing agents,* such as succinylcholine and decamethonium, which bind competitively to nicotinic receptors and cause initial receptor depolarization and muscle contraction

In singly innervated (en plaque) muscle fibers, depolarization and contraction are followed by prolonged unresponsiveness and flaccidity. However, depolarizing agents produce sustained contractions of multiply innervated fibers, which make up one-fifth of the muscle fibers of extraocular muscles. Such contractions of extraocular muscles (a nicotinic agonist action) exert force on the globe.

CLINICAL PEARL

Depolarizing agents should not be used to induce general anesthesia for operations on open globes because the force of extraocular muscle contractions on the eye, occurring with use of these drugs, could expel intraocular contents. In addition, these agents can increase IOP via a similar mechanism and thus should be used with caution for examinations under anesthesia.

Adrenergic Drugs

Several ophthalmic medications affect the activity of adrenergic receptors (also called *adrenoceptors*) in synapses of the peripheral nervous system. These receptors are found in

- the cell membranes of the iris dilator muscle, the superior palpebral smooth muscle of Müller, the ciliary epithelium and processes, the trabecular meshwork, and the smooth muscle of ocular blood vessels (supplied by postganglionic autonomic fibers from the superior cervical ganglion)
- the presynaptic terminals of some sympathetic and parasympathetic nerves, where the receptors have feedback-inhibitory actions

Although adrenergic receptors were originally defined by their response to epinephrine (adrenaline), the transmitter of most sympathetic postganglionic fibers is actually norepinephrine. Adrenergic receptors are subclassified into 5 categories—α_1, α_2, β_1, β_2, and β_3—on the basis of their profile of responses to natural and synthetic catecholamines (Fig 16-4). α_1-Receptors generally mediate smooth muscle contraction, whereas α_2-receptors mediate feedback inhibition of presynaptic sympathetic (and sometimes parasympathetic) nerve terminals. β_1-Receptors are found predominantly in the heart, where they mediate stimulatory effects; β_2-receptors mediate relaxation of smooth muscle in most blood vessels and in the bronchi, whereas β_3-receptors are found on fat cells mediating lipolysis.

Table 16-6 Cholinergic Antagonists

Category	Examples
Muscarinic receptor–blocking drugs	Atropine Scopolamine
Ganglion-blocking drugs	Mecamylamine Nicotine Trimethaphan
Neuromuscular blocking drugs	Gallamine Pancuronium Rocuronium Succinylcholine Tubocurarine Vecuronium

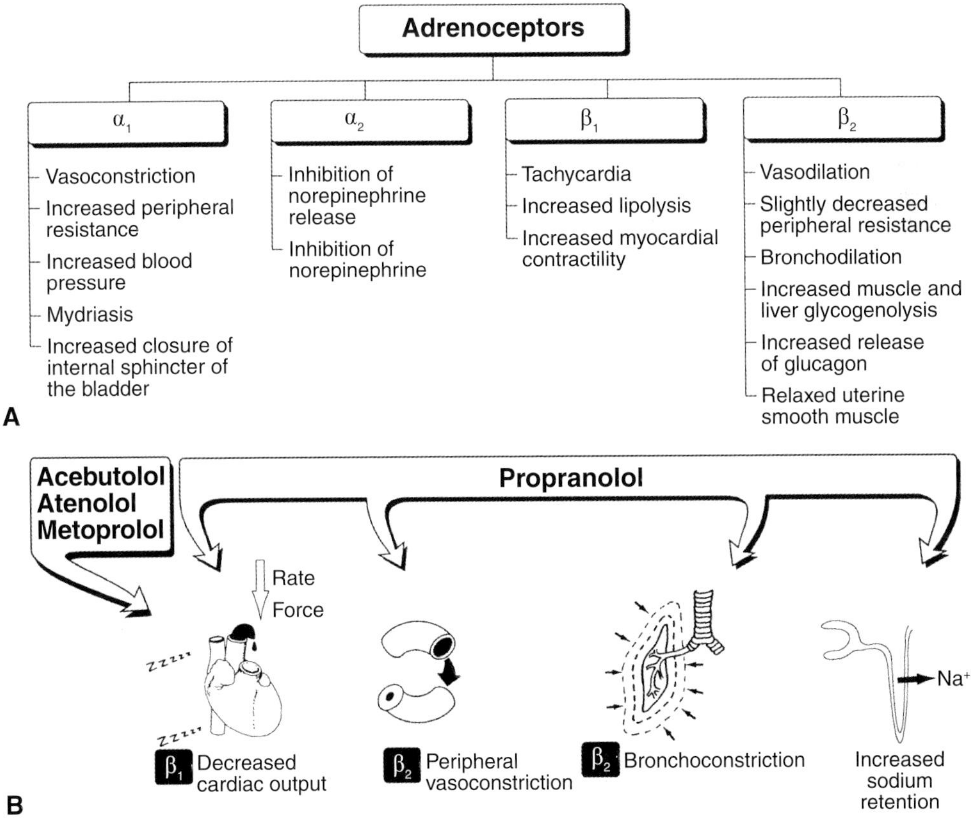

Figure 16-4 **A,** Major effects mediated by α- and β-adrenoceptors. **B,** Actions of propranolol and β_1-blockers. *(Reproduced with permission from Mycek MJ, Harvey RA, Champe PC, eds.* Pharmacology. *2nd ed. Lippincott's Illustrated Reviews. Philadelphia: Lippincott-Raven; 1997:60, 75.)*

Adrenergic drugs may be direct-acting agonists, indirect-acting agonists, or antagonists at one or more of the 5 types of receptors. Systemic absorption of ocular adrenergic drugs is frequently sufficient to cause systemic effects, which are manifested in the cardiovascular system, the bronchial airways, and the brain.

α-Adrenergic Drugs

Direct-acting α_1-adrenergic agonists

The primary clinical use of direct-acting α_1-adrenergic agonists, such as phenylephrine, is stimulation of the iris dilator muscle to produce mydriasis. Because the parasympathetically innervated iris sphincter muscle is much stronger than the dilator muscle, the dilation achieved with phenylephrine alone is largely overcome by the pupillary light reflex during ophthalmoscopy. Co-administration of a cycloplegic drug allows sustained dilatation.

Systemic absorption of phenylephrine may elevate systemic blood pressure. This effect is clinically significant if the patient is an infant or has an abnormally increased sensitivity to α-agonists, which occurs with orthostatic hypotension and in association with the use of drugs that accentuate adrenergic effects (eg, reserpine, tricyclic antidepressants, cocaine, monoamine oxidase [MAO] inhibitors—discussed later). Even with lower doses of phenylephrine (2.5%), infants may exhibit a transient rise in blood pressure because the dose received in an eyedrop is high for their weight.

Phenylephrine, 10%, should be used cautiously, particularly in pledget application and in patients with vasculopathic risk factors. A 10% solution contains 5 mg of drug per drop, and ocular medications passing through the canalicular system are available for systemic absorption through the vascular nasal mucosa (see Chapter 15). In contrast, the typical systemic dose of phenylephrine for hypotension is 50–100 μg given all at once. The ophthalmic use of phenylephrine, 10%, has been associated with stroke, myocardial infarction, and cardiac arrest. Vascular baroreceptors are particularly sensitive to phenylephrine. An increase in blood pressure after topical application may therefore cause a significant drop in pulse rate that can be particularly dangerous in an individual with vasculopathy who is already taking a β-blocking medication for systemic effect.

Intracameral use of phenylephrine to maintain dilatation during cataract surgery has recently been evaluated. The compound Omidria (phenylephrine 1%/ketorolac 0.3%) is added to the irrigating solution and has been approved by the FDA to prevent miosis during cataract surgery and prevent postoperative pain. One study recently demonstrated the efficacy of this compound for management of intraoperative floppy iris syndrome (IFIS) in patients taking tamsulosin.

Hovanesian JA, Sheppard JD, Trattler WB, et al. Intracameral phenylephrine and ketorolac during cataract surgery to maintain intraoperative mydriasis and reduce postoperative ocular pain: integrated results from 2 pivotal phase 3 studies. *J Cataract Refract Surg.* 2015;41(10):2060–2068.

Silverstein SM, Rana VK, Stephens R, et al. Effect of phenylephrine 1.0%-ketorolac 0.3% injection on tamsulosin-associated intraoperative floppy-iris syndrome. *J Cataract Refract Surg.* 2018;44(9):1103–1108.

α_2-Adrenergic agonists

Apraclonidine hydrochloride (*para*-aminoclonidine) is a selective α_2-adrenergic agonist and a clonidine derivative that prevents release of norepinephrine at nerve terminals (Tables 16-7, 16-8). It decreases aqueous production as well as episcleral venous pressure and improves trabecular outflow. However, its true ocular hypotensive mechanism is not fully understood. When administered preoperatively and postoperatively, the drug effectively diminishes the acute increase in IOP that follows argon laser iridotomy, argon or selective laser trabeculoplasty, Nd:YAG laser capsulotomy, and cataract extraction (see BCSC Section 10, *Glaucoma*, for additional information on apraclonidine). Apraclonidine hydrochloride may be effective for the short-term reduction of IOP, but the development of topical sensitivity and tachyphylaxis often limits its long-term use.

> Ligand binding to α_2-receptors in other systems mediates inhibition of the enzyme adenylate cyclase. Adenylate cyclase is present in the ciliary epithelium and is thought to have a role in aqueous production.

Table 16-7 Adrenergic Agonists

Generic Name	Trade Name	Strengths
β_2-Adrenergic agonists		
Dipivefrin HCl	Propine	0.1%
	Available generically	0.1%
Epinephrine HCl	Not available in the United States	0.5%, 1%, 2%
α_2-Selective agonists		
Apraclonidine HCl	Iopidine	0.5%, 1% (single-use container)
Brimonidine tartrate	Alphagan P	0.1%, 0.15%
	Available generically	0.2%
Brimonidine tartrate/timolol maleate	Combigan	0.2%/0.5%

Table 16-8 Mode of Action of Antiglaucoma Drugs That Act Through Receptors

Primary Mechanism of Action	Drug Class	Examples
Decrease aqueous humor production	1. β-Adrenergic antagonists	Timolol, betaxolol, carteolol, levobunolol
	2. α_2-Adrenergic agonists	Apraclonidine, brimonidine
Increase trabecular outflow	1. Miotics	Pilocarpine
	2. Adrenergic agonists	Epinephrine, dipivalyl epinephrine
Increase uveoscleral outflow	1. Prostaglandins	Latanoprost, bimatoprost, travoprost, tafluprost
	2. α_2-Adrenergic agonists	Apraclonidine, brimonidine

Apraclonidine can also be used to diagnose Horner syndrome, characterized by denervation hypersensitivity of the α_1-receptors in the iris. Under normal conditions, as a weak α_1-adrenergic agonist, apraclonidine has no effect on pupil dilation; however, in cases of Horner syndrome, instillation of the drug results in dilation of the affected pupil (see BCSC Section 5, *Neuro-Ophthalmology*, for additional information on the role of apraclonidine in the diagnosis of Horner syndrome).

Brimonidine tartrate is another selective α_2-adrenergic agonist. Compared with apraclonidine, brimonidine tartrate is more α_2 selective, is more lipophilic, and causes less tachyphylaxis during long-term use. The rate of reactions, such as follicular conjunctivitis and contact blepharodermatitis, is also lower (less than 15% for brimonidine but up to 40% for apraclonidine). Cross-sensitivity to brimonidine in patients with known hypersensitivity to apraclonidine is minimal.

Brimonidine's mechanism in lowering IOP is thought to involve both decreased aqueous production and increased uveoscleral outflow. As with β-blockers, a central mechanism of brimonidine, 0.2%, may account for some IOP reduction: A 1-week trial of treatment in a single eye caused a statistically significant reduction of 1.2 mm Hg in the fellow eye.

The peak IOP reduction with brimonidine is approximately 26%. At peak (2 hours postdose), its IOP reduction is comparable to that of a nonselective β-blocker and superior to that of the selective β-blocker betaxolol; however, at trough (12 hours postdose), the reduction is only 14%–15%, which makes brimonidine at trough less effective than the nonselective β-blockers but comparable to betaxolol.

> As shown in animal models of optic nerve and retinal injuries, brimonidine may have neuroprotective properties that are independent of IOP reduction. The proposed mechanism of neuroprotection is upregulation of a neurotrophin, basic fibroblast growth factor, and cellular regulatory genes.

In addition to brimonidine, 0.2%, preserved with benzalkonium chloride, a 0.15% solution preserved with polyquaternium-1 and 0.15% and 0.1% solutions preserved with sodium chlorite are available. Brimonidine tartrate, 0.15%, is comparable to brimonidine, 0.2%, when given 3 times daily.

Ophthalmologists should exercise caution when using apraclonidine or brimonidine in patients taking MAO inhibitors or tricyclic antidepressants and in patients with severe cardiovascular disease. Use of these drugs concomitantly with β-blockers (ophthalmic and systemic), antihypertensives, and cardiac glycosides also requires prudence.

Though effective for rapid lowering of IOP in angle-closure glaucoma, these drugs may also induce vasoconstriction that can prolong iris sphincter ischemia and reduce the efficacy of concurrent miotics. Apraclonidine has a much greater affinity for α_1-receptors than does brimonidine and is therefore more likely to produce vasoconstriction in the eye. Brimonidine does not induce vasoconstriction in the posterior segment or the optic nerve.

Because brimonidine is more lipophilic than apraclonidine, its penetration of the blood–brain barrier is presumably higher. Central nervous system (CNS) adverse effects include fatigue and drowsiness.

CLINICAL PEARL

Severe systemic toxicity, with hypotension, hypothermia, and bradycardia, has been reported in infants treated with topical ocular brimonidine. As a result, this drug is contraindicated in infants and should be used with caution in young children.

Indirect-acting adrenergic agonists

Indirect-acting adrenergic agonists (cocaine, 4% or 10%, and hydroxyamphetamine, 1%, currently available only through compounding pharmacies) are used to test for and localize defects in sympathetic innervation to the iris dilator muscle. Normally, pupil response fibers originating in the hypothalamus pass down the spinal cord to synapse with cells in the intermediolateral columns. In turn, preganglionic fibers exit the cord through the anterior spinal roots in the upper thorax to synapse in the superior cervical ganglion in the neck. Finally, postganglionic adrenergic fibers terminate in a neuroeffector junction with the iris dilator muscle. The norepinephrine released is inactivated primarily by reuptake into secretory granules in the nerve terminal (Fig 16-5). Approximately 70% of released norepinephrine is recaptured (see the discussion of Horner syndrome in BCSC Section 5, *Neuro-Ophthalmology*).

Antagonists

Thymoxamine hydrochloride (moxisylyte), an α_1-adrenergic blocking agent, acts by competitively inhibiting norepinephrine at the receptor site. Thymoxamine inhibits α-adrenergic receptors of the dilator muscle of the iris and causes pupil constriction; however, it has no significant effect on ciliary muscle contraction and therefore does not induce substantial changes in anterior chamber depth, facility of outflow, IOP, or accommodation in POAG. In patients with an increase in IOP secondary to primary angle closure, thymoxamine may widen the peripheral angle and reduce IOP. Thymoxamine is useful in differentiating angle-closure glaucoma from POAG with narrow angles and in reversing the pupil dilation caused by phenylephrine. This drug is not commercially available in the United States, although it has been widely used in Europe for years.

Dapiprazole hydrochloride (no longer available in the United States) is an α-adrenergic blocking agent that reverses, in 30 minutes, the mydriasis produced by phenylephrine and tropicamide but not by cycloplegics. It affects the dilator muscle but not ciliary muscle contraction (anterior chamber depth, facility of outflow, or accommodation).

β-Adrenergic Drugs

β_2-Adrenergic agonists

β_2-Adrenergic agonists lower IOP by improving trabecular outflow and possibly by increasing uveoscleral outflow. The beneficial effect on outflow more than compensates for a small increase in aqueous inflow as detected by fluorophotometry. The effect on outflow facility seems to be mediated by β_2-receptors.

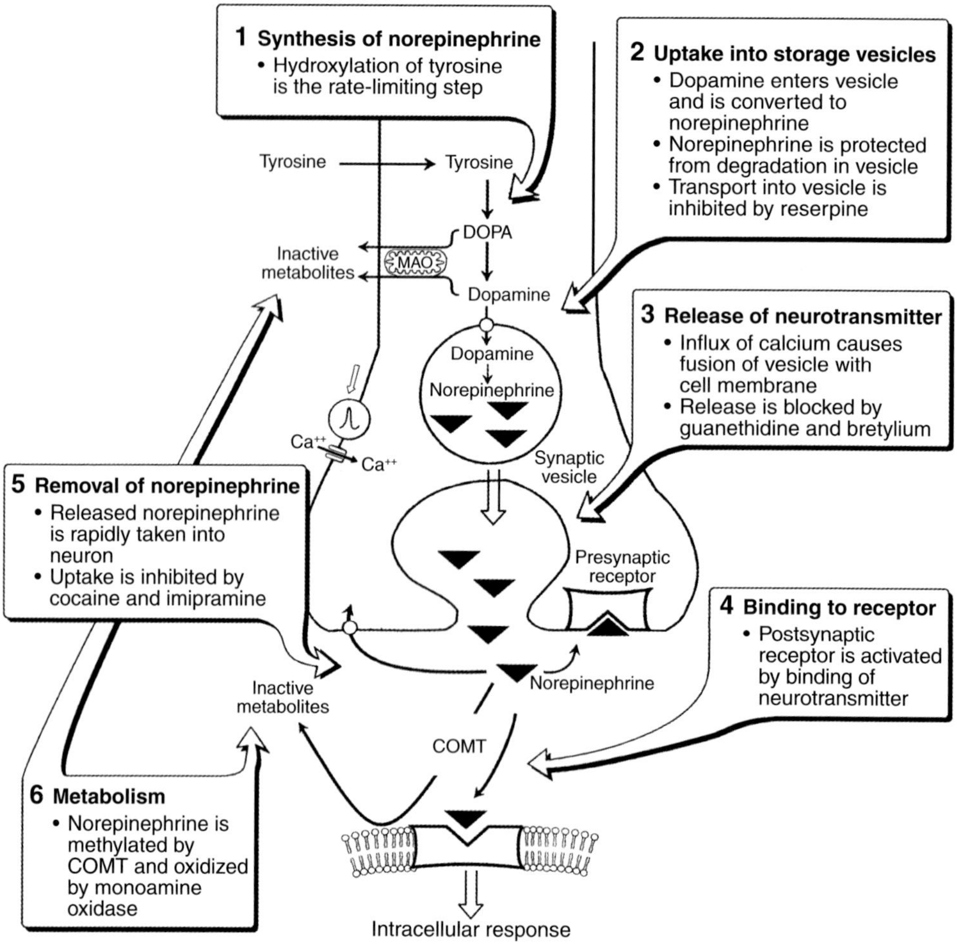

Figure 16-5 Synthesis and release of norepinephrine from the adrenergic neuron. COMT = catechol-O-methyltransferase; DOPA = dihydroxyphenylalanine; MAO = monoamine oxidase inhibitor. *(Reproduced with permission from Mycek MJ, Harvey RA, Champe PC, eds.* Pharmacology. *2nd ed. Lippincott's Illustrated Reviews. Philadelphia: Lippincott-Raven; 1997:57.)*

β_2-Receptors linked to adenylate cyclase are present in the ciliary epithelium and processes as well as in the trabecular meshwork. Treatment with L-epinephrine, a nonselective mixed α- and β-agonist, increases intracellular levels of cyclic adenosine monophosphate (cAMP) in these tissues and in the aqueous humor. In other tissues, β-receptor–mediated generation of cAMP in turn activates cAMP-dependent enzymes, which results in responses such as glycogenolysis and gluconeogenesis in the liver and lipolysis in adipose tissue. However, the biochemical mechanisms responsible for lowering IOP remain to be determined.

Topical L-epinephrine is no longer commercially available in the United States or used in most countries (see Table 16-7). Local and systemic adverse effects are common (see BCSC Section 10, *Glaucoma*). Clinically, nonselective adrenergic drugs have been replaced by the selective α_2-adrenergic agonists because of their improved efficacy and adverse effect profiles. In an animal model, long-term therapy with epinephrine was shown to downregulate the number of β-receptors. This phenomenon may underlie the loss of some of the drug's therapeutic effectiveness over time (tachyphylaxis).

β-Adrenergic antagonists

β-Adrenergic antagonists, also known as *β-blockers,* lower IOP by reducing aqueous humor production by as much as 50% (Table 16-9). Six β-blockers are approved for use in the treatment of glaucoma: timolol maleate, levobunolol, metipranolol, carteolol, betaxolol, and timolol hemihydrate. Although it is likely that the site of action is the ciliary body, it is not known whether the vasculature of the ciliary processes or the pumping mechanism of the ciliary epithelium is primarily affected. A possible mechanism may be an effect on the β-adrenergic receptor–coupled adenylate cyclase of the ciliary epithelium.

Table 16-9 β-Adrenergic Antagonists

Generic Name	Trade Name	Strengths
Betaxolol HCl	Betoptic S	0.25%
	Available generically	0.5%
Carteolol HCl	Ocupress	1%
	Available generically	1%
Levobunolol HCl	Betagan	0.25%, 0.5%
	Available generically	0.25%, 0.5%
Metipranolol HCl	OptiPranolol	0.3%
	Available generically	0.3%
Timolol hemihydrate	Betimol	0.25%, 0.5%
Timolol maleate	Istalol	0.5%
	Timoptic in Ocumeter or Ocumeter Plus container	0.25%, 0.5%
	Available generically	0.25%, 0.5%
	Timoptic-XE in Ocumeter or Ocumeter Plus container (gel)	0.25%, 0.5%
	Available generically as Timolol gel-forming solution	0.25%, 0.5%
Timolol maleate (preservative-free)	Timoptic in OcuDose	0.25%, 0.5%
Brimonidine tartrate/timolol maleate	Combigan	Brimonidine tartrate, 0.2%/ timolol maleate, 0.5%
Dorzolamide HCl/timolol maleate	Cosopt Ocumeter Plus	Dorzolamide, 2%/timolol, 0.5%
	Available generically	Dorzolamide, 2%/timolol, 0.5%
Dorzolamide HCl/timolol maleate (preservative-free)	Cosopt in OcuDose	Dorzolamide, 2%/timolol, 0.5%
	Available generically	Dorzolamide, 2%/timolol, 0.5%

Although systemic administration of β-blockers has been reported to elevate blood lipid levels, such elevation has not been demonstrated with topical β-blockers such as timolol. All β-blockers can inhibit the increase in pulse and blood pressure that is exhibited in response to exertion. For this reason, they may be poorly tolerated in elderly patients during routine activities, as well as in young, physically active individuals. Nonselective β-blockers inhibit the pulmonary β_2-receptors that dilate the respiratory tree. The induced bronchospasm may be significant in patients with asthma or chronic obstructive lung disease. In patients with bradycardia and second- or third-degree atrioventricular block, the underlying cardiac condition may be exacerbated with use of these drugs.

The traditional teaching that topical β-blockers are contraindicated in patients with congestive heart failure is being challenged. Indeed, current cardiologic evidence strongly demonstrates that β-blockage is an important component of treatment for heart failure, except in advanced cases. Therefore, ophthalmologists should maintain continuous communication with patients' internists or cardiologists regarding the systemic effects of ophthalmic therapy.

Timolol maleate, 0.25% or 0.5%, and levobunolol, 0.25% or 0.5%, are mixed β_1-/β_2-antagonists. Tests of more specific β-blockers suggest that β_2-antagonists have a greater effect on aqueous secretion than do β_1-antagonists. For example, comparative studies have shown that the specific β_1-antagonist betaxolol, 0.5%, is approximately 85% as effective as timolol in lowering IOP.

Metipranolol hydrochloride is a nonselective β_1- and β_2-adrenergic receptor–blocking drug. As a 0.3% topical solution, it is similar in effect to other topical nonselective β-blockers, in addition to reducing IOP.

Carteolol hydrochloride demonstrates intrinsic sympathomimetic activity; in other words, while acting as a competitive antagonist, it also causes a slight to moderate activation of receptors. Thus, even though carteolol has β-blocking activity, it may be tempered, reducing the effects on cardiovascular and respiratory systems. Carteolol is also less likely than other β-blockers to adversely affect the systemic lipid profile.

Betaxolol is a selective β_1-antagonist that is substantially safer than the nonselective β-blockers when pulmonary, cardiac, CNS, or other systemic conditions are considered. Betaxolol may be useful in patients with a history of bronchospastic disorders, although other therapies should be tried first because betaxolol's β selectivity is relative and not absolute, and some β_2 effects can therefore remain. In general, the IOP-lowering effect of betaxolol is less than that of the nonselective β-adrenergic antagonists.

Betaxolol is available as a generic 0.5% solution and as a 0.25% suspension. The 0.25% suspension causes less irritation on instillation yet maintains its clinical efficacy compared with the brand-name 0.5% solution (now discontinued), a finding that is generally extrapolated to the currently available generic 0.5% solution.

Prodrugs of nonselective β-blockers are being developed. They may offer higher potency of β_1-/β_2-blocking medications while reducing their systemic adverse effects.

Curiously, both β-agonist and β-antagonist drugs can lower IOP. This paradox is compounded by the observation that β-agonist and β-antagonist drugs have slightly additive effects in lowering IOP.

Carbonic Anhydrase Inhibitors

Systemic carbonic anhydrase inhibitors (CAIs) such as acetazolamide and methazolamide are approved for the treatment of glaucoma and idiopathic intracranial hypertension (IIH, also known as *pseudotumor cerebri*), in addition to other systemic conditions. They may also be effective in treating cystoid macular edema (CME). See Table 16-10.

Systemic CAIs are administered orally and/or parenterally. The longer half-life of methazolamide allows it to be used twice daily; acetazolamide is also available in a 500-mg sustained-release form used twice daily. Neither of these compounds has the ideal combination of high potency (low binding affinity, K_i), good ocular penetration (high penetration percentage in the nonionized form and high lipid solubility to facilitate passage through the blood–ocular barrier), high proportion of the drug present in the blood in unbound form, and long plasma half-life. The mechanism of action of this class of medications is via inhibition of carbonic anhydrase.

The amount of carbonic anhydrase present in tissues is much higher than that needed to supply the amount of bicarbonate (HCO_3^-) required. Calculations based on the K_{cat} (catalysis constant) and K_m (apparent affinity constant) of the enzyme and on the concentrations of substrates and product indicate that the amount of enzyme present in the ciliary

Table 16-10 Carbonic Anhydrase Inhibitors

Generic Name	Trade Name	Strengths	Onset of Action	Duration of Action
Systemic				
Acetazolamide	Diamox Sequels	500 mg (time-release)	1–1.5 h, 2 h	8–12 h, 18–24 h
	Available generically	125 mg, 250 mg, 500 mg (time-release)	1–1.5 h	8–12 h
Acetazolamide sodium	Available generically	500 mg, 5–10 mg/kg[3]	2 min	4–5 h
Methazolamide	Available generically	25 mg, 50 mg	2–4 h	10–18 h
Topical				
Brinzolamide	Azopt	1% suspension	2 h	8–12 h
Dorzolamide HCl	Trusopt Ocumeter Plus	2% solution	2 h	8 h
	Available generically	2% solution	2 h	8 h
Combination drugs				
Dorzolamide HCl/ timolol maleate	Cosopt Ocumeter Plus	Dorzolamide HCl, 2%/ timolol, 0.5%	2 h	8–12 h
	Available generically	Dorzolamide HCl, 2%/ timolol, 0.5%	2 h	1 h
Dorzolamide HCl/ timolol maleate (preservative-free)	Cosopt in OcuDose	Dorzolamide HCl, 2%/ timolol, 0.5%	2 h	1 h
	Available generically	Dorzolamide HCl, 2%/ timolol, 0.5%	2 h	1 h

body is 100 times greater than needed. Correspondingly, in clinical use, the enzyme must be more than 99% inhibited to significantly reduce aqueous flow. In contrast, the amount of enzyme in the kidney, which is 1000-fold greater than needed, must be more than 99.9% inhibited to affect the usual pathway for HCO_3^- reabsorption.

In addition to lowering IOP by inhibiting ciliary body carbonic anhydrase, each drug at high doses further lowers IOP by causing renal metabolic acidosis. The mechanism by which acidosis lowers secretion is uncertain, but it probably involves reduction in HCO_3^- formation and activity of Na^+,K^+-ATPase.

At the onset of acidosis, renal effects cause alkaline diuresis, with loss of Na^+, K^+, and HCO_3^-. In patients receiving CAI therapy concurrently with diuretics, steroids, or adrenocorticotropic hormone (ACTH), severe hypokalemia can result. This situation may be dangerous for patients using digitalis, in whom hypokalemia may elicit arrhythmias. When such patients are receiving long-term CAI therapy, they should have their potassium levels checked at regular intervals, preferably by their primary care physician.

Over time, the acidosis prompts a renal mechanism for HCO_3^- reabsorption unrelated to carbonic anhydrase; this mechanism limits the degree of acidosis and halts both the diuresis and K^+ loss after the first few days of treatment.

In certain systemic conditions, CAI therapy may cause or contribute to additional adverse effects. Alkalinization of the urine, present during initial CAI treatment, prevents excretion of ammonium (NH_4^+), a factor to consider in patients with cirrhosis of the liver. Metabolic acidosis may exacerbate diabetic ketoacidosis or precipitate sickle cell crisis. In patients with severe chronic obstructive pulmonary disease, respiratory acidosis may be caused by impairment of CO_2 transfer from the pulmonary vasculature to the alveoli. Elderly patients have physiologically reduced renal function, which predisposes them to severe metabolic acidosis with the use of systemic CAIs.

CLINICAL PEARL

With the inhibitor methazolamide, the difference between the concentrations of carbonic anhydrase in the ciliary body and in the kidney can be exploited to lower IOP without incurring renal HCO_3^- loss, and metabolic acidosis can be limited, resulting in fewer adverse effects. Although renal stone formation has been reported with use of methazolamide, the incidence is substantially lower than with other drugs because methazolamide is metabolized in the liver. In contrast, acetazolamide is actively secreted into the renal tubules, and renal effects are unavoidable.

The use of acetazolamide has been linked to the formation of stones in the urinary tract. A retrospective case-control series showed that the incidence of stones was 11 times higher in patients using this drug than in those not using it. The increased risk occurred primarily during the first year of therapy. Continued use after occurrence of a stone was associated with a high risk of recurrent stone formation. However, a history of spontaneous stone formation more than 5 years prior to acetazolamide therapy did not appear to increase risk. The mechanisms responsible for stone formation may be related to metabolic acidosis and associated pH changes, as well as to decreased excretion of citrate.

Nearly 50% of patients are intolerant of systemic CAIs because of CNS and gastrointestinal adverse effects. They include numbness and tingling of the hands, feet, and lips; malaise; metallic taste when drinking carbonated beverages; anorexia and weight loss; nausea; somnolence; impotence and loss of libido; and depression. When the clinical situation allows, it is wise to begin therapy at low dosages (eg, 125 mg of acetazolamide 4 times daily or 25–50 mg methazolamide twice daily) to reduce the incidence and severity of adverse effects. Patients should be informed of the potential adverse effects of these drugs; otherwise, they may fail to associate their systemic symptoms with the medication prescribed by their ophthalmologists.

Rare adverse effects from this class of drugs include those common to other members of the sulfonamide family, such as transient myopia, hypersensitive nephropathy, skin rash, Stevens-Johnson syndrome, and thrombocytopenia. One potential adverse effect, aplastic anemia, is idiosyncratic. Blood cell counts do not identify susceptible patients. CAIs have also been associated with teratogenic effects (forelimb deformity) in rodents, and their use is not advised during pregnancy. However, these systemic adverse effects are rare with topical CAIs (see the section "Sulfonamides" later in the chapter for discussion of allergies to sulfonamides).

The topical CAIs—dorzolamide and brinzolamide—are also available for long-term treatment of glaucoma. They penetrate the cornea easily and are water soluble. When administered as solution 3 times per day, these drugs effectively inhibit carbonic anhydrase II while avoiding the systemic adverse effects of oral administration. The 2 medications are equally effective and reduce IOP by 14%–17%. Adverse effects of topical CAIs include burning on instillation, punctate keratitis, local allergy, and bitter taste. The hypotensive effects of topical and oral CAIs are probably not additive when adequate doses of each are used.

Prostaglandin Analogues

Currently, 5 prostaglandin (PG) analogues have been approved by the FDA for clinical use (Table 16-11). Latanoprost, bimatoprost, travoprost, and tafluprost are administered once daily, with nighttime dosing; unoprostone is used twice daily. Tafluprost is available preservative-free in single-use containers. Latanoprost, travoprost, tafluprost, and unoprostone are prodrugs that require hydrolyzation before becoming active compounds in the eye. Except for unoprostone, whose exact mechanism of action remains unknown, they interact with the prostaglandin FP receptor. In contrast, bimatoprost is not a prodrug, and it acts on the prostamide receptor.

Latanoprost is a prodrug of prostaglandin $F_{2\alpha}$ ($PGF_{2\alpha}$); it penetrates the cornea and becomes biologically active after being hydrolyzed by corneal tissue esterase. It appears to lower IOP by enhancing uveoscleral outflow and may reduce the pressure by 6–9 mm Hg (25%–35%). In addition to once-daily dosing, other advantages of the drug are a lack of cardiopulmonary adverse effects and additivity to other antiglaucoma medications.

A unique ocular adverse effect associated with this class of drugs is the darkening of the iris and periocular skin as a result of increased numbers of melanosomes (increased melanin content, or melanogenesis) within the melanocytes. The risk of iris pigmentation

Table 16-11 Prostaglandin Analogues

Generic Name	Trade Name	Strengths
Bimatoprost	Lumigan	0.01%, 0.03%
Latanoprost	Xalatan	0.005%
	Available generically	0.005%
Tafluprost	Zioptan in single-use containers (preservative-free)	0.0015%
Travoprost	Travatan	0.004%
	Travatan Z	0.004%
Unoprostone isopropyl	Rescula	0.15%
Bimatoprost/timolol maleate	Ganfort (not available in the United States)	Bimatoprost, 0.03%/timolol, 0.5%
Latanoprost/timolol maleate	Xalacom (not available in the United States)	Latanoprost, 0.005%/timolol, 0.5%
Travoprost/timolol maleate	DuoTrav (not available in the United States)	Travoprost, 0.004%/timolol, 0.5%
Latanoprostene bunod	Vyzulta	0.024%

correlates with baseline iris pigmentation. In 10%–20% of light-colored irides, increased pigmentation may occur in the initial 18–24 months of therapy, whereas nearly 60% of eyes that are light brown or 2-toned may experience increased pigmentation over the same period. The long-term sequelae of this adverse effect, if any, are unknown. Other adverse effects associated with topical PG analogues are conjunctival injection, hypertrichosis of the eyelashes, CME, and uveitis. CME and uveitis are more common in eyes with preexisting risk factors for either condition.

Reported systemic reactions include flulike symptoms, rash, and possible uterine bleeding in postmenopausal women. Reactivation of herpetic keratitis has been reported with use of latanoprost. Topical PGs are classified as category C according to the FDA's use-in-pregnancy ratings. Although their elimination from human plasma is rapid, PGs are known to cause contraction of the uterus. Thus, topical PGs should be used with caution in pregnant patients.

Nitric Oxide Donors

Nitric oxide (NO) is a ubiquitous, versatile, endogenous signaling molecule with diverse biological effects. As a gaseous molecule, NO is highly lipophilic and volatile, able to readily diffuse across cell membranes and function as a paracrine messenger that induces changes in adjacent cells. NO is also a highly reactive free radical. Excessive NO, particularly during ischemia, can result in tissue damage.

Endogenous NO is derived from the amino acid L-arginine by the action of NO synthase (NOS). The enzyme has 3 isoforms: endothelial NOS (eNOS or NOS-3), found mainly in endothelial cells; neuronal NOS (nNOS or NOS-1), expressed in central and peripheral neurons; and inducible NOS (iNOS or NOS-2), expressed primarily in macrophages but potentially in any cell type and induced by inflammatory cytokines or bacterial endotoxins.

In physiologic conditions, eNOS is present in the endothelium of ciliary and retinal vessels, ciliary muscle, and Schlemm canal cells, whereas nNOS is found in the nonpigmented ciliary epithelium and optic nerve head. Under stimulated conditions, iNOS can be detected in the iris, ciliary body, vessels, and optic nerve head. NO generated in the trabecular meshwork (TM) is most likely mediated by iNOS.

Significant clinical and experimental evidence indicates that an endogenous insufficiency of NO bioavailability is linked to POAG, although the exact relationship between the two is unclear. NO is thought to lower IOP by increasing trabecular outflow. Evidence suggests that NO affects trabecular outflow by relaxing the juxtacanalicular TM, altering contractility and cell volume of the TM and Schlemm canal cells. NO may be involved in aqueous secretion through regulation of blood flow, uveoscleral outflow via relaxation of the smooth muscle fibers, and autoregulation of optic nerve head circulation during changes in IOP. Exogenous NO delivered to the anterior eye can facilitate outflow and lower IOP.

Latanoprostene bunod (LBN) ophthalmic solution, 0.024%, is a NO-donating PG analogue that chemically combines an NO-donating moiety with latanoprost. The molecular structure of LBN is nearly identical to that of latanoprost. However, LBN is distinguished by the integration of an NO-donating moiety (a terminal butyl nitrate ester functional group) in lieu of an isopropyl ester. Upon topical administration, LBN is hydrolyzed by endogenous corneal esterases into latanoprost acid and butanediol mononitrate, which is further metabolized to NO and the inactive 1,4-butanediol. The molecule is thought to exert pharmacologic effects, with latanoprost increasing uveoscleral outflow and NO enhancing trabecular outflow.

LBN is dosed once daily at bedtime and has an adverse effect profile similar to that of other PGs in clinical settings. In phase 3 clinical trials, LBN produced a mean IOP reduction of 7.5–9.1 mm Hg and was superior to twice-daily timolol 0.5%; in addition, the IOP-lowering efficacy lasted for 12 months. Notably, in the phase 2 study, reduction in IOP was 1.2 mm Hg greater with LBN treatment for 28 days than with latanoprost.

NO-donating moieties combined with other ocular hypotensive agents are under development. They include introduction of NO-donating moieties to bimatoprost (another PG analogue), to a nonselective β-blocker, and to the CAIs dorzolamide and brinzolamide.

Aliancy J, Stamer WD, Wirostko B. A review of nitric oxide for the treatment of glaucomatous disease. *Ophthalmol Ther.* 2017;6(2):221–232.

Rho Kinase Inhibitors

Rho kinase (ROCK) is a serine/threonine kinase that serves as an important downstream effector of Rho guanosine triphosphate hydrolase (Rho GTPase). The Rho family of GTPases is composed of small (≈21 kDa) signaling G proteins (also known as *guanine nucleotide-binding proteins*) found in the cytosol and has 3 main classes: Rho, Rac, and Cdc42.

The Rho class has 3 isoforms: RhoA, RhoB, and RhoC. RhoA is activated by guanine nucleotide exchange factors. Upon binding to GTP, RhoA activates ROCK, which phosphorylates several downstream substrates involved in a wide variety of cellular functions. Two isoforms, ROCK-I and ROCK-II, have been isolated.

ROCK plays a critical role in regulating the tone of smooth muscle tissues. Animal studies have demonstrated increased ocular blood flow presumably through the relaxation of vascular endothelial smooth muscle, as well as the neuroprotective promotion of retinal ganglion cell survival and axon regeneration. ROCK inhibitors may also reduce scarring after glaucoma filtering surgery by blocking the assembly and contraction of transforming growth factor β-induced stress fibers and inhibiting fibroproliferation and collagen deposition postoperatively.

ROCK inhibitors have also been proposed for the treatment of corneal endothelial decompensation. Topical ROCK inhibitors have promoted cell proliferation in animal models, and pilot clinical research suggests a similar response in humans. ROCK inhibitors are being studied for wound healing in the corneal endothelium, Fuchs endothelial corneal dystrophy, and corneal decompensation after cataract surgery, as well as for enhancing engraftment of corneal endothelial cells onto recipient tissues in tissue engineering therapy.

Selective ROCK inhibitors are thought to increase aqueous humor drainage through the TM, subsequently decreasing IOP. The exact molecular mechanism has not been fully elucidated. ROCK inhibitors appear to have several actin cytoskeletal-related targets that directly affect the contractile properties of TM outflow tissue.

In 2014, the ROCK inhibitor ripasudil, 0.4%, twice-daily ophthalmic solution was approved in Japan for the treatment of glaucoma and ocular hypertension when other therapeutic drugs are not effective or cannot be administered. Another agent, netarsudil, is an inhibitor of both ROCK and the norepinephrine transporter. Netarsudil is thought to work via 3 mechanisms:

- increase of trabecular outflow
- reduction of episcleral venous pressure by ROCK inhibition
- reduction of aqueous production by norepinephrine transporter inhibition

In a phase 3 clinical trial, netarsudil was associated with a 3.3- to 4.6-mm Hg reduction in IOP. In another study, netarsudil, 0.02%, dosed once daily was noninferior to timolol, 0.5%, dosed twice daily. The drug is currently FDA approved for the reduction of IOP. Common adverse effects include hyperemia (up to 53% of study eyes), cornea verticillata (20% of study eyes), irritation, and blurred vision.

Fixed-combination therapy with netarsudil, 0.02%, and latanoprost, 0.005%, is also available.

Okumura N, Okazaki Y, Inoue R, et al. Effect of the rho-associated kinase inhibitor eye drop (ripasudil) on corneal endothelial wound healing. *Invest Ophthalmol Vis Sci*. 2016; 57(3):1284–1292.

Serle JB, Katz LJ, McLaurin E, et al; ROCKET-1 and ROCKET-2 Study Groups. Two phase 3 clinical trials comparing the safety and efficacy of netarsudil to timolol in patients with elevated intraocular pressure: Rho Kinase Elevated IOP Treatment Trial 1 and 2 (ROCKET-1 and ROCKET-2). *Am J Ophthalmol*. 2018;186:116–127.

Tanna AP, Johnson M. Rho kinase inhibitors as a novel treatment for glaucoma and ocular hypertension. *Ophthalmology*. 2018;125(11):1741–1756.

Table 16-12 Fixed-Combination Glaucoma Medications

Generic Name	Trade Name	Strengths
Dorzolamide HCl/timolol maleate solution	Cosopt	Dorzolamide, 2%/timolol, 0.5%
Brimonidine tartrate/timolol maleate solution	Combigan	Brimonidine, 2%/timolol, 0.5%
Brinzolamide/brimonidine tartrate suspension	Simbrinza	Brinzolamide, 1%/brimonidine, 2%
Latanoprost/timolol maleate solution	Xalacom[a]	Latanoprost, 0.005%/timolol, 0.5%
Travoprost/timolol maleate	DuoTrav[a]	Travoprost, 0.004%/timolol, 0.5%
Bimatoprost/timolol maleate	Ganfort[a]	Bimatoprost, 0.03%/timolol, 0.5%
Netarsudil/latanoprost	Rocklatan	Netarsudil, 0.02%/latanoprost, 0.005%

[a] Not available in the United States.

Fixed-Combination Medications

Medications that are combined in a single bottle have the potential benefits of improved efficacy, convenience, and patient compliance, as well as reduced cost. FDA guidelines require the fixed combination to be more efficacious than either drug given alone.

Table 16-12 lists the currently available fixed-combination medications for glaucoma (some are not available in the United States). Before a patient uses the combination drug, each component should be checked for its effect on that patient's IOP (see BCSC Section 10, *Glaucoma*).

Osmotic Drugs

Actions and Uses

Increased serum osmolarity reduces IOP and vitreous volume by drawing fluid across vascular barriers and out of the eye. The osmotic activity of a drug depends on the number of particles in the solution and the maintenance of an osmotic gradient between the plasma and the intraocular fluids. This activity is independent of molecular weight. Low-molecular-weight agents such as urea, which penetrate the blood–ocular barrier, produce a small increase in IOP after an initial reduction because of a reversal of the osmotic gradient when the kidneys clear the blood of excess urea.

Osmotic drugs are FDA approved for the short-term management of acute glaucoma in adults and may be used to reduce vitreous volume before intraocular surgery.

The hyperosmotic drugs glycerin, mannitol, and urea are currently available for ophthalmic use in the United States (Table 16-13). Osmotic drugs should be used with care in patients in whom cardiovascular overload can occur with moderate vascular volume expansion; this includes patients with a history of congestive heart failure, angina, and systemic hypertension or recent myocardial infarction.

Lichter PR. Glaucoma clinical trials and what they mean for our patients. *Am J Ophthalmol.* 2003;136(1):136–145.

Netland PA. *Glaucoma Medical Therapy: Principles and Management.* 2nd ed. Ophthalmology Monograph 13. San Francisco: American Academy of Ophthalmology; 2008.

Table 16-13 Hyperosmotic Drugs

Generic Name	Trade Name	Strengths	Dose	Route	Onset of Action	Duration of Action
Glycerin	Available generically		1–1.5 g/kg	Oral	10–30 min	5 h
Mannitol[a]	Osmitrol	5%–20%	0.25–2 g/kg	Intravenous	30–60 min	4–8 h
	Available generically	5%–25%	0.25–2 g/kg	Intravenous	30–60 min	4–8 h
Urea	Available generically	Powder	0.5–2 g/kg	Intravenous	30–45 min	5–6 h

[a] A single mannitol dose of 0.25–0.5 g/kg is often enough to reduce intraocular pressure (IOP).

Intravenous Drugs

Mannitol must be administered intravenously because it cannot be absorbed from the gastrointestinal tract. This drug may be given as either an intravenous infusion or an intravenous push. For an intravenous infusion, mannitol may be given as a 20% premixed solution (concentration, 200 mg/mL) over 30–60 minutes. For an intravenous push, a 25% solution may be injected over 3–5 minutes. A too-rapid infusion of mannitol may shift intracellular water into the extracellular space, causing cellular dehydration with a high risk of hyponatremia, cardiovascular overload, congestive heart failure, pulmonary edema, and intracranial bleeding.

Urea is unpalatable and thus is used intravenously. Urea has fallen out of favor because of rebound effects (see the earlier section Actions and Uses) and because of its tendency to cause tissue necrosis when it extravasates during administration. However, intravenous administration of urea produces a rapid onset of action, which is usually desirable.

Both mannitol and urea have been associated with subarachnoid hemorrhage attributed to rapid volume overload of the blood vessels and/or rapid shrinkage of the brain with traction of the subarachnoid vessels. This shrinkage is of particular concern in elderly patients, who may already have brain shrinkage from microischemic disease and are therefore at increased risk of bleeding.

These drugs are cleared by the kidneys and produce marked osmotic diuresis that may be troublesome during surgery. Conscious patients should void shortly before surgery, and a urinal or bedpan should be available. If general anesthesia is used, an indwelling urethral catheter may be required to prevent bladder distension.

Oral Drugs

Glycerin, 50%, was discontinued in the United States in 2004; however, it can be compounded by diluting the 100% solution. This frequently used oral osmotic drug is given over cracked ice to minimize its nauseatingly sweet taste. Glycerin is chiefly converted to glucose, glycogen, and other carbohydrates in the liver. Hyperglycemia and glycosuria can result from the oral administration of the agent. The nonmetabolized sugar isosorbide was preferred in patients with diabetes mellitus but has been discontinued in the United States.

Anti-inflammatory Drugs

Ocular inflammation can be treated with medications administered topically, by local injection, by ocular implantation, or systemically. These agents are classified as glucocorticoids, nonsteroidal anti-inflammatory drugs (NSAIDs), mast-cell stabilizers, antihistamines, or antifibrotics.

Glucocorticoids

Corticosteroids, or steroids, are applied topically to prevent or suppress ocular inflammation in trauma and uveitis, as well as after most ocular surgical procedures (Table 16-14). Subconjunctival, sub-Tenon, and intravitreal injections of steroids are used to treat more severe cases of ocular inflammation. Systemic steroid therapy is used to treat systemic immune diseases, such as giant cell arteritis, vision-threatening capillary hemangiomas in childhood, and severe ocular inflammation that is resistant to topical therapy. Intravenous methylprednisolone is sometimes used in short-term management of various orbital and neuro-ophthalmic conditions (see BCSC Section 5, *Neuro-Ophthalmology,* and Section 7, *Oculofacial Plastic and Orbital Surgery*). Corticosteroids are divided into 2 major groups, glucocorticoids and mineralocorticoids, on the basis of their predominant biological activities.

Glucocorticoids induce cell-specific effects on lymphocytes, macrophages, polymorphonuclear leukocytes, vascular endothelial cells, fibroblasts, and other cells. In each of these cells, glucocorticoids must

- penetrate the cell membrane
- bind to soluble receptors in the cytosol
- allow the translocation of the glucocorticoid receptor complex to nuclear-binding sites for gene transcription
- induce or suppress the transcription of specific messenger RNA (mRNA)

The proteins produced in the eye under the control of these mRNAs are not known, and only resultant effects have been described.

At the tissue level, glucocorticoids prevent or suppress local hyperthermia, vascular congestion, edema, and the pain of initial inflammatory responses, whether the cause is traumatic (radiant, mechanical, or chemical), infectious, or immunologic. They also suppress the late inflammatory responses of capillary proliferation, fibroblast proliferation, collagen deposition, and scarring.

At the biochemical level, the most important effect of anti-inflammatory drugs may be the inhibition of arachidonic acid release from phospholipids (see the following section). Liberated arachidonic acid is otherwise converted into PGs, PG endoperoxides, leukotrienes, and thromboxanes, which are potent mediators of inflammation. Glucocorticoids also suppress the liberation of lytic enzymes from lysozymes.

The effects of glucocorticoids on immune-mediated inflammation are complicated. Glucocorticoids do not affect the titers of either immunoglobulin E (IgE), which mediates allergic mechanisms, or immunoglobulin G (IgG), which mediates autoimmune mechanisms. Also, glucocorticoids do not appear to interfere with normal processes in the afferent limb of cell-mediated immunity, as in graft rejection. Instead, they interfere with

Table 16-14 **Topical Anti-inflammatory Drugs**

Generic Name	Trade Name	Strengths
Corticosteroids		
Dexamethasone sodium phosphate	Maxidex	Suspension, 0.1%
	Maxidex, Ocu-Dex	Ointment, 0.05%
	Available generically	Solution, 0.1%
Difluprednate	Durezol	Emulsion, 0.05%
Fluorometholone	FML S.O.P.	Ointment, 0.1%
	FML Liquifilm	Suspension, 0.1%
	FML Forte Liquifilm	Suspension, 0.25%
	Fluor-Op	Suspension, 0.1%
	Available generically	Suspension, 0.1%
Fluorometholone acetate	Flarex	Suspension, 0.1%
Loteprednol etabonate	Alrex	Suspension, 0.2%
	Lotemax	Suspension, 0.5%
	Lotemax	Ointment, 0.5%
Medrysone	HMS	Suspension, 1%
Prednisolone acetate	Econopred Plus	Suspension, 1%
	Omnipred	Suspension, 1%
	Pred Forte	Suspension, 1%
	Available generically	Suspension, 1%
	Pred Mild	Suspension, 0.12%
Prednisolone sodium phosphate	Inflamase Forte	Solution, 1%
	Prednisol	Solution, 1%
	Available generically	Solution, 1%, 0.125%
Rimexolone	Vexol	Suspension, 1%
Nonsteroidal anti-inflammatory drugs		
Bromfenac sodium	Xibrom, Bromday	Solution, 0.09%
	Prolensa	Solution, 0.07%
	Available generically	Solution, 0.09%
Diclofenac sodium	Voltaren	Solution, 0.1%
	Available generically	Solution, 0.1%
Flurbiprofen sodium	Ocufen	Solution, 0.03%
	Available generically	Solution, 0.03%
Ketorolac tromethamine	Acular, Acular PF	Solution, 0.5%
	Acular LS	Solution, 0.4%
	Acuvail	Solution, 0.45%
	Available generically	Solution, 0.5%
Nepafenac	Nevanac	Suspension, 0.1%
	Ilevro	Suspension, 0.3%

the subsequent efferent limb of the immune response. For example, glucocorticoids prevent macrophages from being attracted to sites of inflammation by interfering with the cells' response to lymphocyte-released migration-inhibiting factor. Glucocorticoids administered for systemic effect cause sequestration of lymphocytes, especially the T lymphocytes that mediate cellular immunity. However, the posttranscriptional molecular mechanisms of these responses remain unknown. BCSC Section 9, *Uveitis and Ocular Inflammation,* discusses immune responses in detail.

Adverse effects

Glucocorticoids may cause several adverse effects in the eye and elsewhere in the body.

Complications in the eye include

- glaucoma
- posterior subcapsular cataracts
- exacerbation of bacterial and viral (especially herpetic) infections through suppression of protective immune mechanisms
- fungal infection
- ptosis
- mydriasis
- scleral melting
- eyelid skin atrophy
- pseudohypopyon from intraocular injection
- central serous chorioretinopathy

In the body, oral doses can cause

- suppression of the pituitary–adrenal axis
- gluconeogenesis resulting in hyperglycemia, muscle wasting, and osteoporosis
- redistribution of fat from the periphery to the trunk
- CNS effects, such as euphoria
- insomnia
- aseptic necrosis of the hip
- peptic ulcer
- diabetes mellitus
- occasionally psychosis

Elderly patients have particular difficulty taking long-term systemic steroids. For example, the adverse effect of proximal muscle wasting may make it difficult for these patients to climb stairs. Osteoporosis, another adverse effect of glucocorticoids, exacerbates the risk of falls and fractures for these patients, who are generally at an increased risk of both. Elderly patients with inflammatory diseases may require a steroid-sparing regimen.

Steroid-induced elevation in IOP may occur with topical, intraocular, periocular, nasal, and systemic glucocorticoid therapies. The exact mechanism by which steroids diminish aqueous outflow through the TM remains unknown but may be related to deposition of glycosaminoglycans in the TM.

Individual response to steroids is dependent on the duration, potency, and frequency of therapy and the route of administration of the drug used. Steroid-induced IOP elevation almost never occurs in less than 5 days and is infrequent in less than 2 weeks of use. However, failure of IOP to rise after 6 weeks of therapy does not ensure that a patient will maintain normal IOP after several months of therapy. For this reason, monitoring of IOP at periodic intervals is required throughout the course of long-term steroid therapy to prevent iatrogenic glaucomatous nerve damage. Steroid-induced elevations in IOP are usually reversible by discontinuing therapy if the drug has not been used longer than 1 year; however, if therapy has continued for 18 months or more, permanent elevations of pressure are common.

Table 16-15 lists the anti-inflammatory and IOP-elevating potencies of 6 steroids used in ophthalmic therapy. The anti-inflammatory potencies were determined by an in vitro assay of inhibition of lymphocyte transformation, and the IOP effects were determined by tests in individuals already known to be highly responsive to topical dexamethasone. However, until all these drugs are compared in a model of ocular inflammation relevant to human disease, no conclusion can be reached about the observed dissociation of effects. The lower-than-expected effect on pressure with some of these drugs may be explained by more rapid metabolism of fluorometholone in the eye compared with dexamethasone and by the relatively poor penetration of medrysone. The efficacy of these drugs for intraocular inflammation may be similarly reduced.

CLINICAL PEARL

The rates of IOP spikes for various steroids differ and depend on the potency, formulation, and delivery of the particular drug. When patients are treated with steroids, it is important that ophthalmologists consult the literature for information on individual agents and their effects on IOP.

When a steroid-induced pressure rise is suspected but continued steroid therapy is warranted, the physician faces the following choices:

- continue the same treatment and closely monitor the status of the optic nerve
- attempt to offset the pressure rise with other drugs or treatments
- reduce the potency, concentration, or frequency of the steroid used while monitoring both pressure and inflammation
- consider a steroid-sparing alternative

Table 16-15 Comparison of Anti-inflammatory[a] and IOP-Elevating[b] Potencies

Glucocorticoid	Relative Potency	Rise in IOP, mm Hg
Dexamethasone, 0.1% (equivalent to betamethasone, 0.1%, less than or equivalent to difluprednate, 0.05%)	24.0	22
Fluorometholone, 0.1%[c]	21.0	6
Prednisolone acetate, 1%	2.3	10
Medrysone, 1%[d]	1.7	1
Tetrahydrotriamcinolone, 0.25%	1.4	2
Hydrocortisone, 0.5%	1.0	3

[a] Anti-inflammatory potency determined by in vitro assay of inhibition of lymphocyte transformation. Anti-inflammatory potency of difluprednate, 0.05%, is equal to or stronger than betamethasone, 0.1%, which has a 6-fold anti-inflammatory potency compared with that of prednisolone or equivalent to that of dexamethasone. In clinical trials on uveitis, a significant increase in IOP occurred in 6% of patients treated with difluprednate, 0.05%, emulsion compared with 5% of those treated with prednisolone acetate, 1%.

[b] IOP effects determined in topical dexamethasone responders.

[c] Rapid metabolism of fluorometholone in the eye compared with dexamethasone.

[d] Relatively poor ocular penetration.

Immunomodulatory therapy (IMT) is an important component in the management of ocular inflammation, avoiding the toxicity associated with long-term corticosteroid therapy. IMT drugs are classified as antimetabolites, inhibitors of T-cell signaling, alkylating agents, and biologic response modifiers. Biologic response modifiers inhibit various cytokines, which are active in inflammation. See Table 16-16 for a summary of this class of medications and also BCSC Section 9, *Uveitis and Ocular Inflammation.*

Jabs DA. Immunosuppression for the uveitides. *Ophthalmology.* 2018;125(2):193–202.

Specific drugs and regimens

Appropriate selection from the available corticosteroid drugs, formulations, and dosage regimens are contingent on the clinical situation. Steroids can be administered topically, periocularly, intravenously, or intravitreally (Table 16-17). All corticosteroids may exacerbate infections and lead to ocular adverse effects. Recent research in corticosteroids has focused on medications that can be used intraocularly and periocularly as well as developing drugs with decreased effect on IOP. As a general rule, however, the more potent the steroid, the more prevalent and severe are the adverse events.

Rimexolone, 1%, is a synthetic topical steroid designed to minimize IOP elevations, similar to fluorinated steroids. Elevated IOP has been reported with this medication, but it is rare. Ocular adverse effects still include secondary glaucoma and posterior subcapsular cataracts. Systemic adverse effects, including headache, hypotension, rhinitis, pharyngitis, and taste perversion, occur in fewer than 2% of patients.

Loteprednol etabonate, 0.5%, is structurally similar to other steroids but lacks a ketone group at position 20. Loteprednol etabonate, 0.2%, is marketed for the temporary treatment of allergic conjunctivitis. The combination drug loteprednol etabonate (0.5%)/tobramycin (0.3%) is approved for superficial bacterial infections of the eye with inflammation. Studies have shown that in corticosteroid responders treated with loteprednol, the incidence of clinically significant IOP elevation is low.

Difluprednate is a difluorinated derivative of prednisolone. Its glucocorticoid receptor-binding affinity and corneal penetration are greatly enhanced by modification of the glucocorticoid molecule with the addition of fluorine atoms and ester groups at several carbon positions. Difluprednate is formulated as a stable oil-in-water emulsion to achieve consistent dose uniformity compared with suspensions, regardless of bottle storage position or shaking before use. Although the strong therapeutic potency of difluprednate emulsion is desirable, IOP increase has been reported anecdotally and clinically to be greater than that of other moderate to strong topical steroids.

Fluocinolone acetonide is available in 2 intraocular devices. A nonbiodegradable implant with 0.59 mg of fluocinolone acetonide surgically placed in the pars plana region was approved by the FDA for the treatment of chronic noninfectious posterior uveitis. It is designed to release fluocinolone acetonide at a nominal initial rate of 0.6 µg/d, decreasing over the first month to a steady state between 0.3 and 0.4 µg/d over approximately 30 months. Another 0.19-mg nonbiodegradable implant, delivered by intravitreal injection, was FDA approved for the treatment of diabetic macular edema in patients who are not steroid responders. It releases fluocinolone acetonide at an average rate of 0.2 µg/d for 36 months.

Table 16-16 Immunomodulatory Medications in the Treatment of Uveitis

Class	Medication	Mechanism of Action	Dosage	Potential Complications
Conventional immunosuppressive drugs				
Antimetabolites				
	Methotrexate	Folate analogue; inhibits dihydrofolate reductase	Initial dose: 15 mg/wk by mouth, SQ, or IM Maximum dose: 25 mg/kg by mouth, SQ, or IM	Hepatitis, cytopenias, fatigue/malaise, nausea
	Azathioprine	Alters purine metabolism	Initial dose: 2 mg/kg/d by mouth Maximum dose: 3 mg/kg/d by mouth	Gastrointestinal upset, cytopenias, hepatitis
	Mycophenolate mofetil	Inhibits purine synthesis	Initial dose: 1 g twice a day by mouth Maximum dose: 1.5 g twice a day by mouth	Diarrhea, cytopenias, hepatitis
Alkylating agents				
	Cyclophosphamide	Cross-links DNA	Initial dose: 2 mg/kg/d by mouth Maximum dose: 250 mg/d by mouth	Cytopenias, bladder toxicity
	Chlorambucil	Cross-links DNA	Initial dose: 0.1 mg/kg/d by mouth Maximum dose: 0.2 mg/kg/d by mouth	Cytopenias
T-cell inhibitors				
	Cyclosporine	Inhibits NF-AT activation	Initial dose: 2 mg/kg twice a day by mouth Maximum dose: 2 mg/kg twice a day by mouth	Nephrotoxicity, hypertension, anemia, hirsutism

Table 16-16 *(continued)*

Class	Medication	Mechanism of Action	Dosage	Potential Complications
	Tacrolimus	Inhibits NF-AT activation	Initial dose: 1 mg twice a day by mouth Maximum dose: 3 mg twice a day by mouth	Nephrotoxicity, neurotoxicity (tremors)
	Sirolimus	Inhibits T-lymphocyte activation in G1; blunts T- and B-lymphocyte responses to lymphokines	6-mg loading dose, 2-mg maintenance dose; intravitreal dose in phase 3 study for noninfectious uveitis: 440 μg in 20 μL, repeated in 60 d and 120 d	Diabetes mellitus–like symptoms, lung toxicity, immunosuppression, malignancy, impaired wound healing
Biologic response modifiers				
TNF inhibitors				
	Etanercept	TNF-α receptor blocker	0.4 mg/kg twice weekly SQ given 72–96 hours apart (maximum dose: 25 mg per dose)	Susceptibility to infection; reactivation of tuberculosis, histoplasmosis, hepatitis B, and fungal infection; hypersensitivity reactions; demyelinating disease; lupuslike syndrome; malignancy; thromboembolic events; congestive heart failure
	Infliximab[a]	TNF-α inhibitor	3 mg/kg IV at wk 0, 2, and 6 and then every 6–8 wk	Same as for etanercept
	Adalimumab[a, b]	TNF-α inhibitor	Initial dose: 80 mg SQ Maintenance dose: 40 mg SQ every other week	Same as for etanercept

(Continued)

Table 16-16 *(continued)*

Class	Medication	Mechanism of Action	Dosage	Potential Complications
Lymphocyte inhibitors				
	Abatacept	Binds to CD80 or CD86 molecule and prevents antigen presentation to T cell for T-cell activation	500–1000 mg IV loading, then 125 mg SQ weekly	Susceptibility to infections, allergic reactions, headache, nausea, and malignancy
	Daclizumab	Binds to CD25, the α subunit of the IL-2 receptor of T cells	1–2 mg/kg IV or SQ every 2 or 4 wk	Hypersensitivity reactions, headache, and gastrointestinal disturbance
	Rituximab	Binds to CD20 on B cells, triggering cell death	500–1000 mg IV at wk 0 and 2; may repeat at 6–12 mo thereafter	Susceptibility to infections, infusion reactions, gastrointestinal disturbance, cardiovascular events, muscle spasm, and headache
Specific receptor antagonists				
	Efalizumab	Binds CD11a, the α subunit of lymphocyte function–associated antigen 1	Initial dose of 0.7 mg/kg SQ, then 1 mg/kg weekly (not to exceed 200 mg per dose)	Headaches, fever, nausea, vomiting, progressive multifocal leukoencephalopathy, thrombocytopenia, arthritis
	Tocilizumab	IL-6 receptor inhibitor	4 mg/kg IV every 4 wk, then increase to 8–12 mg/kg every 2–4 wk	Serious infections, hypersensitivity reactions, and gastrointestinal perforation

IL = interleukin; IM = intramuscularly; IV = intravenously; NF-AT = nuclear factor of activated T lymphocyte; SQ = subcutaneously; TNF = tumor necrosis factor.

[a]In uveitis, most of the data on biologics are related to use of agents directed against TNF-α and involve infliximab and adalimumab.

[b]Adalimumab is FDA-approved for the treatment of uveitis.

Table 16-17 Usual Route of Corticosteroid Administration in Ocular Inflammation

Condition	Route
Blepharitis	Topical
Conjunctivitis	Topical
Endophthalmitis	Periocular, systemic, intravitreal
Keratitis	Topical
Macular edema, cystoid	Topical, periocular, intravitreal injection or implant
Macular edema, diabetic	Periocular, intravitreal
Optic neuritis	Systemic
Scleritis	Topical, periocular, systemic
Scleritis-Epi (episcleritis)	Topical
Sympathetic ophthalmia	Topical, periocular, systemic, intravitreal
Temporal arteritis	Systemic
Uveitis, anterior	Topical, periocular, systemic
Uveitis, posterior	Periocular, systemic, intravitreal injection or implant

A 0.7-mg dexamethasone biodegradable polymer matrix for injection into the vitreous cavity was approved for the treatment of macular edema secondary to retinal vein occlusion, noninfectious posterior uveitis, and diabetic macular edema. The polymer dissolves, and dexamethasone is slowly released for up to 6 months, with clinical efficacy lasting at least 3 months.

A 40-mg/mL preservative-free triamcinolone acetonide injectable suspension was FDA approved for intraocular use. Its indications include visualization during vitrectomy and treatment of sympathetic ophthalmia, temporal arteritis, uveitis, and ocular inflammatory conditions that do not respond to topical corticosteroids.

Armaly MF. Effect of corticosteroids on intraocular pressure and fluid dynamics, I: the effect of dexamethasone in the normal eye. *Arch Ophthalmol.* 1963;70(4):482–491.

Armaly MF. Effect of corticosteroids on intraocular pressure and fluid dynamics, II: the effect of dexamethasone in the glaucomatous eye. *Arch Ophthalmol.* 1963;70(4):492–499.

Donnenfeld ED. Difluprednate for the prevention of ocular inflammation postsurgery: an update. *Clin Ophthalmol.* 2011;5:811–816.

Mulki L, Foster CS. Difluprednate for inflammatory eye disorders. *Drugs Today* (Barcelona). 2011;47(5):327–333.

Nonsteroidal Anti-inflammatory Drugs

Derivatives

Derivatives of arachidonic acid, a 20-carbon essential fatty acid, mediate a wide variety of biological functions, including regulation of smooth muscle tone (in the blood vessels, bronchi, uterus, and gut), platelet aggregation, hormone release (growth hormone, ACTH, insulin, renin, and progesterone), and inflammation. The synthetic cascade that produces a wide variety of derivatives (depending on the stimulus and tissue) begins with stimulation of phospholipase A_2. Phospholipase A_2 liberates arachidonic acid from phospholipids of the cell membrane and is a target of steroid therapy (Fig 16-6).

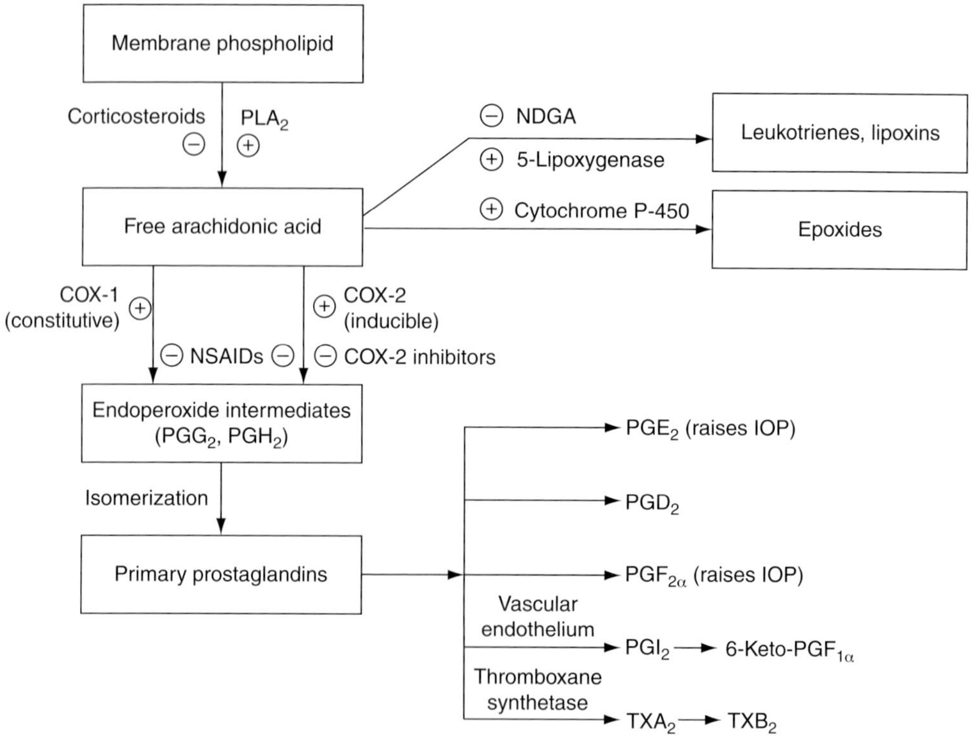

Figure 16-6 An outline of the synthesis of prostaglandins (PGs) and leukotrienes from arachidonic acid. In response to stimulation of a target cell with a relevant stimulus (eg, a cytokine, a neurotransmitter, various pharmacologic agents), phospholipase A_2 (PLA_2) is activated, and arachidonic acid is released from the sn-2 position of membrane phospholipids. Arachidonic acid is then converted by cyclooxygenase-1 (COX-1) or cyclooxygenase-2 (COX-2) to prostaglandin H_2 (PGH_2), and then PGH_2 is isomerized to biologically active prostanoid products. Arachidonic acid can also be metabolized through the 5-lipoxygenase and cytochrome P-450 pathways to generate leukotrienes and epoxides, respectively. PLA_2 can be inhibited by corticosteroids such as dexamethasone; COX-1, by nonsteroidal anti-inflammatory drugs (NSAIDs) such as indomethacin and aspirin; COX-2, by DUP697, SC58125, L-745-337, and NS398; and the 5-lipoxygenase pathway, by nordihydroguaiaretic acid (NDGA). IOP = intraocular pressure; PGD_2 = prostaglandin D_2; PGE_2 = prostaglandin E_2; $PGF_{1\alpha}$ = prostaglandin $F_{1\alpha}$; $PGF_{2\alpha}$ = prostaglandin $F_{2\alpha}$; PGG_2 = prostaglandin G_2; PGI_2 = prostaglandin I_2; TXA_2 = thromboxane A_2; TXB_2 = thromboxane B_2. *(Courtesy of Ata Abdel-Latif, PhD.)*

Arachidonic acid is then converted either into hydroperoxides by lipoxygenase or into cyclic endoperoxides by cyclooxygenase (COX, also called *prostaglandin-endoperoxide synthase*). The hydroperoxides form a chemotactic agent and the leukotrienes C_4, D_4, and E_4, previously known as the slow-reacting substance of anaphylaxis. Like oral antihistamines, oral leukotriene inhibitors are used in the management of seasonal allergies.

Subsequent products of endoperoxides include the PGs, which mediate inflammation and other responses; prostacyclin, a vasodilator and platelet antiaggregant; and thromboxane, a vasoconstrictor and platelet aggregant. PGs have profound effects on inflammation in the eye, aqueous humor dynamics, and blood–ocular barrier functions. When administered intracamerally or topically at high concentrations, arachidonic acid and PGs of the

E and F subtypes cause miosis, an elevation of IOP, an increase in aqueous protein content, and the entry of white cells into the aqueous and tear fluid.

COX has 2 isoforms (ie, COX-2 and COX-1):

- COX-2 is the relevant enzyme in inflammation (it is expressed at low levels under normal physiologic conditions and is regulated only in response to pro-inflammatory signals).
- Constitutively expressed COX-1 (but not COX-2) is present in various tissues (including the inner lining of the stomach).

Previously developed NSAIDs (eg, ibuprofen, naproxen) inhibit both COX-1 and COX-2 and compete with arachidonate in binding to the COX-active site. Although these compounds are effective anti-inflammatory drugs, all of them can produce gastric ulcers when administered systemically. In contrast, COX-2 inhibitors are anti-inflammatory and analgesic, and they lack gastrointestinal toxicity. Moreover, they provide time-dependent, reversible inhibition of the COX-2 enzyme. However, oral COX-2 inhibitors, including rofecoxib, celecoxib, and valdecoxib, increase risks of cardiovascular toxicity and complications (eg, myocardial infarction).

Specific drugs

Table 16-18 lists several NSAIDs along with their initial adult oral dosages. Aspirin and other NSAIDs inhibit the local signs of inflammation (heat, vasodilation, edema, swelling), as well as pain and fever. However, they have complex effects on clotting. At low doses (300 mg every other day), aspirin permanently inhibits the COX in platelets, which is

Table 16-18 Nonsteroidal Anti-inflammatory Drugs (Systemic)

Drug (Generic Name)	Starting Oral Dosage (Adult)
Aspirin	650 mg, 4 times daily
Celecoxib	100 mg, 2 times daily
Diclofenac	50 mg, 3 times daily
Diflunisal	500 mg, 2 times daily
Etodolac	300 mg, 2 times daily
Fenoprofen	200 mg, 4 times daily
Flurbiprofen	300 mg, 3 times daily
Ibuprofen	400 mg, 4 times daily
Indomethacin	25 mg, 3 times daily
Ketoprofen	75 mg, 3 times daily
Ketorolac	10 mg, 4 times daily
Meloxicam	7.5 mg, 4 times daily
Nabumetone	1000 mg, 4 times daily
Naproxen	250 mg, 2 times daily
Oxaprozin	1200 mg, 4 times daily
Piroxicam	20 mg, 4 times daily
Sulindac	150 mg, 2 times daily
Tolmetin	400 mg, 3 times daily

essential for the conversion of arachidonic acid to prostaglandin G_2 and thromboxane. Inhibition of thromboxane production, in turn, prevents coagulation. Although nucleated cells can replenish their COX, anucleate platelets cannot. After aspirin is stopped, COX activity recovers by 10% per day in parallel with platelet turnover. The anticoagulant effect of aspirin therefore lasts for at least 48–72 hours despite discontinuation of aspirin therapy. Other NSAIDs inhibit clotting in a reversible fashion, and their use does not need to be discontinued so far in advance of elective surgery.

When used during febrile viral infections in children, aspirin has been associated with Reye syndrome, although no causal link has been proven. The National Reye's Syndrome Foundation, the US Surgeon General, the FDA, the Centers for Disease Control and Prevention, and the American Academy of Pediatrics recommend that aspirin and combination products containing aspirin not be taken by anyone younger than 19 years during fever-causing illnesses. The British Medicines and Healthcare Products Regulatory Agency recommends that aspirin labels state that the drug is not intended for use in children younger than 16 years unless recommended by a physician. Other NSAIDs are effective antipyretics and are not associated with the constellation of symptoms observed in Reye syndrome.

The relative risks and benefits of aspirin therapy should be assessed for each patient. Aspirin therapy for postoperative pain or for pain associated with traumatic hyphema may increase the risk of hemorrhage because of the antiaggregant effect on platelets. The same side effect may benefit patients with platelet emboli, as in some cases of amaurosis fugax. Diversion of arachidonic acid to the lipoxygenase pathway by inhibition of COX may explain why aspirin is associated with asthma attacks and hypersensitivity reactions (mediated by the leukotrienes C_4, D_4, and E_4) in susceptible people. Systemic acidosis associated with concomitant use of CAIs may shift a higher proportion of aspirin molecules into the more lipid-soluble nonionized form, which penetrates the blood–brain barrier more readily and potentiates CNS toxicity from aspirin. Aspirin and other COX inhibitors are less effective than steroids in the treatment of scleritis and uveitis.

NSAIDs such as indomethacin can be effective for orbital inflammatory diseases. The prophylactic use of indomethacin in patients undergoing cataract surgery has reduced the incidence of angiographically detected CME, but an effect on visually significant CME has yet to be determined. Flurbiprofen sodium, 0.03% (generic available), was the first commercially available topical ocular NSAID. When applied preoperatively, it reduces PG-mediated intraoperative miosis.

In addition to treating ocular inflammation, topical NSAIDs as a class have been reported to prevent and treat CME related to cataract surgery. Topical diclofenac sodium, 0.1% (generic available), has been approved by the FDA for treatment of inflammation and pain following cataract surgery, and ketorolac tromethamine (0.4%, 0.45%, 0.5%, and generic 0.5%) has been approved to treat postoperative pain and irritation. Additional topical NSAIDs with various dosages were approved by the FDA for the treatment of inflammation and reduction of pain after cataract extraction, with dosing initiated 1 day before surgery and continued through the first 2 weeks after surgery. They include nepafenac, 0.1%, 3 times daily, and 0.3%, 1 time daily; and bromfenac sodium, 0.09%, 1 time daily or 2 times daily, and 0.07%, 1 time daily (see Table 16-14).

NSAIDs have been associated with corneal complications, including melting and corneal perforation; these complications have been observed both in postoperative patients and in cases of uveitis, usually in patients with preexisting diabetes mellitus and ocular surface disorders.

Congdon NG, Schein OD, von Kulajta P, Lubomski LH, Gilbert D, Katz J. Corneal complications associated with topical ophthalmic use of nonsteroidal antiinflammatory drugs. *J Cataract Refract Surg.* 2001;27(4):622–631.

Flach AJ. Corneal melts associated with topically applied nonsteroidal anti-inflammatory drugs. *Trans Am Ophthalmol Soc.* 2001;99:205–210.

Antiallergic Drugs: Mast-Cell Stabilizers and Antihistamines

The human eye has approximately 50 million mast cells. Each cell contains several hundred granules that in turn contain preformed chemical mediators. Allergic conjunctivitis is an immediate hypersensitivity reaction in which triggering antigens couple to antibodies (IgE) on the cell surface of mast cells and basophils, causing the release of histamine, PG, leukotrienes, and chemotactic factors from secretory granules. The released histamine causes capillary dilatation and increased permeability and, therefore, conjunctival injection and swelling. It also stimulates nerve endings, causing pain and itching.

Drugs treat ocular allergies by interfering at different points along this pathway. Corticosteroids are very effective, but adverse effects limit their application for this chronic condition. Mast-cell stabilizers and antihistamines (which block histamine receptor-1 [H_1]) have fewer and less dangerous adverse effects and can be used singly or in combination. Table 16-19 lists drugs that relieve allergic conjunctivitis.

Corticosteroids

Corticosteroids are very effective for treating ocular allergies, especially in the acute phase, but they are prone to overuse and have a more dangerous adverse effect profile than other antiallergic drugs (see the section "Adverse effects" under Glucocorticoids). Loteprednol etabonate, 0.2%, a steroid designed to cause less IOP elevation, can be used for temporary treatment of ocular allergies. Recalcitrant cases of severe allergic, vernal, and atopic conjunctivitis may require the short-term use of stronger topical steroids, but these cases should be carefully monitored and patients switched to one of the previously mentioned drugs as soon as clinically prudent.

Antihistamines

Patients may achieve short-term relief of mild allergic symptoms with over-the-counter topical antihistamines such as antazoline and pheniramine, which are usually combined with the decongestant naphazoline. Specific H_1-antagonists include emedastine and levocabastine.

Emedastine difumarate, 0.05%, is a relatively selective H_1-receptor antagonist indicated for temporary relief of signs and symptoms of allergic conjunctivitis. Dosing is 1 drop up to 4 times per day. The most common adverse effect reported is headache (11% of patients). Other adverse effects are unpleasant taste, blurred vision, burning or stinging, corneal infiltrates, dry eye, rhinitis, and sinusitis.

Table 16-19 Drugs for Allergic Conjunctivitis

Generic Name	Trade Name	Class
Alcaftadine	Lastacaft	H_1-antagonist/mast-cell stabilizer
Azelastine HCl	Optivar, available generically	H_1-antagonist/mast-cell stabilizer
Bepotastine besilate	Bepreve	H_1-antagonist/mast-cell stabilizer
Cromolyn sodium	Crolom, available generically	Mast-cell stabilizer
Emedastine difumarate	Emadine	H_1-antagonist
Epinastine HCl	Elestat, available generically	H_1-antagonist/mast-cell stabilizer
Ketotifen fumarate	Zaditor (OTC), Alaway (OTC), available generically	H_1-antagonist/mast-cell stabilizer
Levocabastine HCl	Discontinued in the United States	H_1-antagonist
Lodoxamide tromethamine	Alomide	Mast-cell stabilizer
Loteprednol etabonate	Alrex	Corticosteroid
Naphazoline HCl	Ak-Con, Albalon, available generically	Decongestant
Naphazoline HCl/antazoline phosphate	Vasocon-A (OTC)	Antihistamine/decongestant
Naphazoline HCl/pheniramine maleate	Naphcon-A (OTC), Opcon-A (OTC), Visine-A (OTC)	Antihistamine/decongestant
Nedocromil sodium	Alocril	Mast-cell stabilizer
Olopatadine HCl	Patanol, 0.1%, Pataday, 0.2%	H_1-antagonist/mast-cell stabilizer
Pemirolast potassium	Alamast	Mast-cell stabilizer

OTC = over-the-counter.

Levocabastine hydrochloride, another H_1-receptor antagonist, has an onset of action in minutes and lasts for at least 4 hours. It is as effective as cromolyn sodium for treating allergic conjunctivitis. The usual dosage of levocabastine, 0.05%, is 1 drop 4 times per day for up to 2 weeks. This drug has been discontinued in the United States.

Mast-cell stabilizers

Mast-cell stabilizers are thought to prevent calcium influx across mast-cell membranes, thereby preventing mast-cell degranulation and mediator release. Traditional mast-cell stabilizers such as cromolyn sodium, lodoxamide, and pemirolast prevent mast-cell degranulation but take days to weeks to reach peak efficacy. They have little or no antihistamine effect and do not provide immediate relief from allergic symptoms. Therefore, topical steroids or H_1-antagonists may have to be used concurrently with mast-cell stabilizers for the first several weeks, until these drugs are fully effective.

Lodoxamide stabilizes the mast-cell membrane 2500 times as effectively as cromolyn sodium does. In the treatment of allergic conjunctivitis, its onset of action is more rapid, with less stinging, than that of cromolyn sodium. In addition, a multicenter double-masked study showed that lodoxamide was superior to cromolyn sodium in treating vernal keratoconjunctivitis. The usual dose of lodoxamide, 0.1%, for adults and children older than 2 years is 1 or 2 drops in the affected eye 4 times daily for up to 3 months. The most frequently reported adverse reactions are burning, stinging, and discomfort upon instillation (15% of patients).

> **CLINICAL PEARL**
>
> Comparisons between different mast-cell stabilizers and antihistamines are limited, and no clinical evidence indicates that any particular product is superior to others in treating ocular allergies. Mast-cell stabilizers and antihistamines are used for allergic, vernal, and atopic conjunctivitis.

Combined antihistamine and mast-cell stabilizers

Some drugs, including olopatadine, ketotifen, epinastine, azelastine, and alcaftadine, have a mast cell–stabilizing effect as well as H_1-antagonism. These drugs provide immediate relief against released histamine and prevent the future degranulation of mast cells. Olopatadine hydrochloride, 0.1%, has a rapid onset, and its duration of action is at least 8 hours. Recommended dosing is 1 or 2 drops in the affected eye 2 times per day at an interval of 6–8 hours. This drug is now also available for once-a-day dosing as olopatadine, 0.2%. Adverse reactions of ocular burning, stinging, dry eye, foreign-body sensation, hyperemia, keratitis, eyelid edema, pruritus, asthenia, cold syndrome, pharyngitis, rhinitis, sinusitis, and taste perversion were all reported at an incidence of less than 5% (for each adverse effect). For ketotifen fumarate, 0.025%, the recommended dosing is 1 drop every 8–12 hours. Conjunctival injection, headaches, and rhinitis were reported at an incidence of 10%–25% with use of this drug, which is now available without a prescription.

Greiner JV, Edwards-Swanson K, Ingerman A. Evaluation of alcaftadine 0.25% ophthalmic solution in acute allergic conjunctivitis at 15 minutes and 16 hours after instillation versus placebo and olopatadine 0.1%. *Clin Ophthalmol.* 2011;13(5):87–93.

La Rosa M, Lionetti E, Reibaldi M, et al. Allergic conjunctivitis: a comprehensive review of the literature. *Ital J Pediatr.* 2013;39:18.

Verin P. Treating severe eye allergy. *Clin Exp Allergy.* 1998;28(suppl 6):44–48.

Antifibrotic Drugs

Antiproliferative medications, also known as *antimetabolites,* are used in the treatment of severe ocular inflammatory diseases. They can also be used locally as antiproliferative agents in ocular surface neoplasia and as antifibrotic agents to limit scarring related to ophthalmic procedures, particularly of the ocular surface, as in glaucoma filtering procedures and pterygium surgery. The use of fluorouracil (5-FU) and mitomycin C (MMC) for these purposes, though common, is considered off-label.

Fluorouracil is a fluorinated pyrimidine nucleoside analogue that blocks production of thymidylate synthase and interrupts normal cellular DNA and RNA synthesis. Its primary action may be to cause cellular thymine deficiency and resultant cell death. The effect of 5-FU is most pronounced on rapidly growing cells, and its use as an antiviral drug is related primarily to the destruction of infected cells (eg, warts) by topical application. The drug is also thought to inhibit cellular proliferation that may otherwise occur in response to inflammation.

Two randomized clinical trials compared use of 5-FU infusion with use of low-molecular-weight heparin and placebo during vitrectomy to prevent proliferative vitreoretinopathy (PVR). One trial was conducted in patients at high risk of developing postoperative PVR and the other in unselected cases of rhegmatogenous retinal detachment (ie, including patients who were not viewed as being at risk of postoperative PVR). The results concerning the effects of these 2 agents were inconclusive.

In another study involving high-risk patients, including young patients (≤40 years of age) with glaucoma, the success rate for initial trabeculectomy with adjunctive 5-FU was higher than the rate with surgery without the adjunct. 5-FU was used postoperatively as a subconjunctival injection and intraoperatively as a topical application to the trabeculectomy site.

MMC, another antiproliferative compound, is isolated from the fungus *Streptomyces caespitosus.* The parent compound becomes a bifunctional alkylating agent after enzymatic alteration within the cell; it then inhibits DNA synthesis by DNA cross-linkage. Although mitomycin's immunosuppressive properties are fairly weak, it is a potent inhibitor of fibroblast proliferation. During glaucoma filtering operations, MMC is used topically in a single application to impede scarring and prevent surgical failure (see BCSC Section 10, *Glaucoma*). Complications of therapy are wound leakage, hypotony, and localized scleral melting. In an animal model, severe toxicity was reported with intraocular instillation of MMC, resulting in irreversible progressive bullous keratopathy in 3 of 4 rabbits.

Both mitomycin and 5-FU have been used to treat conjunctival intraepithelial neoplasia. Mitomycin is also commonly used to reduce haze in patients undergoing phototherapeutic keratectomy and has been recommended both as single-dose topical therapy and as postoperative drops to prevent recurrence of pterygia after pterygium excision. The recommended dosage is 0.02%–0.04% 4 times daily for 1–2 weeks after surgery. The reported recurrence rate with this therapy has been as low as 0%–11%. However, several adverse effects, such as corneal edema, corneal and scleral perforation, corectopia, anterior uveitis, cataract, and intractable pain, have been reported. With a primary conjunctival graft after pterygium removal, recurrence rates may be similarly low but without these serious complications. For additional information on uses of mitomycin and 5-FU, see BCSC Section 8, *External Disease and Cornea.*

Anderson Penno E, Braun DA, Kamal A, Hamilton WK, Gimbel HV. Topical thiotepa treatment for recurrent corneal haze after photorefractive keratectomy. *J Cataract Refract Surg.* 2003;29(8):1537–1542.

Khaw PT. Advances in glaucoma surgery: evolution of antimetabolite adjunctive therapy. *J Glaucoma.* 2001;10(5 suppl 1):S81–S84.

Sundaram V, Barsam A, Virgili G. Intravitreal low molecular weight heparin and 5-fluorouracil for the prevention of proliferative vitreoretinopathy following retinal reattachment surgery. *Cochrane Database Syst Rev.* 2010;7:CD006421.

Wormald R, Wilkins MR, Bunce C. Post-operative 5-fluorouracil for glaucoma surgery. *Cochrane Database Syst Rev.* 2001;3:CD001132.

Yamamoto N, Ohmura T, Suzuki H, Shirasawa H. Successful treatment with 5-fluorouracil of conjunctival intraepithelial neoplasia refractive to mitomycin-C. *Ophthalmology.* 2002;109(2):249–252.

Medications for Dry Eye

Artificial tear preparations (demulcents and emollients) form an occlusive film over the corneal surface to lubricate and protect the eye from drying. The active ingredients in demulcent preparations are polyvinyl alcohol, cellulose, and methylcellulose as well as their derivatives: hydroxypropyl cellulose, hydroxyethylcellulose, hydroxypropyl methylcellulose, and carboxymethylcellulose. Other ingredients used include glycerin, polysorbate 80, polyethylene glycol 400, dextran 70, povidone, and propylene glycol.

The viscosity of artificial tears varies in part because of the concentration of the wetting agent. For example, carboxymethylcellulose is available in 0.25%, 0.5%, and 1% solutions; higher-viscosity solutions are used to treat increasingly severe dry eye symptoms.

Some data support the hypothesis that changes in tear osmolality trigger corneal and conjunctival epithelial damage and initiation of dry eye. Artificial tear products with lower osmolality may relieve dry eye symptoms to a greater extent, but clinical results thus far have not been conclusive.

The pH of commercially available artificial tear products also varies widely. A patient may experience a stinging sensation after eyedrop use because of a mismatch between the pH of the instilled eyedrops and that of the patient's tear. Patients who report a stinging sensation following eyedrop use can try another product with a different pH.

Multidose preparations also contain preservatives, including benzalkonium chloride, EDTA (ethylenediaminetetraacetic acid), methylparaben, polyquad (polyquaternium 1), potassium sorbate, propylparaben, sodium chlorite, sodium perborate, and sorbic acid. Although early preservatives such as thimerosal and benzalkonium chloride were highly toxic, the newest generation of ophthalmic preservatives are less harmful to the ocular surface. Nonpreserved unit-dose preparations eliminate the cytotoxic effects of preservatives.

Ocular emollients are ointments prepared with sterile petrolatum, liquid lanolin, mineral oil, methylparaben, and polyparaben. Ophthalmic lubricating ointments help ease the symptoms of severe dry eye and exposure keratopathy and are suitable for nighttime use in dry eye and nocturnal lagophthalmos.

Topical cyclosporine emulsion, 0.05%, targets the inflammatory etiology of dry eye. Because cyclosporine is poorly water soluble, it is prepared in an emulsion composed of glycerin, castor oil, and polysorbate 80. It is available in a multidose bottle and a preservative-free single-use package. The oily vector is marketed separately as a tear supplement. Studies have shown that twice-daily dosing with this drug has negligible systemic absorption and adverse effects. Biopsies have demonstrated a measurable repopulation of goblet cells and a decrease in both conjunctival epithelial cell turnover and the number of lymphocytes. Lifitegrast, 5%, preservative-free topical solution, a lymphocyte function–associated antigen 1 (LFA-1) antagonist administered twice daily, was approved by the FDA in 2016 for treatment of dry eye. It inhibits binding of intercellular adhesion molecule-1 (ICAM-1) to LFA-1 and has been effective in reducing ocular surface inflammation.

Given the wide variety of commercially available products, some principles can help guide the selection of artificial tear preparation for a particular patient. Generally, a more viscous tear lubricant should be used as the severity of the dry eye increases. A trial-and-error approach that involves titration of the frequency of instillation according to the patient's daily activities, the use of tear substitutes with different mechanisms of action or properties, and even a combination of different lubricants may be necessary. Preservative-free products should be utilized if frequent instillation is required, such as for severe dry eye. Nonpreserved preparations are at risk of microbial contamination and therefore should be discarded within a few hours of use, even though the vial may be recapped after opening.

For the treatment of ocular surface diseases such as persistent epithelial defects, superior limbic keratoconjunctivitis, keratoconjunctivitis sicca, and neurotrophic keratopathy, autologous serum eyedrops are beneficial. They are typically formulated by compounding a 20%–100% solution packaged into sterile dropper bottles. Reported complications include peripheral corneal infiltrate and ulcer, eyelid eczema, microbial keratitis, ocular discomfort or epitheliopathy, bacterial conjunctivitis, scleral vasculitis and melting in patients with rheumatoid arthritis, and immune complex deposition with 100% serum.

Two dry eye products currently under investigation are diquafosol tetrasodium and rebamipide. Diquafosol tetrasodium is a $P2Y_2$ purinergic receptor agonist that activates $P2Y_2$ receptors on the ocular surface, causing rehydration through activation of the fluid pump mechanism of the accessory lacrimal glands on the conjunctival surface. It was approved for use in Japan in 2010 for treating dry eye. Rebamipide is a derivative of quinolone-class antibiotics that enhances the secretion of mucin to support tear film adhesion and slow tear film breakup time (also see BCSC Section 8, *External Disease and Cornea*).

Foulks GN, Nichols KK, Bron AJ, Holland EJ, McDonald MB, Nelson JD. Improving awareness, identification, and management of meibomian gland dysfunction. *Ophthalmology.* 2012;119(suppl 10):S1–S12.

Geerling G, MacLennan S, Hartwig D. Autologous serum eye drops for ocular surface disorders. *Br J Ophthalmol.* 2004;88(11):1467–1474.

Kunert KS, Tisdale AS, Gipson IK. Goblet cell numbers and epithelial proliferation in the conjunctiva of patients with dry eye syndrome treated with cyclosporine. *Arch Ophthalmol.* 2002;120(3):330–337. [Erratum appears in *Arch Ophthalmol.* 2002;120(8):1099.]

Kunert KS, Tisdale AS, Stern ME, Smith JA, Gipson IK. Analysis of topical cyclosporine treatment of patients with dry eye syndrome: effect on conjunctival lymphocytes. *Arch Ophthalmol.* 2000;118(11):1489–1496.

Pflugfelder SC. Antiinflammatory therapy for dry eye. *Am J Ophthalmol.* 2004;137(2): 337–342.

Tong L, Petznick A, Lee S, Tan J. Choice of artificial tear formulation for patients with dry eye: where do we start? *Cornea.* 2012;31(suppl 1):S32–S36.

Ocular Decongestants

Common drugs such as naphazoline, oxymetazoline, tetrahydrozoline, and phenylephrine hydrochloride are used as topical drops to cause temporary vasoconstriction of conjunctival vessels. This effect is mediated by α_1-receptors. Other than providing temporal relief of hyperemia, they have no clear therapeutic benefit. Possible adverse effects include rebound vasodilation and conjunctival injection. The mechanisms of the adverse effects are unclear; possibilities include receptor desensitization and damage to the ocular surface as a result of vasoconstriction of arteries, which may involve activation of α_2-receptors, and toxicity of preservatives. These medications can be abused by patients and may cause ocular surface toxicity. Systemic absorption of ocular adrenergic drugs is frequently sufficient to cause systemic effects, which are manifested in the cardiovascular system, the bronchial airways, and the brain (see the earlier section Adrenergic Drugs).

Although ocular decongestants are available as over-the-counter preparations, patients should be instructed not to use them on a long-term basis. Further, all efforts should be made to determine the etiology of the patient's hyperemia and to target the source before use of these medications is considered.

Antimicrobial Drugs

Penicillins and Cephalosporins

The penicillins and cephalosporins are β-lactam–containing antibacterial drugs that react with and inactivate a particular bacterial transpeptidase that is essential for bacterial cell-wall synthesis (Table 16-20). Some bacteria are resistant to the action of penicillins and cephalosporins. The lipopolysaccharide outer coat of many gram-negative bacteria may prevent certain hydrophilic antibiotics from reaching their cytoplasmic membrane sites of action. Furthermore, some bacteria produce β-lactamases (penicillinase), enzymes capable of cleaving the critical amide bond within these antibiotics. The different penicillins and cephalosporins vary in susceptibility to the β-lactamases produced by different bacterial species.

The penicillins and cephalosporins penetrate the blood–ocular and blood–brain barriers poorly and are actively transported out of the eye by the organic-acid transport system of the ciliary body. However, their penetration into the eye increases with inflammation and with coadministration of probenecid.

Serious and occasionally fatal hypersensitivity (anaphylactoid) reactions can occur in association with penicillin and cephalosporin therapy. A history of immediate allergic response (anaphylaxis or rapid onset of hives) to any penicillin is a strong contraindication to the use of any other penicillin. Approximately 10% of people who are allergic to a penicillin will have cross-reactivity to cephalosporins.

Kelkar PS, Li JT. Cephalosporin allergy. *N Engl J Med.* 2001;345(11):804–809.

Penicillins

There are 5 classes of penicillins, which differ in their spectrum of antibiotic activity and in their resistance to penicillinase:

1. Penicillin G, penicillin V, and phenethicillin are highly effective against most gram-positive and gram-negative cocci; many anaerobes; and *Listeria, Actinomyces, Leptospira,* and *Treponema* organisms. However, most strains of *Staphylococcus aureus* and many strains of *Staphylococcus epidermidis,* anaerobes, and *Neisseria gonorrhoeae* are now resistant, often through production of penicillinase. Resistance by enterococci often arises from altered penicillin-binding proteins. Penicillin V and phenethicillin are absorbed well orally, whereas penicillin G is better absorbed when administered intravenously because it is inactivated by stomach

Table 16-20 Principal Antibiotics and Their Administration[a]

Drug Name	Topical	Subconjunctival	Intravitreal	Intravenous (Adult)
Amikacin sulfate	10 mg/mL	25 mg	400 µg	15 mg/kg daily in 2 or 3 doses
Ampicillin sodium	50 mg/mL	50–150 mg	500 µg	4–12 g daily in 4 doses
Bacitracin zinc	10,000 units/mL	5000 units	NA	NA
Carbenicillin disodium	4–6 mg/mL	100 mg	250–2000 µg	8–24 g daily in 4–6 doses
Cefazolin sodium	50 mg/mL	100 mg	2250 µg	2–4 g daily in 3 or 4 doses
Ceftazidime	50 mg/mL	200 mg	2000 µg	1 g daily in 2 or 3 doses
Ceftriaxone sodium	50 mg/mL	125 mg	2000 µg	1–2 g daily
Clindamycin	50 mg/mL	15–50 mg	1000 µg	900–1800 mg daily in 2 doses
Colistimethate sodium	10 mg/mL	15–25 mg	100 µg	2.5–5.0 mg/kg daily in 2–4 doses
Erythromycin	50 mg/mL	100 mg	500 µg	NA
Gentamicin sulfate	8–15 mg/mL	10–20 mg	100–200 µg	3–5 mg/kg daily in 2 or 3 doses
Imipenem/cilastatin sodium	5 mg/mL	NA	NA	2 g daily in 3 or 4 doses
Kanamycin sulfate	30–50 mg/mL	30 mg	500 µg	15 mg/kg daily in 2 or 3 doses
Methicillin sodium	50 mg/mL	50–100 mg	1000–2000 µg	6–10 g daily in 4 doses
Neomycin sulfate	5–8 mg/mL	125–250 mg	NA	NA
Penicillin G	100,000 units/mL	0.5–1.0 million units	300 units	12–24 million units daily in 4 doses
Polymyxin B sulfate	10,000 units/mL	100,000 units	NA	NA
Ticarcillin disodium	6 mg/mL	100 mg	NA	200–300 mg/kg daily
Tobramycin sulfate	8–15 mg/mL	10–20 mg	100–200 µg	3–5 mg/kg daily in 2 or 3 doses
Vancomycin HCl	12.5–50 mg/mL	25 mg	1000 µg	15–30 mg/kg daily in 1 or 2 doses

NA = not applicable.

[a] Most penicillins and cephalosporins are physically incompatible when combined with aminoglycosides in the same bottle or syringe.

acid. These penicillins are excreted rapidly by the kidneys and have short half-lives unless they are given in depot form (ie, procaine penicillin G) or administered with probenecid, which competitively inhibits excretion by the kidneys.

2. The penicillinase-resistant penicillins include methicillin sodium, nafcillin, oxacillin sodium, cloxacillin sodium, dicloxacillin sodium, and floxacillin. They are less potent than penicillin G against susceptible organisms but are the drugs of choice for infections that are caused by penicillinase-producing *S aureus* and that are not methicillin resistant. Methicillin and nafcillin are acid labile; therefore, they are given either parenterally or by subconjunctival injection. The other medications in this group have reasonable oral absorption. When they are given

systemically, coadministration of probenecid reduces renal excretion and outward transport from the eye.

3. The broad-spectrum penicillins such as ampicillin, amoxicillin, and bacampicillin hydrochloride have antibacterial activity that extends to such gram-negative organisms as *Haemophilus influenzae, Escherichia coli, Salmonella* and *Shigella* species, and *Proteus mirabilis.* Resistant strains of *H influenzae* are becoming more common. These drugs are stable in acid and may be given orally. They are not resistant to penicillinase or to the broader-spectrum β-lactamases that are increasingly common among gram-negative bacteria.
4. Carbenicillin and ticarcillin have antimicrobial activity that extends to *Pseudomonas* and *Enterobacter* species and indole-positive strains of *Proteus.* These drugs are given parenterally or subconjunctivally, although the indanyl ester of carbenicillin may be given orally. They are not resistant to penicillinase and are less active against gram-positive bacteria and *Listeria* species.
5. Piperacillin sodium, mezlocillin sodium, and azlocillin are particularly potent against *Pseudomonas* and *Klebsiella* species and retain strong gram-positive coverage and activity against *Listeria* species. They are administered parenterally or subconjunctivally, and they are not resistant to penicillinase.

Cephalosporins

Bacterial susceptibility patterns and resistance to β-lactamases dictate the classification of the cephalosporins as first, second, third, or fourth generation, although fifth- and sixth-generation drugs are under development.

1. *First generation.* Cephalothin, cefazolin, cephalexin, cefadroxil, and cephradine have strong antimicrobial activity against gram-positive organisms, especially *Streptococcus* species and *S aureus.* They retain moderate activity against gram-negative organisms. Of these drugs, cephalothin is the most resistant to staphylococcal β-lactamase and is used in severe staphylococcal infections. Because cephalothin is painful when given intramuscularly, it is used only intravenously. In contrast, cefazolin is more sensitive to β-lactamase but has somewhat greater activity against *Klebsiella* species and *E coli.* Cefazolin also has a longer half-life and is tolerated both intramuscularly and intravenously; thus, it is used more frequently than the other first-generation cephalosporins. Cephalexin, cefadroxil, and cephradine are stable in gastric acid and are available in oral forms.
2. *Second generation.* These medications were developed to expand activity against gram-negative organisms while retaining much of their gram-positive spectrum of activity. Compared with first-generation medications, cefamandole, cefoxitin, and cefuroxime display greater activity against *H influenzae, Enterobacter aerogenes,* and *Neisseria* species. Cefamandole has increased activity against *Enterobacter* and indole-positive *Proteus* species, *H influenzae,* and *Bacteroides* species. Cefoxitin is active against indole-positive *Proteus* and *Serratia* organisms, as well as against *Bacteroides fragilis.* Cefuroxime is valuable in the treatment of penicillinase-producing *N gonorrhoeae* and ampicillin-resistant *H influenzae,* and its penetration of the blood–brain barrier is adequate for initial treatment of suspected pneumococcal, meningococcal, or *H influenzae* meningitis.

3. *Third generation.* The third-generation cephalosporins have further enhanced activity against gram-negative bacilli, specifically the β-lactamase–producing members of the Enterobacteriaceae family, but they are inferior to first-generation cephalosporins with regard to their activity against gram-positive cocci. Commonly used drugs include cefotaxime, cefoperazone sodium, ceftriaxone sodium, ceftazidime, and ceftizoxime sodium. These drugs have a similar spectrum of activity against gram-positive and gram-negative organisms; anaerobes; *Neisseria, Serratia,* and *Proteus* species; and some *Pseudomonas* isolates. Cefoperazone and ceftazidime are particularly effective against *Pseudomonas* but lose more coverage of the gram-positive cocci. Cefotaxime penetrates the blood–brain barrier better than the other cephalosporins can, and it presumably also penetrates the blood–ocular barrier.
4. *Fourth generation.* Cefepime hydrochloride and cefpirome have a spectrum of gram-negative coverage similar to that of the third-generation cephalosporins, but these drugs are more resistant to some β-lactamases.

No cephalosporin provides coverage for enterococci, *Listeria* and *Legionella* species, or methicillin-resistant *S aureus* (MRSA).

Other Antibacterial Drugs

Tables 16-21 and 16-22 list ophthalmic antibacterial drugs and ophthalmic combination anti-inflammatory/antibiotic drugs, respectively.

Fluoroquinolones

Fluoroquinolones are synthetic fluorinated derivatives of nalidixic acid. These drugs are highly effective broad-spectrum antimicrobials with potent activity against common gram-positive and gram-negative ocular pathogens. Their mechanism of action targets bacterial DNA supercoiling through the inhibition of bacterial topoisomerase II (DNA gyrase) and topoisomerase IV, 2 of the enzymes responsible for replication, genetic recombination, and DNA repair. Mutations in the bacterial genes for these enzymes allow the development of resistance to fluoroquinolone drugs, an incidence that is increasing, as well as evidence of cross-resistance among them. Fluoroquinolone resistance has been reported in *Mycobacterium chelonae, S aureus,* coagulase-negative *Staphylococcus* species, *Pseudomonas aeruginosa, Clostridium difficile, Salmonella enterica, E coli,* and *Helicobacter pylori.*

In vitro studies have demonstrated that the fluoroquinolones, especially ciprofloxacin and temafloxacin, inhibit 90% of common corneal bacterial pathogens and have a lower minimum inhibitory concentration than that of the aminoglycosides gentamicin and tobramycin and the cephalosporin cefazolin. They are also less toxic to the corneal epithelium than are the aminoglycosides. Methicillin-susceptible strains of *S aureus* are generally susceptible to fluoroquinolones, but methicillin-resistant strains of staphylococci are often resistant to them.

The older generations of fluoroquinolones have good potency against gram-negative bacteria, and the newer generations were designed to broaden the spectrum of coverage and increase potency against gram-positive bacteria. For example, the second-generation fluoroquinolone ciprofloxacin may be more effective against *P aeruginosa* than the newer drugs.

Table 16-21 Selected Ophthalmic Antibacterial Drugs

Generic Name	Trade Name	Strength
Individual drugs		
Azithromycin	AzaSite	Solution, 1%
Bacitracin zinc	Ak-Tracin, available generically	Ointment (500 units/g)
Besifloxacin	Besivance	Suspension, 0.6%
Chloramphenicol	Powder available for compounding	Solution, 0.5%; ointment, 1%
Ciprofloxacin HCl	Ciloxan, available generically	Solution, 0.3%; ointment, 0.3%
Erythromycin	Romycin, available generically	Ointment, 0.5%
Gatifloxacin	Zymar, Zymaxid	Solution, 0.3%; solution, 0.5%
Gentamicin sulfate	Garamycin	Solution, 0.3%; ointment, 0.3%
	Genoptic	Solution, 0.3%
	Gentasol	Solution, 0.3%
	Gentak	Solution, 0.3%; ointment, 0.3%
	Available generically	Solution, 0.3%; ointment, 0.3%
Levofloxacin	Quixin	Solution, 0.5%
Moxifloxacin HCl	Vigamox, Moxeza	Solution, 0.5%
	Available generically	Solution, 0.5%
Norfloxacin	Norflox	Solution, 0.3%
Ofloxacin	Ocuflox	Solution, 0.3%
	Available generically	Solution, 0.3%
Sulfacetamide sodium	Bleph-10	Solution, 10%; ointment, 10%
	Available generically	Solution, 10%; ointment, 10%
Tobramycin sulfate	Ak-Tob	Solution, 0.3%
	Tobrasol	Solution, 0.3%
	Tobrex	Solution, 0.3%; ointment, 0.3%
	Available generically	Solution, 0.3%
Combination drugs		
Polymyxin B sulfate/bacitracin zinc	Ak-Poly-Bac	Ointment (10,000 units/g, 500 units/g)
	Polycin-B	Ointment (10,000 units/g, 500 units/g)
	Available generically	Ointment (10,000 units/g, 500 units/g)
Polymyxin B sulfate/neomycin sulfate/bacitracin zinc	Available generically	Solution (10,000 units, 1.75 mg, 0.025 mg/mL), ointment (10,000 units/g, 3.5 mg/base, 400 units/g)
Polymyxin B sulfate/neomycin sulfate/gramicidin	Neosporin, available generically	Solution (10,000 units/mL, 1.75 mg base/mL, 0.025 mg/mL)
Polymyxin B sulfate/ oxytetracycline	Terak	Ointment (10,000 units/g, equivalent to 5 mg base/g)
Polymyxin B sulfate/ trimethoprim sulfate	Polytrim, available generically	Solution (10,000 units/mL, equivalent to 1 mg base/mL)

Table 16-22 Combination Ocular Anti-inflammatory and Antibiotic Drugs

Generic Name	Trade Name	Preparation and Concentration
Dexamethasone/neomycin sulfate/polymyxin B sulfate	Ak-Trol, Poly-Dex, Dexacidin, Dexasporin, Maxitrol, available generically	Suspension, 0.1%; equivalent to 3.5 mg base/mL; 10,000 units/mL
	Maxitrol, Ak-Trol, Poly-Dex, available generically	Ointment, 0.1%; equivalent to 3.5 mg base/g; 10,000 units/g
Dexamethasone/tobramycin	Tobradex, available generically	Suspension, 0.1%, 0.3%
	Tobradex	Ointment, 0.1%, 0.3%
Fluorometholone/ sulfacetamide	FML-S	Suspension, 0.1%, 10%
Hydrocortisone/neomycin sulfate/polymyxin B sulfate	Cortisporin suspension, available generically	Suspension, 1%; equivalent to 3.5 mg base/mL; 10,000 units/mL
Hydrocortisone/neomycin sulfate/polymyxin B sulfate/bacitracin zinc	Ak-Spore, Cortisporin ointment, available generically	Ointment, 1%; equivalent to 3.5 mg base/g; 5000 units/g; 400 units/g
Loteprednol etabonate/ tobramycin	Zylet	Suspension, 0.5%, 0.3%
Neomycin sulfate/polymyxin B sulfate/prednisolone acetate	Poly-Pred, available generically	Suspension; equivalent to 0.35% base; 10,000 units/ mL; 0.5%
Prednisolone acetate/ gentamicin sulfate	Pred-G	Suspension; equivalent to 0.3% base; 1%
	Pred-G S.O.P.	Ointment; equivalent to 0.3% base; 0.6%
Prednisolone acetate/ sulfacetamide sodium	Blephamide, available generically	Suspension, 0.2%, 10%
	Blephamide S.O.P.	Ointment, 0.2%, 10%
Prednisolone sodium phosphate/sulfacetamide sodium	Vasocidin, available generically	Solution, 0.25%, 10%
	Ak-Cide	Ointment, 0.5%, 10%

Seven currently available topical fluoroquinolones are ofloxacin ophthalmic solution, 0.3%; ciprofloxacin, 0.3%; levofloxacin, 0.5%; gatifloxacin, 0.3% and 0.5%; moxifloxacin, 0.5%; norfloxacin, 0.3%; and besifloxacin, 0.6%. They are used to treat corneal ulcers caused by susceptible strains of *S aureus, S epidermidis, Streptococcus pneumoniae, P aeruginosa, Serratia marcescens* (efficacy studied in fewer than 10 infections), and *Propionibacterium acnes.* They are also indicated for bacterial conjunctivitis due to susceptible strains of *S aureus, S epidermidis, S pneumoniae, Enterobacter cloacae, H influenzae, P mirabilis,* and *P aeruginosa.* These fluoroquinolones have a high rate of penetration into ocular tissue. Their sustained tear concentration levels exceed the minimum inhibitory concentrations of key ocular pathogens for 12 hours or more after 1 dose. They also deliver excellent susceptibility kill rates; 1 in vitro study confirmed eradication of 87%–100% of indicated pathogenic bacteria, including *P aeruginosa.* Ofloxacin has a high intrinsic solubility that enables formulation at a near-neutral pH of 6.4. Ciprofloxacin is formulated at a pH of 4.5, gatifloxacin at a pH of 6.0, and moxifloxacin at a pH of 6.8.

The most frequently reported drug-related adverse reaction with fluoroquinolones is transient ocular burning or discomfort. Other reported reactions are stinging, redness, itching, chemical conjunctivitis/keratitis, periocular/facial edema, foreign-body sensation, photophobia, blurred vision, tearing, dry eye, and eye pain. Though rare, dizziness has also been reported. Both norfloxacin and ciprofloxacin have caused white, crystalline corneal deposits of medication, which have resolved after discontinuation of the drug.

Case reports of tendonitis and tendon rupture have been associated with systemic fluoroquinolone use. The possibility of damage to growth-plate cartilage poses a safety concern for the use of fluoroquinolones in children. However, larger cohorts and comparative studies did not show an increased risk of musculoskeletal disorders in children treated with systemic fluoroquinolones. There is no evidence that the ophthalmic administration of fluoroquinolones has any effect on weight-bearing joints in the pediatric population.

Sulfonamides

Sulfonamides are derivatives of *para*-aminobenzenesulfonamide. They are structural analogues of *para*-aminobenzoic acid (PABA) and competitive antagonists of dihydropteroate synthase for the bacterial synthesis of folic acid. Unlike mammals, bacteria cannot use exogenous folic acid but must synthesize it from PABA. Sulfonamides are bacteriostatic only and are more effective when administered with trimethoprim or pyrimethamine, each of which is a potent inhibitor of bacterial dihydrofolate reductase; together, they block successive steps in the synthesis of folic acid. For example, sulfadiazine, systemic pyrimethamine, and folinic acid are used in the treatment of toxoplasmosis, with the folinic acid coadministered to minimize bone marrow suppression. A 3-week course of systemic sulfonamide therapy is also useful for chlamydial infection.

Sulfacetamide ophthalmic solution (10%–30%) and ointment (10%) penetrate the cornea well but may sensitize the patient to sulfonamide medication. Susceptible organisms include *S pneumoniae, Corynebacterium diphtheriae, H influenzae, Actinomyces* species, and *Chlamydia trachomatis.* Local irritation, itching, periorbital edema, and transient stinging are common adverse effects from topical administration. As for all sulfonamide preparations, severe sensitivity reactions such as toxic epidermal necrolysis and Stevens-Johnson syndrome have been reported. The incidence of adverse reactions to all sulfonamides is approximately 5%.

The cross-allergenicity between sulfonamide antibiotics and nonantibiotic sulfonamide-containing drugs complicates drug therapy. The immunologic determinant of type I immediate hypersensitivity reaction to sulfonamide antibiotics is the N1 heterocyclic ring. Nonantibiotic sulfonamides do not contain this structural feature. Non–type I hypersensitivity responses to sulfonamide antibiotics are largely attributable to reactive metabolites formed at the N4 amino nitrogen of the sulfonamide antibiotics, a structure that is also absent from nonantibiotic sulfonamide drugs. Therefore, cross-reactivity between sulfonamide antibiotics and nonantibiotic sulfonamide-containing drugs is unlikely. However, a T-cell–mediated immune response to the parent sulfonamide structure appears to be responsible for hypersensitivity that occurs in a small subset of patients. Thus, cross-reactivity remains possible, at least theoretically. There is no cross-allergenicity between sulfonamide and the sulfate group (*sulfate* refers to the bivalent SO_4 group of a compound).

Brackett CC, Singh H, Block JH. Likelihood and mechanisms of cross-allergenicity between sulfonamide antibiotics and other drugs containing a sulfonamide functional group. *Pharmacotherapy.* 2004;24(7):856–870.

Lehmann DF. The metabolic rationale for a lack of cross-reactivity between sulfonamide antimicrobials and other sulfonamide-containing drugs. *Drug Metab Lett.* 2012;6(2):129–133.

Strom BL, Schinnar R, Apter AJ, et al. Absence of cross-reactivity between sulfonamide antibiotics and sulfonamide nonantibiotics. *N Engl J Med.* 2003;349(17):1628–1635.

Tetracyclines

The tetracycline family includes agents produced by *Streptomyces* species (chlortetracycline, oxytetracycline, demeclocycline), as well as the semisynthetically produced medications tetracycline, doxycycline, and minocycline. Tetracyclines enter bacteria by active transport across the cytoplasmic membrane. They inhibit protein synthesis by binding to the ribosomal subunit 30S, thereby preventing access of aminoacyl transfer RNA to the acceptor site on the mRNA–ribosome complex. Host cells are less affected because they lack an active transport system. Doxycycline and minocycline are more lipophilic and thus more active by weight.

Tetracyclines are broad-spectrum bacteriostatic antibiotics that are active against many gram-positive and gram-negative bacteria and against *Rickettsia* species, *Mycoplasma pneumoniae,* and *Chlamydia* species. However, many strains of *Klebsiella* and *H influenzae* and nearly all strains of *Proteus vulgaris* and *P aeruginosa* are resistant. These medications demonstrate cross-resistance. Tetracycline is poorly water soluble but is soluble in eyedrops containing mineral oil; it readily penetrates the corneal epithelium. Chlortetracycline was previously used in ophthalmic preparations, but neither chlortetracycline nor tetracycline is currently available for ophthalmic use in the United States. Oxytetracycline is available in combination with polymyxin as an ophthalmic ointment.

Systemic therapy with the tetracyclines is used to treat chlamydial infections; because these drugs are excreted into oil glands, they are also used to treat staphylococcal infections of the meibomian glands. Tetracyclines have anti-inflammatory properties that include suppression of leukocyte migration, reduced production of NO and reactive oxygen species, inhibition of matrix metalloproteinases, and inhibition of phospholipase A2. In the management of meibomian gland dysfunction and rosacea, they are used mainly for their anti-inflammatory and lipid-regulating properties, rather than for their antimicrobial effects (see BCSC Section 8, *External Disease and Cornea*).

As bacteriostatic drugs, tetracyclines may inhibit bactericidal medications such as the penicillins; therefore, these drugs should not be used concurrently. Tetracyclines also depress plasma prothrombin activity and thereby potentiate warfarin. In addition, the use of tetracyclines may decrease the efficacy of oral contraceptives. Patients should be instructed to use an additional form of birth control during administration of tetracyclines and for 1 month after discontinuation of their use.

Tetracyclines chelate to calcium in milk and antacids and are best taken on an empty stomach. Because tetracyclines may cause gastric irritation, they may be taken with nondairy foods to improve patient compliance. Tetracyclines should not be given to children or pregnant women because they may be deposited in growing teeth, causing permanent discoloration of the enamel, and they may deposit in bone and inhibit bone growth. They can also cause photosensitivity; consequently, patients taking tetracycline should avoid extended exposure to sunlight. Degraded or expired tetracyclines may cause renal toxicity, also called *Fanconi syndrome.* Tetracyclines have been implicated as a cause of idiopathic intracranial hypertension, a condition discussed in BCSC Section 5, *Neuro-Ophthalmology.*

Geerling G, Tauber J, Baudouin C, et al. The international workshop on meibomian gland dysfunction: report of the Subcommittee on Management and Treatment of Meibomian Gland Dysfunction. *Invest Ophthalmol Vis Sci.* 2011;52(4):2050–2064.

Chloramphenicol

Chloramphenicol, a broad-spectrum bacteriostatic drug, inhibits bacterial protein synthesis by binding reversibly to the ribosomal subunit 50S, preventing aminoacyl transfer RNA from binding to the ribosome. Chloramphenicol is effective against *H influenzae, Neisseria meningitidis,* and *N gonorrhoeae,* as well as all anaerobic bacteria. It has some activity against *S pneumoniae, S aureus, Klebsiella pneumoniae, Enterobacter* and *Serratia* species, and *P mirabilis. P aeruginosa* is resistant.

Chloramphenicol penetrates the corneal epithelium well during topical therapy and penetrates the blood–ocular barrier readily when given systemically. However, the use of this medication is limited because it has been implicated in an idiosyncratic and potentially lethal aplastic anemia. Although most cases of this type of anemia have occurred after oral administration, some have been associated with parenteral and even topical ocular therapy. Chloramphenicol is available as a powder for compounding, but it should not be used if an alternative drug with less potential toxicity is available.

Aminoglycosides

The aminoglycosides consist of amino sugars in glycosidic linkage. They are bactericidal agents that are transported across the cell membrane into bacteria, where they bind to ribosomal subunits 30S and 50S, interfering with initiation of protein synthesis. The antibacterial spectrum of these drugs is determined primarily by the efficiency of their transport into bacterial cells. Such transport is energy dependent and may be reduced in the anaerobic environment of an abscess. Resistance to aminoglycosides may be caused by failure of transport, low affinity for the ribosome, or a plasmid-transmitted ability to enzymatically inactivate the drug. The coadministration of drugs such as penicillin that alter bacterial cell-wall structure can markedly increase aminoglycoside penetration, resulting in a synergism of antibiotic activity against gram-positive cocci, especially enterococci. One such aminoglycoside, amikacin, is remarkably resistant to enzymatic inactivation.

Gentamicin, tobramycin, kanamycin, and amikacin have antibacterial activity against aerobic, gram-negative bacilli such as *P mirabilis; P aeruginosa;* and *Klebsiella, Enterobacter,* and *Serratia* species. Gentamicin and tobramycin are also active against gram-positive *S aureus* and *S epidermidis.* Kanamycin is generally less effective than the others against gram-negative bacilli. Resistance to gentamicin and tobramycin has gradually increased as a result of the plasmid-transmitted ability to synthesize inactivating enzymes, as described earlier. Amikacin, which is generally impervious to these enzymes, is particularly valuable in treating these resistant organisms. It is effective against tuberculosis, as well as atypical mycobacteria, and can be compounded for topical use against mycobacterial infection.

Aminoglycosides are not absorbed well orally but are given systemically, either intramuscularly or intravenously. They do not readily penetrate the blood–ocular barrier but may be administered as eyedrops, ointments, or periocular injections. Gentamicin and carbenicillin should not be mixed for intravenous administration because carbenicillin inactivates gentamicin over several hours. Similar incompatibilities exist in vitro between gentamicin and other penicillins and cephalosporins.

The use of streptomycin is now limited to *Streptococcus viridans* bacterial endocarditis, tularemia, plague, and brucellosis. Neomycin is a broad-spectrum antibiotic that is effective against *Enterobacter* species, *K pneumoniae, H influenzae, N meningitidis, C diphtheriae,* and *S aureus.* It is given topically in ophthalmology and orally as a bowel preparation for surgery. Topical allergy to ocular use of neomycin occurs in approximately 8% of cases. Neomycin can cause punctate epitheliopathy and retard re-epithelialization of abrasions.

All aminoglycosides can cause dose-related vestibular and auditory dysfunction and nephrotoxicity when they are given systemically. Dosage adjustments must be made to prevent accumulation of drugs and toxicity in patients with renal insufficiency.

Miscellaneous antibiotics

Vancomycin is a tricyclic glycopeptide produced by *Streptococcus orientalis.* It is bactericidal for most gram-positive organisms through the inhibition of glycopeptide polymerization in the cell wall. Vancomycin is useful in the treatment of staphylococcal infections in patients who are allergic to or have not responded to the penicillins and cephalosporins. It can also be used in combination with aminoglycosides to treat *S viridans* or *Streptococcus bovis* endocarditis. Oral vancomycin is poorly absorbed but is effective in the treatment of pseudomembranous colitis caused by *C difficile.* Vancomycin resistance has increased in isolates of *Enterococcus* and *Staphylococcus,* and antibiotic resistance is transmitted between pathogens by a conjugative plasmid.

Vancomycin may be used topically or intraocularly to treat sight-threatening infections of the eye, including infectious keratitis and endophthalmitis caused by MRSA or multidrug-resistant streptococci. It has been used within the irrigating fluid of balanced salt solution during intraocular surgery. The contribution of this prophylactic use of vancomycin to the emergence of resistant bacteria, as well as to an increased risk of postoperative CME, is controversial. Vancomycin is a preferred substitute for a cephalosporin used in combination with an aminoglycoside in the empirical treatment of endophthalmitis. See BCSC Section 8, *External Disease and Cornea,* and Section 9, *Uveitis and Ocular Inflammation,* for further discussion.

Topical vancomycin may be compounded and given in a concentration of 50 mg/mL in the treatment of infectious keratitis. Intravitreal vancomycin combined with amikacin has been used for initial empirical therapy for exogenous bacterial endophthalmitis. Ceftazidime has largely replaced amikacin in clinical practice, primarily because of concerns about potential aminoglycoside retinal toxicity. A vancomycin dose of 1 mg/0.1 mL establishes intraocular levels that are significantly higher than the minimum inhibitory concentration for most gram-positive organisms. The intravenous dosage of vancomycin in adults with normal renal function is 500 mg every 6 hours or 1 g every 12 hours. Dosing must be adjusted in patients with renal impairment.

Unlike systemic treatment with vancomycin, topical and intraocular vancomycin has not been associated with ototoxicity or nephrotoxicity. Hourly use of 50 mg of vancomycin per milliliter delivers a dose of 36 mg per day, which is well below the recommended systemic dose. In addition to the ototoxicity and nephrotoxicity associated with systemic therapy, possible complications include chills, rash, fever, and anaphylaxis. Furthermore, rapid intravenous infusion may cause "red man syndrome" due to flushing.

Erythromycin is a macrolide (many-membered lactone ring attached to deoxy sugars) antibiotic that binds to subunit 50S of bacterial ribosomes and interferes with protein synthesis. The drug is bacteriostatic against gram-positive cocci such as *Streptococcus pyogenes* and *S pneumoniae,* gram-positive bacilli such as *C diphtheriae* and *Listeria monocytogenes,* and a few gram-negative organisms such as *N gonorrhoeae* and *C trachomatis.* In sufficient dosing, it may be bactericidal against susceptible organisms.

Drug resistance to erythromycin is rising and is as high as 40% among *Streptococcus* isolates. There are 4 mechanisms of resistance:

1. esterases from Enterobacteriaceae
2. mutations that alter the ribosomal subunit 50S
3. enzyme modification of the ribosomal binding site
4. active pumping to extrude the drug

Macrolide antibiotics such as erythromycin are the treatment of choice for *Legionella pneumophila,* the agent of legionnaires' disease, as well as for *M pneumoniae.* Erythromycin is administered orally as enteric-coated tablets or in esterified forms to avoid inactivation by stomach acid. It can also be administered parenterally or topically as an ophthalmic ointment. The drug penetrates the blood–ocular and blood–brain barriers poorly.

Clarithromycin and azithromycin are semisynthetic macrolides with a spectrum of activity similar to that of erythromycin. Clarithromycin is more effective against staphylococci, streptococci, and *Mycobacterium leprae,* whereas azithromycin is more active against *H influenzae, N gonorrhoeae,* and *Chlamydia* species. Both drugs have enhanced activity against *Mycobacterium avium-intracellulare,* atypical mycobacteria, and *Toxoplasma gondii.* Azithromycin, 1%, has been approved by the FDA for bacterial conjunctivitis caused by coryneform group G, *H influenzae, S aureus,* the *Streptococcus mitis* group, and *S pneumoniae.*

Polymyxin B sulfate is a mixture of basic peptides that function as cationic detergents to dissolve phospholipids of bacterial cell membranes, thereby disrupting cells. It is used topically or by local injection to treat corneal ulcers. Gram-negative bacteria including *Enterobacter* and *Klebsiella* species and *P aeruginosa* are susceptible; bacterial sensitivity is related to the phospholipid content of the cell membrane, and resistance may occur if a cell wall prevents access to the pathogen cell membrane. Systemic use of this medication has been abandoned because of severe nephrotoxicity. Topical hypersensitivity is uncommon. One commercially available topical antibiotic contains polymyxin B sulfate and trimethoprim sulfate. Sulfonamide allergy does not preclude the use of products with trimethoprim or with a sulfate group.

Bacitracin is a mixture of polypeptides that inhibits bacterial cell-wall synthesis. It is active against *Neisseria* and *Actinomyces* species, *H influenzae,* most gram-positive bacilli and cocci, and most but not all strains of MRSA. It is available as an ophthalmic ointment either alone or in various combinations with polymyxin, neomycin, and hydrocortisone. The primary adverse effect is local hypersensitivity, although it is not common.

Topical povidone-iodine solution, 5%, exhibits broad-spectrum antimicrobial activity when used to prepare the surgical field and to rinse the ocular surface; it is approved by the FDA for this purpose. It is the only drug that has had a significant effect on the development of postsurgical endophthalmitis. Povidone-iodine scrub may be used periocularly, but it is contraindicated in the eye because it is damaging to the corneal epithelium.

> Povidone-iodine is the only compound that has been demonstrated to reduce the risk of postoperative endophthalmitis following cataract surgery.

Topical povidone-iodine solution has been incorrectly considered contraindicated in patients with hypersensitivity to iodine or to intravenous contrast dye. Reported allergies to seafood or contrast media are not a contraindication to the use of topical povidone-iodine solution. Iodine is not thought to be the eliciting factor in iodinated contrast media reactions or in those related to shellfish, for which tropomyosin has been implicated. Iodine, a ubiquitous element (eg, iodized salt), is a simple molecule that is widely believed to lack the complexity required for antigenicity. Instead, patients probably develop hypersensitivity reactions to specific proteins of the food itself (eg, seafood) or to the contrast medium, rather than to the iodine in the compound. Cases of hypersensitivity to povidone, another common substance, have been reported. It is important to carefully discuss the ramifications of not using povidone-iodine with patients before intraocular procedures. One can also ask, "Have you ever had a reaction to Betadine?" or refer patients for allergy testing. This is especially important in patients who may need repeated procedures, such as intravitreal injections.

Ciulla TA, Starr MB, Masket S. Bacterial endophthalmitis prophylaxis for cataract surgery: an evidence-based update. *Ophthalmology.* 2002;109(1):13–24.

Isenberg SJ, Apt L, Yoshimori R, Khwarg S. Chemical preparation of the eye in ophthalmic surgery, IV: comparison of povidone-iodine on the conjunctiva with a prophylactic antibiotic. *Arch Ophthalmol.* 1985;103(9):1340–1342.

Kollef MH. Limitations of vancomycin in the management of resistant staphylococcal infections. *Clin Infect Dis.* 2007;45(suppl 3):S191–S195.

Modjtahedi BS, van Zyl T, Pandya HK, et al. Endophthalmitis after intravitreal injections in patients with self-reported iodine allergy. *Am J Ophthalmol.* 2016;170:68–74.

Schabelman E, Witting M. The relationship of radiocontrast, iodine, and seafood allergies: a medical myth exposed. *J Emerg Med.* 2010;39(5):701–707.

Scoper SV. Review of third- and fourth-generation fluoroquinolones in ophthalmology: in-vitro and in-vivo efficacy. *Adv Ther.* 2008;25(10):979–994.

Werner G, Klare I, Fleige C, Witte W. Increasing rates of vancomycin resistance among *Enterococcus faecium* isolated from German hospitals between 2004 and 2006 are due to wide clonal dissemination of vancomycin-resistant enterococci and horizontal spread of VanA clusters. *Int J Med Microbiol.* 2008;298(5–6):515–527.

Wykoff CC, Flynn HW, Han DP. Allergy to povidone-iodine and cephalosporins: the clinical dilemma in ophthalmic use. *Am J Ophthalmol.* 2011;151(1):4–6.

Antifungal Drugs

Table 16-23 summarizes common antifungal drugs encountered in ophthalmology practice.

Polyenes

The polyene antibiotics are named for a component sequence of 4–7 conjugated double bonds. That lipophilic region allows these antibiotics to bind to sterols in the cell membrane of susceptible fungi, an interaction that results in damage to the membrane and leakage of essential nutrients. Other antifungals (such as flucytosine and the imidazoles) and even other antibiotics (such as tetracycline and rifampin) can enter through the damaged membrane, yielding synergistic effects.

Natamycin and amphotericin B are 2 examples of polyene macrolide antibiotics. Natamycin is available as a 5% suspension for topical ophthalmic use (once per hour). Local hypersensitivity reactions of the conjunctiva and eyelid and/or corneal epithelial toxicity may occur. Amphotericin B may be reconstituted at 0.25%–0.5% in sterile water (with deoxycholate to improve solubility) for topical use (every 30 minutes). It may also be administered systemically for disseminated disease, although careful monitoring for renal and other toxicities is required. Both drugs penetrate the cornea poorly. They have been used topically against various filamentous fungi, including species of *Aspergillus, Cephalosporium, Curvularia, Fusarium,* and *Penicillium,* as well as the yeast *Candida albicans.* Systemic amphotericin B has been reported as useful in treating systemic *Aspergillus, Blastomyces, Candida, Coccidioides, Cryptococcus,* and *Histoplasma* infections. Amphotericin can also be administered intravitreally; however, it has been associated with retinal toxicity.

Imidazoles and triazoles

The imidazole- and triazole-derived antifungal drugs also increase fungal cell-membrane permeability and interrupt membrane-bound enzyme systems. These antifungals act against various species of *Aspergillus, Coccidioides, Cryptococcus,* and *Candida,* among others. The triazoles have less effect on human sterol synthesis, as well as a longer half-life, than the imidazoles, and they are being more actively developed. The imidazole miconazole is available in a 1% solution that may be injected subconjunctivally (5 mg/0.5 mL, once or twice daily) or applied topically. Miconazole penetrates the cornea poorly.

Ketoconazole is available in 200-mg tablets for oral therapy (once or twice daily). Ketoconazole normally penetrates the blood–brain barrier and, presumably, the blood–ocular barrier poorly, but therapeutic levels can be achieved in inflamed eyes. The triazole itraconazole, with an expanded antifungal spectrum and less systemic toxicity, has largely replaced ketoconazole. However, there is an extensive and growing list of potentially dangerous drug interactions with itraconazole that should be consulted before instituting systemic therapy. Fluconazole, another triazole, has good bioavailability but limited spectrum and may also increase the plasma concentrations of other medications. Oral

Table 16-23 Antifungal Drugs

Generic (Trade) Name	Route	Dosage	Indication (Additional Reports of Use)
Polyenes			
Amphotericin B (Fungizone, available generically)	Topical	0.1%–0.5% solution; dilute with water for injection or dextrose 5% in water	*Aspergillus* *Candida* *Cryptococcus* *(Blastomyces)* *(Coccidioides)* *(Colletotrichum)* *(Histoplasma)*
	Subconjunctival	0.8–1.0 mg	
	Intravitreal	5 µg	
	Intravenous	Because of possible adverse effects and toxicity, dose needs to be carefully adjusted	
Natamycin (Natacyn)	Topical	5% suspension	*Fusarium* *(Aspergillus)* *(Candida)* *(Cephalosporium)* *(Curvularia)* *(Penicillium)*
Imidazoles			
Ketoconazole (Nizoral, available generically)	Oral	200 mg daily, up to 400 mg for severe or incomplete response	*Blastomyces* *Candida* *Coccidioides* *Histoplasma*
Miconazole nitrate (available as powder for compounding)	Topical Subconjunctival Intravitreal	1% solution 5 mg 10 µg	*Aspergillus* *Candida* *Cryptococcus*
Triazoles			
Fluconazole (Diflucan)	Oral	200 mg daily	*Candida* *Cryptococcus* *(Acremonium)*
	Subconjunctival	10 mg/0.5 mL	
	Intravenous	Same as oral dose	
Itraconazole (Sporanox)	Oral Intravenous	200 mg daily	*Aspergillus* *Blastomyces* *Histoplasma* *(Candida)* *(Curvularia)* (nonsevere *Fusarium*)
Voriconazole (Vfend)	Topical	1% (made from intravenous solution)	*Aspergillus* *Blastomyces* *Candida* *Cryptococcus* *Fusarium* *Histoplasma* *Penicillium* *Scedosporium*
	Oral	200 mg orally twice daily	
	Intravenous	3–6 mg/kg intravenously every 12 h	
	Intravitreal	50–100 µg	

Table 16-23 *(continued)*

Generic (Trade) Name	Route	Dosage	Indication (Additional Reports of Use)
Fluorinated pyrimidine			
Flucytosine (Ancobon)	Oral	50–150 mg/kg daily divided every 6 h	*Candida* *Cryptococcus*
	Topical	1% solution	*(Aspergillus)*
Echinocandins			
Caspofungin	Intravenous	Loading dose of 50–70 mg, maintenance dose of 50 mg	*Candida* *Aspergillus*
Micafungin	Intravenous	100–150 mg	*Candida* *Aspergillus*
Anidulafungin	Intravenous	Loading dose of 100–200 mg, maintenance dose of 50–100 mg	*Candida* *Aspergillus*

voriconazole is rapidly replacing other antifungals because of its excellent bioavailability, intraocular penetration, and broad-spectrum coverage.

Echinocandins

This class of antifungals inhibits a component (glucan) of the fungal cell wall. Caspofungin and micafungin are the 2 most commonly used agents. Their primary activity is against *Candida* and *Aspergillus* species, and they are used prophylactically in stem cell recipients and in patients with candidemia, for whom an ophthalmologist is frequently consulted to rule out ocular involvement.

Patil A, Majumdar S. Echinocandins in antifungal pharmacotherapy. *J Pharm Pharmacol.* 2017;69(12):1635–1660.

Flucytosine

Flucytosine (5-fluorocytosine) is converted by some species of fungal cells to 5-FU by cytosine deaminase and then to 5-fluorodeoxyuridylate. This last compound inhibits thymidylate synthase, an important enzyme in DNA synthesis. Host cells lack cytosine deaminase activity and are less affected. Only fungi that have both a permease to facilitate flucytosine penetration and a cytosine deaminase are sensitive to flucytosine. Flucytosine is taken orally at 50–150 mg/kg daily, divided every 6 hours. Although the drug is well absorbed and penetrates the blood–ocular barrier well, most *Aspergillus* and half of *Candida* isolates are resistant to it. Flucytosine is used primarily as an adjunct to systemic amphotericin B therapy.

Antiviral Drugs

Table 16-24 summarizes information on common antiviral drugs.

Table 16-24 Common Antiviral Drugs

Generic Name	Trade Name	Topical Concentration/ Ophthalmic Solution	Systemic Dosage/Intravitreal Dosage
Trifluridine	Viroptic, available generically	1%	NA
Idoxuridine	Available as powder for compounding	0.1%	NA
Vidarabine monohydrate	Vira-A, available as powder for compounding	3% (ointment)	NA
Acyclovir sodium[a]	Zovirax, available generically	NA	Oral: herpes simplex virus (HSV) keratitis 200–400 mg 5 times daily for 7–10 d Oral: herpes zoster ophthalmicus 600–800 mg 5 times daily for 10 d; intravenous if patient is immunocompromised Intravenous for necrotizing herpetic retinopathy: 13 mg/kg per dose divided every 8 h for 7 days, followed by oral therapy Intravitreal: 10–40 μg/0.1 mL
	Zovirax ointment (not available in the United States)	3% (ointment)	NA
Zidovudine	Retrovir, available generically	NA	Dosage variable per source consulted; dosing per internal medicine consultation recommended
Cidofovir[a, b]	Vistide	NA	Intravenous induction: 5 mg/kg constant infusion over 1 h once weekly for 2 consecutive weeks Maintenance: 5 mg/kg constant infusion over 1 h administered every 2 wk
Famciclovir[a, b]	Famvir HZV	NA	500 mg 3 times daily for 7 d
Foscarnet sodium	Foscavir, available generically	NA	Intravenous induction: By controlled infusion only, either by central vein or by peripheral vein induction: 60 mg/kg (adjusted for renal function) given over 1 h every 8 h for 14–21 d Maintenance: 90–120 mg/kg given over 2 h once daily Intravitreal injection: 2.4 mg/0.1 mL or 1.2 mg in 0.05 mL

Table 16-24 *(continued)*

Generic Name	Trade Name	Topical Concentration/ Ophthalmic Solution	Systemic Dosage/Intravitreal Dosage
Ganciclovir	Vitrasert (discontinued)	NA	Intravitreal: 4.5 mg sterile intravitreal insert designed to release the drug over a 5- to 8-mo period
Ganciclovir sodium[a, b]	Cytovene IV	NA	Intravenous induction: 5 mg/kg every 12 h for 14–21 d Intravenous maintenance: 5 mg/kg daily (7 d per wk) or 6 mg/kg once daily (5 d per wk) Intravitreal: Induction: 2 mg/0.1 mL, 0.1-mL injection 2 times per week for 3 weeks; maintenance: 0.1 mL once per week
	Zirgan	0.15% gel	NA
Valacyclovir HCl[a, c]	Valtrex HZV	NA	Oral: 1 g 3 times daily for 7–14 d
Valganciclovir	Valcyte	NA	Oral: Induction: 900 mg every 12 h for 21 d Maintenance: 900 mg once a day

NA = not applicable.

[a] Dose adjustment is needed for elderly patients and those with renal disease or with concomitant nephrotoxic medications.

[b] Because of potential adverse and toxic effects with systemic dosage, the possible dosage adjustments and warnings should be followed properly.

[c] At high doses, valacyclovir has been associated with thrombotic thrombocytopenic purpura/hemolytic uremic syndrome in immunocompromised patients.

Topical antiviral drugs

Idoxuridine, ganciclovir, trifluridine, and vidarabine compete with natural nucleotides for incorporation into viral and mammalian DNA and have been used to treat herpes simplex virus (HSV) keratitis. Idoxuridine (5-iodo-2′-deoxyuridine) and trifluridine are structural analogues of thymidine and work in a similar manner; vidarabine is an analogue of adenine. Trifluridine (1% drops, every 2–4 hours) is more soluble than the other drugs and can be used in drop form, providing adequate penetration of diseased corneas to treat herpetic epithelial keratitis. Trifluridine is currently marketed in the United States, but vidarabine ophthalmic ointment (3%) is not. Idoxuridine and vidarabine powder are available for compounding. Vidarabine can be used when a drug with a different mechanism of action is required. Cross-resistance does not seem to occur among these medications.

Acyclovir is activated by HSV thymidine kinase to inhibit viral DNA polymerase. The 3% ophthalmic ointment is not commercially available in the United States, and the

5% dermatologic ointment is not approved for ophthalmic use. Ganciclovir is activated by triphosphorylation to inhibit viral DNA polymerase. It is available as 0.15% ophthalmic gel approved for treatment of HSV keratitis. It has been moderately effective in treating cytomegalovirus (CMV) corneal endotheliitis and anterior uveitis.

Systemic antiviral drugs

Acyclovir is a synthetic guanosine analogue. Because the viral thymidine kinase in HSV types 1 and 2 has much more affinity to acyclovir than does host thymidine kinase, high concentrations of acyclovir monophosphate accumulate in infected cells. Acyclovir monophosphate is then further phosphorylated to the active compound acyclovir triphosphate, which cannot cross cell membranes and accumulates further.

Acyclovir-resistant thymidine kinase HSVs have evolved. They occur primarily in patients receiving multiple courses of therapy or in patients with human immunodeficiency virus (HIV) infection. Thymidine kinase mutants are susceptible to vidarabine and foscarnet. Changes in viral DNA polymerase structures can also mediate resistance to acyclovir.

Oral acyclovir is only 15%–30% bioavailable, and food does not affect absorption. For unknown reasons, bioavailability is lower in patients with transplants. The drug is well distributed; cerebrospinal fluid (CSF) and brain concentrations equal approximately 50% of serum values. Concentrations of acyclovir in zoster vesicle fluid are equivalent to those in plasma. Aqueous humor concentrations are 35% those of plasma, and salivary concentrations are 15%. Vaginal concentrations are equivalent to those of plasma, and breast milk concentrations exceed them.

For adults and neonates with normal renal function, the plasma half-lives of acyclovir are 3.3 and 3.8 hours, respectively. The half-life increases to 20 hours in patients who are anuric. Acyclovir may interfere with the renal excretion of drugs that are eliminated through the renal tubules (eg, methotrexate); probenecid significantly decreases the renal excretion of acyclovir. This drug is effectively removed by hemodialysis (60% decrease in plasma concentrations following a 6-hour dialysis period) but only minimally removed by peritoneal dialysis.

Acyclovir is used off-label for ocular HSV and herpes zoster virus (HZV) but has proven effective in preventing the recurrence of HSV epithelial and stromal keratitis with twice-daily oral doses of 400 mg. Although this prophylactic dosage was originally studied over a 1-year treatment period, clinicians are using this dosage indefinitely to decrease the likelihood of disease recurrence. Similar dosing of acyclovir has proven beneficial in reducing the likelihood of recurrent herpetic eye disease after corneal transplantation. However, oral acyclovir was not beneficial when used with topical steroids and trifluridine in the treatment of active HSV stromal keratitis. The addition of oral acyclovir to a regimen of topical antiviral drugs may be considered for patients with HSV iridocyclitis. Although the benefit of this drug did not reach statistical significance in one study, participant enrollment had been halted because of inadequate numbers of patients.

Acyclovir is well tolerated in oral form, but parenteral acyclovir can cause renal toxicity due to crystalline nephropathy. Neurotoxicity may also occur with intravenous use. A commonly used intravenous dosage for acyclovir is 1500 mg/m^2 per day.

Valacyclovir is currently approved for management of HZV infections in immunocompetent persons but not for HSV. It is an amino-acid ester prodrug of acyclovir; its bioavailability is much higher than that of acyclovir (54% vs 20%, respectively). Valacyclovir has been associated with nephrotoxicity and thrombocytopenia in immunocompromised patients.

Famciclovir is the oral prodrug of penciclovir and is currently approved for the management of uncomplicated acute HSV. Penciclovir, like acyclovir, requires phosphorylation by viral thymidine kinase to become active. It has demonstrated efficacy in relieving acute zoster signs and symptoms and reducing the duration of postherpetic neuralgia when administered during acute HZV.

Ganciclovir (9-2-hydroxypropoxymethylguanine) is a synthetic guanosine analogue active against many herpesviruses. It is approved for CMV retinitis and for CMV prophylaxis in patients with advanced HIV infection and in patients undergoing a transplant. Like acyclovir, it must be phosphorylated to become active. Infection-induced kinases, viral thymidine kinase, or deoxyguanosine kinase of various herpesviruses can catalyze this reaction. After monophosphorylation, cellular enzymes convert ganciclovir to the triphosphorylated form, and the triphosphate inhibits viral DNA polymerase rather than cellular DNA polymerase. Because of ganciclovir's toxicity and the availability of acyclovir for treatment of many herpesvirus infections, the use of ganciclovir is currently restricted to treatment of CMV.

Systemic ganciclovir is used primarily intravenously because less than 5% of an oral dose is absorbed. CSF concentrations are approximately 50% of plasma concentrations; peak plasma concentrations reach 4–6 μg/mL. The plasma half-life is 3–4 hours in people with normal renal function, increasing to more than 24 hours in patients with severe renal insufficiency. More than 90% of systemic ganciclovir is eliminated unchanged in urine, and dose modifications are necessary for individuals with compromised renal function. Approximately 50% of ganciclovir is removed by hemodialysis. Bone marrow suppression is the primary adverse effect of systemic therapy. Periodic complete blood counts and platelet counts are required during the course of treatment. Ganciclovir can also be administered intravitreally.

Valganciclovir is a prodrug for ganciclovir that offers significantly higher bioavailability (60%) than ganciclovir (9%) when taken orally. After oral administration, it is rapidly converted to ganciclovir by intestinal and hepatic esterases. It can be used during the induction and/or maintenance phase of treatment in patients with CMV retinitis, affording them an outpatient alternative to ganciclovir.

CLINICAL PEARL

Oral administration of the prodrugs valacyclovir and valganciclovir has greatly improved the bioavailability of acyclovir and ganciclovir, respectively. In many cases, this has facilitated outpatient management of ophthalmic conditions that previously required hospital admission for induction therapy and placement of peripherally inserted central catheters (PICCs) (ie, acute retinal necrosis (ARN) and CMV retinitis).

Foscarnet (phosphonoformic acid) inhibits DNA polymerases, RNA polymerases, and reverse transcriptases. In vitro, it is active against herpesviruses, the influenza virus, and HIV. Foscarnet is approved for the treatment of HIV-infected patients with CMV retinitis and for acyclovir-resistant mucocutaneous HSV infections in immunocompromised patients. It also inhibits CMVs that are resistant to acyclovir and ganciclovir. Foscarnet acts by blocking the pyrophosphate receptor site of CMV DNA polymerase. Viral resistance is attributable to structural alterations in this enzyme.

Foscarnet bioavailability is approximately 20%. Because it can bind with calcium and other divalent cations, foscarnet becomes deposited in bone and may be detectable for many months; 80%–90% of the administered dose appears unchanged in the urine. It is administered intravenously in doses adjusted for renal function and with hydration to establish sufficient diuresis. Treatment may be limited by nephrotoxicity in up to 50% of patients; other adverse effects include hypocalcemia and neurotoxicity. To limit systemic adverse effects, foscarnet can also be administered intravitreally.

Cidofovir is the third medication approved by the FDA for the treatment of CMV retinitis, and it is approved only for that use. Cidofovir is a cytidine nucleoside analogue that is active against herpesviruses, poxviruses, polyomaviruses, papillomaviruses, and adenoviruses. The drug is the second-line therapy for complications after smallpox vaccination (vaccinia virus) and has been used in selected studies for varicella-zoster retinitis, as well as adenoviral keratoconjunctivitis.

The mechanism of action of cidofovir is inhibition of DNA synthesis, and resistance is achieved through mutations in DNA polymerase. The prolonged intracellular half-life of an active metabolite allows once-weekly dosing during induction, with dosing every 2 weeks thereafter. Cidofovir does not have direct cross-resistance with acyclovir, ganciclovir, or foscarnet, although some virus isolates may have multiple resistances and may even develop triple resistance. In a small series of patients, cidofovir inhibited CMV replication when administered intravitreally. Long-lasting suppression of CMV retinitis was observed; the average time to progression was 55 days.

The primary adverse effect of cidofovir is renal toxicity, which can be decreased by intravenous prehydration and by both pretreatment and posttreatment with high-dose probenecid. Ocular adverse effects include uveitis and irreversible hypotony.

Zidovudine is a thymidine nucleoside analogue with activity against HIV. Zidovudine becomes phosphorylated to monophosphate, diphosphate, and triphosphate forms by cellular kinases in infected and uninfected cells. It has 2 primary methods of action:

1. The triphosphate acts as a competitive inhibitor of viral reverse transcriptase.
2. The azido group prevents further chain elongation and acts as a DNA chain terminator.

Zidovudine inhibits HIV reverse transcriptase at much lower concentrations than needed to inhibit cellular DNA polymerases.

Since the introduction of zidovudine in the 1980s, numerous antiretroviral drugs have been approved for the treatment of HIV infection. They are divided into 6 classes: nucleoside reverse transcriptase inhibitors, non-nucleoside reverse transcriptase inhibitors, protease inhibitors, fusion inhibitors, entry inhibitors, and integrase strand transfer inhibitors. The current standard antiretroviral therapy (ART) consists of a combination of antiretroviral drugs.

Herpetic Eye Disease Study Group. Acyclovir for the prevention of recurrent herpes simplex virus eye disease. *N Engl J Med.* 1998;339(5):300–306.

Herpetic Eye Disease Study Group. Oral acyclovir for herpes simplex virus eye disease: effect on prevention of epithelial keratitis and stromal keratitis. *Arch Ophthalmol.* 2000;118(8):1030–1036.

Martin DF, Sierra-Madero J, Walmsley S, et al. A controlled trial of valganciclovir as induction therapy for cytomegalovirus retinitis. *N Engl J Med.* 2002;346(15):1119–1126.

Schoenberger SD, Kim SJ, Thorne JE, et al. Diagnosis and treatment of acute retinal necrosis: a report by the American Academy of Ophthalmology. *Ophthalmology.* 2017; 124(3):382–392.

Medications for *Acanthamoeba* Infections

Acanthamoeba is a genus of ubiquitous, free-living amoebae that inhabit soil, water, and air. Their appearance as corneal pathogens has increased because of several factors, including increased use of contact lenses. The species responsible for corneal infections, which include *Acanthamoeba polyphaga, Acanthamoeba castellanii, Acanthamoeba hatchetti,* and *Acanthamoeba culbertsoni,* exist as both trophozoites and double-walled cysts. Because of variations among species of *Acanthamoeba,* no single drug is effective in treating all cases of *Acanthamoeba* keratitis. Polyhexamethylene biguanide (0.02% solution) is a non–FDA-approved disinfectant and the first-line agent with the lowest minimal amebicidal concentration. Effective medications include chlorhexidine; neomycin; polymyxin B–neomycin–gramicidin mixtures; natamycin, 5%, topical suspension; imidazoles such as miconazole (powder compounded to 1% topical solution); systemic imidazoles and triazoles; propamidine isethionate, 0.1%, drops (not approved in the United States); and topical dibromopropamidine, 0.15%, ointment (not approved in the United States). Combination therapy is commonly required. See BCSC Section 8, *External Disease and Cornea,* for further discussion of treatment.

Dart JK, Saw VP, Kilvington S. Acanthamoeba keratitis: diagnosis and treatment update 2009. *Am J Ophthalmol.* 2009;148(4):487–499.

Seal DV. *Acanthamoeba* keratitis update: incidence, molecular epidemiology and new drugs for treatment. *Eye* (London). 2003;17(8):893–905.

Local Anesthetics

Overview

Local anesthetics are used extensively in ophthalmology. Topical preparations yield corneal and conjunctival anesthesia for comfortable performance of examination techniques, such as tonometry, gonioscopy, removal of superficial foreign bodies, corneal scraping for bacteriologic studies, and paracentesis, as well as for use of contact lenses associated with fundus examination and laser procedures. Topical and intracameral anesthesia has gained increasing acceptance in cataract, pterygium, and glaucoma surgery. Local retrobulbar, peribulbar, and eyelid blocks yield excellent anesthesia and akinesia for intraocular and orbital surgery (Tables 16-25, 16-26).

The local anesthetic drugs used in ophthalmology are tertiary amines linked by either ester or amide bonds to an aromatic residue. Because the protonated form is far more soluble and these compounds undergo hydrolysis more slowly in acidic solutions, local anesthetic drugs are supplied in the form of their hydrochloride salts. When exposed to tissue fluids at pH 7.4, approximately 5%–20% of the anesthetic agent's molecules will be in the unprotonated form, as determined by the pK_a value (8.0–9.0) of the individual drug. The more lipid-soluble unprotonated form penetrates the lipid-rich myelin sheath and cell membrane of axons. Once inside, most of the molecules are again protonated. The protonated form gains access to and blocks the sodium channels on the inner wall of the cell membrane and increases the threshold for electrical excitability. As increasing numbers of sodium channels are blocked, nerve conduction is impeded and finally blocked.

After administration of a local anesthetic, small or unmyelinated nerve fibers are blocked the most quickly because their higher discharge rates open sodium channel gates more frequently and because conduction can be prevented by the disruption of a shorter axon. In unmyelinated fibers, the action potential spreads continuously along the axon. In myelinated fibers, the action potential spreads by saltation. Thus, only a short length of an unmyelinated fiber needs to be functionally interrupted, whereas one or more nodes must be blocked in a myelinated fiber. In larger myelinated fibers, the nodes are farther apart.

Table 16-25 Regional Anesthetics

Generic Name (Trade Name)	Concentration (Maximum Dose)	Onset of Action	Duration of Action	Major Advantages/ Disadvantages
Bupivacaine[a] (Marcaine, Sensorcaine)	0.25%–0.75%	5–11 min	480–720 min (with epinephrine) 480 min (without epinephrine)	Long duration of action/increased toxicity to the extraocular muscles
Lidocaine[a] (Anestacaine, Xylocaine)	0.5%–2% (500 mg)	4–6 min	40–60 min; 120 min (with epinephrine)	Spreads readily without hyaluronidase
Mepivacaine[a] (Carbocaine)	1%–3% (500 mg)	3–5 min	120 min	Duration of action greater without epinephrine
Procaine[b] (Novocain)	1%–2% (500 mg)	7–8 min	30–45 min; 60 min (with epinephrine)	Short duration; poor absorption from mucous membranes

[a] Amide-type compound.
[b] Ester-type compound.

Table 16-26 Topical Anesthetic Drugs

Generic Name	Trade Name	Strength
Cocaine		1%–4%
Fluorescein sodium/benoxinate (oxybuprocaine)	Fluress	0.25%/0.4%
	Flurox	0.25%
	Available generically	0.25%
Fluorescein sodium/proparacaine	Fluoracaine	0.25%/0.1%
	Flucaine	0.25%/0.1%
Lidocaine	Xylocaine	4%
	Akten	2%
Proparacaine	Alcaine	0.5%
	Parcaine	0.5%
	Ophthetic	0.5%
	Available generically	0.5%
Tetracaine	Altacaine	0.5%
	TetraVisc	0.5%
	Available generically	0.5%

Clinically, local anesthetics first block the poorly myelinated and narrow parasympathetic fibers (as evidenced by pupil dilation) and sympathetic fibers (vasodilation), followed by the sensory fibers (pain and temperature), and finally the larger and more myelinated motor fibers (akinesia). The optic nerve, enclosed in a meningeal lining, is often not blocked by retrobulbar injections.

For retrobulbar blocks, amide local anesthetics are preferred to ester drugs because the amides have a longer duration of action and less systemic toxicity. Amide local anesthetics are not metabolized locally but are inactivated in the liver primarily by dealkylation; thus, their duration of action is partly determined by diffusion from the site of injection.

Ester anesthetics are susceptible to hydrolysis by serum cholinesterases in ocular vessels as well as by metabolism in the liver. When serum cholinesterase levels are low because of treatment with echothiophate eyedrops or a hereditary serum cholinesterase deficiency, toxicity may occur at lower doses of ester anesthetics.

The toxic manifestations of local anesthetics are generally related to the dose. However, patients with severe hepatic insufficiency may have symptoms of toxicity even at lower doses of either amide or ester local anesthetics. These manifestations include restlessness and tremor that may proceed to convulsions and respiratory and myocardial depression. CNS stimulation can be counteracted by intravenous diazepam; respiratory depression calls for ventilatory support.

Because local anesthetics block sympathetic vascular tone and dilate vessels, a 1:200,000 concentration of epinephrine is frequently added to shorter-acting drugs to retard vascular absorption. Such use of epinephrine raises circulating catecholamine levels and may cause systemic hypertension and cardiac arrhythmias.

Topically applied anesthetics disrupt intercellular tight junctions, increasing corneal epithelial permeability to subsequently administered drugs (ie, dilating drops). They also interfere with corneal epithelial metabolism and repair and thus cannot be used for long-term pain relief. Because topical anesthetics can become drugs of abuse that can eventually lead to chronic pain syndromes and vision loss, they should not be dispensed to patients.

Specific Drugs

Lidocaine is an amide local anesthetic used in strengths of 0.5%, 1%, and 2% (with or without epinephrine) for injection; 2% as a gel, and 4% as a solution for topical mucosal anesthesia. It yields a rapid (4–6-minute) retrobulbar or eyelid block that lasts about an hour (2 hours with epinephrine). The topical solution, applied to the conjunctiva with a cotton swab for 1–2 minutes, reduces the discomfort of subconjunctival injections. Topical lidocaine is preferable to cocaine or proparacaine for conjunctival biopsy because it has less effect on epithelial morphology. Lidocaine is also extremely useful for suppressing a cough during ocular surgery. For local injection in adults, the maximum safe dose of the 2% solution is 15 mL. A common adverse effect is drowsiness.

Mepivacaine is an amide drug used in strengths of 1%–3% (with or without a vasoconstrictor). It has a rapid onset and lasts approximately 2 hours; 2% is the most commonly used strength and has a maximum safe dose of 25 mL.

Bupivacaine is an amide anesthetic with a slower onset of action than lidocaine. It may yield relatively poor akinesia but has the advantage of a long duration of action, up to 8 hours without epinephrine. It is available in 0.25%–0.75% solutions (with or without epinephrine) and is frequently administered in a mixture with lidocaine or mepivacaine to achieve a rapid, complete, and long-lasting effect. The maximum safe dose of a 0.75% solution is 25 mL.

Hyaluronidase can be combined with local injection of anesthetics to increase the dispersion of the anesthetic drug(s) for intraocular, adnexal, or orbital surgery. Hyaluronidase catalyzes the hydrolysis of hyaluronic acid, a constituent of the extracellular matrix; it temporarily lowers the viscosity of the extracellular matrix and increases tissue permeability. Increased dispersion of the anesthetic drug may reduce the IOP rise in the limited orbital space, minimize distortion of the surgical site, decrease the risks of postoperative strabismus and myotoxicity, and increase akinesia of the globe and eyelid; lower volumes of anesthetic may be used.

Hyaluronidase products approved by the FDA include those derived from bovine and ovine sources, as well as a recombinant human product. Because of a lack of reliable animal sources and a shortage of supply from manufacturers, compounded formulations of hyaluronidase from animal-derived active pharmaceutical ingredients are only occasionally used. FDA regulations for compounding pharmacies are not as stringent as are regulations for pharmaceutical products, and concerns have been raised about the potency and purity of compounded hyaluronidase products from animal sources. There have been reports of hypersensitivity reactions to retrobulbar or peribulbar blocks associated with use of animal-derived hyaluronidase. For retrobulbar or peribulbar injection, 1 mL of hyaluronidase (150 USP U/mL; single-dose vial of recombinant human product) can be added to a syringe of the anesthetic to be administered.

Several other drugs are commonly used for topical anesthesia of the ocular surface. Because of their higher lipid solubilities, these medications have a more rapid onset than other topical anesthetics; thus, the initial discomfort caused by the drops is reduced. Proparacaine is an ester anesthetic available as a 0.5% solution. The least irritating of the topical anesthetics, it has a rapid onset of approximately 15 seconds and lasts approximately 20 minutes. Its structure is different enough from that of other local anesthetics that cross-sensitization apparently does not occur.

CLINICAL PEARL

Used without a preservative, proparacaine reportedly does not inhibit the growth of *Staphylococcus, Candida,* or *Pseudomonas,* so it may be preferred to other drugs for corneal anesthesia before obtaining a scraping for culture from a corneal ulcer.

Benoxinate (also known as *oxybuprocaine*) is an ester anesthetic available in a 0.4% solution with fluorescein for use in tonometry. Its onset and duration are similar to those of proparacaine. Benoxinate is also available alone as a topical anesthetic in Europe.

Tetracaine is an ester anesthetic available in 0.5% solution and approved for short-duration ocular surface procedures. Its onset of action and duration of action are longer than those of proparacaine, and it causes more extensive corneal epithelial toxicity.

Anesthetics in Intraocular Surgery

Topical

The first modern application of topical anesthetics was Koller's use of cocaine in 1884. Since then, synthetic drugs have become available; cocaine is no longer used because of the potential risk of adverse effects and drug abuse. Tetracaine, 0.5% or 1% (amethocaine), and proparacaine, 0.5%, are short-acting (20 minutes) drugs and are the least toxic of the regional and topical anesthetics to the corneal epithelium. Lidocaine, 4%, for injection can be used topically, as can lidocaine jelly, 2%. Bupivacaine, 0.5% and 0.75%, has a longer duration of action but an increased risk of associated corneal toxicity.

The aim of topical anesthetics is to block the nerves that supply the superficial cornea and conjunctiva—namely, the long and short ciliary nerves. Patients should be warned that they will experience some stinging upon application of the drops onto the surface of the cornea.

Topical anesthetics may be combined with subconjunctival anesthetics. Such combinations are well tolerated by patients and allow subconjunctival and scleral manipulations to be carried out. The surgeon can use both topical and sub-Tenon anesthesia initially. Alternatively, topical anesthesia can be achieved and, if not sufficient, it can be supplemented intraoperatively with a sub-Tenon infusion of anesthetic using a blunt cannula.

In a retrospective series involving a large sample size, application of lidocaine, 2%, gel before povidone-iodine preparation was one of the potential risk factors for acute-onset endophthalmitis after temporal clear cornea incision phacoemulsification, but it did not significantly alter rates of endophthalmitis after intravitreal injection.

Intraocular lidocaine

Intraocular lidocaine has been used to provide analgesia during surgery. The solution used is 0.3 mL of 1% isotonic nonpreserved lidocaine administered intracamerally. No adverse effects have been reported, except for possible transient retinal toxicity when lidocaine was injected posteriorly in the absence of a posterior capsule. Intracameral lidocaine obviates the need for intravenous and regional anesthetic supplementation in most patients. Adequate anesthesia is obtained in approximately 10 seconds. As with topical techniques, patient cooperation during surgery is desirable. Contrasting studies have shown no difference in the degree of cooperation regardless of whether intracameral lidocaine was used as a supplement to topical anesthetics. Because of unreliable patient cooperation, topical and intracameral anesthetics should be used cautiously, if at all, in patients with deafness, dementia, and severe photophobia.

Peribulbar and retrobulbar anesthesia

As stated previously, a mixture of lidocaine and bupivacaine in equal ratio is commonly used for peribulbar or retrobulbar anesthesia. This can be supplemented with hyaluronidase depending on technique and surgeon preference. Before injecting, it is important to pull back on the plunger to ensure that no blood or clear fluid is aspirated into the needle hub. The presence of blood indicates possible intravascular entry, where injection could lead to cardiac arrhythmia. Aspiration of clear fluid suggests the presence of CSF, meaning injection could lead to respiratory depression and seizures. The latter is more likely with the retrobulbar technique. For further discussion of peribulbar and retrobulbar anesthesia and other techniques, see BCSC Section 11, *Lens and Cataract.*

> Peribulbar and retrobulbar injections of anesthetics frequently consist of mixtures of lidocaine, bupivacaine, and hyaluronidase. The lidocaine provides rapid onset and the bupivacaine provides sustained anesthesia. The hyaluronidase promotes diffusion of the block and may reduce the volume of anesthetic delivered into the orbit.

Crandall AS. Anesthesia modalities for cataract surgery. *Curr Opin Ophthalmol.* 2001; 12(1):9–11.

Kansal S, Moster MR, Gomes MC, Schmidt CM Jr, Wilson RP. Patient comfort with combined anterior sub-Tenon's, topical, and intracameral anesthesia versus retrobulbar anesthesia in trabeculectomy, phacotrabeculectomy, and aqueous shunt surgery. *Ophthalmic Surg Lasers.* 2002;33(6):456–462.

Mindel JS. Pharmacology of local anesthetics. In: Tasman W, Jaeger EA, eds. *Duane's Foundations of Clinical Ophthalmology.* Vol 3. Philadelphia: Lippincott Williams & Wilkins; 2006: chapter 35.

Purified Neurotoxin Complex

Botulinum toxin type A is produced from cultures of the Hall strain of *Clostridium botulinum*. It blocks neuromuscular conduction by binding to receptor sites on motor nerve terminals, entering the nerve terminals and inhibiting the release of acetylcholine. Botulinum toxin type A injections provide effective relief of the excessive, abnormal contractions associated with benign essential blepharospasm and hemifacial spasm. Cosmetic use of botulinum toxin, specifically in the treatment of glabellar folds, is popular as well. Botulinum is FDA approved for the treatment of strabismus; it may function by inducing atrophic lengthening of the injected muscle and corresponding shortening of the muscle's antagonist (see also BCSC Section 6, *Pediatric Ophthalmology and Strabismus,* and Section 7, *Oculofacial Plastic and Orbital Surgery*).

Harrison AR. Chemodenervation for facial dystonias and wrinkles. *Curr Opin Ophthalmol.* 2003;14(5):241–245.

Issaho DC, Carvalho FRS, Tabuse MKU, Carrijo-Carvalho LC, de Freitas D. The use of botulinum toxin to treat infantile esotropia: a systematic review with meta-analysis. *Invest Ophthalmol Vis Sci.* 2017;58(12):5468–5476.

Khan JA, Steinsapir KD, McCracken M. Facial fillers, botulinum toxin, and facial rejuvenation. *Focal Points: Clinical Modules for Ophthalmologists.* San Francisco: American Academy of Ophthalmology; 2011: module 1.

Hyperosmolar Drugs

Hyperosmolar drugs are used to decrease corneal and epithelial edema. One such drug is sodium chloride, which is available without a prescription in a 2% or 5% solution or as an ointment. These products are used to treat corneal edema from Fuchs endothelial corneal dystrophy, other causes of endothelial dysfunction, postoperative prolonged edema, and recurrent erosion syndrome.

Irrigating Solutions

Sterile isotonic solutions are available for general ophthalmic use. Depending on the solution, nonprescription ocular irrigating solutions may contain sodium chloride, potassium chloride, calcium chloride, magnesium chloride, sodium acetate, sodium citrate, boric acid, sodium borate, and sodium phosphate. They are preserved with EDTA, benzalkonium chloride, and sorbic acid. Sterile, physiologically balanced, preservative-free salt solutions are isotonic to eye tissues and are used for intraocular irrigation during surgical procedures. Postoperatively, a glucose, glutathione, and bicarbonate solution causes the least change in the corneal endothelial morphology and augments endothelial pump function. It is not routinely used because of cost concerns, but it may be used in patients who have compromised corneas preoperatively.

McDermott M, Snyder R, Slack J, Holley G, Edelhauser H. Effects of intraocular irrigants on the preserved human corneal endothelium. *Cornea.* 1991;10(5):402–407.

Diagnostic Agents

Solutions commonly used in the examination and diagnosis of external ocular diseases include fluorescein, 2%; lissamine green, 1%; and rose bengal staining as impregnated paper strips. The first 2 stains outline defects of the conjunctival and corneal epithelium, whereas rose bengal staining indicates abnormal devitalized epithelial cells. A stinging sensation with instillation of these eyedrops is common.

Rose bengal has significant antiviral activity. Therefore, diagnostic use of rose bengal before viral culture may preclude a positive result, and its use to grade keratitis in the study of new antiviral drugs is discouraged.

For the study of retinal and choroidal circulation as well as abnormalities in the retinal pigment epithelium (RPE), sodium fluorescein solution in a concentration of 5%, 10%, or 25% is injected intravenously. Fundus fluorescein angiography is helpful in diagnosing various vascular diseases and neoplastic disorders. Adverse effects range from localized skin reactions to hypersensitivity and allergic reactions. The most common adverse effect is nausea, occurring in up to 10% of patients.

Indocyanine green (ICG), a tricarbocyanine dye, is approved for the study of choroidal vasculature in a variety of choroidal and retinal disorders. ICG angiography is particularly helpful in identifying and delineating poorly defined choroidal neovascular membranes in age-related macular degeneration (AMD). ICG angiography can also be used to evaluate patients with anterior scleritis. Typically, 25 mg of dye is injected as an intravenous solution. ICG is mildly toxic; adverse effects include localized skin reactions, sore throat, and hot flushes. Individual cases of severe adverse effects, such as anaphylactic shock, hypotension, tachycardia, dyspnea, and urticaria, have been reported.

ICG and trypan blue dye are useful for delineating the anterior capsule during phacoemulsification of mature cataracts. Although the FDA has approved trypan blue as an anterior capsule stain during surgery, administration of ICG for this purpose constitutes an off-label use.

ICG, trypan blue, brilliant blue G (BBG), and triamcinolone acetonide are also utilized to facilitate internal membrane peeling in macular-hole repair, although their use in this way is off-label. The preservative-free formulation of triamcinolone acetonide is FDA approved for intraoperative visualization of the vitreous. Despite considerable literature raising concerns about the toxicity of ICG dye in the retina and RPE, good surgical and visual results have been reported. The toxicity of ICG on cultured RPE cells may be related to the hypoosmolarity of the solvent. Short exposure of trypan blue has not had a toxic effect on cultured RPE cells. However, trypan blue does not appear to stain the internal limiting membrane as effectively as ICG does. Exposure of the retina to the dye and pooling at the macular hole should be minimized to reduce concerns about toxicity to the retina.

Haritoglou C, Gandorfer A, Gass CA, Schaumberger M, Ulbig MW, Kampik A. The effect of indocyanine-green on functional outcome of macular pucker surgery. *Am J Ophthalmol.* 2003;135(3):328–337.

Korb DR, Herman JP, Finnemore VM, Exford JM, Blackie CA. An evaluation of the efficacy of fluorescein, rose bengal, lissamine green, and a new dye mixture for ocular surface staining. *Eye Contact Lens.* 2008;34(1):61–64.

Saini JS, Jain AK, Sukhija J, Gupta P, Saroha V. Anterior and posterior capsulorhexis in pediatric cataract surgery with or without trypan blue dye: randomized prospective clinical study. *J Cataract Refract Surg.* 2003;29(9):1733–1737.

Shimada H, Nakashizuka H, Hattori T, Mori R, Mizutani Y, Yuzawa M. Double staining with brilliant blue G and double peeling for epiretinal membranes. *Ophthalmology.* 2009; 116(7):1370–1376.

Werner L, Pandey SK, Escobar-Gomez M, Hoddinott DS, Apple DJ. Dye-enhanced cataract surgery, part 2: learning critical steps of phacoemulsification. *J Cataract Refract Surg.* 2000;26(7):1060–1065.

Ophthalmic Viscosurgical Devices

Ophthalmic viscosurgical devices (OVDs) protect ocular tissues, such as the corneal endothelium and epithelium, from surgical trauma; help maintain the intraocular space; and facilitate tissue manipulation. Thus, they are indispensable tools in cataract and glaucoma surgery, penetrating keratoplasty, anterior segment reconstruction, and retinal surgery. Chemical and physical properties of OVDs include the capacity to resist flow and deformation. OVDs for ophthalmic use must also be inert, isosmotic, sterile, nonpyrogenic, nonantigenic, and optically clear. In addition, they must be sufficiently hydrophilic to allow easy dilution and irrigation from the eye. Naturally occurring and synthetic compounds available in various concentrations include sodium hyaluronate, chondroitin sulfate, hydroxypropyl methylcellulose, and polyacrylamide. Combined chondroitin sulfate/sodium hyaluronate materials are also available.

The 2 basic categories of OVDs are cohesive and dispersive. A cohesive OVD has a higher molecular weight and surface tension and tends to cohere to itself. A dispersive OVD has a lower molecular weight and surface tension and tends to coat intraocular structures. Available OVDs form a continuum on the basis of their cohesive and dispersive properties. The Healon, Healon GV, and Healon-5 products are mostly cohesive, and Ocucoat and Viscoat are mostly dispersive. There are also single agents with both cohesive and dispersive properties. (See also BCSC Section 11, *Lens and Cataract.*)

Riedel PJ. Ophthalmic viscosurgical devices. *Focal Points: Clinical Modules for Ophthalmologists.* San Francisco: American Academy of Ophthalmology; 2012: module 7.

Fibrinolytic Agents

Tissue plasminogen activator (tPA), urokinase, and streptokinase are all fibrinolytic agents. tPA is a naturally occurring serine protease with a molecular mass of 68 kD. Because tPA is normally present at a higher concentration in the aqueous humor of the human eye than in blood, it is less toxic to ocular tissues than other fibrinolytic agents and is specific for dissolution of fibrin clots. tPA has been used successfully to resolve fibrin clots after intraocular surgery, vitrectomy, keratoplasty, glaucoma filtering procedures, and sub-retinal hemorrhage due to choroidal neovascularization. These drugs are not approved by the FDA for ocular use and are therefore used off-label.

Chang W, Garg SJ, Maturi R, et al. Management of thick submacular hemorrhage with subretinal tissue plasminogen activator and pneumatic displacement for age-related macular degeneration. *Am J Ophthalmol.* 2014;157(6):1250–1257.
Dotan A, Kaiserman I, Kremer I, Ehrlich R, Bahar I. Intracameral recombinant tissue plasminogen activator (r-tPA) for refractory toxic anterior segment syndrome. *Br J Ophthalmol.* 2014;98(2):252–255.
Zalta AH, Sweeney CP, Zalta AK, Kaufman AH. Intracameral tissue plasminogen activator use in a large series of eyes with valved glaucoma drainage implants. *Arch Ophthalmol.* 2002;120(11):1487–1493.

Thrombin

Thrombin, a sterile protein substance, is approved for the control of hemorrhage from accessible capillaries and small venules, as observed with standard surface incisions. Its use in maintaining hemostasis during complicated intraocular surgery is off-label because such use requires injection. Intravitreal thrombin has been used to control intraocular hemorrhage during vitrectomy. The addition of thrombin (100 U/mL) to the vitrectomy infusate significantly shortens intraocular bleeding time, and thrombin produced by DNA recombinant techniques minimizes the degree of postoperative inflammation. Thrombin causes significant ultrastructural corneal endothelial changes when human corneas are exposed to 1000 U/mL.

Fibrin sealant is a biological tissue adhesive that includes a fibrinogen component and a thrombin component, both of which are prepared from pooled human plasma. When activated by thrombin, a solution of human fibrinogen imitates the final stages of the coagulation cascade. Fibrin sealant has been used widely in ophthalmic surgeries, including as a substitute for suturing in conjunctival or corneal wound closures, in fixing conjunctival autografts during pterygium surgery, for closing or preventing corneal perforation, during amniotic membrane transplantation, and in a variety of oculoplastic surgeries. It also has the advantage of reducing the total surgical time. However, the use of fibrin sealant in ophthalmic surgery is off-label.

The tissue sealant is applied as a thin layer to ensure that it covers the entire intended application area. Preparation of this product for application must adhere to the manufacturer's instructions. The incidence of allergic reactions is low, but anaphylactic reactions have been reported after its application.

Antifibrinolytic Agents

Antifibrinolytic drugs, such as ε-aminocaproic acid and tranexamic acid, inhibit the activation of plasminogen. These medications may be used systemically to treat patients with hemorrhage secondary to excessive fibrinolysis and to prevent recurrent hyphema, which most commonly occurs 2–6 days after the original hemorrhage. These agents are contraindicated in the presence of active intravascular clotting, such as diffuse intravascular coagulation, because they can increase the risk of thrombosis. They should not be used in pregnant patients, in patients with coagulopathies or who are receiving platelet inhibition therapy, or in patients with renal or hepatic disease. Patients with larger hyphemas and those with delayed presentation are at high risk of rebleeding, but patients with early presentation and those with smaller hyphemas are at low risk of rebleeding. ε-Aminocaproic acid is usually reserved for patients at higher risk of rebleeding.

ε-Aminocaproic acid is used in a dosage of 50–100 mg/kg every 4 hours, up to 30 g daily. Possible adverse reactions include nausea, vomiting, muscle cramps, conjunctival suffusion, nasal congestion, headache, rash, pruritus, dyspnea, tonic toxic confusional states, cardiac arrhythmias, and systemic hypotension. Gastrointestinal adverse effects are similar with doses of either 50 or 100 mg/kg. The drug should be continued for a full 5–6 days to achieve maximal clinical effectiveness. Topical ε-aminocaproic acid may be an attractive alternative to systemic delivery in the treatment of traumatic hyphema, but the efficacy of topical treatment has been questioned. Optimal topical concentration to maximize aqueous levels and minimize corneal epithelial toxicity is 30% ε-aminocaproic acid in 2% carboxypolymethylene.

Tranexamic acid is used off-label to reduce the incidence of rebleeding after traumatic hyphema. It is 10 times more potent in vitro than ε-aminocaproic acid. The usual dosage is 25 mg/kg of tranexamic acid 3 times daily for 3–5 days. Gastrointestinal adverse effects are rare.

Karkhaneh R, Naeeni M, Chams H, Abdollahi M, Mansouri MR. Topical aminocaproic acid to prevent rebleeding in cases of traumatic hyphema. *Eur J Ophthalmol.* 2003;13(1):57–61.

Vitamin Supplements and Antioxidants

Nonprescription vitamin supplements have enjoyed increased popularity because of their antioxidant properties and are used for intermediate to severe AMD. The Age-Related Eye Disease Studies 1 and 2 are discussed in depth in BCSC Section 12, *Retina and Vitreous.* In addition, omega-3 fatty acid supplements seem to have some benefit in treating meibomian gland dysfunction (see BCSC Section 8, *External Disease and Cornea*).

Interferon

A naturally occurring species-specific defense against viruses, interferon is synthesized intracellularly and increases resistance to viral infection. Synthetic analogues such as polyinosinic acid–polycytidylic acid have induced patients to form their own interferon.

Topically administered interferon (off-label) is ineffective in the treatment of epidemic keratoconjunctivitis caused by adenovirus. Likewise, interferon alone has little effect on herpes simplex keratitis. In combination, however, it seems to act as a topical adjuvant to traditional antiviral therapy in resistant herpes simplex keratitis. In one study of patients with herpes simplex keratitis, interferon used in conjunction with acyclovir yielded significantly faster healing time than treatment with acyclovir alone (5.8 vs 9.0 days, respectively). Interferon also speeds the healing of epithelial defects when used in combination with trifluridine. The dosage of interferon (30 million IU/mL) is 2 drops per day for the first 3 days of treatment.

Interferon also has been shown to inhibit vascular endothelial cell proliferation and differentiation. It is particularly effective in the treatment of juvenile pulmonary hemangiomatosis, which was fatal before the development of interferon. Interferon alfa-2b (off-label), administered subconjunctivally, intralesionally, and/or topically, is a treatment option for conjunctival intraepithelial neoplasia and invasive squamous cell carcinoma (see BCSC Section 8, *External Disease and Cornea*). Intralesional administration of interferon is reported to be especially effective in ocular Kaposi sarcoma.

Growth Factors

Growth factors are a diverse group of proteins that act at autocrine and paracrine levels to affect various cellular processes, including metabolic regulation, tissue differentiation, cell growth and proliferation, maintenance of viability, and changes in cell morphology. Growth factors are synthesized in a variety of cells and have a spectrum of target cells and tissues. The following growth factors have been found in retina, vitreous humor, aqueous humor, and corneal tissues:

- epidermal growth factor
- fibroblast growth factors
- transforming growth factor βs
- vascular endothelial growth factor (VEGF)
- insulin-like growth factors

These growth factors are capable of diverse, synergistic, and sometimes antagonistic biological activities.

Under normal physiologic conditions, the complex and delicate coordination of both the effects of and the interactions among growth factors maintains the homeostasis of intraocular tissues. The net effect of a growth factor depends on its bioavailability, which is determined by its concentration; its binding to carrier proteins; the level of its receptor in the target tissue; and the presence of complementary or antagonistic regulatory factors.

Pathologically, the breakdown of the blood–ocular barrier disrupts the balance among growth factors in the ocular media and tissues and may result in various abnormalities. Disruption in the balance among isoforms of transforming growth factor βs, basic fibroblast growth factor, VEGF, and insulin-like growth factors is thought to cause ocular neovascularization. Transforming growth factor βs and platelet-derived growth factor are also implicated in the pathogenesis of proliferative vitreoretinopathy and in the excessive proliferation of Tenon capsule fibroblasts, which can result in scarring of the glaucoma filtration bleb. Increased concentrations of insulin-like growth factors in plasmoid aqueous humor may be responsible for the abnormal hyperplastic response of the lens epithelium and corneal endothelium observed in inflammatory conditions and in ocular trauma.

Identifying growth factors and understanding their mechanisms of action in the eye can provide the ophthalmologist with new methods for manipulation of and intervention in ocular disorders. Epidermal and fibroblast growth factors can accelerate corneal wound repair after surgery, chemical burns, or ulcers and can increase the number of corneal endothelial cells. Fibroblast growth factor also was shown to delay the process of retinal dystrophy in Royal College of Surgeons rats.

VEGF, also known as *vasculotropin,* deserves special mention. It is a dimeric, heparin-binding, polypeptide mitogen with 4 isoforms that are generated from alternative splicing of mRNA. The *VEGF* gene is widely expressed in actively proliferating vascular tissue and is implicated in the pathogenesis of various retinovascular conditions.

Intravitreal injections of VEGF inhibitors are used to treat neovascular ("wet") AMD. Patients with choroidal neovascularization who were treated with anti-VEGF showed a slower loss of vision than occurred in controls, especially moderate (>3 lines of vision lost) to severe (>6 lines lost) vision loss, and in many cases, an improvement in vision (≥3 lines of visual acuity). Pegaptanib, the first approved drug for choroidal neovascularization, requires intravitreal injections every 6 weeks for up to 2 years. Newer drugs have largely supplanted pegaptanib.

Bevacizumab, a full-length antibody against VEGF approved for the intravenous treatment of advanced carcinomas, has been used extensively in ophthalmology for neovascular AMD, diabetic retinopathy, retinal vein occlusions, retinopathy of prematurity, and other chorioretinal vascular disorders. Ranibizumab is a monoclonal antibody fragment (Fab) derived from the same parent mouse antibody as bevacizumab and demonstrates similar efficacy. Pegaptanib and ranibizumab were developed for intraocular use, for which they are approved by the FDA, whereas the use of bevacizumab remains off-label. Although these drugs exhibit excellent safety profiles, ocular and systemic complications, particularly thromboembolic events, remain a concern for patients receiving therapy.

Aflibercept is a novel recombinant fusion protein engineered to bind all isoforms of VEGF A, VEGF B, and placental growth factor. It has been approved for the treatment of neovascular AMD, retinal vein occlusions, and diabetic macular edema. It may have a longer duration of action than other anti-VEGF therapies; a monthly loading dose is administered for 3 months, after which the drug can be given every 2 months depending on the condition (see BCSC Section 12, *Retina and Vitreous*).

PART VI

Imaging and Digital Ophthalmology

CHAPTER 17

Principles of Radiology for the Comprehensive Ophthalmologist

This chapter includes related activities, which can be accessed by scanning the QR codes provided in the text or going to www.aao.org/bcscactivity_section02.

Highlights

- Computed tomography (CT) is the modality of choice when patients are being evaluated for acute hemorrhage, calcification, and diseases of the bone and orbit and in patients for whom magnetic resonance imaging (MRI) is contraindicated.
- MRI is the modality of choice for assessing the central nervous system.
- Administration of contrast material improves the sensitivity and specificity of both CT and MRI in diagnosing a disease and should be requested unless there is a contraindication to contrast agents or it is not required.
- Vascular lesions can be evaluated by CT angiography and/or magnetic resonance angiography. The sensitivity of these studies varies by institution and should be compared with that of cerebral angiography.
- Ultrasonography uses high-frequency sound waves for evaluation of structures in the eye and orbit. The frequency of ultrasound is directly proportional to its resolution and inversely proportional to its depth of penetration.

Overview

Computed tomography (CT) and magnetic resonance imaging (MRI) are the most common imaging studies ordered by an ophthalmologist to evaluate the orbit, brain, and sometimes the eye. The ophthalmologist also relies on ultrasonography to provide biometrics, facilitate diagnosis, and evaluate the extent of ocular and orbital diseases. This chapter focuses on the basic principles of these imaging modalities, identification of normal anatomical structures, and recognition of the modality that is best suited to evaluate a certain clinical condition. For more specific indications for radiographic studies in particular diseases, consult BCSC volumes covering those entities. See also BCSC Section 5, *Neuro-Ophthalmology.*

Computed Tomography

Computed tomography technology is widely available and provides rapid acquisition of images. The scanners generate cross-sectional images of the body as an x-ray tube continuously rotates around the patient. Current-generation scanners can image body slices as thin as 0.5 mm, which may be reformatted in multiple anatomical planes. In addition, the acquired sections can be reconstructed in varying thicknesses from the source data, depending on the study and anatomical region examined. Studies are conducted with or without intravenous contrast material enhancement depending on the clinical situation. Although contrast-enhanced studies can increase the sensitivity and specificity of CT scans in disease diagnosis, contrast is not always required. Table 17-1 presents some of the advantages and disadvantages of CT, as well as contraindications. CT scans are very useful for identifying acute intracranial/orbital hemorrhage and osseous abnormalities, where the ease of CT and rapidity in obtaining images make it the method of choice for evaluating trauma involving the face and orbit.

Generally, for evaluation of orbital conditions, thin-section (ie, high-resolution) studies are critical to delineate the small anatomical structures of the orbit (Fig 17-1):

- lacrimal gland
- extraocular muscles
- globe
- paranasal sinuses around the orbit

Axial scans are always performed during orbital studies. However, coronal reformations, which provide optimal evaluation of the orbital roof and floor, should also be a standard part of these examinations. Sagittal reformations may be added to help further characterize and localize lesions.

Further, CT is an excellent modality for evaluating the vascular system. CT angiography (CTA) combines intravenous contrast enhancement with high-resolution imaging to produce high-quality, noninvasive scans of arterial and venous pathologies. Three-dimensional reformations that mimic catheter angiography are routinely produced and can detect cerebral aneurysms measuring 3–5 mm with high sensitivity and specificity. Additional series acquired at later times (CT venography) can be used to evaluate the cerebral venous system, especially in suspected cases of venous thrombosis or obstruction.

When additional diagnostic information is needed, CT scans can be combined with nuclear medicine imaging, as in single-photon emission computed tomography (SPECT) and positron emission tomography (PET-CT). These modalities use radiolabeled molecules to help evaluate metabolic activity in a wide range of diseases. SPECT is commonly used to evaluate myocardial perfusion and brain function, whereas PET-CT scans are typically used to diagnose and stage tumors, as well as to diagnose degenerative diseases of the brain. In ophthalmology, PET-CT has been used to assess ocular adnexal lymphoma and cortical blindness. In addition, PET-CT scans of the body are utilized in evaluation of patients with sarcoidosis and for metastatic screening of patients with uveal melanoma.

Table 17-1 Comparison of Magnetic Resonance Imaging and Computed Tomography

	Advantages	Disadvantages	Contraindications
MRI	Better able to distinguish white matter from gray matter Better visualization of posterior fossa pathology Better visualization of soft tissue Better resolution of optic nerve and orbital apex Ability to establish evolution of intraparenchymal hemorrhage No ionizing radiation	Contrast dye reactions and systemic nephrogenic fibrosis Greater cost Susceptibility artifacts from metal (eg, braces) or air–tissue interfaces Longer acquisition time	Cochlear implants Ferromagnetic implants/foreign bodies Metallic cardiac valves Non–MRI-compatible intracranial aneurysm clips Pacemakers Pregnancy (ie, gadolinium is Category C for pregnant patients) Renal insufficiency Other considerations: claustrophobia/patient too large for the bore
CT	Assessment of bony abnormalities Assessment of orbital and hyperacute intracranial hemorrhage Detection of calcification in lesions Evaluation of globe and orbital trauma (includes high-resolution bone algorithms)	Exposure to ionizing radiation (CT head radiation dose = 1.5 mGy[a]) Reaction to iodine-based contrast agents Lack of direct sagittal imaging Limited resolution in the posterior fossa Poor resolution of the orbital apex	Renal insufficiency (ie, if estimated GFR is <30 mL/min/1.73 m^2)
MRA/MRV	Less invasive than catheter angiography	Limited resolution (in aneurysms ≤3 mm) Possible overestimation of carotid stenosis or venous sinus stenosis	Same as for MRI
CTA/CTV	Less invasive than catheter angiography	Artifacts from superimposed bone and adjacent vessels, especially where aneurysms lie within or close to bone Limited resolution (in aneurysms ≤3 mm)	Same as for CT

CT = computed tomography; CTA = computed tomography angiography; CTV = computed tomography venography; GFR = glomerular filtration rate; MRA = magnetic resonance angiography; MRI = magnetic resonance imaging; MRV = magnetic resonance venography.

[a] *Milligray (mGy)* refers to the total dose of ionizing radiation delivered to a tissue and is not the same as millisievert (mSv), the SI unit that takes into account the type of imaging study and the biological effects of the radiation dose. The biological effect of the total mGy delivered varies depending on the tissue being examined. Some tissues (eg, gonads, eye) are more radiosensitive than others (eg, the skin), and the differing effects of a similar mGy dose on these organ systems are taken into account by reporting radiation doses in the unit mSv.

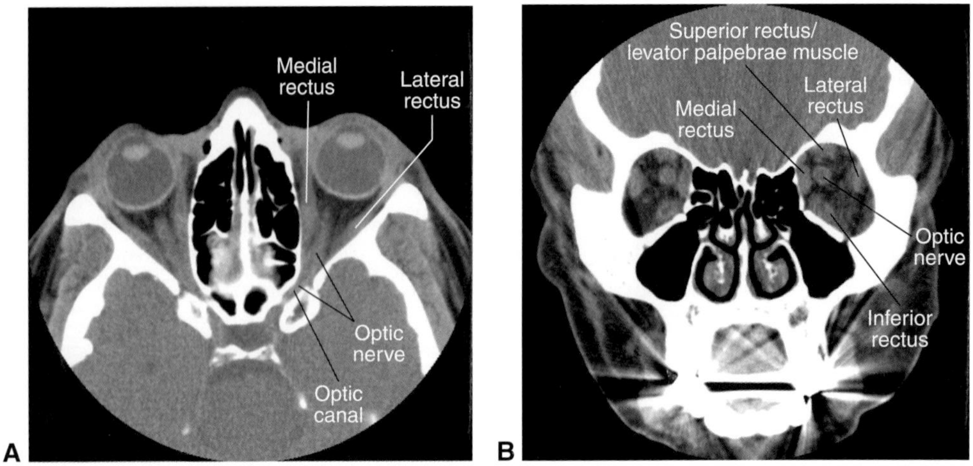

Figure 17-1 Computed tomography (CT) scans. **A,** Axial orbital view of a healthy subject. Note the orbital and intracanalicular portions of the optic nerve. **B,** Coronal orbital view of a healthy subject. *(Courtesy of Rod Foroozan, MD.)*

Betts AM, O'Brien WT, Davies BW, Youssef OH. A systematic approach to CT evaluation of orbital trauma. *Emerg Radiol.* 2014;21(5):511–531.

Yang ZL, Ni QQ, Schoepf UJ, et al. Small intracranial aneurysms: diagnostic accuracy of CT angiography. *Radiology.* 2017;285(3):941–952.

Disadvantages

Although CT is a transformational noninvasive technology for evaluating orbital and central nervous system diseases, ophthalmologists should be aware of the limitations of this imaging modality and safety concerns. CT scans employ ionizing radiation, a potential concern especially in pediatric cases and pregnant patients. In general, CT scans expose the patient to higher doses of radiation than conventional x-ray studies do. CT scans of the brain are typically oriented to avoid imaging of the globe, which is a more radiosensitive organ. In the International System of Units, millisievert (mSv) is the unit used to determine the amount of tissue damage expected from the absorbed dose of ionizing radiation. Millisievert is technically different from milligray (mGy), which refers to the total dose of ionizing radiation delivered to a tissue during a particular scan sequence. The US Food and Drug Administration has estimated that 10 mSv of radiation may cause an additional case of cancer in 1/2000 patients. However, the impact of a single (or even serial) CT scan(s) of the brain in relation to the risk of cancer development is typically outweighed by the clinical need for diagnostic information; nonetheless, ordering clinicians should be aware of this safety consideration when ordering a CT scan, particularly in children.

While CT scans are very useful in studying bony structures, visibility of the posterior fossa may be reduced because of streak artifact from the skull base. Further, in evaluation of the central nervous system, CT scans provide lower spatial resolution than does MRI, although the intravenous administration of iodinated contrast material improves the soft-tissue imaging capabilities of CT.

Iodinated contrast agents pose another potential safety concern for patients undergoing CT, mostly related to allergic reactions and potential nephrotoxicity in those with underlying renal insufficiency. Allergic reactions have ranged from 1% to 12%, depending on the type of contrast material used, with symptoms ranging from relatively mild (eg, pruritus, nausea, and vomiting) to severe (eg, anaphylaxis). The rate of severe allergic reactions has been reduced to less than 0.1% with the use of newer low osmolar contrast agents. Nephrotoxicity has been reported in 2%–7% of patients receiving contrast media, with higher rates in those with preexisting kidney disease and/or diabetes mellitus. The American College of Radiology (ACR) currently recommends limiting intravenous contrast agent administration in patients with an estimated glomerular filtration rate less than 30 mL/min/1.73 m^2, and considering alternative imaging methods (eg, MRI) or hydrating before the examination. Because recommendations for the use of contrast agents vary by institution, consultation with a diagnostic radiologist is advised before ordering contrast-enhanced CT examinations in at-risk patients.

American College of Radiology, ACR Committee on Drugs and Contrast Media. ACR Manual on Contrast Media. 2021. www.acr.org/-/media/ACR/Files/Clinical-Resources/Contrast_Media.pdf. Accessed November 14, 2021.

Meinel FG, De Cecco CN, Schoepf UJ, Katzberg R. Contrast-induced acute kidney injury: definition, epidemiology, and outcome. *Biomed Res Int.* 2014;2014:859328.

Magnetic Resonance Imaging

Because of its superior contrast resolution, MRI is the imaging modality of choice for evaluation of the central nervous system (see Table 17-1). In addition, the technology does not use ionizing radiation, which is a relative advantage over CT. Instead, MRI uses a strong magnetic field that causes hydrogen atoms found in water and fat to align themselves with the field. Once the atoms are aligned, protons within a selected imaging section/volume are exposed to a series of radiofrequency (RF) and/or magnetic gradient pulses and become excited. As the protons relax again to a steady state, they emit radio waves, which are detected by a receiver coil in the MRI system. The time it takes for the signal to reach the MRI machine following the applied RF (or gradient) pulse is known as the *echo time (TE),* which varies by type of tissue. The time between RF pulses is known as the *repetition time (TR).* The TE and TR can be adjusted to modify the contrast between images and thus enhance visualization of different tissues.

The energy given off by the rotating protons is expressed by 2 aspects: the longitudinal relaxation constant, or T1, and the transverse relaxation constant, or T2. T1-weighted images (T1WIs), which are generated with shorter TEs and TRs, are typically used for contrast-enhanced studies. In a T1WI, water appears dark (hypointense) and fat appears bright (hyperintense). Melanin shows an intrinsically elevated T1 signal, which can be helpful in providing a diagnosis in patients with melanoma. Sometimes, however, fat suppression is required in T1WIs to improve contrast enhancement and characterization of tissues, such as the optic nerve and other orbital structures. In comparison, T2-weighted images (T2WIs) use a longer TE to depict differences in water content, thus revealing inflammatory, ischemic, and neoplastic-related edematous changes. On T2WIs, vitreous, cerebrospinal, and other fluids are bright.

On both T1WIs and T2WIs, gray matter is hypointense compared with white matter (Table 17-2, Fig 17-2). In fluid-attenuated inversion recovery (FLAIR) images, the fluid signal is suppressed on T2WIs, facilitating visualization of signal abnormalities associated with changes in the periventricular white matter (eg, as in multiple sclerosis).

Gadolinium-based contrast medium is administered intravenously and used to enhance T1WIs, especially for assessment of inflammatory and neoplastic lesions. Gadolinium may also be administered during high spatial and temporal resolution MRI sequences of large and medium-sized vessels (ie, MR angiography [MRA]), when dynamic contrast enhancement can be assessed more practically than with CTA. The decision to use MRA versus CTA for evaluation of intracranial and orbital blood vessels is often complex and varies depending on the patient and clinical question being asked; consultation with a neuroradiologist may be required in complex cases.

Diffusion-weighted imaging (DWI) is another form of MRI that is relevant to the ophthalmologist, as this sequence is the most sensitive for the detection of acute ischemic changes (eg, cerebrovascular accident). DWI can detect changes within minutes compared with potentially hours with other MRI methods. A quantitative metric of DWI sequences, the apparent diffusion coefficient, can be used to further characterize edema as cytotoxic versus vasogenic (eg, posterior reversible encephalopathy syndrome) (Table 17-3).

Disadvantages

Adverse effects are occasionally associated with the gadolinium chelates used for contrast-enhanced imaging in MRI, though at a lower frequency than with iodinated contrast agents in CT. Common symptoms are sweating, pruritus, and rash. Although gadolinium agents do not adversely affect renal function at the doses administered for clinical imaging, certain gadolinium chelates may be restricted in patients with severe end-stage renal disease because of the risk of nephrogenic systemic fibrosis, a rare and potentially fatal multiorgan fibrosing disorder. In addition, gadolinium has been shown to collect in certain neurologic structures after repeated administration; however, no clinical features have been attributed to this deposition. Recommendations for the use of gadolinium-based contrast agents vary by institution; thus, the ophthalmologist is advised to consult with a diagnostic radiologist before ordering such studies in at-risk patients.

Because MRI uses strong magnetic fields to generate pictures, patients with metallic foreign bodies or implants should also be carefully screened before undergoing imaging. Ophthalmologists may be consulted to assess patients for foreign bodies on the ocular surface, within the eye, and/or in the orbit. The incidence of damage from undetected ocular foreign bodies during MRI is low, restricted to a few case reports; however, it is not zero. This is an important consideration when counseling patients before their scans. Patients are also screened at the imaging center before MRI.

The following list highlights general and ophthalmic concerns in patients scheduled to undergo MRI. The reader is also directed to the ACR safety guidelines (see reference list) for further details.

Table 17-2 Signal Characteristics of Normal Ocular Structures in Different Imaging Sequences

Ocular Structure	Signal Intensity on T1-Weighted Images[a]	Signal Intensity on T2-Weighted Images[a]	Enhancement on Postcontrast Images[a]	Additional Comments
Sclera, choroid, retina (seen as a single coat)	Hyperintense (bright/white)	Hypointense (dark/black)	None	The 3 coats cannot be distinguished separately on routine imaging
Aqueous	Hypointense (dark/black)	Hyperintense (bright/white)	None	
Lens	Hyperintense (bright/white)	Low (gray)	None	Typically has a biconvex appearance
Vitreous	Hypointense (dark/black)	Hyperintense (bright/white)	None	
Extraocular muscles	Intermediate (gray)	Intermediate (gray)	Enhances brightly	
Orbital fat	Hyperintense (bright/white)	Intermediate (gray)	None	Typically has a homogeneous appearance
Optic nerve	Isointense to cerebral white matter (gray)	Isointense to cerebral white matter (gray)	Does not typically enhance; it can be compared with the extraocular muscles	
Optic nerve sheath with cerebral spinal fluid around the optic nerve	Hypointense (dark/black)	Hyperintense (bright/white)	None	
Lacrimal gland	Isointense with gray matter (gray)	Isointense with gray matter (gray)	Enhances brightly	
Bone	Signal void (dark)	Signal void (dark)	None	Better studied with computed tomography
Cerebral spinal fluid	Hypointense (dark/black)	Hyperintense (bright/white)	None	

[a] Signal intensity (hypointense/hyperintense) is described in comparison with the reference tissue. Intracranially, the reference tissue is the gray matter of the brain; extracranially, it is the skeletal muscle.

Modified with permission from Simha A, Irodi A, David S. Magnetic resonance imaging for the ophthalmologist: a primer. *Indian J Ophthalmol.* 2012;60(4):308.

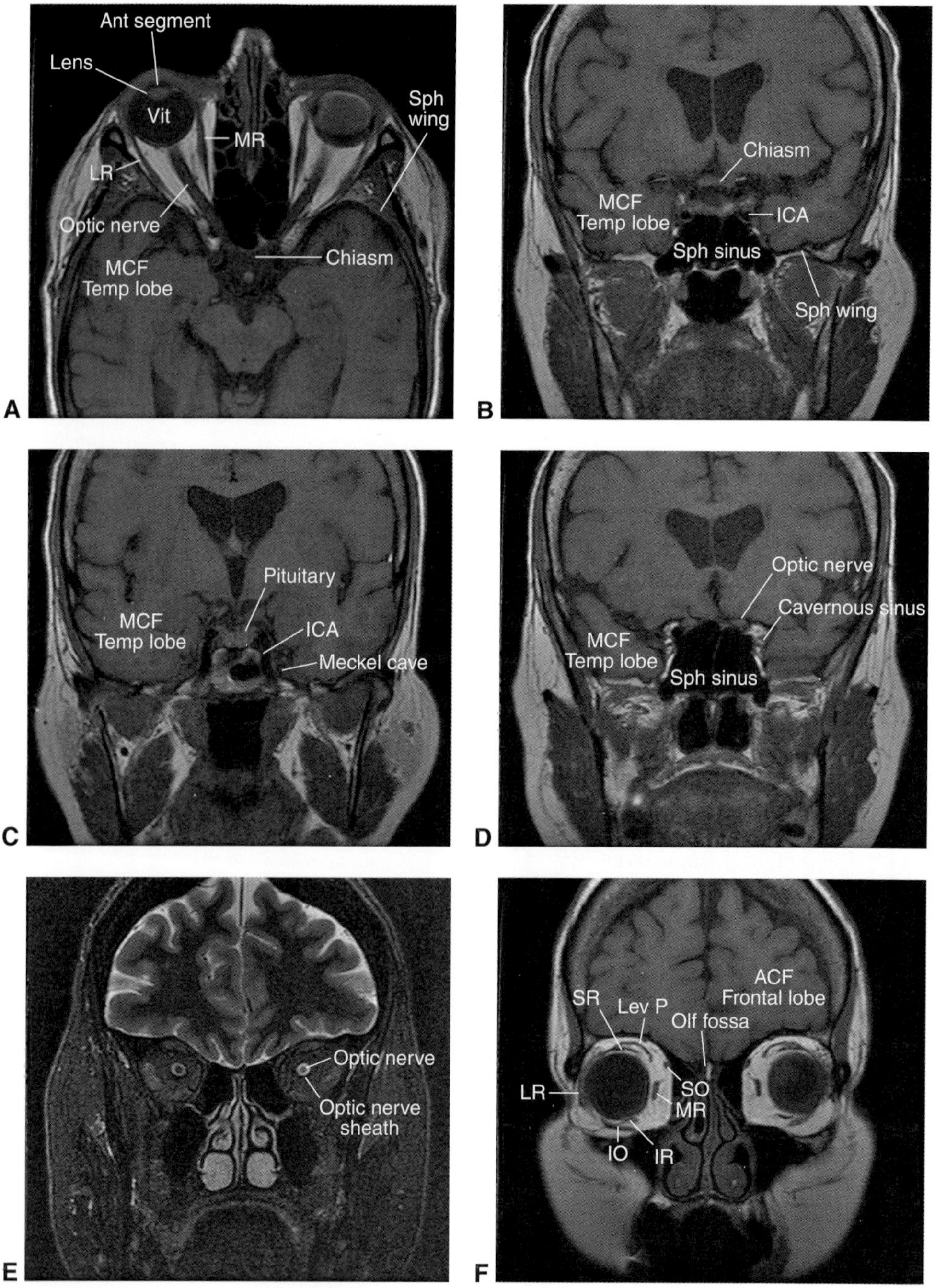

Figure 17-2 Brain and orbital magnetic resonance (MR) images showing the anatomy of visual and orbital structures from the chiasm to the anterior orbit. (The left-globe abnormality is not pertinent to the figure's objective.) **A,** T1-weighted axial image. **B–D,** T1-weighted coronal images. **E,** T2-weighted coronal image with fat saturation. **F,** T1-weighted coronal image. ACF = anterior cranial fossa; Ant segment = anterior segment; ICA = internal carotid artery; IO = inferior oblique muscle; IR = inferior rectus muscle; LR = lateral rectus muscle; Lev P = levator palpebrae superioris muscle; MCF = middle cranial fossa; MR = medial rectus muscle; Olf fossa = olfactory fossa; SO = superior oblique muscle; Sph sinus = sphenoid sinus; Sph wing = sphenoid wing; SR = superior rectus muscle; Temp lobe = temporal lobe; Vit = vitreous. *(Courtesy of M. Tariq Bhatti, MD.)*

Table 17-3 Edema: DWI and ADC

Type of Edema	DWI Signal	ADC Signal
Cytotoxic	Bright (high or restricted diffusion)[a]	Dark (low)
Vasogenic	Dark (low)	Normal (sometimes bright)

ADC = apparent diffusion coefficient; DWI = diffusion-weighted imaging.
[a] Bright signal on DWI represents restricted diffusion or decreased water movement.

Considerations when ordering an MRI:

- Metal in the body, including metallic intraocular or orbital foreign bodies
  - Screening radiography or CT may be helpful in detecting intraocular and orbital foreign bodies.
  - Consultation with a diagnostic radiologist is advised regarding the safety of some metals (eg, MRI-compatible aneurysm clips).
  - Gold weight and titanium mesh orbital floor implants have shown no movement when placed in a magnetic field. Some clinicians prefer to wait for fibrosis to secure the implant before obtaining an MRI.
- Cardiac pacemaker or defibrillator
  - Consultation with a diagnostic radiologist regarding all implantable devices is advised.
- Allergy to gadolinium-based contrast media

Activities 17-1 and 17-2 demonstrate normal structures identified on axial and coronal orbital imaging, respectively, with CT and MRI.

ACTIVITY 17-1 Axial imaging of the normal orbit with computed tomography and magnetic resonance imaging.
Developed by Vikram S. Brar, MD. Figures reproduced with permission from Dutton JJ. Atlas of Clinical and Surgical Orbital Anatomy. *2nd ed. Elsevier/Saunders; 2011: Figs 11-1 to 11-6.*
Access all Section 2 activities at www.aao.org/bcscactivity_section02.

ACTIVITY 17-2 Coronal imaging of the normal orbit with computed tomography and magnetic resonance imaging.
Developed by Vikram S. Brar, MD. Figures reproduced with permission from Dutton JJ. Atlas of Clinical and Surgical Orbital Anatomy. *2nd ed. Elsevier/Saunders; 2011: Figs 11-7 to 11-12.*

Expert Panel on MR Safety; Kanal E, Barkovich AJ, Bell C, et al. ACR guidance document on MR safe practices: 2013. *J Magn Reson Imaging.* 2013;37(3):501–530.

Lawrence DA, Lipman AT, Gupta SK, Nacey NC. Undetected intraocular metallic foreign body causing hyphema in a patient undergoing MRI: a rare occurrence demonstrating the limitations of pre-MRI safety screening. *Magn Reson Imaging.* 2015;33(3): 358–361.

Marra S, Leonetti JP, Konior RJ, Raslan W. Effect of magnetic resonance imaging on implantable eyelid weights. *Ann Otol Rhinol Laryngol.* 1995;104(6):448–452.

Modjtahedi BS, Rong A, Bobinski M, McGahan J, Morse L. Imaging characteristics of intraocular foreign bodies: a comparative study of plain film X-ray, computed tomography, ultrasound, and magnetic resonance imaging. *Retina.* 2015;35(1):95–104.

Seidenwurm DJ, McDonnell CH III, Raghavan N, Breslau J. Cost utility analysis of radiographic screening for an orbital foreign body before MR imaging. *Am J Neuroradiol.* 2000;21(2):426–433.

Sullivan PK, Smith JF, Rozzelle AA. Cranio-orbital reconstruction: safety and image quality of metallic implants on CT and MRI scanning. *Plast Reconstr Surg.* 1994;94(5):589–596.

Williamson MR, Espinosa MC, Boutin RD, Orrison WW Jr, Hart BC, Kelsey CA. Metallic foreign bodies in the orbits of patients undergoing MR imaging: prevalence and value of radiography and CT before MR. *AJR Am J Roentgenol.* 1994;162(4):981–983.

Ultrasonography

Ultrasound refers to sound waves with frequencies above the audible range. Ultrasonography uses echoes, much like light-based optical coherence tomography uses reflections, to image and differentiate tissues. During ultrasonography, electrical energy is converted into sound waves by means of a piezoelectric crystal. The resultant waves are emitted by the ultrasound probe, which is placed as close as possible to the tissue being studied. When the sound waves encounter tissues, their speed changes depending on the density of the surface/interface, and some of the waves bounce back to the probe; on the basis of their amplitude, frequency, and travel time, these echoes are then converted into a signal. For example, during ultrasonography, a sound wave traversing the cornea encounters the aqueous of the anterior chamber and then the lens–iris diaphragm. As the tissue density changes at the posterior cornea and then again at the lens–iris diaphragm, signals are generated. The distance between the 2 signal spikes is then used to determine the anterior chamber depth.

The frequency of the ultrasound determines the depth of penetration and the resolution. These 2 variables are inversely related. High-frequency ultrasound, which provides greater detail, is used to evaluate smaller objects such as the eye. Low-frequency ultrasound provides less resolution but can penetrate deeper. For example, it is useful in obstetrics to traverse through the abdominal wall and uterus to image a fetus.

Ophthalmic ultrasonography utilizes high-frequency sound waves (8–80 MHz) for safe, effective, noninvasive imaging of the anterior and posterior segments of the eye and orbit using equipment routinely found in most practices. Indications for ophthalmic ultrasonography include biometry and evaluation of the following structures and conditions:

- intraocular structures with media opacities
- posterior sclera
- extraocular muscles and the surrounding orbit
- intraocular tumors

Three main ultrasound devices are used to evaluate the eye: the A-scan probe, the B-scan probe, and the ultrasound biomicroscopy (UBM) probe (Fig 17-3).

Singh AD, Hayden BC. *Ophthalmic Ultrasonography.* Philadelphia: Elsevier/Saunders; 2012.

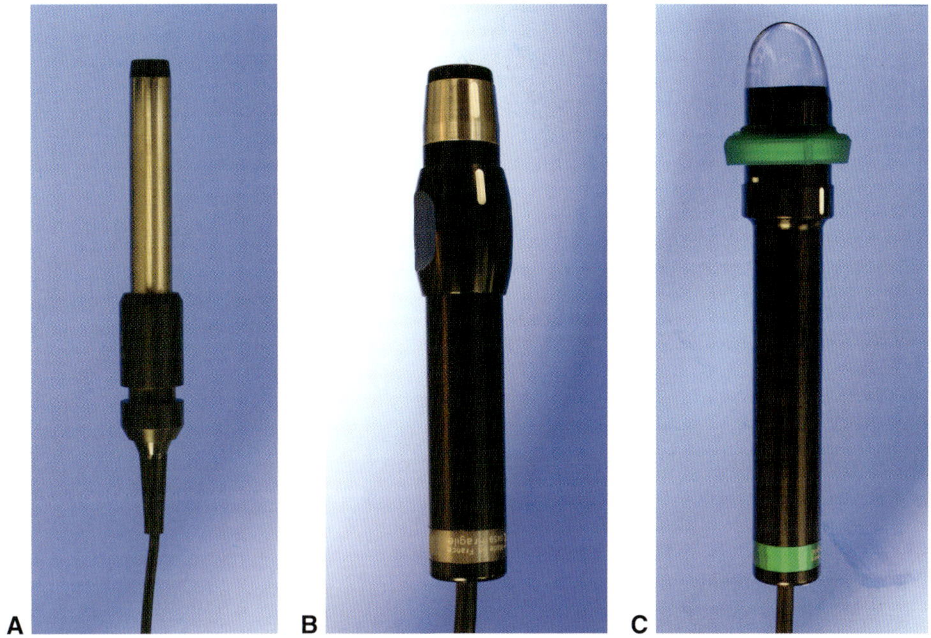

Figure 17-3 Ophthalmic ultrasound probes. **A,** A-scan probe. **B,** B-scan probe. **C,** Ultrasound biomicroscopy (UBM) probe. *(Courtesy of Vikram S. Brar, MD.)*

Table 17-4 A-Scan: Quantification of Reflectivity

Grade	A-Scan Spike Height, %
Low	0–33
Medium	34–66
High	67–100

Reproduced with permission from Singh AD, Hayden BC. *Ophthalmic Ultrasonography.* Philadelphia: Elsevier/Saunders; 2012:20.

A-Scan

Biometry of the eye with an A-scan probe (eg, for measuring axial length) uses frequencies between 8 and 12 MHz. After a topical anesthetic agent is applied, the probe makes direct contact with the cornea, or it can be applied via immersion. The latter eliminates the possibility of altering the measurement with compression of the cornea.

When operating at 8 MHz, the A-scan probe can also enable demonstration of intralesional characteristics within the eye and orbit, known as *internal reflectivity.* Reflectivity within a lesion may be low, medium, or high depending on the relative percentage of the internal spike compared with that of the initial spike of the lesion (Table 17-4). The reflectivity within a tissue is inversely proportional to its homogeneity. Less-organized tissue, as in a vascular lesion (ie, a choroidal hemangioma), will demonstrate high internal reflectivity compared with homogenous tissue (ie, a choroidal melanoma).

B-Scan

B-scan ultrasonography commonly uses 10 MHz, with axial resolution of 100 μm, to provide 2-dimensional images of the eye and orbit. Combining data from 2 orthogonal scans at a given point yields 3-dimensional information: shape, location, and extent. Three types of B-scans—axial, transverse, and longitudinal—are obtained depending on the position of the probe on the eye and the orientation of the linear white marker on its surface (Fig 17-4). These scans are best performed with direct contact on an anesthetized ocular surface, facilitated by a coupling agent such as methylcellulose. This improves image resolution and allows the examiner to monitor the position of the patient's eyes. The probe marker indicates the direction of the scan and corresponds to the top of the 2-dimensional B-scan image.

Axial scans

Axial scans are performed by placing the probe directly on the cornea with the patient looking straight ahead and the probe marker oriented vertically at 12 o'clock or horizontally

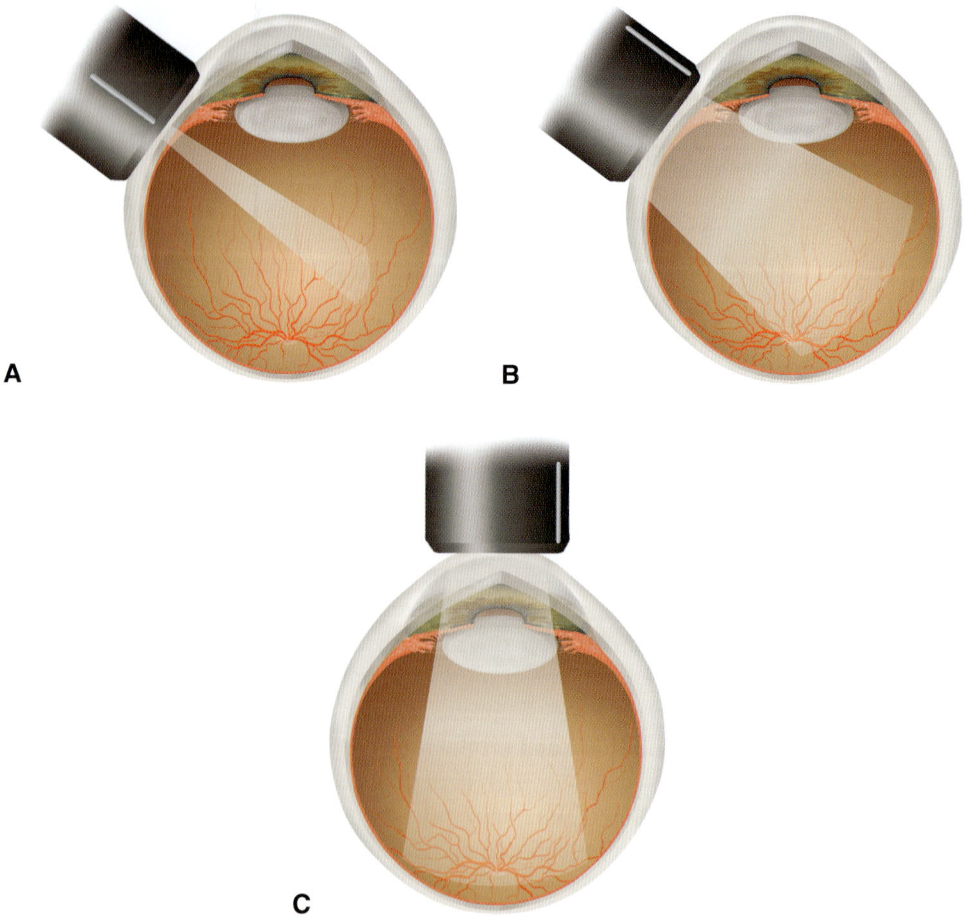

Figure 17-4 Three primary scans used in B-scan ultrasonography. **A,** Transverse scan. **B,** Longitudinal scan. **C,** Axial scan. *(Illustration by Cyndie C.H. Wooley.)*

A B

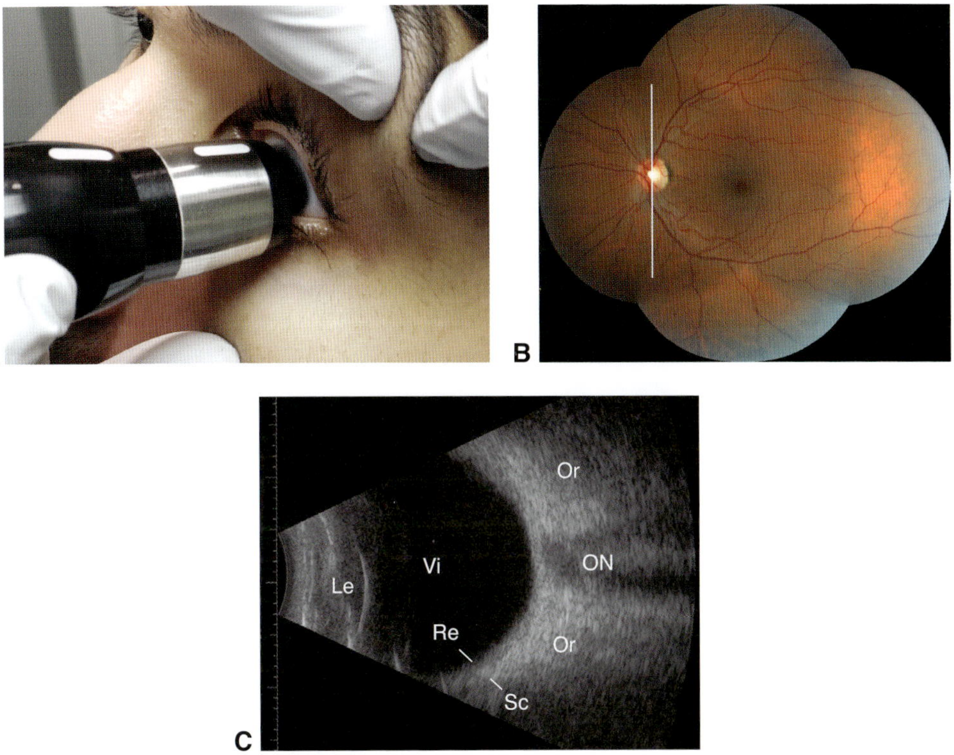

C

Figure 17-5 Vertical axial B-scan ultrasonography of the left eye. **A,** The probe is placed directly on the cornea and oriented vertically. **B,** Corresponding fundus photograph. The white line indicates the corresponding section of the fundus being imaged at the posterior aspect of the scan. **C,** Two-dimensional B-scan image. Based on the orientation of the probe, the top of the scan is the superior retina. Le = lens; ON = optic nerve; Or = orbit; Re = retina; Sc = sclera; Vi = vitreous. *(Courtesy of Vikram S. Brar, MD.)*

with the probe marker oriented nasally (Fig 17-5). This allows visualization of the posterior pole and the optic nerve. The posterior sclera and underlying Tenon space can also be examined, as in cases of posterior scleritis. Attenuation of the signal by the cornea and lens limits the resolution of these scans.

Transverse scans

During B-scan ultrasonography, transverse scans cover the greatest area of the posterior segment of the eye. The probe is placed on the sclera, avoiding image degradation from the anterior segment, and is oriented parallel to the limbus, providing a circumferential scan of the opposing retina (ie, when imaging the nasal quadrant, the probe is placed on the temporal sclera with the patient adducting his or her eye; Fig 17-6). The farther the probe traverses posteriorly from the limbus, the more the anterior part of the eye is imaged (ie, with the patient looking just nasal to midline, the probe is touching the edge of the limbus, and the back of the 2-dimensional image is posterior to the equator). As the patient looks farther nasally, the probe slides posteriorly on the surface of the globe

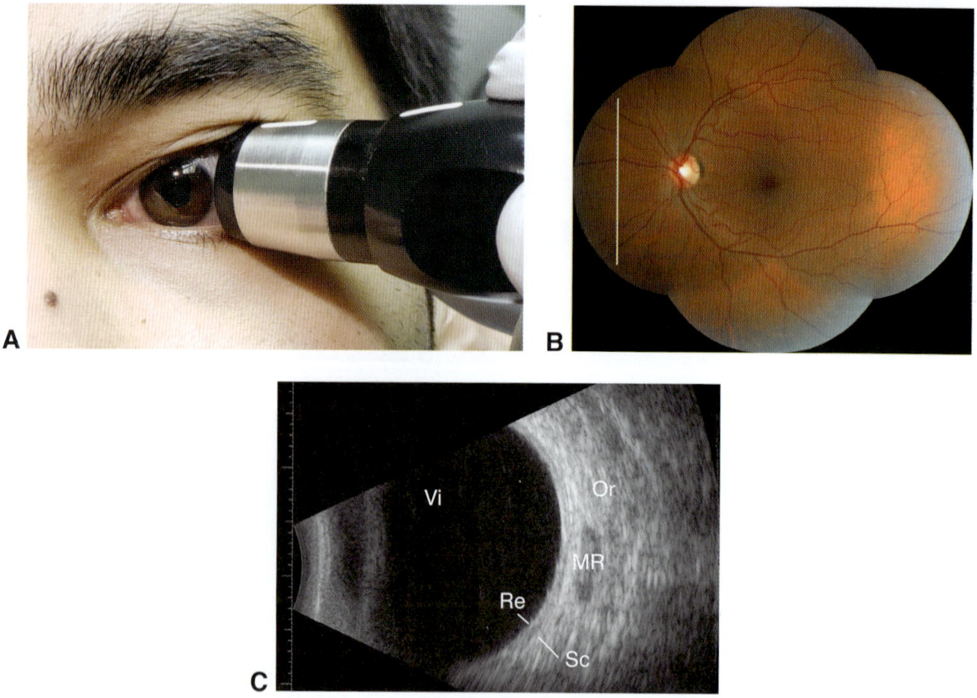

Figure 17-6 Lateral transverse B-scan ultrasonography of the left eye. **A,** The probe is on the temporal sclera (left eye) with the patient looking to his right and the marker oriented up. **B,** Corresponding fundus photograph is shown. The white line indicates the corresponding section of the fundus being imaged at the posterior aspect of the scan. **C,** The back of the scan is the nasal retina, and the top is the superior retina. MR = medial rectus muscle; Or = orbit; Re = retina, Sc = sclera; Vi = vitreous. *(Courtesy of Vikram S. Brar, MD.)*

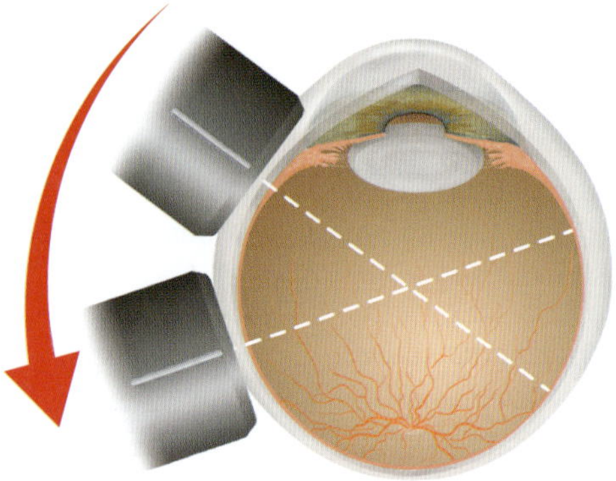

Figure 17-7 When transverse scans are performed, anterior-to-posterior excursion of the B-scan probe maximizes visualization of the desired quadrant. *(Illustration by Cyndie C.H. Wooley.)*

and the scan is directed more anteriorly (Fig 17-7). This maximizes visualization of that quadrant.

When the posterior segment cannot be visualized, 4 transverse scans (ie, superior, inferior, nasal, and temporal) in addition to the axial scan are typically performed as part of the screening B-scan. The nasal and temporal scans are known as the *lateral transverse*

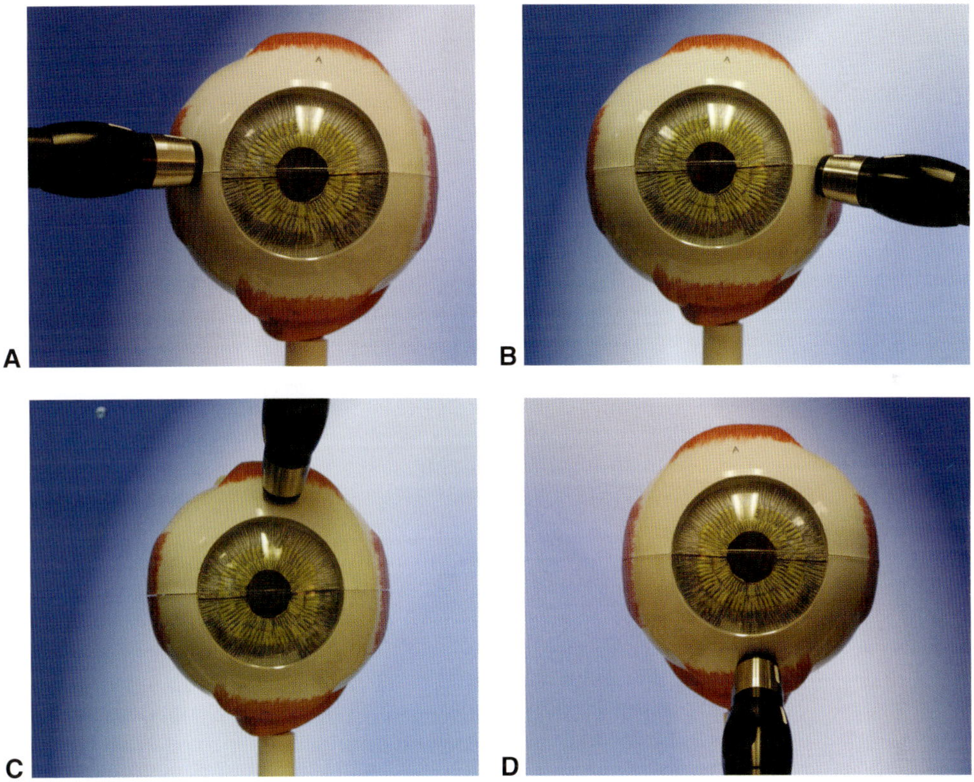

Figure 17-8 Model of the left eye, showing positioning of the probe and orientation of the probe marker in the 4 primary transverse scans performed in a screening B-scan. The probe marker is oriented up for lateral transverse scans (**A,** temporal; **B,** nasal) and nasally for inferior **(C)** and superior **(D)** scans. *(Courtesy of Vikram S. Brar, MD.)*

scans (see Fig 17-6). By convention, when the superior or inferior eye is imaged, the probe marker is oriented nasally. In all other positions, the probe marker is oriented superiorly. Figure 17-8 demonstrates the appropriate positioning of the probe and the orientation of the marker for the 4 primary transverse scans.

Longitudinal scans

Similar to transverse scans, longitudinal scans are performed with the probe placed on the sclera, with the marker oriented perpendicular to the limbus. These scans are performed when a lesion is identified on a screening B-scan and describe the anterior-posterior extent. The optic nerve should be visualized below the center on longitudinal scans (Fig 17-9). Longitudinal scans can also be used to visualize the macula (Fig 17-10).

Dynamic B-scan

B-scan ultrasonography is not a static process. Already, we have discussed the anterior-to-posterior excursion of the ultrasound probe to increase the area imaged during transverse scans. In addition, the patient can be asked to look up and down during lateral transverse

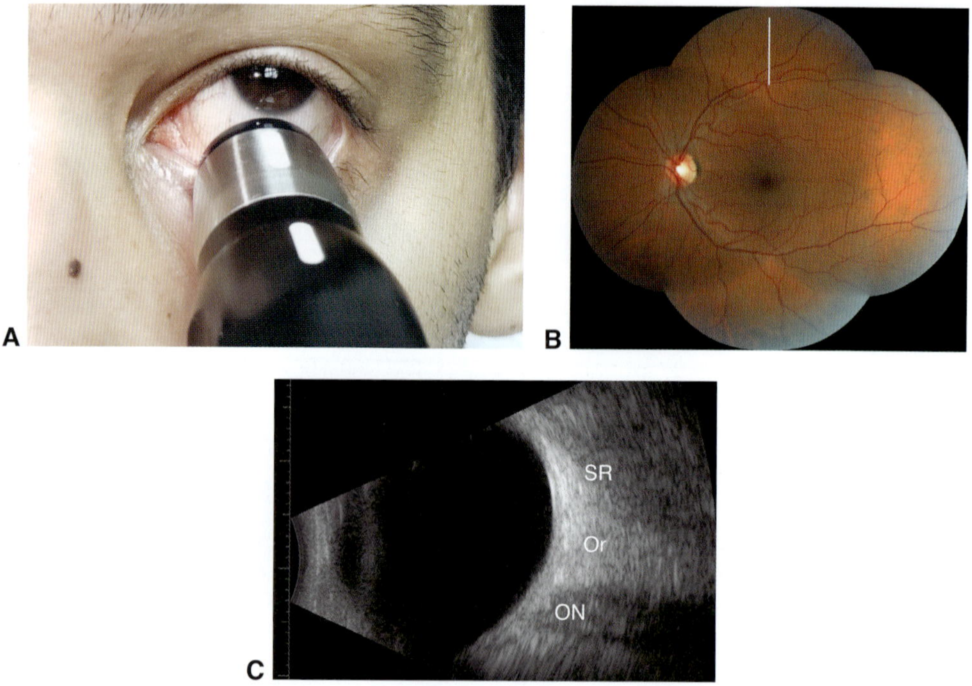

Figure 17-9 Superior longitudinal B-scan ultrasonography of the left eye. **A,** The probe is placed directly on the sclera (left eye) with the patient looking up and the marker oriented vertically, perpendicular to the limbus. **B,** Corresponding fundus photograph is shown. The white line indicates the corresponding section of the fundus being imaged at the posterior aspect of the scan. These scans demonstrate the anterior-posterior extent of a lesion. **C,** In the 2-dimensional B-scan image, the back of the scan represents the superior fundus. Note the positioning of the optic nerve, which is found toward the bottom of longitudinal scans. ON = optic nerve; Or = orbit; SR = superior rectus muscle. *(Courtesy of Vikram S. Brar, MD.)*

scans and right and left during superior/inferior transverse scans to study movement of the vitreous/posterior hyaloid face and a detached retina. Furthermore, the gain of the scan can be adjusted to enhance visualization of particular structures (Table 17-5).

Figures 17-11, 17-12, and 17-13 highlight the differential diagnoses requiring ophthalmic ultrasonography and their diagnostic features.

Ultrasound Biomicroscopy

Ultrasound biomicroscopy (UBM) utilizes the highest frequency available in ophthalmic ultrasonography, usually 50 MHz, with axial resolution of 37 μm, and is used to evaluate the anterior segment of the eye. It requires topical anesthesia and a fluid reservoir, which is placed in direct contact with the cornea and/or anterior sclera depending on which structures need to be evaluated. Two types of scans are obtained with UBM depending on the orientation of the probe. *Axial* UBM scans are generated by placing the probe on the cornea positioned horizontally (Fig 17-14). This allows visualization of the cornea, the anterior chamber, the iris with the pupil in the center of the iris plane, and the lens. *Radial*

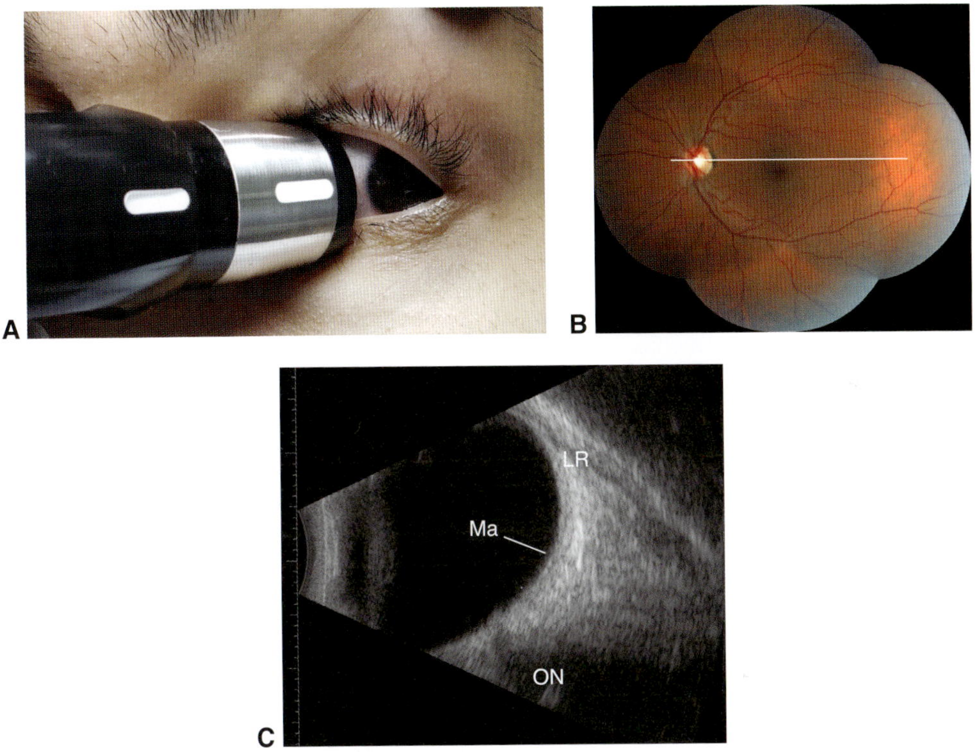

Figure 17-10 Longitudinal B-scan ultrasonography demonstrating the macula in the left eye. **A,** The patient is asked to abduct his or her eye. The probe is placed directly on the nasal sclera with the marker oriented perpendicular to the limbus. **B,** Corresponding fundus photograph is shown. The white line indicates the corresponding section of the fundus being imaged at the posterior aspect of the scan. **C,** In this 2-dimensional image, the top of the scan demonstrates the lateral rectus muscle; the optic nerve is toward the bottom of longitudinal scans. The intervening retina includes the macula. LR = lateral rectus muscle; Ma = macula; ON = optic nerve. *(Courtesy of Vikram S. Brar, MD.)*

Table 17-5 B-Scan: Tissue-Specific Gain Setting

Tissue	Decibel Value, dB	Gain Setting
Vitreous	75–100	High
Retina/choroid	55–75	Medium
Sclera/orbit/calcification	35–55	Low

Modified with permission from Singh AD, Hayden BC. *Ophthalmic Ultrasonography.* Philadelphia: Elsevier/Saunders; 2012:18.

UBM scans are generated by centering the probe at the limbus, with the marker oriented perpendicular to the limbus. The anterior chamber angle, iris, and ciliary body can be evaluated with this scan (Fig 17-15).

Fledelius HC. Ultrasound in ophthalmology. *Ultrasound Med Biol.* 1997;23(3):365–375.

Diagnosis		Ultrasonographic Findings
Myositis Graves orbitopathy	1	Thickened extraocular muscles
Periorbital space-occupying lesions	2	Change in the relief of the orbital wall, sound propagation into perinasal sinuses
Orbital neoplasm	3	Directly evident (it may be difficult to demonstrate a small cavernous hemangioma because of its high acoustic reflectivity)
Inflammatory orbital pseudotumor	4	Widening of normal orbital structures, low acoustic reflectivity, Tenon space may be demonstrated
Disc edema	5	Widened dural diameter of the optic nerve
Axial hyperopia	6	Axial length below 22 mm, ocular walls concentrically thickened
Ocular hypotony	7	Ocular walls concentrically thickened
Macular degeneration		Thickening of the ocular walls in the area of the macula, high acoustic reflectivity
Scleritis	8	Circumscribed widening of the ocular walls, Tenon space apparent

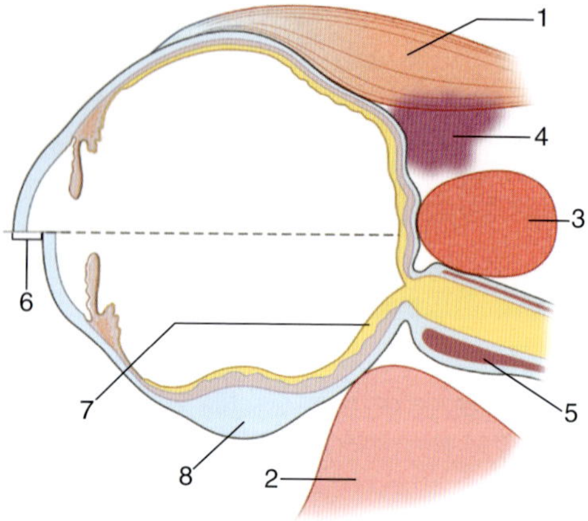

Figure 17-11 Schematic of ultrasonographic findings. The dotted line separates the top half of the eye from the bottom half, which is shorter (demonstrating hyperopia) and where different disease processes are depicted. *Inset:* Differential diagnosis for choroidal folds. *(Adapted with permission from Schachat AP, Wilkinson CP, Hinton DR, Sadda SR, Wiedemann P, eds.* Ryan's Retina. *6th ed. Philadelphia: Elsevier; 2017:321, Table 11.3 and Fig 11.85.)*

Diagnosis		Ultrasonographic Findings
Normal axial length for the patient's age		
Retinoblastoma	1	Widening of the ocular walls, extremely high acoustic reflectivity, shadowing effect, atypical findings possible
Congenital cataract	2	Increased reflectivity from the posterior lens surface, vitreous space empty, ocular walls normal
Shortened axial length		
Retinopathy of prematurity	3	In stages IV and V, beginning or complete traction detachment (normal findings in stages I–III)
PFV	4	Dense strand of tissue between optic nerve head and posterior lens pole; formes frustes may occur (posterior or anterior PFV)
Retinal anomalies		Membranes in the vitreous, atypical detachment, which in part appears solid (no typical echogram)
Fundus coloboma	5	Directly demonstrable protrusion of ocular wall, sometimes with orbital cyst (microphthalmos with cyst)
Coats disease	6	Floating crystals in the vitreous and subretinal space (fast-flickering spikes on A-mode)

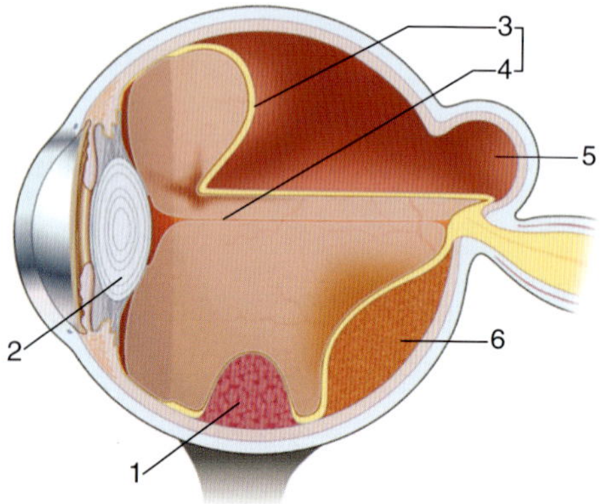

Figure 17-12 Schematic of ultrasonographic findings. *Inset:* Differential diagnosis for leukocoria. PFV = persistent fetal vasculature. *(Adapted with permission from Schachat AP, Wilkinson CP, Hinton DR, Sadda SR, Wiedemann P, eds.* Ryan's Retina. *6th ed. Philadelphia: Elsevier; 2017:322, Table 11.4 and Fig 11.86.)*

Diagnosis		Ultrasonographic Findings
Symptomatic posterior vitreous detachment	1	Thickened detached posterior hyaloid membrane, occasionally early retinal detachment
Recently formed retinal break with torn vessel	2	Blood-covered vitreous strands converge toward the retinal break; occasionally a high-floating operculum may be detected
Proliferative retinopathy	3	Strands or membranes extending from the optic nerve head or the posterior pole, high acoustic reflectivity
Terson syndrome (vitreous hemorrhage after subchoroidal bleeding	4	Vitreous opacities in front of the optic nerve head or behind the detached vitreous
Disciform macular degeneration	5	Widening of the ocular walls in the macular area, high acoustic reflectivity, vitreous strands extending from the macula
Choroidal melanoma	6	Biconvex thickening of the ocular wall, low acoustic reflectivity, sometimes mushroom-shaped; accompanying retinal detachment distant from the tumor

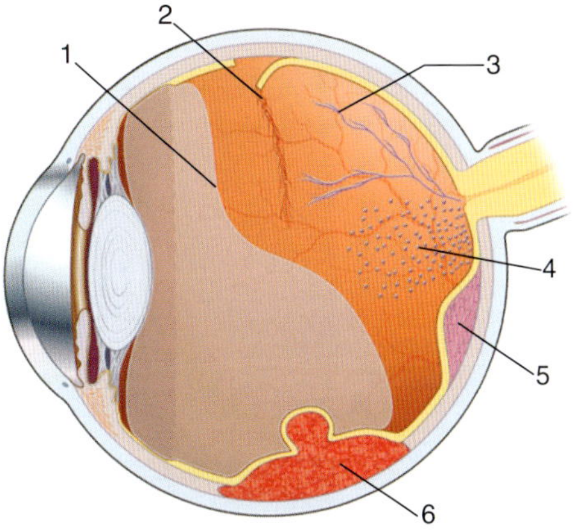

Figure 17-13 Schematic of ultrasonographic findings. *Inset:* Differential diagnosis for vitreous hemorrhage. *(Adapted with permission from Schachat AP, Wilkinson CP, Hinton DR, Sadda SR, Wiedemann P, eds.* Ryan's Retina. *6th ed. Philadelphia: Elsevier; 2017:322, Table 11.5 and Fig 11.87.)*

A

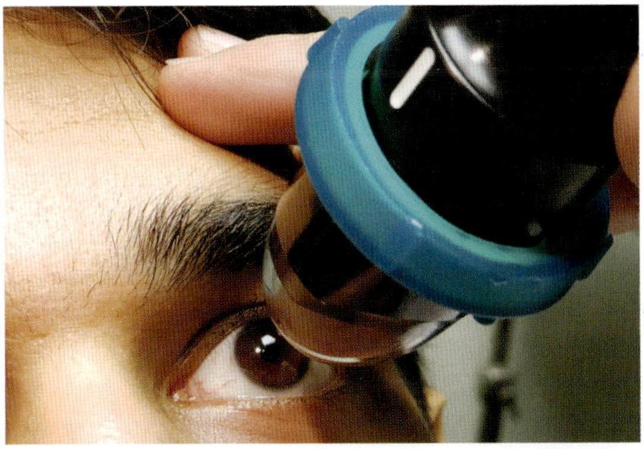

B

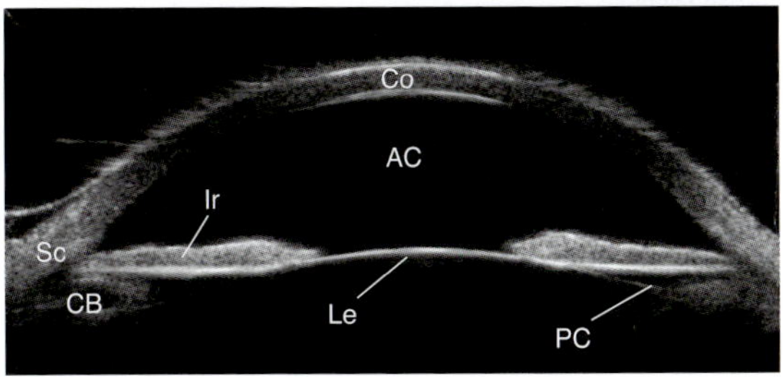

Figure 17-14 Ultrasound biomicroscopy (UBM). **A,** After the eye is anesthetized, the probe is placed directly on the cornea, in this case, oriented horizontally. **B,** Axial scan of the anterior segment. AC = anterior chamber; CB = ciliary body; Co = cornea; Ir = iris; Le = lens anterior capsule; PC = posterior chamber; Sc = sclera. *(Courtesy of Vikram S. Brar, MD.)*

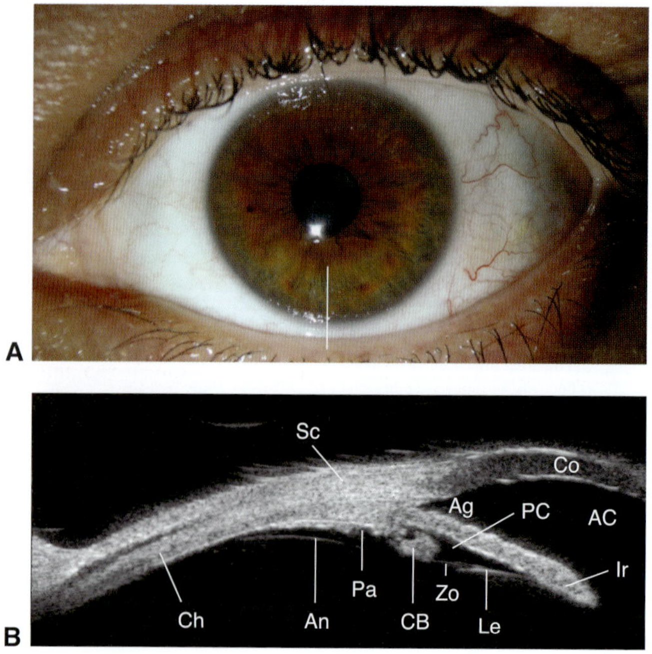

Figure 17-15 Radial UBM. **A,** Slit-lamp photograph. The white line demonstrates the location and orientation of the probe. **B,** Radial scan demonstrates the structures. AC = anterior chamber; Ag = angle; An = anterior hyaloid face; CB = ciliary body; Ch = choroid; Co = cornea; Ir = iris; Le = lens anterior capsule; Pa = pars plicata; PC = posterior chamber; Sc = sclera; Zo = zonular fibers. *(Courtesy of Vikram S. Brar, MD.)*

Ordering Imaging Studies

Requesting the correct study is imperative for arriving at the correct diagnosis. Imaging orders should include clinical information regarding the patient, the location or perceived location of the pathology to be studied, use of a contrast agent, and urgency. The more detail provided with the order, the higher the likelihood of obtaining the desired information. Communication with the diagnostic radiologist can facilitate this process and increase the yield. Table 17-6 provides recommendations for ordering a study. Tables 17-7 and 17-8 cover specific disease entities, recommended imaging modality, and use of contrast material for common neuro-ophthalmic and orbital conditions, respectively.

Kruger JM, Lessell S, Cestari DM. Neuro-imaging: a review for the general ophthalmologist. *Semin Ophthalmol.* 2012;27(5-6):192–196.

Lee AG, Brazis PW, Garrity JA, White M. Imaging for neuro-ophthalmic and orbital disease. *Am J Ophthalmol.* 2004;138(5):852–862.

Lee AG, Johnson MC, Policeni BA, Smoker WR. Imaging for neuro-ophthalmic and orbital disease: a review. *Clin Exp Ophthalmol.* 2009;37(1):30–53.

Simha A, Irodi A, David S. Magnetic resonance imaging for the ophthalmologist: a primer. *Indian J Ophthalmol.* 2012;60(4):301–310.

Table 17-6 Recommendations for Ordering Imaging Studies in Ophthalmology

Decide whether a CT or MR scan is indicated. In most cases, MRI is superior to CT for neuro-ophthalmic indications. CT is superior to MRI for visualizing calcifications, bone, and acute hemorrhage and when an emergent scan is needed. CT is also used when the patient cannot undergo MRI.

Decide whether contrast-material enhancement is needed. In most cases, contrast material should be ordered for all studies. Contrast enhancement may not be necessary in acute hemorrhage, thyroid ophthalmopathy, and trauma cases.

Localize the lesion clinically ("Where is the lesion?"), and then order a study tailored to the location (eg, head, orbit, neck). To obtain the correct study, take the time to fill out the radiographic order form personally with sufficient clinical details for the radiologist. Do not just order a "brain MRI" for every case.

Depending on the clinical indication, consider ordering special imaging sequences (eg, fat suppression for an orbital postcontrast study, fluid attenuation inversion recovery for white matter lesions, gradient echo for hemorrhage).

Call the radiologist and tell him or her the differential diagnosis ("What is the lesion?") and the location ("Where is the lesion?").

If the imaging shows either no abnormality or an abnormality that does not match the clinical location, call the radiologist or, better yet, review the films directly with him or her. Ask the radiologist if the area of interest has been adequately imaged, if artifact might be obscuring the lesion, or if additional studies might show the lesion.

If the clinical picture suggests a specific lesion or location and initial imaging is "normal," consider repeating the imaging study with thinner sections and higher magnification of the area of interest, especially if the clinical signs and symptoms are progressive.

Recognize that the lack of an abnormality on imaging does not exclude pathology.

CT = computed tomography; MRI = magnetic resonance imaging.

Modified with permission from Lee AG, Brazis PW, Garrity JA, White M. Imaging for neuro-ophthalmic and orbital disease. *Am J Ophthalmol.* 2004;138(5):855.

Table 17-7 Neuro-Ophthalmic Indications and Recommended Imaging Study

Indication	Imaging Study	Contrast Material	Comment
Optic nerve drusen	CT scan of the orbit (may show calcification) B-scan ultrasonography (axial)	Not necessary	Ultrasonography is less costly and more sensitive than a CT scan for drusen.
Papilledema	MRI of the head (with MRV)	Yes	Consider contrast MRV to exclude venous sinus thrombosis, especially in atypical patients with idiopathic intracranial hypertension (IIH, formerly known as *pseudotumor cerebri*) and who are thin, male, or elderly.

(Continued)

Table 17-7 *(continued)*

Indication	Imaging Study	Contrast Material	Comment
Transient vision loss (amaurosis fugax)	MRA or CTA of the neck for carotid stenosis or dissection	Depends on clinical situation	An adjunctive carotid Doppler study or catheter angiography may be required.
Demyelination optic neuritis	MRI of the head and orbit	Yes	Consider FLAIR to look for demyelinating white matter lesions; MRI has prognostic significance for the development of multiple sclerosis.
Inflammatory, infiltrative, or compressive optic neuropathy	MRI of the head and orbit	Yes	Fat suppression will exclude intraorbital optic nerve enhancement; CT is superior in traumatic optic neuropathy for canal fractures.
Junctional scotoma (ie, optic neuropathy in 1 eye and superotemporal visual field loss in fellow eye)	MRI of the head (attention to the sella)	Yes	
Bitemporal hemianopia	MRI of the head (attention to the chiasm and sella)	Yes	Consider CT of the sella if an emergent scan is needed (eg, pituitary or chiasmal apoplexy) or when imaging for calcification (eg, meningioma, craniopharyngioma, or aneurysm).
Homonymous hemianopia	MRI of the head	Yes	Retrochiasmal pathway. DWI may be useful with acute ischemic infarct. If structural imaging is negative and there is organic loss, consider functional imaging.

Table 17-7 *(continued)*

Indication	Imaging Study	Contrast Material	Comment
Cortical vision loss or visual association cortex (eg, cerebral achromatopsia, alexia, prosopagnosia, simultagnosia, optic ataxia, Balint syndrome)	MRI of the head	Yes	Retrochiasmal pathway. DWI may be useful with acute ischemic infarct. If structural imaging is negative and there is organic loss, consider functional imaging (eg, PET, SPECT, MRS).
Third, fourth, or sixth nerve palsy or cavernous sinus syndrome	MRI of the head with attention to the skull base; isolated vasculopathic cranial neuropathies may not require initial imaging	Yes	Rim calcification in aneurysm, calcification in tumors, and hyperostosis may be better seen on CT.
Internuclear ophthalmoplegia (INO), supranuclear or nuclear gaze palsies, dorsal midbrain syndrome, skew deviation	MRI of the head (brainstem)	Yes	Rule out demyelinating or other brainstem lesion; include a FLAIR sequence.
Nystagmus	MRI of the brainstem	Yes	Localize nystagmus.
Hemifacial spasm	MRI of the brainstem (with or without MRA)	Yes	Compression of the facial nerve root near its exit from the brainstem by adjacent artery, eg, anterior/posterior inferior cerebellar artery.
Horner syndrome: preganglionic	MRI of the head and neck to the second thoracic vertebra (T2) in the chest with neck MRA	Yes	Rule out lateral medullary infarct, apical lung neoplasm, carotid dissection, etc.
Horner syndrome: postganglionic	MRI of the head and neck to the level of the superior cervical ganglion (C4 level) with MRA of the neck	Yes	Rule out carotid dissection; isolated postganglionic lesions are often benign.

CT = computed tomography; CTA = CT angiography; DWI = diffusion-weighted imaging; FLAIR = fluid attenuation inversion recovery; MRA = magnetic resonance angiography; MRI = magnetic resonance imaging; MRS = magnetic resonance spectroscopy; MRV = magnetic resonance venography; PET = positron emission tomography; SPECT = single-photon emission computed tomography.

Modified with permission from Lee AG, Brazis PW, Garrity JA, White M. Imaging for neuro-ophthalmic and orbital disease. *Am J Ophthalmol.* 2004;138(5):854.

Table 17-8 Orbital Indications and Recommendations for Imaging

Orbital Lesion	Imaging Study	Contrast Enhancement	Comment
Thyroid eye disease	CT or MRI of the orbit	Iodinated contrast medium may interfere with evaluation and treatment of systemic thyroid disease	Bone anatomy is better seen on a CT scan, especially if orbital decompression is being considered.
Orbital cellulitis and orbital disease secondary to sinus disease (eg, silent sinus syndrome, sinusitis)	CT of the orbit and sinuses	Depends on clinical situation	MRI may be a useful adjunct to a CT scan, especially if concomitant cavernous sinus thrombosis is present.
Nonspecific orbital inflammation	CT or MRI of the orbit (with fat suppression)	Yes	Beware of fat suppression artifact.
Orbital tumor (eg, proptosis or enophthalmos, gaze-evoked vision loss)	CT or MRI of the orbit	Yes	Include head imaging if lesion could extend intracranially (eg, optic nerve sheath meningioma); CT scan may be superior if looking for hyperostosis or calcification (eg, sheath meningioma).
Orbital trauma (eg, fracture, subperiosteal hematoma, orbital foreign body, orbital emphysema)	CT scan of the orbit with axial and direct coronal imaging	Not generally necessary	CT is superior for visualizing a fracture or bone fragment; MRI may be superior for optic nerve sheath hemorrhage.
Carotid cavernous sinus or dural fistula (eg, orbital bruit, arterialization of conjunctival and episcleral vessels, glaucoma)	CT or MRI of the head and orbit (with contrast-enhanced MRA)	Yes	CT or MRI may show an enlarged superior ophthalmic vein and may require a catheter angiogram for final diagnosis and therapy. Color flow Doppler studies may be useful for detecting reversal of orbital venous flow.

CT = computed tomography; MRA = magnetic resonance angiography; MRI = magnetic resonance imaging.

Modified with permission from Lee AG, Brazis PW, Garrity JA, White M. Imaging for neuro-ophthalmic and orbital disease. *Am J Ophthalmol.* 2004;138(5):857.

CHAPTER 18

Digital Ophthalmology

Highlights

- Artificial intelligence (AI) algorithms exploit the complex spatial, temporal, and other relationships in digital data derived from the eye.
- In ophthalmology, the ubiquitous use of images and well-established prognostic standards provide many opportunities to employ AI in clinical care and research.
- AI in ophthalmology is more than just machine learning algorithms: its goals, design, development, and implementation need to be carefully considered.

Glossary

Artificial intelligence (AI) Systems that perform tasks mimicking human cognitive capabilities through the use of machine learning or other optimization techniques.

Artificial intelligence bias AI that performs differently for some groups (eg, different races and ethnicities) than others, as a result of concept, design, development, or implementation.

Coherence A measure of similarity, such as neighboring pixels in an image of the retina having similar color.

Machine learning algorithm An algorithm whose parameters are adjusted in a stepwise fashion during training to increase accuracy or another metric.

Deep learning algorithm A specific type of machine learning with a large number of parameters, typically millions.

Training set A set of images or other data, in which each image contains its "truth."

Truth The best estimate for what the image or other data represent, such as a disease.

The Role of Digital Ophthalmology

The term *digital ophthalmology* broadly encompasses health information technology, including electronic health records, clinical repositories such as the American Academy of Ophthalmology (AAO) IRIS Registry (Intelligent Research in Sight), teleophthalmology, and AI, on which this chapter focuses. Digital ophthalmology has been driving a revolution in our profession and has shown evidence of its potential to improve quality of care and clinical outcomes, reduce health disparities, and improve access, while lowering cost. It can also improve physician satisfaction and patient autonomy at both individual and population levels. Finally, it contributes to the discovery of new disease mechanisms and treatment for eye diseases.

Artificial Intelligence

Artificial intelligence describes systems that perform tasks mimicking human cognitive capabilities through the use of machine learning or other optimization techniques. AI leverages imaging and clinical data that reflect highly cognitive tasks, such as imaging interpretation and clinical decision making. In ophthalmology, AI has been applied to the diagnosis and staging of many diseases, including diabetic retinopathy, retinopathy of prematurity, age-related macular degeneration, glaucoma, and keratoconus, as well as in ocular oncology. AI allows analysis of large amounts of data for a single patient, thus improving ophthalmologists' effectiveness in using this information. It also allows for large-scale analysis of many patients' data, thus improving ophthalmologists' productivity. Ophthalmology is particularly well suited to AI because of the widespread use of objective imaging data, as well as widely accepted evidence-based clinical standards.

Clinical Application of AI: An Example

Consider the development of an AI system for diagnosing diabetic retinopathy and diabetic macular edema from retinal images. There is substantial evidence that examining a patient with diabetes annually for diabetic retinopathy, before symptoms occur, helps prevent vision loss. However, for various reasons—including social determinants of health—many people with diabetes are not getting consistent eye examinations. The goal of such an AI system would be to improve visual outcomes for people with diabetes by making the diabetic eye examination more accessible and increasing ophthalmologists' productivity.

The outputs of this proposed AI system would be the identification of "disease present" when the patient has at least a defined level of disease, and "disease absent" otherwise, based on established guidelines, in this case, the AAO *Diabetic Retinopathy Preferred Practice Pattern* guidelines. The outputs need to be accurate for the AI to be safe. Because the US population of patients with diabetes is diverse, AI bias—such as differing levels of accuracy in assessing different races, ethnicities, and genders—must be avoided.

The AI system uses digital retinal images as inputs. Each pixel in such an image measures the property of a small region of the retina, such as color reflectance in the case of fundus images. Reflectance characterizes physiologic and pathologic processes, such as the local amount of hemoglobin. Blood vessels, hemorrhages, and exudates determine the color of multiple adjoining pixels in different ways. For example, groups of pixels representing a hemorrhage are more likely to have a similar (reddish) color than the rest of the retina. Such similarities can be measured and are described as *spatial coherence*. An AI system can be made to associate such characteristics with a diagnosis using machine learning, as explained in the following section.

Machine Learning

The highest AI accuracy is typically achieved by means of machine learning algorithms. Explicitly programming an algorithm, without machine learning, to recognize the coherences requires them to be defined mathematically, which so far has been elusive. Instead, machine learning algorithms have thousands or more parameters that are not explicitly programmed but are adjusted step by step during a training phase. *Deep learning algorithms* are an advanced type of machine learning algorithm, incorporating millions of parameters grouped in complex ways. During the training phase, an algorithm learns to associate spatial coherences in a set of examples with the desired output. The set of examples is called the *training set,* which, in this case, is a set of retinal images of people with diabetes. This set requires the disease state, or diagnosis, for each such image—often called the *truth.*

Machine learning uses the power of statistics to differentiate between relevant and irrelevant coherences in the training images so that spurious coherences are discarded. The process is performed step by step, image by image. To start, an algorithm that is initially not very accurate is presented with the first image of the training set as input. The algorithm uses its parameters to calculate the output. If this output is different from the truth for that image, the algorithm was incorrect, and some of its parameters are adjusted. If the output is accurate, the parameters are typically left unchanged. Over many iterations, accuracy improves, and the process continues until a desired level of accuracy has been achieved.

Machine learning generalizes step by step from the training set; it does not memorize each training example. This enables the algorithm to give a correct output for a previously unseen image. This process demonstrates the importance of accurate truth in the training set: if an image has incorrect truth, the accuracy goes down rather than up for that step.

This explanation clarifies how larger and more diverse training sets, with accurate truths, lead to better algorithm accuracy with less AI bias. The relevant coherences will dominate the irrelevant, spurious ones. Unfortunately, in ophthalmology, obtaining such large training sets is an expensive, laborious process, within narrow ethical and legal constraints. Such fundamental data scarcity limits the direct translation of AI algorithms widely used outside ophthalmology.

Design and Bias

The distribution of the training set explains how racial and ethnic bias can unwittingly be introduced into AI. Some machine learning algorithms, so-called *black box AI,* do not have any built-in prior knowledge. Black box algorithms can learn to associate any information in the image with the desired output, even information that is irrelevant to the disease. This can be an advantage when the goal of AI is to discover new, previously unknown associations, such as research into a potential new disease mechanism. If the goal of the AI is to accurately identify patients with diabetic retinopathy, however, racial and ethnic bias can be introduced.

For example, consider a training set that is inadvertently skewed toward images of darkly pigmented patients with a lower incidence of disease than lightly pigmented patients. After machine learning from this training set, a black box AI will associate a lightly pigmented retina more with a "disease" output than a darkly pigmented retina. After all, it has no other information to learn that this association is incorrect. This biased AI is more likely to diagnose a previously unseen darkly pigmented patient as not having disease than a lightly pigmented patient.

Such bias can be mitigated by AI design, by careful development and analysis of the training set, and by validation. Prior knowledge can be introduced, such as the fact that diabetic retinopathy is characterized by hemorrhages, exudates, or new vessels, independent of race or ethnicity. Using machine learning to create lesion detectors can result in AI systems that are better understood, more robust to noisy inputs, and protected against racial and ethnic bias.

Validation

An AI system, once developed and validated, may be used on hundreds of millions of patients. Such large-scale AI has the potential for both patient benefit and risk of harm. Thus, safety, equity, and other ethical issues of the AI need to be prioritized; they are as important as, or more important than, the AI system's technical details. It is essential to understand what the AI output was validated against—from a single clinician's diagnosis (which can vary by clinician) to patient outcomes—and how any biases were identified and addressed. There are multiple examples of an AI system that was determined to be safe in a laboratory setting but when deployed in clinical practice was found to worsen rather than improve patient outcomes. Our profession is tasked with ensuring that ophthalmological AI systems are designed, developed, validated, and introduced in a safe and equitable manner.

The Future of AI in Ophthalmology

Ophthalmology remains at the leading edge of AI in medicine. If AI is implemented appropriately, it has the potential to lead to better quality of care, decrease health disparities, improve access for disadvantaged populations, lower cost, enhance job satisfaction for ophthalmologists, and enable more effective research.

Abràmoff MD, Cunningham B, Patel B, et al; Collaborative Community on Ophthalmic Imaging Executive Committee and Foundational Principles of Ophthalmic Imaging and Algorithmic Interpretation Working Group. Foundational considerations for artificial intelligence using ophthalmic images. *Ophthalmology.* 2022;129(2):e14–e32.

American Medical Association. Policy Statement. Augmented intelligence in healthcare. 2019. Accessed November 15, 2021. https://www.ama-assn.org/system/files/2019-08/ai-2018-board-policy-summary.pdf

Artificial intelligence. American Academy of Ophthalmology. Accessed November 15, 2021. https://www.aao.org/artificial-intelligence

APPENDIX

Genetics Glossary

AAV (adeno-associated virus) vector gene therapy A form of gene therapy in which the target gene is inserted into the cell by an AAV vector.

Allele Alternative form of a gene that may occupy a given locus on a pair of chromosomes. Clinical traits, gene products, and disorders are said to be *allelic* if their genes are determined to be at the same locus and *nonallelic* if they are determined to reside at different loci.

Allelic heterogeneity Refers to the capability of different alleles at the same locus to produce an abnormal phenotype.

Aneuploidy An abnormal number of chromosomes.

Anticipation The occurrence of a dominantly inherited disease at an earlier age (often with greater severity) in subsequent generations. Now known to occur with expansion of trinucleotide repeats. Observed, for example, in fragile X syndrome, myotonic dystrophy, and Huntington disease.

Antisense strand of DNA The strand of double-stranded DNA that serves as a template for RNA transcription. Also called the *noncoding,* or *transcribed,* strand.

Apoptosis The process by which internal or external messages trigger expression of specific genes and their products, resulting in the initiation of a series of cellular events that involve fragmentation of the cell nucleus, dissolution of cellular structure, and orderly cell death. Unlike traumatic cell death, apoptosis results in the death of individual cells rather than clusters of cells and does not lead to the release of inflammatory intracellular products. Also called *programmed cell death (PCD).*

Assortative mating Mating between individuals with a preference for or against a specific phenotype or genotype; that is, nonrandom mating.

Autosome Any chromosome other than the sex (X and Y) chromosomes. The normal human has 22 pairs of autosomes.

Barr body Inactive X chromosome found in the nucleus of some female somatic cells.

Base pair (bp) Two complementary nitrogen bases that are paired in double-stranded DNA. Used as a unit of physical distance or length of a sequence of nucleotides.

Biobank A repository that stores biological samples for use in research. The UK Biobank is a collection of DNA samples from more than 500,000 people and, for many participants, ophthalmic phenotype data.

Carrier An individual who has a pair of genes consisting of 1 normal and 1 abnormal, or *mutant,* gene. Usually, such individuals are by definition phenotypically "normal," although in certain disorders biochemical evidence of a deficient or defective gene product may be present. Occasionally, carriers of an X-linked disorder may show partial expression of a genetic trait.

Cell-free fetal DNA (cffDNA) Fetal DNA that circulates freely in the maternal blood and can be sampled by phlebotomy, providing a noninvasive method of prenatal diagnosis. Sometimes called *noninvasive prenatal screening.*

Centimorgan (cM) A measure of the crossover frequency between linked genes; 1 cM equals 1% recombination and represents a physical distance of approximately 1 million bp.

Centromere The constricted region of a chromosome where sister chromatids are joined. It is also the site of attachment to spindle fibers during mitosis and meiosis and is important in the movement of chromosomes to the poles of the dividing cell.

Chorionic villus sampling (CVS) Transcervical procedure in which chorionic villi are retrieved with a flexible suction catheter and used in studies to establish a prenatal diagnosis.

Chromatid One of the duplicate arms (also called *sister chromatids*) of chromosomes that are created after DNA replication during mitosis or the first division of meiosis.

Chromatin The complex of DNA and proteins that is present in chromosomes. Chromatin is found in 2 varieties: euchromatin and heterochromatin. Euchromatin is a lightly packed form of chromatin that is often under active transcription. Heterochromatin consists primarily of genetically inactive satellite sequences such as centromeres, telomeres, and the Barr body.

Clinical heterogeneity The production of different phenotypes by different mutations at the same locus. Examples include macular dystrophy and retinitis pigmentosa from differing mutations of peripherin/*RDS* and Crouzon, Pfeiffer, and Apert syndromes from differing mutations of *FGFR2.* See *Genetic heterogeneity.*

Clinical Laboratory Improvement Amendments (CLIA) A federal program that sets standards for clinical laboratory testing in the United States. Clinicians are advised to use a CLIA-certified laboratory to provide results to their patients.

Codominance Simultaneous expression of both alleles of a heterozygous locus (eg, ABO blood groups).

Codon A sequence of 3 adjacent nucleotides that forms the basic unit of the genetic code. The DNA molecule is a chain of nucleotide bases read in units of 3 bases *(triplets),* each of which will translate through messenger RNA (mRNA) into an amino acid. Thus, each triplet codon specifies a single amino acid.

Complementary DNA (cDNA) DNA created by the action of reverse transcriptase from mRNA. In contrast to genomic DNA, cDNA does not have introns.

Complex genetic disorder (multigene disorder) A trait or medical disorder (eg, age-related macular degeneration) that does not follow mendelian patterns of inheritance. Close relatives have a higher risk of the disorder, suggesting that the state is determined by genes at multiple loci (and that environmental factors may be involved).

Compound heterozygote An individual with 2 different, abnormal alleles at the same locus, 1 on each homologous chromosome.

Congenital Present at birth. The term has no implications about the origin of the congenital feature, which could be genetic or environmental.

Consanguinity The genetic relationship between individuals who are the descendants of a sexual union between blood relatives; in other words, individuals who share a recent common ancestor (eg, offspring of a marriage between cousins).

Conservation Refers to the presence of a similar genetic sequence or nucleotide position among different species at 1 gene or related genes of similar sequence. In such cases, the sequence or position is said to be *conserved* or to show conservation.

Copy number variation A structural variation in the genome resulting from deleted or inserted nucleotides, exons, or genes (also referred to as *indels*). Indels have been used as DNA markers to locate genes but may also cause disease by adding amino acids (eg, in triplet repeat disorders) or may affect gene expression (eg, the expression of color opsins on the X chromosome).

CRISPR–Cas9 (clustered, regularly interspaced, short palindromic repeats–CRISPR-associated protein 9) A new form of genome editing technology used to modify genes in organisms.

Crossing over A process in which matching segments of homologous chromosomes (chromatids) break and are exchanged to the other chromosome, where they are reconnected to the other chromosome by repair of the breaks. Crossing over is a regular event in meiosis but occurs only rarely in mitosis. See *Recombination.*

Database of Genotypes and Phenotypes (dbGaP) Funded by the US National Institutes of Health, a catalog of genetic information (genotypes) linked to clinical information (phenotypes) from results of genome-wide association studies (GWAS).

Degeneracy of genetic code The redundancy of the genetic code stemming from the fact that most of the 20 amino acids are coded for by more than 1 of the 64 possible triplet codons. The genetic code is termed *degenerate.*

Digenic inheritance Simultaneous inheritance of 2 nonallelic mutant genes, giving rise to a genetic disorder in which inheritance of only 1 of the 2 is insufficient to cause disease. Digenic inheritance is the simplest form of polygenic inheritance. An example is retinitis pigmentosa caused by simultaneous inheritance in the heterozygous state of otherwise tolerable mutations of both the *ROM1* and peripherin/*RDS* genes.

Diploid Refers to the number of chromosomes in most somatic cells, which in humans is 46. The diploid number is twice the haploid number (the number of chromosomes in gametes).

Direct-to-consumer genetic tests Genetic tests marketed directly to consumers. An individual orders a test kit directly from a genetic testing laboratory and mails a tissue sample (saliva or blood) back to the laboratory, which runs a series of DNA tests, usually single nucleotide polymorphisms (SNPs) or, in some cases, sequencing. These DNA tests may be specific to certain genes or diseases or may involve a large panel of genes and diseases. Lack of counseling, quality control, and appropriate scientific interpretation of data are major challenges to direct-to-consumer testing.

Dizygotic (DZ) twins Occur when 2 individual ova (eggs) are fertilized by separate sperm, resulting in nonidentical (fraternal) twins, who share 50% of their DNA sequence.

DNA code The sequences of DNA trinucleotides corresponding to the amino acids.

Dominant Refers to an allele that is expressed in the phenotype when inherited along with a normal allele. See *Recessive.*

Dominant medical disorder A distinctive disease state that occurs in an individual with a genotype that is heterozygous for a dominant disease-producing allele. Homozygotes for dominant disease-producing alleles are rare and are usually more severely affected than heterozygotes.

Dominant negative mutation An autosomal dominant mutation that disrupts the function of the normal or wild-type allele in the heterozygous state, producing a phenotype approaching that of the homozygous mutant.

ENCODE (Encyclopedia of DNA Elements) A catalog of functional elements in the human genome (see https://www.genome.gov/encode/).

Endonuclease A phosphodiester-cleaving enzyme, usually derived from bacteria, that cuts nucleic acids at internal positions. Restriction endonucleases cut at specific recognition sites determined by the occurrence of a specific recognition sequence of 4, 5, or 6 bp. Endonuclease specificity may also be confined to substrate conformation, nucleic acid species (DNA, RNA), and the presence of modified nucleotides.

Enhancer Any sequence of DNA upstream or downstream of the coding region that acts in *cis* (ie, on the same chromosome) to increase (or, as a negative enhancer, to decrease) the rate of transcription of a nearby gene. Enhancers may display tissue specificity and act over considerable distances.

Epigenetics/epigenomics The study of modifications of the expression of the genetic code by factors that may themselves be genetically or environmentally influenced. In these cases, gene expression is affected without alteration of the DNA sequence. Examples of such factors include cytosine methylation and histone formation.

Eukaryote Organisms whose DNA is located within a nucleus (includes all multicellular and higher unicellular organisms).

Exome sequencing A strategy to selectively sequence the coding regions of the genome as a less expensive alternative to whole-genome sequencing. Approximately 180,000 exons constitute 1% of the human genome, or approximately 30 megabases (Mb).

Exon A coding sequence of DNA is represented in the mature mRNA product. See *Intron.*

Expressed-sequence tag (EST) A partial sequence of a gene that uniquely identifies the gene's message. These tags are useful in reverse transcriptase polymerase chain reaction (RT-PCR) detection for determining the expression levels of large numbers of genes in parallel reactions.

Expressivity The variation in clinical manifestation among individuals with a particular genotype, usually a dominant medical disorder. The variability may be a difference in either age at onset (manifestation) or severity. See *Penetrance.*

Fragile sites Reproducible sites of secondary constrictions, gaps, or breaks in chromatids. Fragile sites are transmitted as mendelian codominant traits and are not usually associated with abnormal phenotype. The most notable exceptions are the association of fragile X chromosomes with X-linked cognitive impairment and with postpubertal macroorchidism (fragile X syndrome). See *Trinucleotide repeat expansion/contraction.*

Frameshift mutation (framing error, frameshift) A deletion or insertion of a nucleotide or a number of nucleotides not divisible by 3 that results in a loss of the normal sequences of triplets, causing the new sequence to code for entirely different amino acids from the original. The mutation usually leads to the eventual chance formation of a *stop codon.*

Gene The segment of DNA and its associated regulatory elements coding for a single trait, usually a single polypeptide or mRNA. The definition was expanded to include any expressed sequence of nucleotides that has functional significance, including DNA sequences that govern the transcription of a gene (promoter sequences immediately upstream of the gene or enhancer sequences that may be more distantly located).

Genetic heterogeneity The production of a phenotype (or apparently similar phenotypes) by different genetic entities. Refers to genetic disorders that are found to be two or more fundamentally distinct entities. See *Clinical heterogeneity.*

Genetic Information Nondiscrimination Act (GINA) A law enacted by the US Congress in 2008 to prohibit the improper use of genetic information by health insurance providers and employers.

Genome The sum of the genetic material of a cell or an organism.

Genome-wide association studies (GWAS) Research studies that examine the associations between single nucleotide polymorphisms (SNPs) and traits or diseases by comparing the DNA of a group of people with a particular disease (cases) and another, similar group without that disease (controls). Hundreds of thousands of SNPs are read on arrays in studies designed to find common ancestral mutations that contribute risk for disease.

Genomic imprinting Imprinting is an epigenetic phenomenon that causes genes to be expressed in a parent-of-origin-specific manner. It involves DNA methylation and histone methylation without altering the genetic sequence. These epigenetic marks are established *(imprinted)* in the germline (sperm or egg cells) of the parents and are maintained through mitotic cell divisions in the somatic cells of an offspring. Appropriate imprinting of certain genes is important for normal development. Diseases resulting from abnormalities of genomic imprinting include Angelman syndrome and Prader-Willi syndrome.

Genomics The study of the genome. Names for the fields of *transcriptomics, proteomics,* and *metabolomics* were coined in a similar fashion.

Genotype The genetic constitution of an organism. Also, the specific set of 2 alleles inherited at a locus.

Germinal mosaicism The occurrence of 2 populations of gametes in an individual, 1 population with a normal allele and the other with a disease-producing mutant gene. Of new cases of some autosomal dominant diseases (eg, osteogenesis imperfecta), 5%–10% are thought to result from germinal mosaicism; offspring of the affected parent are at significant risk for the same disease.

Haploid Half the number of chromosomes in most somatic cells; equal to the number of chromosomes in gametes. In humans, the haploid number is 23. Also used to denote the state in which only 1 of a pair or set of chromosomes is present. See *Diploid.*

Haploid insufficiency (haploinsufficiency) The condition of dominant genetic disease caused by a reduction in the gene product to levels that are insufficient to produce the desired function of the protein. For example, aniridia and Waardenburg syndrome result from insufficiency of the single functional copy of the *PAX6* and *PAX3* genes, respectively, to activate transcription of the genes that they normally control.

Haplotype A series of contiguous alleles along the length of a single chromosome that may be inherited as a block. Also referred to as a *haploblock.*

HapMap The haplotype map of the human genome describing the common patterns of human genetic variation. A key resource in finding variants affecting health and disease.

Hemizygous (hemizygote) Having only 1 allele at a locus; usually refers to X-linked loci in males, who normally have only 1 set of X-linked genes. An individual who is missing an entire chromosome or a segment of 1 chromosome is considered hemizygous for the genes on the homologous chromosome. See *Heterozygous, Homozygous.*

Hereditary Genetically transmitted or capable of being genetically transmitted from parent to offspring. Not quite synonymous with *heritable,* which implies the ability to be transmitted to the next generation but does not intrinsically connote inheritance from the prior generation.

Heteroplasmy The presence of two or more different populations of mitochondria within a cell, each population carrying a different allele (or the presence or absence of a mutation) at a given locus.

Heterozygous (heterozygote) Having 2 unlike alleles at a particular locus. See *Hemizygous, Homozygous.*

Homeobox A conserved 180-bp sequence of DNA, first detected within homeobox genes (also known as *homeotic selector genes*), that helps determine the cell's fate.

Homeobox genes Transcription factor genes that regulate the activity or expression of other genes, eventually guiding the embryonic development of cells into body segments, body parts, and specialized organ systems. Examples are the *HOX* and *PAX* families of developmental genes. Whereas *HOX* genes are involved in early body plan organization, *PAX* genes are involved in somewhat later organ and body part development. See the discussion of homeobox genes in Chapter 4.

Homologous chromosomes The 2 members of a matched pair of (sister) chromosomes, 1 derived from each parent, that have the same gene loci, but not necessarily the same alleles, in the same order.

Homoplasmy The presence of a single population of mitochondria within a cell, each carrying the same allele (or the same presence or absence of a mutation) at a given locus.

Homozygous (homozygote) Having 2 identical alleles at a particular locus in the diploid genome. The term is sometimes misused to refer to *compound heterozygote* (see earlier entry).

Human Genome Project (HGP) The international scientific research project that identified and mapped the approximately 20,000–25,000 human genes. A working draft of the genome was announced in 2000, and the genome was completed in 2003.

Hybridization The bonding (by Watson-Crick base pairing) of single-stranded DNA or RNA into double-stranded DNA or RNA. The ability of stretches of DNA or RNA to hybridize with one another is highly dependent on complementarity of the base-pair sequence.

Induced pluripotent stem cells (iPSCs) Adult cells such as skin fibroblasts can be induced to produce pluripotent stem cells by using transcription factors. iPSCs hold great promise in the field of regenerative medicine and can be used to create every type of cell (eg, retinal cells that could be used to replace cells lost to damage or disease). Because iPSCs are derived from adult tissues, they not only bypass the need for embryos but also can be made in a patient-matched manner, which means that each individual could have his or her own pluripotent stem cell line. These autologous cells reduce the risk of immune rejection. iPSCs are also used for research purposes; for example, retinal cells that are difficult to obtain from patients can be created for research purposes ("disease in a dish").

Intron A noncoding segment of DNA that is transcribed into heterogeneous RNA but is ultimately removed from the transcript by splicing together the sequences on either side of it (exons) when mature mRNA is produced. See *Exon.*

Karyotype An image of an individual's chromosome set obtained from a single somatic cell and arranged in a standard pattern in pairs by size, shape, band pattern, and other identifiable physical features.

Kilobase (kb) 1000 bp of DNA or 1000 bases of single-stranded RNA.

Library A complete set of clones presumably including all genetic material of interest from an organism, tissue, or specific cell type at a specified stage of development. A *genomic library* contains cloned DNA fragments from the entire genome; a *cDNA library* contains fragments of cloned DNA generated by reverse transcription from mRNA. Genomic libraries are useful sources to search for genes, whereas cDNA libraries provide information about expression within the source cell or tissue.

Linkage A concept that refers to loci rather than to the alleles that reside on those loci. Exists when the loci of 2 genes or DNA sequences are physically close enough to each other on the same chromosome that alleles at the 2 loci do not assort independently at meiosis but tend to be inherited together.

Linkage disequilibrium Alleles residing at loci that are close together in the genome are inherited together through many generations because the close physical distance makes crossover between the loci extremely unlikely. Alleles in linkage disequilibrium are present in subpopulations (eg, those with a given disease) at a frequency higher or lower than expected based on chance alone.

Locus The physical site on a chromosome occupied by a particular gene. The term is often colloquially used interchangeably with *gene.*

Locus heterogeneity The production of a similar disease or trait (phenotype) by mutations in genes at different chromosomal loci, for example, X-linked retinitis pigmentosa resulting from *RP2* at 1 locus, Xp11, and *RP3* at another locus, Xp21. However, only 1 mutant *locus* is needed for the phenotype to manifest.

LOD (*lo*garithm of *od*ds, or logarithm of the likelihood ratio) A statistical method that tests whether a set of linkage data indicates that 2 loci are linked or unlinked. The *LOD score* is the logarithm to the base 10 of the odds favoring linkage. By convention, an LOD score greater than 3 (1000:1 odds in favor of linkage) is generally accepted as proof of linkage.

Lyonization Inactivation of genes on either the maternally or the paternally derived X chromosome in somatic cells. The timing of inactivation is variable but may occur around the time of implantation. First proposed by geneticist Mary Lyon.

Manhattan plot A type of plot used in genome-wide association studies (GWAS). Genomic coordinates are displayed along the x-axis, with the negative logarithm of the association *P* value for each single nucleotide polymorphism (SNP) displayed on the y-axis. The strongest associations appear as peaks, calling to mind the skyline of New York City.

Meiosis The special form of cell division that occurs in germ cells by which gametes of haploid chromosomal number are created. Each of the chromatids, which are clearly visible by prophase, contains a long double helix of DNA associated with histones and other chromosomal proteins. At anaphase, the chromatids separate at the centromere and migrate to each half of the dividing cell; thus, each daughter cell receives an identical set of chromatids (which become the chromosomes for that cell). During the first, or *reduction,* division of meiosis, the chromatids of homologous chromosomes undergo crossover (during the diplotene phase), and the number of chromosomes is reduced to the haploid number by the separation of homologous chromosomes (with duplicate chromatids) to each daughter cell. During the second division of meiosis, the sister chromatids separate to form the haploid set of chromosomes of each gamete.

Mendelian disorder (single-gene disorder) A trait or medical disorder that follows patterns of inheritance suggesting the state is determined by a gene at a single locus (eg, autosomal dominant, autosomal recessive, or X-linked recessive inheritance).

Methylation The attachment of methyl groups to DNA at CpG (cytosine-phosphate-guanine) sites. CpG islands are associated with the promoters of many genes, and there is an inverse relationship between CpG methylation and transcriptional activity.

MicroRNA (miRNA) Small single-stranded RNA fragment (of approximately 22 nucleotides) that directly interacts with target mRNA through complementary base pairing and inhibits translation of the target genes. miRNA modifies gene expression at transcriptional and posttranscriptional levels.

Microsatellites (eg, dinucleotide or trinucleotide repeats) Tandemly repeated segments scattered throughout the genome of varying numbers of 2–4 nucleotides in a row, for example, a stretch of consecutive CA combinations of bases (NNNCACACACACACACACACACANNN or $[CA]_{10}$, where N is any base) in a DNA strand. The repeats are inherently unstable and can undergo mutation at a rate of up to 10%. Defects of some microsatellites are associated with cancer and insulin-dependent diabetes mellitus, although most have no known biological significance. Other terms used are *variable number of tandem repeats (VNTR)* and *variable tandem repeats (VTR).* The highly variable nature of the number of repeats provides information useful as markers for establishing linkage to disease loci.

Missense mutation A mutation, often the change of a single nucleotide, that results in the substitution of 1 amino acid for another in the final gene product.

Mitosis The ordinary form of cell division, which results in daughter cells identical in chromosomal number to the parent cell.

Monozygotic (MZ) twins Identical twins who share 100% of their DNA sequence.

Mosaicism The presence of two or more populations of cells with different genotypes in 1 individual who has developed from a single fertilized egg. Mosaicism can occur in the cells of 1 part of the body (eg, the retina) or in all cells of an individual.

Multifactorial inheritance The combined operation of several unspecified genetic and environmental factors in the inheritance of a particular trait or disease. See *Polygenic inheritance.*

Mutation Any alteration of a gene or genetic material from its "natural" state, regardless of whether the change has a positive, neutral, or negative effect.

Next-generation sequencing (massively parallel DNA sequencing) Sequencing technology that speeds the process, producing thousands or millions of DNA sequences at once. This technology has allowed rapid, large-scale DNA sequencing at much lower cost.

Nondisjunction Failure of 2 chromosomes to separate during meiosis or mitosis.

Nonsense mutation Any mutation that either results directly in the formation of a stop codon or creates a stop codon in the downstream sequence after a frameshift mutation. This typically results in a truncated nonfunctional protein.

Nucleoside The combination of a nitrogen-containing base and a 5-carbon sugar. The 5 nucleosides are adenosine (A), guanosine (G), cytidine (C), uridine (U), and thymidine (T). Note that the abbreviations are the same as those for the nitrogen bases that characterize the nucleoside.

Nucleosome The primary unit of chromatin, consisting of a 146-bp sequence of DNA wrapped twice around a core composed of 8 histone molecules.

Nucleotide The combination of a nucleoside and one or more phosphate groups. *Purine nucleotides* have a nitrogen-containing base of adenine (A) and guanine (G) in DNA or RNA. *Pyrimidine nucleotides* have a nitrogen-containing base of thymine (T) and cytosine (C) in DNA and uracil (U) in RNA.

OMIM (Online Mendelian Inheritance in Man) An online database of genes and genetic disorders (see https://omim.org).

Oncogene A gene that, when dysregulated, is capable of transforming cells into a neoplastic phenotype characterized by loss of growth control and/or tumorigenesis in a suitable host or site. In many cases, cancer is caused by the growth-stimulating effects of increased expression, protein activation, or aberrant regulation of transcription factors required for normal growth. Certain oncogenes are produced by chromosomal translocations of normal transcription factor genes to regions adjacent to more abundantly expressed genes, causing inappropriate excessive expression. See *Tumor suppressor genes.*

1000 Genomes Project An international collaboration, launched in 2008, to compile the most detailed public catalog of human genetic variation.

Open reading frame (ORF) Any part of the genome that could be translated into a protein sequence starting with an initiation (start) codon and ending with a stop codon.

p arm The short arm of a chromosome in relation to the centromere. From *petit*. See *q arm*.

Penetrance The probability of detecting the clinical expression of a gene or combination of genes when they are present. If the penetrance of a particular condition is less than 100%, not all individuals who carry the responsible gene variant will develop the condition. Nonpenetrance is the lack of phenotypic evidence of the genotype. See *Expressivity.*

Personalized genetics The use of personal genomic data to determine care, including drug treatment, for an individual patient.

Pharmacogenetics The study of the influence of genetic variation on drug efficacy or toxicity, focusing on single genes. The term is often used interchangeably with *pharmacogenomics.*

Pharmacogenomics The study of how the genetic makeup of an individual affects his or her response to drugs; in other words, the focus is on many genes.

Phenocopy The occurrence of a particular clinical phenotype as a result of either a non-mutagenic environmental factor (eg, exposure to a drug or virus) or an atypical genetic defect, when the more usually associated genetic defect is absent.

Phenotype The observable or manifest physical, physiologic, biochemical, or molecular characteristics of an individual, either in whole or with regard to one or more traits, which are determined by the genotype but can be modified by the environment.

Pleiotropism Refers to multiple end effects (in different organ systems) arising from a single mutant gene or gene pair.

Polygenic inheritance Inheritance determined by the operation of two or more genes. See *Multifactorial inheritance.*

Polymerase chain reaction (PCR) A technique by which segments of DNA or RNA can be amplified by use of flanking oligonucleotides called *primers* and repeated cycles of amplification with DNA polymerase. The steps involve

- heating to separate the molecules into single-stranded DNA
- repeated annealing to the complementary target DNA sequences or primers specifically designed to delimit the beginning and ending of the target segment
- extension of the primer sequences with the enzyme DNA polymerase, creating double-stranded DNA
- separation of the products into single-stranded DNA

In effect, the amount of DNA is doubled with each cycle. Often, 30 or more cycles are used to obtain sufficient amplification for further testing.

Real-time PCR, or *quantitative PCR (qPCR),* is used to simultaneously amplify and quantify a targeted DNA molecule. *Digital PCR (dPCR)* is a refinement used to directly quantify and clonally amplify nucleic acids. It is a more precise method than qPCR because it allows for more reliable collection and more sensitive measurement of nucleic acid amounts. qPCR is useful for studying variations in gene sequences (eg, copy number variations and point mutations) and is routinely used to amplify samples for *next-generation sequencing.*

Polymorphism The occurrence of two or more alleles at a specific locus with a frequency greater than 1% each in a given population.

Posttranslational modifications Biochemical changes to or modifications of gene products after translation, including removal of amino acids from the end of the peptide, addition or removal of sugars, and addition of lipid side chains or phosphate groups to specific sites in the protein. Often, such changes are essential for proper protein localization or function.

Preimplantation genetic diagnosis (PGD) A genetic test used with in vitro fertilization when one or both parents have a known genetic abnormality. Testing is performed on cells removed from embryos in order to select one or more embryos that are free of the genetic condition.

Prenatal diagnosis (PND) Genetic testing performed during pregnancy using amniocentesis, chorionic villus sampling (CVS), or cell-free fetal DNA (cffDNA) to determine whether a fetus carries a genetic abnormality and allow parents to make reproductive choices.

Proband The affected person whose disorder, or concern about a disorder, brings a family or pedigree to be genetically evaluated. Also called the *propositus* (male), *proposita* (female), or *index case.*

Promoter The sequence of nucleotides upstream (5′) from the coding sequence of a gene that determines the site of binding of RNA polymerase and, hence, initiation of transcription. Different promoters for the same gene may exist and can result in alternately spliced gene products and tissue-specific expression. The promoter may contain the consensus DNA sequence (the so-called TATA box) approximately 25–30 bp (5′) upstream from the transcription start site.

Pseudodominance The appearance of vertical transmission of a recessive genetic disorder from 1 generation to the next due to an unusually high carrier frequency of a recessive allele and the resultant mating of an affected homozygote with an unaffected heterozygote, which results in 50% of offspring being affected. Pseudodominance implies recessive disease that has the appearance of dominant inheritance.

Pseudogene A defective copy of a gene that often lacks introns and is rarely, if ever, expressed. Some pseudogenes are thought to arise by reverse transcription of mRNA that has had the introns spliced out. Others, such as globin pseudogenes, arise from silencing of a tandem duplicate. Because they are released from conservation (the maintenance of essential DNA sequences necessary for function) through selection, pseudogenes often contain numerous base-pair changes and other mutational events (compared with the original functional gene).

q arm The long arm of a chromosome. See *p arm.*

Recessive Classically, describes a gene that results in a phenotype only in the homozygous or compound heterozygous state. See *Dominant.*

Recessive medical disorder A disease state whose occurrence requires a homozygous (or compound heterozygous) genotype—that is, a double "dose" of the mutant allele. Heterozygotes are typically clinically normal.

Recombinant An individual with a combination of genes on a single chromosome unlike that in either parent. Usually applied to linkage analysis, in which *recombinant* refers to a haplotype (a set of alleles on a specific chromosome) that is not present in either parent because of a recombination crossover.

Recombinant DNA DNA that has been cut out of a single organism, reinserted into the DNA of a vector (plasmid or phage), and then reimplanted into a host cell. Also, any DNA that has been altered for further use.

Recombination The formation of a new set of alleles on a single chromosome unlike that in either parent. Due to crossover during meiosis. See *Crossing over.*

Reference genomes DNA sequences from control subjects in selected populations including the International HapMap and 1000 Genomes Projects.

Relatives, first-degree Individuals who share on average half of their genetic material with the proband: parents, siblings, offspring.

Relatives, second-degree Individuals who share on average one-fourth of their genetic material with the proband: grandparents, aunts and uncles, nieces and nephews, grandchildren.

Replication Creation of a new linear DNA copy by the enzyme DNA polymerase, proceeding from the 5′ side of bound primer to the 3′ end of the DNA sequence. Replication of DNA occurs during chromosomal duplication.

Replication slippage An error of DNA replication or copying. Because of the similarity of repeated base-pair sequences, one or more repeats may be skipped over and not represented in the copied DNA sequence.

Replicative segregation The process by which, through partitioning of copies of mitochondrial DNA (mtDNA) to each daughter cell during division, some cells receive a preponderance of normal or mutant copies. Replicative segregation tends to result in conversion of heteroplasmy to homoplasmy with associated development of disease within the affected tissue, if the tissue becomes homoplasmic for the mutant mtDNA. This phenomenon explains the development of new organ-system involvement in multisystem mitochondrial diseases.

Reverse transcription The process, performed by the enzyme reverse transcriptase, in which mRNA is converted back to DNA. If the introns have already been spliced out of the precursor mRNA, the product of this process is cDNA.

Sanger sequencing The chain-termination method of sequencing DNA based on incorporating dideoxynucleotide molecules.

Segregation The separation of pairs of alleles at meiosis.

Sex-linked Refers to genes on the X or Y (sex) chromosome. The term is often used improperly to mean X-linked.

Short interfering RNA (siRNA) A double-stranded RNA molecule (of 20–25 nucleotides) that plays a role in the RNA interference pathway, where it interferes with the expression of genes with complementary nucleotide sequences. Also known as *small interference RNA.*

Simplex A term denoting that only 1 individual within a given family is affected by a condition known to have a heritable component. Thus, a single male or female with a genetic disease is called a *simplex case.* The term *isolated* is also sometimes used.

Single nucleotide polymorphism (SNP) Variation in a single base pair in a nucleotide sequence in the genome that occurs in more than 1% of the population. SNPs are rarely mutations that cause disease, are occasionally linked to disease-causing mutations, and usually are of unknown significance.

Single-nucleotide variant (SNV) A single-nucleotide difference (substitution). The definition of SNV does not imply how often the variant occurs in a population.

Southern blotting A method used in molecular biology for detection of a specific DNA sequence. Southern blotting combines transfer of electrophoresis-separated DNA fragments to a filter membrane and subsequent fragment detection by probe hybridization. Northern blotting is a similar process performed with RNA and Western blotting with protein.

Splice junction site The DNA region that demarcates the boundaries between exons and introns. The specific sequence determines whether the site acts as a 5′ donor or a 3′ acceptor site during splicing. Single-base-pair changes or mutations that involve splice junction sites may result in skipping of the following exon or incorporation of part of the adjacent intron into the mature mRNA.

Splicing Process by which the introns are removed from the precursor mRNA and the exons are joined together as mature mRNA prior to translation. Takes place within *spliceosomes,* specialized structures composed of RNA and proteins.

Sporadic A trait that occurs in a single member of a kindred with no other family members affected. The term has been used by some geneticists to imply that the trait is nongenetic.

Stop codon (termination codon) The DNA triplet that causes translation to end when the translation is coded into mRNA. The DNA stop codons are TAG, TAA, and TGA. Expressed as mRNA, these are UAG, UAA, and UGA.

Telomeric DNA A type of highly repetitive satellite DNA that forms the tips of chromosomes and prevents them from fraying or joining. It decreases in size as a consequence of the normal mechanisms of DNA replication in mitosis and may be important in cellular senescence. Defects in the maintenance of telomeres may play a role in cancer formation.

Threshold In polygenic or multifactorial inheritance, a relatively sharp qualitative difference beyond which individuals are considered affected. The threshold is presumed to have been reached by the cumulative effects of the polygenic and multifactorial influences.

Transcription The synthesis, as catalyzed by a DNA-dependent RNA polymerase, of a single-stranded RNA molecule from the antisense strand of a double-stranded DNA template in the cell nucleus.

Translation The process by which a polypeptide is synthesized from a sequence of specific mRNA.

Translocation The transfer of a part of 1 chromosome to a nonhomologous chromosome.

Trinucleotide repeat expansion/contraction The process by which long sequences of multiple triplet codons (see *Microsatellites*) are lengthened or shortened in the course of gene replication. The process of expansion of trinucleotide repeats over consecutive generations results in the genetic phenomenon of *anticipation.* The underlying mechanisms for expansion (or contraction) appear to be replication slippage and unequal crossing over in the region of the repeats. Most disorders involving trinucleotide repeats are dominant in inheritance (eg, fragile X syndrome, myotonic dystrophy, Huntington disease, and Kennedy disease), but 1 is autosomal recessive (Friedreich ataxia). See *Fragile sites.*

Tumor suppressor genes Genes that must be present in 1 fully functional copy to prevent uncontrolled cell proliferation. Two "hits" (mutations) of the gene, one for each allele, must occur in a given cell for tumor formation to occur. Examples include the genes for retinoblastoma, Wilms tumor, tuberous sclerosis, p53, ataxia-telangiectasia, and von Hippel–Lindau syndrome. Also called *antioncogenes.* See *Oncogene.*

Unequal crossing over An error in the events of chromosomal duplication and cell division occurring during meiosis and, in rare cases, during mitosis. Probably because of similar sequences or repeated segments, chromosomal exchange occurs between nonhomologous regions of the chromosome, resulting in duplication and deletion of genetic material in the daughter cells.

Uniparental disomy The conveyance to an offspring of 2 copies of an abnormal gene or chromosome by only 1 parent (the other parent makes no contribution). The child can be affected with autosomal recessive disease even if only 1 of the parents is a carrier of the abnormal gene. This occurrence has been reported in Stargardt disease, cystic fibrosis, Prader-Willi syndrome, and Angelman syndrome.

Untranslated region (UTR) The region upstream (5′ UTR) or downstream (3′ UTR) of the open reading frame (ORF) of a gene. The 5′ UTR contains the promoter and part or all of the regulatory regions of the gene. The 3′ UTR also serves important functions in regulation and mRNA stability.

Variant A change in the DNA sequence. Historically, a variant that affects function or causes disease (pathogenic variant) is called a *mutation.*

Variant of unknown significance A DNA change found in an individual that has not yet been reliably characterized as benign or pathogenic and/or whose functional consequences are uncertain.

Vector A viral, bacteriophage, or plasmid DNA molecule into which a stretch of genomic DNA or cDNA or a specific gene can be inserted. The λ-bacteriophage can accept segments of DNA up to 25 kb long. Cosmid vectors can accommodate a segment 40 kb long. BAC (bacterial artificial chromosome) and YAC (yeast artificial chromosome) vectors can accept much larger fragments of DNA. Viral vectors such as *adeno-associated virus (AAV)* have been used in gene therapy trials.

Whole-exome sequencing (WES) A laboratory technique for sequencing all the known protein-coding genes in an organism's genome (known as the *exome*).

Whole-genome sequencing (WGS) A laboratory process to determine the complete DNA sequence of an organism's genome.

Wild type A normal phenotype of an organism. Also, a normal allele as compared with a mutant allele.

X-linked Refers to genes on the X chromosome.

Y-linked Refers to genes on the Y chromosome.

Basic Texts

General Ophthalmology

Forrester JV, Dick AD, McMenamin PG, Roberts F, Pearlman E. *The Eye: Basic Sciences in Practice*. 5th ed. Edinburgh: Elsevier; 2021.

Anatomy and Histology

Bron AJ, Tripathi RC, Tripathi BJ, eds. *Wolff's Anatomy of the Eye and Orbit*. 8th ed. London: Chapman & Hall; 1997.

Dutton JJ. *Atlas of Clinical and Surgical Orbital Anatomy*. 2nd ed. Philadelphia: Saunders; 2011.*

Hogan MJ, Alvarado JA, Weddell JE. *Histology of the Human Eye: An Atlas and Textbook*. Philadelphia: Saunders; 1971.

Miller NR, Newman NJ, eds. *Walsh & Hoyt's Clinical Neuro-Ophthalmology, Volume 1*. 6th ed. Philadelphia: Lippincott Williams & Wilkins; 2005.*

Snell RS, Lemp MA. *Clinical Anatomy of the Eye*. 2nd ed. Malden, MA: Wiley-Blackwell; 1998.*

Spalton DJ, Hitchings RA, Hunter PA, eds. *Atlas of Clinical Ophthalmology*. 3rd ed. Oxford: Elsevier; 2005.

Tasman W, Jaeger EA, eds. *Duane's Ophthalmology on DVD-ROM, 2013 Edition*. Philadelphia: Lippincott Williams & Wilkins; 2013.

Zide BM, ed. *Surgical Anatomy Around the Orbit: The System of Zones*. Philadelphia: Lippincott Williams & Wilkins; 2006.

Embryology and Genetics

Couser NL. *Ophthalmic Genetic Diseases: A Quick Reference Guide to the Eye and External Ocular Adnexa Abnormalities*. St Louis: Elsevier; 2019.

Jakobiec FA, ed. *Ocular Anatomy, Embryology, and Teratology*. Philadelphia: Harper & Row; 1982.

Merin S. *Inherited Eye Diseases: Diagnosis and Management*. 2nd ed. Boca Raton, FL: Taylor & Francis; 2005.

Nussbaum RL, McInnes RR, Willard HF. *Thompson & Thompson Genetics in Medicine*. 8th ed. Philadelphia: Elsevier/Saunders; 2016.

Schoenwolf GC, Bleyl SB, Brauer PR, Francis-West PH, eds. *Larsen's Human Embryology*. 5th ed. Philadelphia: Elsevier/Churchill Livingstone; 2015.

Traboulsi EI, ed. *Genetic Diseases of the Eye*. 2nd ed. New York: Oxford University Press; 2012.

* Also see the embryology section in this book.

Biochemistry and Metabolism

Levin LA, Nilsson SFE, Ver Hoeve J, Wu SM, eds. *Adler's Physiology of the Eye*. 11th ed. Philadelphia: Elsevier/Saunders; 2011.

Whikehart DR. *Biochemistry of the Eye*. Boston: Butterworth-Heinemann; 2003.

Ocular Pharmacology

Bartlett JD, Jaanus SD, eds. *Clinical Ocular Pharmacology*. 5th ed. St Louis: Elsevier/Butterworth-Heinemann; 2008.

Brunton LL, Hilal-Dandan R, Knollman BC, eds. *Goodman & Gilman's The Pharmacological Basis of Therapeutics*. 13th ed. New York: McGraw-Hill Education; 2018.

Zimmerman TJ, Karanjit K, Mordechaie S, Fechtner RD, eds. *Textbook of Ocular Pharmacology*. 3rd ed. Philadelphia: Lippincott Williams & Wilkins; 1997.

Imaging

Bhatti MT, Schmalfuss I. *Handbook of Neuroimaging for the Ophthalmologist*. London: JP Medical; 2014.

Dutton JJ. *Radiology of the Orbit and Visual Pathways*. Philadelphia: Elsevier/Saunders; 2010.

Müller-Forell WS. *Imaging of Orbital and Visual Pathway Pathology*. New York: Springer; 2006.

Singh AD, Hayden BC. *Ophthalmic Ultrasonography*. Philadelphia: Elsevier/Saunders; 2012.

Related Academy Materials

The American Academy of Ophthalmology is dedicated to providing a wealth of high-quality clinical education resources for ophthalmologists.

Print Publications and Electronic Products

For a complete listing of Academy products related to topics covered in this BCSC Section, visit our online store at https://store.aao.org/clinical-education/topic/comprehensive-ophthalmology.html. Or call Customer Service at 866.561.8558 (toll free, US only) or +1 415.561.8540, Monday through Friday, between 8:00 AM and 5:00 PM (PST).

Online Resources

Visit the Ophthalmic News and Education (ONE®) Network at https://www.aao.org/comprehensive-ophthalmology to find relevant videos, online courses, journal articles, practice guidelines, self-assessment quizzes, images, and more. The ONE Network is a free Academy-member benefit.

Access free, trusted articles and content with the Academy's collaborative online encyclopedia, EyeWiki, at aao.org/eyewiki.

Get mobile access to the *Wills Eye Manual,* watch the latest 1-minute videos, and set up alerts for clinical updates relevant to you with the AAO Ophthalmic Education App. Download today: Search for "AAO Ophthalmic Education" in the Apple app store or in Google Play.

Requesting Continuing Medical Education Credit

The American Academy of Ophthalmology is accredited by the Accreditation Council for Continuing Medical Education (ACCME) to provide continuing medical education for physicians.

The American Academy of Ophthalmology designates this enduring material for a maximum of 15 *AMA PRA Category 1 Credits*™. Physicians should claim only the credit commensurate with the extent of their participation in the activity.

To claim *AMA PRA Category 1 Credits*™ upon completion of this activity, learners must demonstrate appropriate knowledge and participation in the activity by taking the posttest for Section 2 and achieving a score of 80% or higher.

This activity meets the Self-Assessment CME requirements defined by the American Board of Ophthalmology (ABO). Please be advised that the ABO is not an accrediting body for purposes of any CME program. ABO does not sponsor this or any outside activity, and ABO does not endorse any particular CME activity. Complete information regarding the ABO Self-Assessment CME Maintenance of Certification requirements is available at https://abop.org/maintain-certification/cme-self-assessment/.

To take the posttest and request CME credit online:

1. Go to www.aao.org/cme-central and log in.
2. Click on "Claim CME Credit and View My CME Transcript" and then "Report AAO Credits."
3. Select the appropriate media type and then the Academy activity. You will be directed to the posttest.
4. Once you have passed the test with a score of 80% or higher, you will be directed to your transcript. *If you are not an Academy member, you will be able to print out a certificate of participation once you have passed the test.*

CME expiration date: June 1, 2023. *AMA PRA Category 1 Credits*™ may be claimed only once between June 1, 2019, and the expiration date.

For assistance, contact the Academy's Customer Service department at 866-561-8558 (US only) or +1 415-561-8540 between 8:00 AM and 5:00 PM (PST), Monday through Friday, or send an e-mail to customer_service@aao.org.

Study Questions

Please note that these questions are not part of your CME reporting process. They are provided here for your own educational use and identification of any professional practice gaps. The required CME posttest is available online (see "Requesting CME Credit"). Following the questions are a blank answer sheet and answers with discussions. Although a concerted effort has been made to avoid ambiguity and redundancy in these questions, the authors recognize that differences of opinion may occur regarding the "best" answer. The discussions are provided to demonstrate the rationale used to derive the answer. They may also be helpful in confirming that your approach to the problem was correct or, if necessary, in fixing the principle in your memory. The Section 2 faculty thanks the Self-Assessment Committee for developing these self-assessment questions.

1. The annulus of Zinn consists of superior and inferior orbital tendons and is the origin of which extraocular muscles?
    a. inferior and superior oblique muscles
    b. inferior rectus and inferior oblique muscles
    c. levator palpebrae and superior oblique muscles
    d. inferior and superior rectus muscles

2. In the evaluation of a scleral wound following trauma, it is important to measure the full extent of the lesion. What external landmark of the eye gives the approximate location of the ora serrata?
    a. entrance of the anterior ciliary arteries through the sclera
    b. insertion of the 4 rectus muscle tendons
    c. insertion of the superior oblique tendon
    d. insertion of the inferior oblique tendon

3. Symptoms relating to dry eye are among the most common reasons patients seek medical attention for their eyes. The precorneal tear film (ie, tear film) consists of secretions from the lacrimal glands, goblet cells, and meibomian glands. The meibomian glands release their product via which secretory mechanism?
    a. endocrine
    b. eccrine
    c. apocrine
    d. holocrine

4. Alterations in glucose metabolism can result in cataract formation. Under normal physiologic conditions, what is the primary pathway by which glucose is converted into adenosine triphosphate (ATP) in the human lens?
   a. aerobic metabolism
   b. glycolysis
   c. hexose monophosphate shunt (also called *pentose phosphate pathway*)
   d. polyol pathway (sorbitol-aldose reductase pathway)

5. Durring cataract surgery, capsulorrhexis is performed on the anterior lens capsule. The lens capsule is composed of what type of collagen?
   a. type I
   b. type II
   c. type III
   d. type IV

6. Where are the oldest proteins in the lens located?
   a. in the nucleus
   b. in the cortex
   c. in the subcapsular region
   d. at the equator

7. Traumatic cataracts form rapidly because of a violation of the lens capsule and secondary hydration of the lens, which is due to the oncotic pressure of the lens. Proteins constitute what percentage of the weight of the lens?
   a. 11%
   b. 22%
   c. 33%
   d. 44%

8. The vitreoretinal interface is the site of many conditions affecting the retina, such as idiopathic macular holes and retinal detachment. The rigidity of the vitreous gel is greatest in regions with the highest concentration of what substance?
   a. hyaluronan
   b. water
   c. collagen
   d. fibronectin

9. A mutation in a gene encoding type II collagen, leading to premature liquefaction of vitreous with peripheral condensation that may induce retinal detachment, is seen in what genetic disease?
   a. Marfan syndrome
   b. Stickler syndrome
   c. retinitis pigmentosa
   d. familial exudative vitreoretinopathy

10. What type of collagen is the major structural component of vitreous collagen fibers?
    a. type I
    b. type II
    c. type III
    d. type XII

11. Rods are significantly more senstive to light stimulus than are cones. What is the effect of a light stimulus on the membrane potential of rods and cones?
    a. depolarization
    b. hyperpolarization
    c. no change in polarization
    d. depolarization followed by hyperpolarization

12. What class of retinal cells functions as the resident macrophages and is activated under stress?
    a. microglia
    b. macroglia
    c. pericytes
    d. amacrine cells

13. Mutations in the various proteins involved in the visual cycle and phototransduction are responsible for a number of inherited retinal diseases. Phototransduction in rods begins with rhodopsin. Once activated by light, rhodopsin is finally inactivated by what chemical process?
    a. breaking of the 11-*cis*-retinal double bond
    b. phosphorylation by rhodopsin kinase and binding of arrestin
    c. inflow of cations into the outer segment
    d. release of glutamate from the synaptic terminal

14. Imaging modalities utilize the property of fundus autofluorescence to study diseases of the retina. What is the source of fundus autofluorescence?
    a. melanin in retinal pigment epithelium (RPE)
    b. lipofuscin in RPE
    c. rhodopsin in photoreceptors
    d. retinal vasculature

15. What gene is the cause of Leber congenital amaurosis (LCA) and now utilized in a treatment that uses adeno-associated virus delivery?
    a. *RPE65*
    b. guanylate cyclase
    c. *TIMP3*
    d. *ABCR*

16. Electrophysiologic tests are important because they provide objective data regarding the function of various parts of our visual system. What electrophysiologic test evaluates the RPE?
    a. electro-oculogram
    b. multifocal electroretinogram
    c. pattern electroretinogram
    d. visual evoked potential

17. The lens is susceptible to damage from various reactive oxygen species because it contains trace amounts of what transition metals?
    a. copper and iron
    b. lead and arsenic
    c. gold and silver
    d. magnesium and germanium

18. Oxidative mechanisms have been described in the etiology of diseases that are the leading causes of irreversible blindness worldwide. What characteristic of the retina makes it more vulnerable to damage from lipid peroxidation?
    a. high number of mitochondria in the rod inner segments
    b. high levels of saturated fatty acids in the rod outer segments
    c. poor oxygen supply through the choroid
    d. low light exposure at night

19. The adverse effects of reactive oxygen species have been repeatedly proposed as causal factors in what ocular disease?
    a. cataract
    b. conjunctivitis
    c. strabismus
    d. posterior capsule opacification

20. What property potentially decreases the bioavailability of a topical ocular drug?
    a. isotonicity
    b. high viscosity
    c. low lipid solubility
    d. mildly basic pH

21. Hemorrhagic occlusive retinal vasculitis develops in a patient 5 days after uneventful cataract surgery. What medication does the ophthalmologist suspect was administered intracamerally during the procedure?
    a. cefuroxime
    b. moxifloxacin
    c. triamcinolone acetonide
    d. vancomycin

22. An ophthalmologist is designing a research project to test the hypothesis that variants in a particular gene affect the efficacy of anti–vascular endothelial growth factor (anti-VEGF) therapies for diabetic macular edema. What discipline does the study fall within?
    a. pharmacodynamics
    b. pharmacokinetics
    c. pharmacogenetics
    d. pharmacogenomics

23. Topical medications can achieve significant systemic concentrations. What ophthalmic topical medication is contraindicated in infants?
    a. timolol
    b. brimonidine
    c. pilocarpine
    d. latanoprost

24. On the basis of their efficacy and dosing regimen, prostaglandin analogues are commonly used in the management of open-angle glaucoma. What is a potential adverse effect of topical prostaglandin analogues?
    a. darkening of the iris
    b. central nervous system depression
    c. bronchospasm
    d. elevated blood pressure

25. What imaging study is best to evaluate a patient with homonymous hemianopia?
    a. magnetic resonance imaging (MRI) with contrast
    b. MRI without contrast
    c. computed tomography (CT) with contrast
    d. CT without contrast

26. An orbital floor fracture is suspected in a 23-year-old patient examined in the emergency department following trauma. What imaging modality is best suited to evaluate the orbit in this case?
    a. ultrasound biomicroscopy
    b. MRI
    c. CT
    d. optical coherence tomography

27. What layer of the retina is responsible for causing the macular star seen in neuroretinitis?
    a. inner plexiform layer
    b. outer plexiform layer
    c. inner nuclear layer
    d. outer nuclear layer

28. Vascular injury to cranial nerve (CN) III (oculomotor nerve) can sometimes affect only 1 of its 2 divisions, resulting in partial cranial nerve palsy. Where does CN III typically separate into superior and inferior divisions?
    a. within the posterior cavernous sinus
    b. within the optic canal
    c. within the superior orbital fissure
    d. within the inferior orbital fissure

29. In what quadrant is a chorioretinal coloboma most likely to be found?
    a. inferonasal
    b. superonasal
    c. inferotemporal
    d. superotemporal

30. The site of primary resistance in open-angle glaucoma is the juxtacanalicular component of the trabecular meshwork. What embryonic tissue is the juxtacanalicular tissue derived from?
    a. neuroectoderm
    b. cranial neural crest
    c. surface ectoderm
    d. mesoderm

31. A 45-year-old woman reports blurry vision all day that is worse upon waking. She has photophobia and a foreign-body sensation that worsen when she is vacationing in Florida. During the examination, the patient has a best-corrected visual acuity of 20/40 in the right eye and 20/30 in the left eye; corneal pachymetry measurements are 602 µm in the right eye and 575 µm in the left eye. Endothelial cell count is decreased, and guttae are noted. The layer of cells that is defective in this patient forms with which wave of neural crest cells in differentiation of the anterior chamber?
    a. first wave
    b. second wave
    c. third wave
    d. fourth wave

32. What information can be given to a male with Leber hereditary optic neuropathy who is planning to have children?
    a. The disease is more prevalent in female offspring.
    b. There is a 50% chance that his offspring will be affected.
    c. The trait will be passed to virtually all his offspring.
    d. The trait will not be transmitted to his offspring.

33. The gene product that is defective in cases of retinoblastoma has what cellular function?
    a. transports cell wall proteins
    b. regulates the cell cycle
    c. contributes to cellular structure
    d. produces energy

34. A 28-year-old female patient has 4+ guttae and visually significant corneal edema in both eyes, requiring surgery. During the initial intake and examination, the ophthalmologist discovers that her mother and grandmother have Fuchs endothelial corneal dystrophy, but they have not had symptoms or required surgery. What is the most likely explanation for the proband's early and advanced presentation of this disease?
    a. penetrance
    b. anticipation
    c. pleiotropism
    d. haploinsufficiency

35. The traditional 3-layer concept of the precorneal tear film has been replaced by a 2-layer model consisting of a lipid layer and a mucoaqueous layer. The mucin component of the tear film is secreted primarily by what ocular structure?
    a. conjunctival goblet cells
    b. lacrimal gland
    c. meibomian glands
    d. glands of Moll

36. Levels of what enzyme have been shown to be elevated in patients with severe disorders affecting the ocular surface, including Sjögren syndrome and graft-vs-host disease, as well as in patients after laser in situ keratomileusis (LASIK)?
    a. matrix metalloproteinase 9
    b. lysozyme
    c. hexosaminidase A
    d. lipase

37. A 62-year-old woman reports chronic dry eyes. When she uses artificial tears, her symptoms are relieved for only a few minutes. What glands produce the outermost layer of the tear film to help retard tear film evaporation?
    a. meibomian and Zeis
    b. lacrimal and Krause
    c. accessory lacrimal and Wolfring
    d. lacrimal and accessory lacrimal

38. What is the physiologic rate of endothelial cell loss with normal aging?
    a. 0.4% per year
    b. 0.6% per year
    c. 0.8% per year
    d. 1.0% per year

39. Soft contact lenses with low oxygen permeability cause corneal edema via the accumulation of what substance?
    a. carbon dioxide
    b. lactic acid
    c. aldehyde dehydrogenase
    d. proteoglycans

40. Breakdown of the blood–aqueous barrier alows entry of high-molecular-weight proteins into the aqeuous humor. In addition to the iris vasculature and inner wall endothelium of the Schlemm canal, what structure maintains the blood–aqueous barrier?
    a. RPE
    b. corneal endothelium
    c. nonpigmented ciliary epithelium
    d. pigmented ciliary epithelium

Answer Sheet for Section 2
Study Questions

Question	Answer	Question	Answer
1	a b c d	21	a b c d
2	a b c d	22	a b c d
3	a b c d	23	a b c d
4	a b c d	24	a b c d
5	a b c d	25	a b c d
6	a b c d	26	a b c d
7	a b c d	27	a b c d
8	a b c d	28	a b c d
9	a b c d	29	a b c d
10	a b c d	30	a b c d
11	a b c d	31	a b c d
12	a b c d	32	a b c d
13	a b c d	33	a b c d
14	a b c d	34	a b c d
15	a b c d	35	a b c d
16	a b c d	36	a b c d
17	a b c d	37	a b c d
18	a b c d	38	a b c d
19	a b c d	39	a b c d
20	a b c d	40	a b c d

Answers

1. **d.** The annulus of Zinn consists of superior and inferior orbital tendons. The upper tendon gives rise to the entire superior rectus muscle, as well as portions of the lateral and medial rectus muscles. The inferior tendon gives rise to the entire inferior rectus muscle and portions of the medial and lateral rectus muscles. The levator palpebrae superioris muscle arises from the lesser wing of the sphenoid bone, at the apex of the orbit, just superior to the annulus of Zinn. The superior oblique muscle originates from the periosteum of the body of the sphenoid bone, above and medial to the optic foramen. The inferior oblique muscle originates anteriorly, from a shallow depression in the orbital plate of the maxillary bone, at the anteromedial corner of the orbital floor, near the lacrimal fossa.
2. **b.** The 4 rectus muscles insert anteriorly on the globe. The medial rectus tendon inserts most anteriorly, approximately 5.5 mm from the limbus, followed by the inferior rectus tendon (6.5 mm) and the lateral rectus tendon (6.9 mm). The superior rectus inserts most posteriorly, approximately 7.7 mm from the limbus. An imaginary line drawn externally between the rectus muscle insertions forms the spiral of Tillaux and approximates the internal location of the ora serrata. This is clinically important because a suture passed through the full thickness of the sclera posterior to this line could penetrate the retina. Further, a scleral laceration or rupture that extends beyond the muscle insertion corresponds with a worse visual prognosis.

   The superior oblique tendon inserts superotemporally, below the superior rectus, just posterior to the globe equator. The inferior oblique tendon also inserts in the posterior sclera (behind the equator) in the inferotemporal quadrant, overlying the macula. The anterior ciliary arteries branch from the ophthalmic artery. The branches pass through the belly of each rectus muscle, penetrate the sclera, anastomose with the major arterial circle, and contribute to the blood supply of the anterior segment. These arteries enter the sclera just outside the limbus.
3. **d.** The meibomian glands are oriented vertically in parallel rows within the tarsus. Their duct orifices open just posterior to the gray line of the eyelid margin. Meibomian glands are holocrine sebaceous glands. Holocrine is a type of glandular secretion in which the gland epithelium loses an entire cell to release its secretory product. The secretion of sebaceous glands is oily and lipid rich. The sebaceous secretion of meibomian glands, *meibum,* contributes an oily layer to the tear film.

   The sweat glands in eyelid skin release their products via apocrine and eccrine secretory mechanisms. In apocrine secretion, the gland epithelium loses the apical (top) portion of the cell with the secretion. In eccrine secretion, cytoplasmic vacuoles release the secretion from the cell; no part of the cell is lost. Apocrine sweat glands in the eyelid skin are called *glands of Moll.* Endocrine glands secrete directly into the bloodstream and are part of the body's endocrine system. Exocrine glands, including eccrine, apocrine, and holocrine glands, secrete their products into a duct. The lacrimal and accessory lacrimal glands are examples of exocrine glands.
4. **b.** Normally, glucose enters the lens via diffusion from the aqueous humor and is phosphorylated to glucose-6-phosphate before passing through glycolysis to generate ATP. Due to the poor oxygen saturation in the lens, aerobic metabolism is not possible. A small amount of glucose-6-phosphate enters the hexose monophosphate shunt (also called

pentose phosphate pathway). This pathway is responsible for replenishing nicotinamide adenine dinucleotide phosphate (NADPH) stores, which are depleted by redox reactions. The polyol pathway (also called *sorbitol-aldose reductase pathway*) becomes important in the setting of hyperglycemia, in which glucose is metabolized through the polyol pathway and sorbitol is generated. Sorbitol does not readily traverse cell membranes, and its accumulation is thought to play a role in the development of sugar cataracts.

5. **d.** The human lens capsule (as well as the corneal epithelial basement membrane and Descemet membrane) is composed primarily of type IV collagen. Patients with Alport syndrome (abnormal type IV collagen caused by mutations in *COL4A3, COL4A4,* and *COL4A5* genes) may present with anterior lenticonus, a bowing forward or "ectasia" of the anterior capsule. Type I collagen is the primary type of collagen found in the corneal stroma and sclera. Type II collagen contributes to the structure of the vitreous gel. Type III collagen does not contribute to many ocular structures but has been demonstrated in the lamina cribrosa.
6. **a.** Fibers in the lens nucleus are laid down from embryogenesis through adolescence. Fibers are formed from epithelial cells at the lens equator; therefore, the closer the fibers are to the periphery, the younger they are.
7. **c.** Proteins constitute 33% of the weight of the lens. This is an unusually high protein content for any tissue in the body. The lens has 2–3 times more protein by weight than any other tissue in the body.
8. **c.** Collagen (mostly type II) allows the vitreous to have plasticity and permits resistance to tensile forces. The amount of collagen present determines whether the vitreous is a liquid or a gel. Hyaluronan contributes to the viscosity of the vitreous humor and is thought to help stabilize the collagen network. The vitreous is approximately 98% water and 0.15% macromolecules. Interaction between the cortical collagen fibers and the internal limiting membrane (ILM) occurs via several macromolecules, including laminin and fibronectin.
9. **b.** Stickler syndrome is due to a mutation in *COL2A1,* which codes for type II collagen. Patients have an optically empty vitreous due to premature liquefaction centrally with peripheral condensation, which may induce retinal detachment. Marfan syndrome is an inherited disease caused by mutations in the gene that encodes fibrillin-1; ocular manifestations are ectopia lentis, high myopia, scleral thinning, and retinal detachments. Retinitis pigmentosa is a group of inherited diseases characterized by diffuse, progressive dysfunction of predominantly rod photoreceptors. Familial exudative vitreoretinopathy is an inherited disease that leads to abnormal retinal angiogenesis and incomplete vascularization of the peripheral retina.
10. **b.** Type II fibrils are the major structural component of vitreous collagen fibers and are also found in cartilage. Types I, III, and XII are commonly found in scar tissue and are not major components in the vitreous.
11. **b.** Light hyperpolarizes cones and rods. The cone response is rapid; it turns off while the light is still on. The rod response is more prolonged and turns off very slowly. Depolarization occurs in the dark. Changes in the light flux on the retina produce electrical changes in all the retinal cells.
12. **a.** Microglia are a class of retinal cells that are related to tissue macrophages and activated when retinal homeostasis is disturbed. Macroglia provide physical support, regulate

the ionic and chemical composition of the extracellular milieu, participate in the blood–retina barrier, form the myelin sheath of the optic nerve, guide neuronal migration during development, and exchange metabolites with neurons. Pericytes surround the endothelial cells and are modified smooth muscle cells that play a role in autoregulation of retinal blood vessels. Amacrine cells are inhibitory interneurons that mediate interactions among bipolar and ganglion cells.

13. **b.** Rhodopsin is inactivated by its phosphorylation by rhodopsin kinase and subsequent binding of arrestin. Activation of rhodopsin causes the 11-*cis*-retinal double bond to be reconfigured, creating all-*trans*-retinal. This activates transducin, leading to a cascade that stops the inflow of cations by closing a sodium/calcium channel. The subsequent hyperpolarization of the rod stops the release of the inibitory neurotransmitter glutamate to the corresponding bipolar cell. A signal is then generated in the bipolar cell and passed on to the ganglion cell. Within the rod photoreceptor outer segment, closure of the channel results in reduction of calcium, which activates calcium-regulated proteins and eventually rhodopsin kinase. Rhodopsin kinase phosphorylates rhodopsin, which is then bound by arrestin, which deactivates rhodopsin.
14. **b.** *Autofluorescence* refers to intrinsic fluorescence emitted by a substance after stimulation by excitation energy. RPE phagocytosis of the photoreceptor outer segments produces oxidative by-products of retinoids, fatty acids, and proteins, which form lipofuscin. The RPE accumulates lipofuscin, which is responsible for the background fluorescence of the retina. Melanin is the source of pigmentation in the RPE but does not contribute to autofluorescence. Rhodopsin and the retinal vasculature do not contribute to fundus autofluorescence.
15. **a.** Homozygous defects in the gene *RPE65,* which encodes the RPE65 isomerohydrolase, cause Leber congenital amaurosis (LCA). This protein is the target of a treatment, approved by the US Food and Drug Administration (FDA), that uses an adeno-associated virus to deliver the gene to the RPE of patients with LCA. Mutations of the guanylate cyclase gene also cause LCA but are not treatable using an adeno-associated virus delivery system. *TIMP3* gene mutations result in Sorsby macular dystrophy. *ABCR* mutations cause Stargardt disease. Neither of these is treatable at this time with gene delivery.
16. **a.** The electro-oculogram (EOG), an electrophysiologic test for evaluating the RPE, measures the trans-RPE potential. The electroretinogram (ERG) measures electrical changes in the retina in response to a light stimulus. The a-waves and b-waves, 2 of the major components of the ERG waveform, correspond to the electrical response in the outer retina (photoreceptors) and inner retina (bipolar and Müller cells), respectively. The c-wave of the ERG can be used to study the RPE but is not typically employed clinically. Oscillatory potentials, seen on the ERG, are responses from the inner retina that are used in the evaluation of retinal vascular disease. Multifocal ERG is used to evaluate individual areas of the macula, and the pattern ERG focuses on retinal ganglion cell function. Visual evoked potential (VEP) measures the changes that occur at the occipital cortex following light stimulation and assesses the afferent visual system.
17. **a.** The lens is susceptible to damage by various reactive oxygen species (ROS) because it contains low levels of molecular oxygen and trace amounts of transition metals such as copper and iron. It is thought that metal-catalyzed auto-oxidation reactions of various reducing agents in the lens can lead to the production of potentially damaging oxidants, which can go on to produce hydroxyl radicals.

18. **a.** The retina has several distinctive characteristics that make it vulnerable to damage from lipid peroxidation. (1) Rod inner segments are rich in mitochondria, which may leak activated oxygen species. (2) Rod outer segments possess high levels of polyunsaturated fatty acids (PUFAs), making them susceptible to damage by oxygen. PUFAs are sensitive to peroxidation in proportion to their number of double bonds. (3) The abundant oxygen supply through the choroid and retinal vessels elevates the risk of oxidative damage. (4) There are many chromophores in the outer retina. Light exposure may trigger photooxidative processes mediated by singlet oxygen, and the RPE may play a key role.

19. **a.** The adverse effects of ROS have been repeatedly proposed as causal factors in many vision-threatening diseases, including cataract, age-related macular degeneration (AMD), diabetic retinopathy, and glaucoma. Lipid peroxides are formed when ROS react with unsaturated fatty acids. The oxidation of membrane phospholipids has been hypothesized to increase the permeability of cell membranes, which contributes eventually to cell malfunction and potentially to cell lysis.

20. **c.** Lipid solubility is important for drug penetration of cell membranes, and topical ocular drugs with higher levels of lipid solubility typically have better corneal penetration. Topical drugs that are isotonic and have slightly alkaline pH (tear pH 7.4) are better tolerated on the ocular surface and less quickly eliminated by reflex tearing. Similarly, the addition of a high-viscosity substance to a drug to achieve a viscosity in the range of 1–15 cP can increase drug retention in the inferior cul-de-sac and delay washout.

21. **d.** Hemorrhagic occlusive retinal vasculitis (HORV) is a rare but potentially visually devastating condition that can occur after the intraocular injection of vancomycin. A similar complication has not been observed with other antibiotics administered intracamerally, and triamcinolone is routinely used intravitreally. Any antibiotic solutions prepared for intracameral use should be preservative-free, as toxic anterior segment syndrome (TASS) has been reported after intracameral injection of antibiotics containing preservatives.

22. **c.** *Pharmacogenetics* is the study of the influence of genetic variation on drug efficacy or toxicity, focusing on single genes, whereas *pharmacogenomics* is the study of how an individual's genome affects drug response. *Pharmacodynamics* is defined as the study of the biochemical and physiological effects of drugs/agents on a biological system, including the mechanisms of their actions. *Pharmacokinetics* is the study of the absorption, distribution, metabolism, and excretion of drugs/agents in a biological system.

23. **b.** Brimonidine can affect the central nervous system (CNS) and cause fatigue and drowsiness. Severe systemic toxicity, with hypotension, hypothermia, and bradycardia, has been reported in infants treated with topical brimonidine. Therefore, its use is contraindicated in infants, and it should be used with caution in young children.

24. **a.** Prostaglandin analogues, such as latanoprost, can cause darkening of the iris and periocular skin. Other adverse effects include conjunctival injection (hyperemia), hypertrichosis of the eyelashes, cystoid macular edema, and uveitis. α_2-Adrenergic agonists, such as brimonidine, can cause CNS depression, especially in infants. β-Blockers can cause bronchospasm, which may be significant in patients with asthma or chronic obstructive lung disease. Direct-acting α_1-adrenergic agonists, such as phenylephrine, may elevate blood pressure.

25. **a.** Magnetic resonance imaging (MRI) is the modality of choice for evaluation of the CNS. For neuro-ophthalmic conditions, the best imaging study is MRI with gadolinium-based contrast medium, which enhances T1-weighted images, especially in neoplastic and

inflammatory conditions. Computed tomography is the modality of choice for assessment of bony abnormalities and acute hemorrhages and for detection of calcification.

26. **c.** CT is the modality of choice for assessing bony abnormalities. MRI is better suited for assessment of soft-tissue abnormalities than is CT. Ultrasound biomicroscopy and optical coherence tomography are useful for assessing ocular structures but not the orbit.

27. **b.** Photoreceptor nuclei are located in the outer nuclear layer (ONL). The radial fibers in the outer plexiform layer (OPL) in the perifoveal region are known as the *Henle fiber layer.* The OPL comprises synapses between the photoreceptors and bipolar cells. At the edge of the foveola, the synaptic fiber layer lies approximately parallel to the internal limiting membrane (ILM), resulting in a petaloid or star-shaped pattern when these extracellular spaces are filled with fluid (postoperative cystoid macular edema) or exudate (neuroretinitis). Outside the fovea, the radial fibers maintain an orthogonal orientation to the ILM. The inner nuclear layer (INL) contains nuclei of the bipolar, Müller, horizontal, and amacrine cells. The inner plexiform layer (IPL) comprises axons of the bipolar and amacrine cells and dendrites of the ganglion cells and their synapses.

28. **c.** Cranial nerve III (CN III) usually separates into superior and inferior divisions after passing through the annulus of Zinn in the orbit. Both the superior and inferior divisions pass through the superior orbital fissure within the annulus. However, in some individuals, CN III divides within the anterior cavernous sinus. The optic canal carries the optic nerve through the annulus of Zinn. CN III maintains a topographic organization even in the midbrain, so lesions almost anywhere along its course may cause a divisional nerve palsy. The superior division of CN III innervates the superior rectus and levator palpebrae muscles. The larger inferior division splits into 3 branches to supply the medial rectus, inferior rectus, and inferior oblique muscles. Parasympathetic pupillary fibers also course along the inferior division of CN III to enter the orbit and synapse with the ciliary ganglion.

29. **a.** During embryonic development, invagination of the optic cup leaves a fissure. Failure of the fissure to close leads to a coloboma. The location of the fissure closure correlates with the inferonasal quadrant, which is where colobomas are typically found. Therefore, bilateral optic nerve and/or chorioretinal coloboma should be considered in the differential diagnosis of bitemporal hemianopsia.

30. **b.** The trabecular meshwork, and therefore the juxtacanalicular component, is derived from cranial neural crest cells. The neuroectoderm, surface ectoderm, and mesoderm do not differentiate into trabecular meshwork.

31. **a.** The patient in this clinical scenario has Fuchs corneal endothelial dystrophy. In the differentiation of the anterior segment of the eye, 3 successive waves of neural crest–derived cell migration occur. The first wave gives rise to the corneal endothelium, and abnormalities in this layer can lead to the condition described. The second wave contributes to the iris stroma and part of the pupillary membrane. The third wave forms keratocytes (stroma). There is no fourth wave.

32. **d.** Leber hereditary optic neuropathy, a mitochondrial inherited disease, is more prevalent in males than in females. The trait is not transmitted to the offspring of affected males; however, it is transmitted to both sons and daughters of affected females. The mutations are characterized as missense or nonsense mutations. The most common mutation (≈50% of affected patients) occurs at nucleotide position 11778. The location of the mutation can influence potential visual recovery.

33. **b.** The retinoblastoma protein regulates the cell cycle at the G_1 checkpoint and functions as a tumor suppressor. Mutations in the retinoblastoma gene *(RB1)* are found not only in other related tumors, such as osteoscarcoma, but also in unrelated tumors such as breast cancer and lung cancer. The hereditary pattern of familial retinoblastoma is autosomal dominant. However, at the cellular level, it is autosomal recessive; a mutation on both chromosomes in a given cell is required in order for tumorigenesis to occur.

34. **b.** *Anticipation*—the phenomenon of apparently earlier and more severe onset of a disease in successive generations within a family—may explain why the proband requires surgical correction of her corneal edema at a young age. Fuchs endothelial corneal dystrophy, like Huntington disease, is characterized by trinucleotide tandem-repeat expansions; cases such as this are being investigated for the possibility of anticipation as a cause for earlier and more severe onset of disease.

    Penetrance is an all-or-nothing concept, whereby a gene is considered either penetrant (the gene generates evidence of phenotypic features, no matter how minimal) or nonpenetrant (the gene does not generate phenotypic change at any level of detection). *Penetrance* represents the statistical proportion of individuals carrying a given gene that manifests any evidence of the specific trait.

    Pleiotropism refers to the presentation of multiple phenotypic abnormalities in different organ systems produced by a single mutant gene. Examples include Marfan syndrome, Bardet-Biedl syndrome, and Alport syndrome.

    Haploinsufficiency is the situation in which a single active allele is present but unable to fully execute its normal function (gene product); an example of this phenomenon is *PAX6* mutations and aniridia.

35. **a.** The mucin component of the ocular tear film coats the microplicae of the superficial corneal epithelial cells and forms a fine network over the ocular surface. It contains mucins, proteins, electrolytes, water, and carbohydrates in a polar glycocalyx. The mucins are secreted primarily by the conjunctival goblet cells. Goblet cells produce mucin at a rate of 2–3 μL per day. The 2 primary types of mucins are membrane-spanning and secreted. Two varieties of secreted mucins exist: gel-forming and soluble. The lacrimal gland is complex and secretes many tear film constituents but only a small amount of mucin. The meibomian glands' principal secretion is lipid, forming the superficial lipid layer. The glands of Moll are apocrine sweat glands found on eyelid skin and do not contribute to the tear film.

36. **a.** Matrix metalloproteinase 9 (MMP-9) levels in the tear film have been shown to be elevated in patients with severe disorders affecting the ocular surface, including Sjögren syndrome and graft-vs-host disease, as well as in patients after laser in situ keratomileusis (LASIK). Lysozyme is an important tear antimicrobial constituent. Hexosaminidase is any of the enzymes involved in cleaving hexosamine or *N*-acetylhexosamine residues from gangliosides or other glycosides. Hexosaminidase A deficiency leads to Tay-Sachs disease; the enzyme is not found in the tear film. Lipase is a pancreatic enzyme that catalyzes the breakdown of fats to fatty acids and glycerol or other alcohols.

37. **a.** The meibomian glands and the sebaceous glands of Zeis secrete lipids to produce the outermost, or lipid, layer of the tear film. The lacrimal, accessory lacrimal, Krause, and Wolfring glands all contribute to the mucoaqueous layer.

38. **b.** The corneal endothelium, located posterior to the Descemet membrane, is a monolayer of hexagonal cells with a diameter of 20 μm. In young adults, the normal endothelial cell count is approximately 3000/mm^2 centrally. The number of endothelial cells is higher in

the periphery and decreases with age. There is a concomitant spreading and thinning of the remaining cells. The rate of physiologic corneal endothelial cell loss with normal aging has been reported to be 0.6% per year.

39. **b.** Under anaerobic (low-oxygen) conditions, glucose, the main metabolic substrate for the cornea, is converted to pyruvic acid and then to lactic acid. Lactic acid accumulation in the stroma increases the osmotic load, which draws water into the cornea and causes corneal edema. Carbon dioxide, aldehyde dehydrogenase, and proteoglycans do not accumulate in the cornea in hypoxic conditions. Carbon dioxide is a product of glucose metabolism via glycolysis under aerobic conditions. Aldehyde dehydrogenase is a soluble protein found in the cornea that absorbs ultraviolet B (UVB) light. Proteoglycans confer hydrophilic properties to the corneal stroma and interact with collagen fibrils to provide corneal clarity.

40. **c.** The blood–aqueous barrier restricts the entry of plasma proteins into the aqueous humor. The blood–aqueous barrier is composed of the tight junctions of the nonpigmented ciliary epithelium (NPE), the iris vasculature, and the inner wall endothelium of the Schlemm canal. Normal aqueous contains approximately 0.02 g of protein per 100 mL, as compared with the typical plasma level of 7 g per 100 mL. With compromise of the blood–aqueous barrier, the protein content of the aqueous humor may increase 10–100 times, especially in high-molecular-weight polypeptides. The RPE contributes to the blood–retina barrier. The corneal endothelium and the pigmented ciliary epithelium do not contribute to the blood–aqueous barrier.

Index

(f = figure; t = table)